# CHANGING THE
# U.S. HEALTH CARE SYSTEM

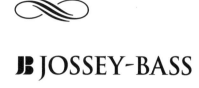

## JB JOSSEY-BASS

# CHANGING THE U.S. HEALTH CARE SYSTEM

## Key Issues in Health Services Policy and Management

### THIRD EDITION

Ronald M. Andersen
Thomas H. Rice
Gerald F. Kominski
Editors

Foreword by Abdelmonem A. Afifi
and Linda Rosenstock

BICENTENNIAL
1807
WILEY
2007
BICENTENNIAL

John Wiley & Sons, Inc.

Published by Jossey-Bass
A Wiley Imprint
989 Market Street, San Francisco, CA 94103-1741    www.josseybass.com

Jossey-Bass books and products are available through most bookstores. To contact Jossey-Bass directly call our Customer Care Department within the U.S. at 800-956-7739, outside the U.S. at 317-572-3986, or fax 317-572-4002.

Jossey-Bass also publishes its books in a variety of electronic formats. Some content that appears in print may not be available in electronic books.

**Library of Congress Cataloging-in-Publication Data**

Changing the U.S. health care system : key issues in health services policy and management / edited by Ronald M. Andersen, Thomas H. Rice, and Gerald F. Kominski.—3rd ed.
   p. ; cm.
 Includes bibliographical references and index.
 ISBN-13: 978-0-7879-8524-0 (cloth)
 ISBN-10: 0-7879-8524-4 (cloth)
1. Health care reform—United States. 2. Medical policy—United States. 3. Medical care—United States. I. Andersen, Ronald. II. Rice, Thomas H. III. Kominski, Gerald F.
 [DNLM: 1. Health Care Reform—United States. 2. Delivery of Health Care—United States. 3. Health Policy—United States. WA 540 AA1 C385 2007]
 RA395.A3C478 2007
 362.10973—dc22                                  2006032155

Printed in the United States of America
THIRD EDITION
*HB Printing*   10  9  8  7  6  5  4

# CONTENTS

# FIGURES AND TABLES

## Figures

# Tables

# FOREWORD

The book you hold in your hand is a gift. With his wife, Audrey, the late Samuel J. Tibbitts gave generously to the Department of Health Services in the UCLA School of Public Health to commission a study of key issues in health policy and management challenging the U.S. health care system. The leadership, scholarship, and charity that Sam exhibited in making this gift typified his life in a number of ways.

Sam changed the health care system in California and the nation, perhaps as much as anyone else of his generation. After receiving a B.S. in public health from the University of California, Los Angeles, in 1949 and an M.S. in public health and hospital administration from the University of California, Berkeley in 1950, he pioneered the development of integrated health care delivery and financing systems. His career course trajectory led in 1988 to the creation of the nonprofit UniHealth America, where he was chairman of the board until his death in 1994.

Along the way, Sam founded and chaired both PacifiCare Health Systems, one of the first major health maintenance organizations, and American Health Care Systems, a group of thirty-two hospital systems across the country that organized the nation's first preferred provider system, PPO Alliance. Both a leader and a scholar, he served as chairman of the board of trustees of the American Hospital Association and published more than one hundred articles. Sensing the need to establish a corporate conscience in a changing health care environment, he was founding chairman of Guiding Principles for Hospitals, the first program to delineate ethical and quality principles in the industry.

Even while he entered the twilight of a long and storied career, his concern for the future of health care remained. For this reason, he invested in the school that had nurtured him and asked its faculty to address the challenges that are crucial to the future of health care in the United States: those relating to cost, quality, and access.

To achieve Sam Tibbitts's vision, the editors sought to gather, in a single book, "a comprehensive, yet readable" account of these issues. We believe that they succeeded remarkably in the first two editions, published in 1996 and 2001, as well as in their efforts to update those issues in this new edition. In particular, the addition of four new chapters covering such issues as disparities in health and health care, the nursing shortage, and information technology make the volume especially useful in confronting key issues for the new millennium and beyond.

The chapter authors in this volume—the third edition of this highly successful book—are gifted scholars. As the current dean and a former dean in the UCLA School of Public Health, we know them well and have followed closely their scholarly contributions. As anticipated by Sam, the book first addresses three key components of health care policy: improving access, controlling costs, and ensuring quality. As noted in Chapter Four, access to health care remains central to the health care reform debate; the chapter authors identify that "the United States cannot escape the need for fundamental reforms that will extend coverage to its entire population." Cost—often pitted against adequate access and improved quality—will continue to be a major force in health care policy making. Chapter Six explores various ways of containing health care costs and emphasizes the need for better data in order to make sensible policy decisions about alternative types of health care reform. Chapter Eight examines the measurement of health outcomes and health-related quality of life (HRQL), concluding that we need "careful and appropriate inclusion of HRQL outcomes in traditional health services research."

A number of subsequent chapters are devoted to segments of the population with special needs for health care. Topics include long-term care for the elderly, providing services for the growing HIV/AIDS community, multidisciplinary coordination of the fragmented child health care system, improving access to primary health care for low-income women, and increasing services to the growing homeless population. Various authors advance proposals that might improve the prognosis for these vulnerable populations.

The final section of the volume contains discussion of the fundamental challenges now facing health care researchers, policy makers, and managers, including the appropriate role of competitive markets and the regulatory role of government. Other topics covered include Medicare reform and the much-publicized new prescription drug benefit, the role of public health agencies in delivering personal health services, medical malpractice liability, and the ethics of public health and health care services. Rather than offer simplistic solutions, here and throughout the book the authors identify key research questions that, if addressed, will advance our tackling these complex issues. The collective message sent to the reader is clear: the time for health care reform is ripe, and effective research in this area is urgently needed to support this fundamental change.

This updated and comprehensive account of critical issues facing the nation in health policy and management is a valuable asset for health care policy researchers and analysts, as well as managers of health care services, providers, and practitioners. Moreover, students in health care policy and management or related fields will appreciate it as a guideline to many subject areas in health care today. Finally, this book can serve as a readable guide to health care professionals and policy makers on health care reform during the next decade.

We commend this volume to you, sharing the hope of Sam and Audrey Tibbitts that training and discourse shall result, in turn leading to innovations in policy and management that enable the gift of health to be shared by all.

*January 2007*                                   Abdelmonem A. Afifi
*Los Angeles*                                    Dean emeritus and professor of biostatistics
                                                 UCLA School of Public Health

                                                 Linda Rosenstock
                                                 Dean, UCLA School of Public Health

# THE EDITORS

*Ronald M. Andersen* is the Wasserman Professor Emeritus in the UCLA Departments of Health Services and Sociology. Previously he was professor at the University of Chicago and director of the Center for Health Administration Studies. Professor Andersen has studied access to medical care for his entire professional career of forty-five years. He developed the Behavioral Model of Health Services Use, which has been extensively used nationally and internationally as a framework for medical care use studies. He has directed three national surveys of access to care and has led numerous evaluations to promote access to care. Of the twenty-five books and 225 articles he has authored, a large proportion deal with issues of access. He is a fellow of the Institute of Medicine and has been chair of the Medical Sociology Section of the American Sociological Association.

*Gerald F. Kominski* is professor in the Department of Health Services, associate dean for academic programs, and associate director of the Center for Health Policy Research at the UCLA School of Public Health. Professor Kominski teaches classes in research methods, health economics, and cost-effectiveness analysis. His research focuses on evaluating the costs and cost-effectiveness of health care programs and technologies, improving access and health outcomes among ethnic and vulnerable populations, and developing models for forecasting population health. Prior to joining the faculty at UCLA, he served as a staff member for the Prospective Payment Assessment Commission (ProPAC) in Washington, D.C., a congressional agency that monitored and developed Medicare hospital payment policy. He currently serves as vice chair for cost impact analysis for the California Health Benefits Review Program, a multicampus project that conducts cost, medical effectiveness, and public health impact analyses for the California legislature regarding proposed health benefit mandates.

*Thomas H. Rice* is vice chancellor for academic personnel at UCLA, and professor of health services, UCLA School of Public Health. He served as department chair from 1996 to 2000 and 2003–04. Professor Rice received his doctorate in economics at the University of California at Berkeley in 1982. Prior to joining the faculty at UCLA in 1991, he was a faculty member at the University of North Carolina School of Public Health. His areas of interest include health insurance, cost containment, Medicare, and the role of competition and regulation in health care markets.

From 1994 to 2000, Rice served as the editor of the *Medical Care Research and Review.* The second edition of his book *The Economics of Health Reconsidered* was published in 2003. In 2005–06, he was chair of the board of directors of Academy-Health, which represents the profession of health services research in the United States. Rice was chair of the 2003 AcademyHealth Annual Research Meeting. Previously he was a recipient of its Young Investigator Award (1988) and Article of the Year Award (1998).

# THE AUTHORS

*Emily K. Abel* is professor of health services and women's studies at UCLA. She teaches courses on the history of public health and aging health policy. Her most recent books are *Hearts of Wisdom: American Women Caring for Kin, 1850–1940* and *Suffering in the Land of Sunshine: A Los Angeles Illness Narrative*.

*John L. Adams* is a senior statistician in the health program at RAND. His current work focuses on improved quantitative methods in quality assessment. His interests include statistical methods for profiling managed care organizations, provider groups, and providers. With Elizabeth McGlynn, he has worked on the QA Tools quality measurement system. He is currently involved in the development of a quality measurement system for cancer care and the validation of patient self-reports of quality of care.

*Lisa Arangua* is senior research analyst in the Department of Family Medicine, UCLA School of Medicine. She has been a health services researcher and policy analyst for more than a decade. She was a fellow in the Woodrow Wilson Public Policy and International Affairs program. Prior to her appointment at UCLA, she was on the research staff at UC Data Archive and Technical Assistance at the University of California, Berkeley, where she evaluated health and welfare programs for the state and federal government. Her professional activities include social justice and health, epidemiology, and concurrent behavior change of severely underserved health populations. She received her M.P.P. from UCLA in 1999.

*Roshan Bastani* is professor of health services and associate dean for research in the School of Public Health at UCLA, codirector of its Center to Eliminate Health Disparities, and associate director of the Division of Cancer Prevention and Control Research. She is a social/health psychologist and studies access to health care among low-income, ethnic minority, and other underserved groups. She is a nationally recognized leader in this field and has conducted numerous patient and health care system directed-intervention trials designed to evaluate the most effective and efficient means of reducing disparities.

*Jeanne T. Black* received her Ph.D. in health services research from UCLA and currently is a Fellow in Reimbursement and Outcomes Planning at Advanced Bionics. Her research interests include racial and ethnic disparities and the cross-cultural validity of health outcomes measures. She was formerly associate director of the Health Policy Institute at the University of Pittsburgh's Graduate School of Public Health, where she conducted research on employer-sponsored health insurance. She received her M.B.A. from the Kellogg Graduate School of Management at Northwestern University in 1977, and she has extensive experience in strategic planning and management of health services organizations.

*Lester Breslow* received his M.D. from the University of Minnesota in 1938 and his public M.P.H. from the University of Minnesota in 1941. Before coming to UCLA in 1968, he was director of the California Department of Health. He served as dean of the UCLA School of Public Health from 1972 to 1980 and now is professor emeritus. He has also served as president of the American Public Health Association, the International Epidemiological Association, and the Association of Schools of Public Health. Dr. Breslow received the American Public Health Association's Sedgwick Medal and is a member of the Institute of Medicine and recipient of its Lienhard Award.

*E. Richard Brown* is professor in the Department of Health Services and the Department of Community Health Sciences in the UCLA School of Public Health. He is also the director of the UCLA Center for Health Policy Research, a leading national health policy research center and the premier source of health-related information and analysis on California's population. His research and publications cover a range of issues and policies affecting access of disadvantaged populations to health care. He also is the principal investigator of the California Health Interview Survey (CHIS), one of the nation's largest ongoing health surveys. He received his Ph.D. in the sociology of education at the University of California, Berkeley.

*William S. Comanor* is professor of health services at UCLA and also professor of economics at UC Santa Barbara. At UCLA, he is director of the Research Program in Pharmaceutical Economics and Policy. His doctoral dissertation at Harvard was entitled *The Economics of Research and Development in the Pharmaceutical Industry,* and this subject remains a primary topic of his research. He has written many articles on facets of the pharmaceutical industry and lectured throughout the world on related issues.

*William E. Cunningham,* M.D., is professor in the Department of Health Services, School of Public Health, and in the Division of General Internal Medicine, Department of Medicine, UCLA School of Medicine. He has authored more than seventy scientific papers, many of which address access to care, barriers to medical care, use of HIV services, racial disparities, HIV prevention, and health outcomes. He teaches courses on race, ethnicity, and health; health services organization and outcomes; and effectiveness research.

*Pamela L. Davidson* is associate professor in the UCLA Department of Health Services. Her major research activities focus on determinants of medical care access, leadership and organizational development for health care professionals, and clinical translational research. She spends most of her professional time conducting research and evaluation studies and teaching health program evaluation to graduate, postdoctoral, and executive students. Her current research activities involve directing two national evaluation studies and participating in the design of the UCLA Clinical Translational Science Institute.

*Linda Delp* is director of the UCLA Labor Occupational Safety and Health Program (UCLA-LOSH) and a graduate of the Community Health Sciences doctoral program in the UCLA School of Public Health. Her research addresses job conditions of home care workers in California's In-Home Supportive Services Program. She initiated and cochaired the California Home Care Research Working Group and has testified at the state and local levels in support of policies to improve home care working conditions. She was previously Western Region director of health and safety for the Service Employees International Union, which represents long-term care workers.

*Susan L. Ettner* is professor in the Division of General Internal Medicine and Health Services Research in the UCLA Department of Medicine and Department of

Health Services in the School of Public Health. After obtaining her Ph.D. in economics at Massachusetts Institute of Technology in 1991, she was on the faculty of the Harvard Department of Health Care Policy prior to joining UCLA in 1999. A recipient of AcademyHealth's Alice Hersch New Investigator Award, Ettner's research interests include mental health and substance abuse services, health and labor market outcomes, insurance markets, managed care, disability, and postacute and long-term care.

*Jonathan E. Fielding*, M.D., is professor of health services and pediatrics at UCLA and director of public health for Los Angeles County. He has written more than 175 original articles, chapters, and editorials on health policy, prevention, and public health. He is a member of the Institute of Medicine, chair of Partnership for Prevention and of the Community Preventive Services Task Force, and a board member of the American Legacy Foundation. He is editor of the *Annual Review of Public Health* and former president of the American College of Preventive Medicine. He received his M.D., M.P.H., and M.A. (history of science) from Harvard University and an M.B.A. from the Wharton Business School.

*Paul Fu Jr.*, M.D., is associate professor of pediatrics and health services at David Geffen School of Medicine at UCLA and UCLA School of Public Health, and chief medical information officer for the Los Angeles County Department of Health Services. Dr. Fu is a graduate of Boston University School of Medicine and completed postgraduate medical training in pediatrics, followed by an HRSA MCHB fellowship in Maternal and Child Health at the UCLA Center for Healthier Children, Families, and Communities at UCLA School of Public Health, and a General Academic Pediatrics fellowship at Harbor-UCLA Medical Center, where he continues as a faculty member in the division of General and Academic Pediatrics.

*Patricia A. Ganz*, M.D., is a medical oncologist who has been a member of the faculty of the UCLA School of Medicine since 1978 and the UCLA School of Public Health since 1992, with current appointments as professor of medicine (hematology and oncology) and professor of health services. Since 1993 she has served as the director of the Jonsson Comprehensive Cancer Center's Division of Cancer Prevention and Control Research. Dr. Ganz is a pioneer in assessment of quality of life in cancer patients, leading the quality-of-life studies in several major cancer prevention and treatment trials. Her other major areas of research are cancer survivorship and late effects of cancer treatment, cancer in the elderly, and quality of care for cancer patients.

*Lillian Gelberg*, M.D., is professor and vice chair for academic affairs in the UCLA School of Medicine. She is a health services researcher and family physician who conducts community-based research on the health, access to care, and quality of care of homeless and other vulnerable populations. She has studied homeless adults living in shelters and outdoor areas, and the health and use of health services among homeless and low-income housed patients. Dr. Gelberg attended Harvard Medical School and completed her internship and residency at Montefiore Hospital in the Bronx, New York City. She earned an M.S.P.H. in health services research from the UCLA School of Public Health. She has been a member of the UCLA School of Medicine faculty since 1986.

*Beth A. Glenn* is adjunct assistant professor in the Department of Health Services at the UCLA School of Public Health and assistant researcher in the UCLA Division of Cancer Prevention and Control Research. Her main research interests are in the area of cancer prevention and control among ethnic minority and underserved populations. She has been involved in a variety of research projects since she joined UCLA in 2001, including surveys focused on understanding factors that predict cancer prevention behaviors and intervention studies aimed at promoting cancer screening and lifestyle changes. She received her Ph.D. in clinical health psychology from Finch University of Health Sciences and the Chicago Medical School in 2001.

*Neal Halfon,* M.D., is director of the UCLA Center for Healthier Children, Families, and Communities and the National Center for Infant and Early Childhood Health Policy. He is also professor of pediatrics in the David Geffen School of Medicine at UCLA, health services in the UCLA School of Public Health, and policy studies in the UCLA School of Public Affairs. Dr. Halfon was a member of the Board on Children, Youth, and Families of the National Research Council and Institute of Medicine from 2001 to 2006. In 2006, the Ambulatory Pediatric Association awarded him its annual Research Award in recognition of his lifetime achievement in the field of pediatric research.

*Ron D. Hays* is professor of medicine at UCLA and a senior health scientist at RAND. He has contributed to the development of research instruments to assess patient evaluations of health care, health-related quality of life, and other health outcomes. He has published 317 research articles, eleven review papers, ten commentaries, and twenty-eight book chapters. He is the current editor-in-chief of *Quality of Life Research* and former deputy editor of *Medical Care.*

*Moira Inkelas* is assistant professor in the Department of Health Services, UCLA School of Public Health, and assistant director of the UCLA Center for Healthier Children, Families, and Communities. She received her M.P.H. in 1993 and her doctorate in public policy analysis at the Frederick S. Pardee RAND Graduate School in 2000. Research interests include systems of care for children with special health care needs, tailoring managed care and health care financing policies to the needs of children with chronic illness, impact of systems on quality and performance, measuring quality of care, and quality improvement.

*Robert M. Kaplan* is professor and chair of the UCLA Department of Health Services and professor of medicine at the David Geffen School of Medicine at UCLA. He is a past president of several organizations, including the American Psychological Association Division of Health Psychology, the International Society for Quality of Life Research, the Society for Behavioral Medicine, and the Academy of Behavioral Medicine Research. He is editor-in-chief of *Health Psychology* and former editor-in-chief of the *Annals of Behavioral Medicine.* In 2005 he was elected to the Institute of Medicine of the National Academies of Sciences.

*Kenneth W. Kizer,* M.D., is CEO and chairman of Medsphere Systems, the leading provider of open source health care information technology. He previously served as founding president and CEO of the National Quality Forum; undersecretary for Health, U.S. Department of Veterans Affairs; and director, California Department of Health Services. Board-certified in six specialties and subspecialties, he graduated from Stanford University and UCLA and holds an honorary doctor of science from the State University of New York. He is a member of Alpha Omega Alpha National Honor Medical Society, Delta Omega National Honorary Public Health Society, and the Institute of Medicine of the National Academy of Sciences.

*Ellen T. Kurtzman* is senior program director for the National Quality Forum (NQF). In this capacity, she has led national efforts to establish voluntary consensus standards for hospital, nursing, and home health quality. Prior to joining NQF, she was vice president of quality improvement for the American Health Care Association and served in a senior capacity for large, national health services organizations that include the National PACE Association, the American Red Cross, and the Partnership for Behavioral Healthcare. Kurtzman holds a bachelor's degree in nursing from the University of Pennsylvania and a master's in public health from Johns Hopkins University.

*Shana Alex Lavarreda* is project manager for the UCLA Center for Health Policy Research and a doctoral student in the UCLA School of Public Health. She currently works with the State of Health Insurance in California (SHIC) project, using data from the California Health Interview Survey (CHIS) to study health insurance in the state. She has coauthored numerous works regarding public health insurance and multicultural health issues, including the book *Health Communication: A Multicultural Perspective*. She received her M.P.H. from UCLA, specializing in health policy.

*Janet C. Link* received her B.A. in economics from the University of North Carolina, Chapel Hill. She is currently a Ph.D. student in the Department of Health Services at UCLA, specializing in economics. Her research interests include understanding the enabling factors and barriers to the mental health care help-seeking processes. Drawing on theory from economics and sociology, she is particularly interested in examining whether contextual factors such as community-level socioeconomic resources and the racial and ethnic composition of communities influence the help-seeking behavior of individuals in need of mental health care.

*Mark S. Litwin*, M.D., is professor of urology and health services, Schools of Medicine and Public Health, University of California, Los Angeles. Dr. Litwin holds degrees from Duke University in economics, Emory University in medicine, and UCLA in public health. He completed his urology training at Harvard. He has authored numerous original articles, reports, reviews, and book chapters in urologic oncology and outcomes research. His research includes quality of care, medical outcomes assessment, health-related quality of life, urologic oncology, resource utilization, and patient preferences. His current grants include a program that provides free prostate cancer treatment to low-income uninsured men in California. He teaches in the UCLA Schools of Medicine and Public Health and practices urologic oncology at UCLA.

*Jeff Luck* is associate professor of health services at the UCLA School of Public Health. His informatics research focuses on aggregation, analysis, and dissemination of data to support research, management, and policy analysis in public health, quality measurement, cancer research, and integrated health care systems. He also studies applications of new management practices in these settings. Luck teaches courses in health care information systems and management strategy. He received his M.B.A. from the Anderson Graduate School of Management at UCLA and his Ph.D. in public policy analysis from the Frederick S. Pardee RAND Graduate School of Policy Studies.

*Elizabeth A. McGlynn* is associate director for RAND Health and holds the RAND Corporate Chair in Health Care Quality. She is an internationally known expert on methods for assessing and reporting on quality of health care delivery at various levels within the health care system and has published extensively in the area. She is a member of the Institute of Medicine and serves on a number of national advisory committees. McGlynn serves on the editorial boards for *Health Services Research* and the *Milbank Memorial Fund Quarterly* and is a reviewer for many leading journals.

*Glenn A. Melnick* is professor of public administration at the University of Southern California and a consultant at RAND. He specializes in health economics and finance. Melnick joined the School of Public Administration faculty in 1996. Previously, he served as a faculty member of the UCLA School of Public Health and an expert witness to the Federal Trade Commission. He has published in the *American Journal of Public Health, Health Affairs, Medical Care, Journal of Health Politics, Policy and Law, Health Policy Reform: Competition and Controls,* and *Journal of Ambulatory Care Management.* He has been principal investigator for a number of funded projects in Jakarta, Indonesia, and in Taiwan.

*Leo S. Morales,* M.D., is associate professor, UCLA Schools of Medicine and Public Health, and affiliated staff at RAND. Dr. Morales recently received a Robert Wood Johnson Foundation Health Policy Investigator Award to study the effects of acculturation on the health of Mexican immigrants. He also directs the methods cores for two federally funded centers on minority health and health disparities. In addition to his research activities, he is a practicing physician at UCLA, where sees patients and supervises internal medicine residents at the UCLA Internal Medicine Clinic and UCLA Hospital.

*Jack Needleman* is associate professor, Department of Health Services, UCLA School of Public Health. His research on nurse staffing and patient outcomes in hospitals received the AcademyHealth Health Services Research Impact Award in 2006. He currently serves on the Nursing Advisory Council of the Joint Commission for the Accreditation of Healthcare Organizations. Other research has examined the quality of care for Medicaid beneficiaries with diabetes, changes in access to inpatient care for psychiatric conditions and substance abuse, safety net hospitals, and nonprofit and public hospital conversions to for-profit status.

*Alexander N. Ortega* is associate professor of health services in the UCLA School of Public Health. He has conducted federally funded studies on the physical and mental health of Latinos. Prior to joining the UCLA faculty, he was senior research associate at the W. M. Krogman Center for Research in Child Growth and Development at the University of Pennsylvania, assistant professor of health policy and administration at Yale University, and associate professor of public health at the Ohio State University. At UCLA, he teaches graduate seminars in health services research methods and health care disparities.

*Nadereh Pourat* is adjunct associate professor of health services at the UCLA School of Public Health and senior research scientist at the UCLA Center for Health Policy Research. Her primary research interest is disparities in access and utilization of health care for underserved populations, including the elderly and members of various racial and ethnic groups. She has numerous publications on aspects of elder care that include long-term care, satisfaction with care of the chronically ill, predictors of supplemental Medicare coverage, and determinants of alternative care. She received her Ph.D. in health services at UCLA.

The late *Ruth Roemer* joined the UCLA faculty in 1962 and was professor emerita in the Department of Health Services in the UCLA School of Public Health from 1980 to 2005. She taught courses in health law, ethical issues, and tobacco epidemic and public policy. In a career spanning more than sixty years, her research involved studies of mental hospital admission law, education and legal regulation of health personnel, laws governing abortion and family planning, organization of health services, and legislation for tobacco control. Roemer received the J.D. degree from Cornell Law School in 1939.

*Pauline Vaillancourt Rosenau* is professor at the University of Texas-Houston School of Public Health. She was previously professor at the University of Quebec in Montreal for two decades. She was awarded a Ph.D. and a master's in public health from the University of California. She is the author of seven books and three dozen articles on the topics of comparative international health policy, public-private policy partnerships, competition, the implications of investor status for provision of health services, pharmacy policy, philosophy, and postmodernism. She is a citizen of both Canada and the United States, is fluent in English and French, and speaks some Spanish.

*Mark A. Schuster,* M.D., is professor of pediatrics and health services at UCLA and co-director for maternal, child, and adolescent health at RAND. His research focuses on child, adolescent, and family health and spans the fields of health services, behavior change, and policy analysis. He received his M.D. from Harvard Medical School, his M.P.P. from the Kennedy School of Government, and his Ph.D. from Frederick S. Pardee RAND Graduate School. He is the 2003 winner of the Nemours Child Health Services Research Award from AcademyHealth. He practices pediatrics at Mattel Children's Hospital at UCLA.

*Stuart O. Schweitzer* is professor of health services at the UCLA School of Public Health. He served as senior health policy advisor to President Carter's Commission for a National Agenda for the Eighties. His interests have been health economics and policy analysis, including health care financing, technology assessment, and industrial policy toward health. In recent years, he has focused his research on the pharmaceutical and biotech industries, writing numerous papers on innovation, drug pricing, and cost containment. He co-directs UCLA's Program in Pharmaceutical Economics and Policy. The second edition of his book *Pharmaceutical Economics and Policy* is being published in 2006.

*Beatriz M. Solís* most recently was director of Cultural and Linguistic Services, L. A. Care Health Plan, and is now pursuing her Ph.D. in the School of Public Health at UCLA. Following nearly ten years with UCLA, she acted most recently as a researcher for the UCLA Center for Healthy Policy Research. She is currently teaching at California State University, Northridge, in the Chicano/Central American Studies Department. She is currently serving on several boards and councils: the Office of Women's Health, Guttmacher Institute, California, Pan Ethnic Health Network, and Vision y Compromiso.

*Steven P. Wallace* is professor at the UCLA School of Public Health and associate director of the UCLA Center for Health Policy Research. He is a leading scholar on aging in communities of color, including access to long-term care for diverse elderly, disparities in the consequences of health policy changes, and the politics of aging. His current research is identifying gaps in health policy for underserved elders in California and examining access to health care for Mexicans on both sides of the border. He is past chair of the Gerontological Health Section of the American Public Health Association.

*David Lee Wood*, M.D., is board-certified in both pediatrics and preventive medicine, with a fellowship in health services research from RAND. He has served on the faculty at the David Geffen School of Medicine at UCLA, as associate medical director for Shriners Hospital, and most recently as chief, Division of Community Pediatrics, and associate professor in the Department of Pediatrics, University of Florida, Jacksonville campus. His research focuses on provision of immunizations, comprehensive care in a medical home to children with special health care needs, and health services to persons with developmental disabilities.

*Roberta Wyn* is associate director of the UCLA Center for Health Policy Research. She conducts research in several health care policy areas, with a particular focus on access to health insurance coverage and health care for women, ethnic populations, and low-income groups. Her work has focused on groups historically underserved in the health care system. Her current work examines women's health insurance coverage and use of the health care system. Her background includes provision of social and health-related services in community-based organizations and hospitals. She received her doctorate in health services from UCLA.

*Antronette K. Yancey*, M.D., is currently associate professor in the Department of Health Services, UCLA School of Public Health, with primary research interests in chronic disease prevention and adolescent health promotion. She returned to academia full-time in 2001 after five years in public health practice, first as director of public health for the city of Richmond, Virginia, and, until recently, as director of chronic disease prevention and health promotion, Los Angeles County Department of Health Services. Dr. Yancey has authored more than seventy-five scientific publications, including briefs, book chapters, health promotion videos, and more than fifty peer-reviewed journal articles.

*David S. Zingmond*, M.D., is assistant professor in the Division of General Internal Medicine and Health Services Research at UCLA. He obtained his M.D. at Stanford University and his Ph.D. in health services at UCLA, and completed a National Research Service Award Fellowship at UCLA. He is a board-certified internist and regularly sees patients at the UCLA Medical Center. Dr. Zingmond has expertise in the organization, delivery, and epidemiology of clinical care in California, with special interests in HIV care and policy, quality of care for the elderly, and quality of surgical care.

To the late Samuel J. Tibbitts and to Audrey Tibbitts, whose generosity made this work possible.

And to our departed friend and colleague, Ruth Roemer— contributor to all three editions of this work and tireless scholar and advocate for the public's health.

# INTRODUCTION AND OVERVIEW

Ronald M. Andersen
Thomas H. Rice
Gerald F. Kominski

The U.S. health care system continues to face many momentous challenges. Since the movement away from heavy-handed managed care, expenditures have risen quickly again, and the number of uninsured individuals has followed suit; it is now estimated that about forty-six million Americans are uninsured.[1] New medical technologies and pharmaceuticals are in great demand, with much anticipation for future genetic therapies. The population continues to age, putting more pressure on Medicare, and state budgetary crises—in part brought about by Medicaid—have resulted in nearly all states making significant cutbacks in programs for the poor. Employers have hardly been immune: job-based coverage is down, and in a sense so are benefits, as employee cost-sharing requirements have burgeoned. Although we are much better at measuring quality, most assessments of the quality of care in the United States show a high error rate and, at best, uneven quality. Authors of this volume have estimated that Americans are getting, on average, only 55 percent of the care that they should.[2] But if we improve this number, costs are likely to rise as well.

These challenges and pressures for change are tempered by a political environment fundamentally opposed to comprehensive change. The defeat of comprehensive health reform in the early 1990s shaped the directions for changing the U.S. health care system in the years since, making it clear that (1) many, if not most, of the problems we face in ensuring access to affordable, high-quality health care would have to be dealt with incrementally rather than through comprehensive reform; and (2) greater reliance would be placed on private markets than on additional governmental regulation.

These conditions remain as true today as they were when the first edition of this book was published, in 1996. Thus, for the foreseeable future, the goals of improving access, ensuring quality, and controlling costs will continue to be addressed mainly through private market initiatives or through enactment of piecemeal legislation. The one ostensible exception—Medicare's new drug benefit—is being implemented through private insurance markets. Not only is there no standard benefit (it varies by insurer) but government is prohibited from negotiating pharmaceutical prices even though the benefit is subsidized, at a 75 percent level, through federal revenues.

This third and expanded edition follows the general format of the first two. Our goal is to take a comprehensive and careful look at current issues in health care policy and management. To carry this out, we have assembled a group of talented and experienced researchers and asked them to take stock of the past, present, and future in their particular area of expertise. For a specific topic, we asked the authors of each chapter to present the most current research and policy issues facing that topic, summarize existing empirical evidence, and discuss research and management strategies that can be used to address current problems. Because of continual change in the health care system since the first two editions were published, we asked authors of revised chapters in this third edition to emphasize recent developments in their area of expertise. Further, to make the third edition even more comprehensive, we have added four much-needed new chapters, on disparities in health, disparities in health care access and delivery, information systems, and performance in the area of nursing.

This book continues to aim at providing, in a single source, a comprehensive yet readable account of the issues facing the United States in health care policy and management. We expect that it will continue to benefit a variety of audiences:

- Students, whether specializing in health care policy and management or in other fields, who will benefit from having a thorough and up-to-date review of the literature in many subject areas in the health care field
- Health service researchers and policy analysts, who will find it useful to have ready access to the state-of-the-art in research, as well as analysis of policy options relevant to many aspects of the health care market
- Health care managers, who will benefit from having a single source of information on how to promote quality and better health outcomes while controlling expenditures
- Practitioners and providers, especially doctors and nurses, who will find issues of special interest addressed in various chapters

# Organization and Summary of the Volume

The volume is divided into five parts. Each section contains three or more chapters relevant to that particular topic. The first three parts are on the three key components of health care policy: access, costs, and quality. In each section, there are chapters on measurement and trends, as well as chapters on policy options. The fourth part addresses special populations, with individual chapters on long-term care and the elderly, AIDS, children's health, mental health, women's health, and the homeless. The fifth and final part concerns proposals for reform, with chapters on managed care, Medicare reform, public and personal health, medical malpractice, and ethical issues in public health and health services management.

Here we briefly summarize some of the key material contained in these chapters.

## Access to Health Care

It is particularly appropriate to start with this topic. Understanding access is essential to addressing major challenges to our health care system today: health and health care disparities. Despite the tremendous attention they have received, both in research and in policy, there are more uninsured people in the country now than in previous decades. The United States holds the dubious distinction of being the only developed country that does not ensure access to health care through guaranteed coverage. Furthermore, many analysts—we are included—believe that one of the major barriers to controlling health care costs is exactly this lack of universal coverage. This is not only because it is difficult for poor and sick people to seek preventive care but also because it fragments the financing system, requiring the existence of an expensive safety net as well as aggravating the problem of cost shifting.

Chapter One, by Ronald M. Andersen and Pamela L. Davidson, is a comprehensive examination of access to health care. The authors argue that understanding access is the key to understanding the health policy because the access framework (1) predicts and measures health service use, (2) can be used to promote social justice, and (3) can be used to promote health outcomes. The chapter explains the multiple dimensions of access using a revised version of the behavioral model that emphasizes contextual as well as individual determinants of health services utilization. It goes on to discuss how access can be measured and presents data on the levels of access and trends in the United States. Certain trends emerge from this analysis: though an increasing number of people are being covered by Medicaid, there has been a decline in the number covered by private insurance in the last twenty years and an overall increase in the proportion without any health insurance coverage; and low-income and black populations appear to have achieved equity of access according to gross measures of hospital and physician utilization not taking into account their greater need for medical care in the United States. Minorities and those with low income continue to lag considerably in receipt of dental care, and equity has certainly not been achieved according to health insurance coverage, what with the proportion uninsured 50 percent higher for blacks and more than twice as high for Hispanics and the low-income population compared to the uninsured rate for non-Hispanic whites.

Chapter Two is new to this third edition; it is by Antronette K. Yancey, Roshan Bastani, and Beth A. Glenn. They describe current health status disparities, review the potential determinants of observed disparities, and outline future directions for policy and practice, with specific emphasis on the contribution of chronic diseases. They show socioeconomic status is a major contributor to ethnic disparities in health. However, income inequality may also be an important contributor to poorer health, and economic indicators demonstrate that the gap between rich and poor is increasing dramatically while opportunities for upward social mobility are decreasing. They suggest that discrimination is the primary social environmental contribution to health disparities. Health services policy and health care organizations must reach beyond their accustomed boundaries of medical care delivery to address the physical, social, and economic environmental conditions underlying health disparities.

Leo S. Morales and Alex N. Ortega, in the new Chapter Three, have added another perspective on racial and ethnic disparities, switching the focus from *health* to *health care* disparities. They begin by defining disparities in care and reviewing some of the historical factors that have contributed to the pattern of disparity we observe today. In the next sections, they summarize some of the evidence documenting racial and ethnic disparities in the treatment of specific disease diseases and discuss some ongoing initiatives to reduce disparities in care. They show that disparities in health care are prevalent, with racial and ethnic minorities receiving lower-quality care in a variety of health care settings and across a range of medical conditions. A variety of factors contribute to disparities in care, among them legal and structural factors as well as patient and provider factors. The authors discuss multiple, ongoing efforts to address racial and ethnic disparities in care. They conclude that if current care disparities are not overcome, minority patients can be expected to continue to have suboptimal health status, which will in turn negatively affect labor market productivity and increase national health care spending.

Chapter Four, by E. Richard Brown and Shana Alex Lavarreda, examines alternative public policies for covering the uninsured and improving access. The authors discuss the successes and failures of Medicare, Medicaid, and the Children's Health Insurance Program (CHIP), with regard to giving their beneficiaries access to affordable, high-quality coverage. The chapter discusses the pros and cons of alternative policy options to extend coverage through the private sector, including consideration of small-group and individual health insurance reform, employer mandates, purchasing cooperatives, and subsidies for small-group and individual coverage. It also discusses options for expanding public coverage through incremental changes in Medicaid as well as universal coverage through social insurance, with a focus on the political barriers that have prevented the United States from achieving universal coverage. In spite of these barriers, the authors conclude that the United States cannot escape the need for fundamental reforms that will extend coverage to its entire population.

## Costs of Health Care

Health care costs were controlled rather well in the United States during the middle to late 1990s, but they have risen quickly since then. There is no shortage of culprits, although most analysts identify a variety of factors—especially the movement away from heavy-handed managed care and continued development of expensive medical and pharmaceutical technologies. At the same time, more Americans than ever lack insurance coverage, and concerns about overall quality persist. It is the trade-offs between costs on the one hand and access and quality on the other that will continue to be the major tension in health care policy for the foreseeable future.

Chapter Five, by Thomas H. Rice, focuses on measuring health care costs and presenting their trends. With regard to measurement, the chapter distinguishes between expenditures and costs, focusing thereafter on the more easily measured concept of expenditures. It also discusses the advantages and disadvantages of various measures of alternative health care prices and expenditures, and the reliability of the data sources that are used to measure expenditures in the United States and throughout the world. The chapter also lays out a discussion of the need for better data in the United States, concluding that requiring private insurers to collect and release data on expenditures is essential for making sensible policy decisions about alternative types of health care reform. As a lead-in to Chapter Six, it concludes with a look at the reasons that cost control is important and is likely to be on the forefront of health policy for years to come.

Chapter Six, by Thomas H. Rice and Gerald F. Kominski, focuses on alternative ways of containing health care costs. It begins by developing a conceptual framework that allows cost-containment methods to be divided into two categories: those based on fee-for-service, and those based on capitation. Within fee-for-service, strategies fall into one of three groups: price controls, volume controls, and expenditure controls. Most of the remainder of the chapter reviews the literature and experiences, both in the United States and in other developed countries, regarding the success and failure of the many strategies employed to contain costs: hospital rate setting programs, diagnosis-related groups, certificate-of-need programs, utilization review, technology controls, physician fee controls, practice guidelines, expenditure controls, health maintenance organizations, patient cost sharing, and managed competition. Although no conclusions are warranted as to the best way to control costs, the chapter indicates that it is important to continually assess the domestic and international experience regarding the success and failures of both market and government strategies to control health care costs.

Chapter Seven, by Stuart O. Schweitzer and William S. Comanor, examines a particular aspect of health care costs: pharmaceuticals. The costs of pharmaceuticals have been an important policy issue for decades, with concern among many consumer advocates that they are too high and should be controlled. The authors analyze the causes of increasing pharmaceutical costs, by critiquing studies conducted by others and then by conducting their own review of drug prices and expenditures over time in the United States and in other countries, adjusting for improvements in quality. They also review the many public policies that have been employed to control these costs, which have been aimed at consumers, physicians, and manufacturers. Although the authors do not reach any definitive conclusion about which policy levers are best, they are particularly concerned whether success can be achieved without sacrificing the vitality and viability of the industry, whose hallmark is a large investment in research and development for new products.

## Quality of Health Care

There is little question that establishing and preserving quality in health care has become the leading issue for health care managers. With tremendous competitive pressures to control health care costs, managers are faced with the task of formulating financial incentives and other mechanisms that will help ensure that a high-quality, cost-effective product is provided to patients. The advent of health care report cards and wider dissemination of information on health care quality, especially over the Internet, symbolize consumers' need for easily digestible information on the relative quality of their alternative insurance choices. This interest is paralleled on the research front, where a great deal of effort is being expended to produce reliable measures of health care outcomes.

Chapter Eight, by Patricia A. Ganz, Mark S. Litwin, Ron D. Hays, and Robert M. Kaplan, examines the measurement of health outcomes and quality of life. After providing an historical perspective on the health outcomes movement, the authors present an overview of the concept of health-related quality of life (HRQL), which focuses on the patient's own perception of health and the ability to function as a result of health status or disease experience. Much of the remainder of the chapter is devoted to the challenging goal of measuring HRQL and to presenting health services research studies that have attempted to measure it. An important conclusion is that patients are most concerned not with prolonging their lives per se but rather with improving the quality of their remaining years. Therefore, the authors argue, consumers are anxious to have information about the HRQL impact of new treatments. What is needed is careful and appropriate inclusion of HRQL outcomes in traditional health services.

Chapter Nine, by Elizabeth A. McGlynn, focuses on ensuring quality of care. The chapter begins by considering criteria for selecting topics for quality assessment. Next, it presents a conceptual framework useful for organizing evaluations of the quality. The definitions, methods, and state-of-the-art in assessing the structure, process, and outcomes of care are then discussed. The bottom line to this chapter is that scientifically sound methods exist for assessing quality and that they must be employed systematically in the future to guard against deterioration in quality that might otherwise occur as an unintended result of organizational and financial changes in the health services system.

Elizabeth A. McGlynn and John L. Adams observe in Chapter Ten that routine public reports on the quality of health care are being demanded thanks to changes in the organization and financing of care. In the unrestricted-choice model characterized by fee-for-service, individual providers were accountable for ensuring the delivery of high-quality health care. However, as third parties began to use financial incentives to control costs and restrict choices, the perception (if not the reality) was that physicians could no longer act solely in the patient's interest. We have moved from assuming that adequate mechanisms of accountability exist in the health system to demanding proof that various levels within the health system are accountable for the decisions that are made regarding resource allocation. Routine reports to the public on the quality of health care are one response to concerns about accountability. This chapter describes the type of information that is currently being publicly released; it discusses some of the methodological issues that arise in producing information for public release and summarizes what is known about the use of information on quality for consumer choice and quality. The authors conclude that the evidence on use of report cards by various audiences—consumers, purchasers, providers—suggests that the information is not widely used and appears to have only a small effect on performance. However, it is premature to declare this experiment a failure. Increased attention to the methods that are used to construct report cards, better use of communication techniques known to be effective, and more formal evaluations of such efforts are required before we have the information necessary to draw conclusions about the utility of public reporting.

## Special Populations

The problems of access, cost, and quality have varied historically for segments of the U.S. population because of their special needs and how the health care system has responded to those needs. It is likely that the nature of the problems faced by numerous groups will continue to change in the face of major alterations in how health services are organized and financed. All of the authors in Part Four have suggestions for health services research and policy implementation that might improve the prognosis for these vulnerable populations.

Chapter Eleven, by Jeff Luck and Paul Fu, Jr., is new to the third edition of the book. It carries out a much-need examination of health care information systems. The authors argue that such systems have the potential to boost both the efficiency and the quality of the health care system. The chapter begins by defining and presenting examples of the many types of health insurance systems. It goes on to examine how these systems can be applied to public health systems. The chapter also discusses several emerging applications of health insurance systems: imaging, telemedicine, and bioinformatics. It ends with recognition of the increasing importance being placed on privacy and security with the advent of electronic medical records.

Chapter Twelve, by Jack Needleman, Ellen T. Kurtzman, and Kenneth W. Kizer, is also new to this edition of the book. This chapter reviews recent efforts and issues involved in identifying a set of nursing-sensitive performance measures. It examines the scope of nursing's contribution to hospital care, priorities for measuring nursing care, and current initiatives to develop and implement systems for measuring nursing care, with special emphasis on the National Quality Forum's endorsement of national voluntary consensus standards. The authors conclude that developing effective performance measurement systems will enable stakeholders to better understand and monitor the degree to which nursing care influences patient safety and quality.

Chapter Thirteen, by Steven P. Wallace, Emily K. Abel, Nadereh Pourat, and Linda Delp, is a comprehensive overview of the long-term care system as a response to the rapidly increasing number of elderly in the United States and their needs for treatment of chronic and disabling illness. This chapter reviews the recent literature on long-term care, showing how financial considerations have framed the dominant policy debates and research agenda. It offers up-to-date information on nursing homes, the range of community based care, informal long-term care, and workers in the long-term care system. The authors emphasize that long-term care includes social as well as medical services, is furnished overwhelmingly by family and friends, and is financed primarily by Medicaid and out-of-pocket payments. After documenting that the driving force in policy and research in long-term care for the past twenty years has been cost containment and efficiency, the authors identify as the most critical policy and research question how to provide adequate high-quality long-term services to a growing and diverse older population. Policy makers frequently view nursing homes as a low-cost alternative to hospitals and consider community services and family care as less expensive substitutes for nursing homes, neglecting quality-of-life issues. The chapter concludes that the limited financial resources of many older persons, especially racial and ethnic minorities, widows, and the working class, create a need for a universal Medicare type of social insurance.

In Chapter Fourteen, David Zingmond and William E. Cunningham argue that the characteristics of HIV/AIDS—contagious, chronically disabling, fatal, and emerging in epidemic proportions—will increasingly force health care policy makers and managers to reevaluate the organization, delivery, and financing of health services for the HIV population. They state that in 2003 between 34.6 million and 42.3 million people were living with HIV infection worldwide, and more than 20 million had died of AIDS. In the United States, an estimated 1.5 million Americans are living with HIV infection, and there have been 524,060 deaths from AIDS. The authors review what is known and the research needs concerning the changing epidemiology and treatment of AIDS, including use of new and expensive antiretroviral drugs; measures of access, costs, and quality; and the range of services needed to treat AIDS, including not only formal medical services but also prevention, psychosocial services, and community-based health and social services. They discuss the growing challenges in providing and paying for services as the HIV/AIDS epidemic spreads from its initial geographic epicenters of Caucasian, homosexual men to much broader communities of socially and economically disadvantaged populations of women, children, adolescents, and minority groups.

Chapter Fifteen, by Moira Inkelas, Neal Halfon, David Lee Wood, and Mark A. Schuster, examines the key issues underlying the incongruities between the needs of children and families and the current and evolving structure of the health services organization in the United States. The authors review the health needs of children and families by examining children's unique vulnerabilities, current health risks and conditions, and service needs. Next, they describe the characteristics of the health care system that influence children's access to care and the overall efficiency of health care for children. They find the organization of services to be disjointed, with multiple financial and structural barriers to children's receipt of care, despite recent enactment of the federally supported SCHIP. They note that the movement to manage care to rationalize delivery of personal medical services may substantially improve children's access to basic medical care, but many of their health needs—especially for complex medical or socially based health problems—may not be sufficiently addressed. The authors conclude that adequate response to the health care needs of at-risk children requires greater effort to expand coverage for the uninsured, including greater effort to enroll eligible children in current programs and development of multidisciplinary coordination that integrates the fragmented child health system.

Chapter Sixteen, by Susan L. Ettner and Janet C. Link, examines mental health services, with emphasis on public policy toward their use. The authors note the substantial access barriers facing those with mental health problems: for example, that only about 40 percent of Americans with a serious mental health disorder receive treatment in a given year. After an overview of the mental health service system in the United States, the authors grapple with a number of difficult issues, among them the stigma associated with mental illness, lack of use of appropriately trained mental health providers, and gaps in both public and private insurance coverage for mental health conditions. Ettner and Link assert that several population groups—the elderly, children, minorities, and those living in rural areas—tend to underuse mental health services relative to their needs. The chapter concludes with a discussion of several actions that can be taken by federal and state government to improve the mental health care system, including support for safety net providers such as public hospitals, tailoring mental health benefits to meet the need of publicly insured patients, and requiring that all insurers offer mental health benefits at parity with other medical services.

Chapter Seventeen, by Roberta Wyn and Beatriz M. Solís, examines how women's health status, socioeconomic status, and multiple role responsibilities interact with their access to and use of services. Although women and men share the same need for affordable, accessible, and high-quality care, there are specific health concerns and patterns of use unique to women that are often overlooked. Many health conditions are particular to women, occur with greater frequency among women, or have different consequences for women than for men. The chapter examines the adequacy of women's access to health insurance coverage and the ability of that coverage to protect against the costs of health services, explores how health insurance coverage affects women's access to care, and looks beyond financial barriers to other aspects of the health care system that influence access. Women have a lower uninsured rate and higher utilization than men, but the authors call attention to women's more limited health insurance options and large discrepancies among women in coverage rates and health care use according to income, education, and ethnicity. They also document women's differential access to procedures and outcomes after they gain access to the system. The authors conclude that particular consideration of low-income women is required in formulating new health policy regarding the financing of services. They have the lowest rate of screening for certain clinical preventive services, have the poorest health status, and are the most vulnerable to the effects of costs.

In Chapter Eighteen, Lisa Arangua and Lillian Gelberg describe the sociodemographic characteristics of homeless adults and children as well as their health status, risk factors for illness, barriers to care, quality of care, and current medical programs available to homeless individuals. They estimated that 3.5 million in the United States are currently without a home and that 14 percent of the U.S. population (26 million people) have been homeless at some time in their lives. The homeless constitute a heterogeneous population that includes families, runaway youths, the physically and mentally ill, and substance abusers. The homeless population experiences a high rate of acute and chronic illness but has limited access to medical care as reflected by high inpatient utilization and low ambulatory service use relative to their level of need. The medical care they do receive is limited in terms of availability, continuity, and comprehensiveness. The authors find the homeless particularly vulnerable in the policy arena because of the absence of strong advocates, a tendency on the part of the public to accept large-scale homelessness as inevitable, and commonly held beliefs that the homeless are responsible for their status. Still, their plight could be improved by stabilizing funding for health care, funding respite care, medical education reform, and more affordable housing options. They conclude that the best way to help the homeless is for the United States to address more fundamental issues concerning alleviation of poverty.

## Directions for Change

The defeat of comprehensive health care reform at the national level in the early 1990s created a unique opportunity to reexamine, in Part Five, the goals of health care reform and the methods for achieving those goals in a political environment that remains strongly polarized over the need for such reform. Health services research has clearly played an influential role in developing policy options at the local, state, and national levels during the past two decades. What significant contributions will health services researchers make in the future? The remainder of this volume addresses some of the fundamental challenges facing health care researchers, policy makers, and managers, now that we are well into the first decade of the twenty-first century.

Perhaps the most basic challenge involves determining the appropriate role of markets versus the role of governments in addressing issues of access, cost, and quality. Chapter Nineteen, by Gerald F. Kominski and Glenn A. Melnick, evaluates the growth of managed care and price competition and the empirical evidence regarding the ability of competition to control health care costs. The chapter describes the various models of managed care that have evolved from the traditional model of prepaid group practice. It then summarizes the growth in managed care during the past three decades and the factors that have contributed to its growth. The authors argue that because California is considered to be the most mature managed care market in the country, it has served as a laboratory to inform policy makers on what might be expected in other parts of the country as managed care expands nationally. But because of the managed care backlash that began in the late 1990s and continues through this decade, managed care is no longer viewed as the centerpiece in market-based efforts to reform health care. Political support has shifted instead toward new forms of market-based reform and price competition in the form of high-deductible health plans and health savings accounts. They conclude that perhaps the time has come for a new paradigm of managed care that focuses on improved health promotion, disease prevention, quality, and outcomes, without necessarily the expectation of lower costs.

Chapter Twenty, by Gerald F. Kominski, Jeanne T. Black, and Thomas H. Rice, examines the federal government's largest health insurance program, Medicare, and the challenges facing its future. They review the political conditions leading to enactment of Medicare, which was widely viewed as a compromise on the road to national health insurance when it was enacted in 1965. Forty years later, Medicare faces several significant challenges, including ongoing cost increases and a rapidly expanding eligible population, that threaten its public support. These challenges have led to a gradual transformation of Medicare during the past decade toward greater reliance on private markets and managed care. The authors examine the nature of the "crisis" in Medicare and efforts to reform the program, including recent introduction of a prescription drug benefit. This major expansion of benefits has already created additional financial demands that are likely to lead to calls for further modification of the program before the end of the decade.

In Chapter Twenty-One, Lester Breslow and Jonathan E. Fielding reexamine the significant role of public health agencies in delivery of personal health services in the United States. They find that these agencies have a vital interest in health care delivery because a substantial portion of the population has inadequate access to services or unstable health benefits. Public health has traditionally been directed at ensuring a safe environment and at addressing behavioral influences on health. Access to quality personal health services made available by the public health system, they argue, is also an important determinant of health. The ability of public health agencies to perform all their core public health functions, however, requires greater commitment to public health and health promotion.

Chapter Twenty-Two, by the late Ruth Roemer, deals with the continuing issue of medical malpractice liability. The author first raises the politically sensitive issue of whether patients should be able to sue their managed care plan. She then steps back and explores the history of malpractice insurance crises of the 1970s and 1980s, state legislative responses, and the impact of those responses. The chapter addresses major potential reforms to the tort system, including alternative dispute resolution, enterprise liability, no-fault insurance, and medical accident compensation. Reviewing U.S. and international experience with these options, the author concludes that despite the soundness of the no-fault approach political realities seem to mitigate against adoption of this alternative. Instead, the climate may be favorable for rationalizing our handling of medical injury compensation through adopting an administrative system that is more equitable and less costly than the tort system.

Finally, Chapter Twenty-Three, by Pauline Vaillancourt Rosenau and Ruth Roemer, deals with the ethics of public health and health care services. The cardinal principles of medical ethics—autonomy, beneficence, and justice—apply in public health ethics, but in a somewhat altered form. The authors contrast these principles as usually applied in medical ethics (where individual rights and autonomy prevail) with a broader social perspective in which individual rights may be subsumed by consideration of social welfare. At a time when we continue moving toward market-based solutions, the authors construct a framework for reexamining some of the ethical and social issues related to resource development, economic support, organization, management, delivery, and quality of care. Ethical issues in public health and health services management are likely to become increasingly complex in the future. The authors conclude, however, that even in the absence of agreement on ethical assumptions and in the face of diversity and complexity that prohibit easy compromise, mechanisms for resolving ethical dilemmas in public health do exist.

# Conclusion

We have asked the authors of this volume to explore what health services research has to tell us about making fundamental changes so as to ensure access to affordable high-quality health care. We have added new chapters in this third edition, and all of the authors of revised chapters have extensively updated their work. We think that as an informed reader you will find the authors have met the challenge of comprehensive review of key policy and management issues regarding problems of access, costs, and quality as well as of serving special populations and assessing strategies for reform. Unfortunately, neither the authors of this volume (nor any other possible set of authors, for that matter) have answers for all the major challenges facing our health care system, but you will find that they delineate the critical questions clearly and propose a number of informed, innovative solutions.

# Notes

1. "Income Stable, Poverty Rate Increases, Percentage of Americans Without Health Insurance Unchanged." *U.S. Census Bureau News.* Aug. 30, 2005. [http://www.census.gov/PressRelease/www/releases/archives/income_wealth/005647.html].
2. McGlynn, E. A., and others. "The Quality of Health Care Delivered to Adults in the United States." *New England Journal of Medicine,* June 26, 2003, *348*(26), 2635–2645.

# ACKNOWLEDGMENTS

The authors of this volume have once again met their obligations effectively and expediently. Their rewards for substantial contributions to this third edition were largely the intangible ones of providing service to the students and practitioners of health services policy and research. We are particularly thankful to the new authors who have contributed to this volume.

Charles Doran, administrative specialist for the Department of Health Services UCLA School of Public Health, once again performed the essential tasks of organizing the efforts of the authors, formatting their work, and facilitating communication with our publisher, Jossey-Bass.

Alyssa Schabloski deserves special thanks for her support on developing the Instructor's Guide for Chapter 22 on behalf of our dear departed colleague Ruth Roemer.

Finally, Andy Pasternack, senior editor, public health and health service evaluation and research at Jossey-Bass once again supported us in undertaking this revision and providing high-quality publishing support to complete the task.

*January 2007*
*Los Angeles*

Ronald M. Andersen
Thomas H. Rice
Gerald F. Kominski

# CHANGING THE
# U.S. HEALTH CARE SYSTEM

PART ONE

## ACCESS TO HEALTH CARE

CHAPTER ONE

# IMPROVING ACCESS TO CARE IN AMERICA

## Individual and Contextual Indicators

Ronald M. Andersen
Pamela L. Davidson

This chapter presents basic trends as well as research and policy issues related to health care access. We define *access* as actual use of personal health services and everything that facilitates or impedes their use. It is the link between health services systems and the populations they serve. Access means not only visiting a medical care provider but also getting to the right services at the right time to promote improved health outcomes. Conceptualizing and measuring access is the key to understanding and making health policy in a number of ways: (1) predicting use of health services, (2) promoting social justice, and (3) improving effectiveness and efficiency of health service delivery.

The chapter presents a conceptual framework for understanding the multiple dimensions of access to medical care. The various types of access are considered and related to their policy purposes. Examples of key access measures are given, and trend data are used to track changes that have occurred over time in these access indicators. The chapter addresses the questions: Is access improving or declining in the United States? for whom? according to what measures? It concludes by discussing future access indicators and research directions.

## Understanding Access to Health Care

This section proposes a conceptual framework based on a behavioral model of health services use that emphasizes contextual as well as individual determinants of access to medical care. Also reviewed are the dimensions of access defined according to components of the framework and how access might be improved for each dimension.

## Conceptual Framework

The framework presented in Figure 1.1 stresses that improving access to care is best accomplished by focusing on contextual as well as individual determinants.[1] By contextual, we point to the circumstances and environment of health care access. Context includes health organization and provider-related factors as well as community characteristics.[2] Contextual factors are measured at some aggregate rather than individual level. These aggregate levels range from units as small as the family to those as large as a national health care system. In between are workgroups and teams, provider organizations, health plans, neighborhoods, local communities, and metropolitan statistical areas. Individuals are related to these aggregate units through membership (family, workgroup, provider institutions, health plan) or residence (neighborhood, community, metropolitan area, national health system).

The model suggests that the major components of contextual characteristics are divided in the same way as individual characteristics determining access: (1) existing conditions that predispose people to use or not use services even though these conditions are not directly responsible for use, (2) enabling conditions that facilitate or impede use of services, and (3) need or conditions that laypeople or health care providers recognize as requiring medical treatment.[3] The model emphasizes contextual factors in recognition of the importance of community, the structure and process of providing care,[4] and the realities of a managed care environment.[5] Still, the ultimate focus of the model remains on health behavior of individuals (especially their use of health services) and resulting outcomes regarding their health and satisfaction with services.

We now turn to brief consideration of each major component of the model shown in Figure 1.1.

***Contextual Predisposing Characteristics.*** Demographic characteristics include the age, gender, and marital status composition of a community. Thus a community populated primarily by older persons might well have a different mix of available health services and facilities from one in which the majority are younger parents and children.

Social characteristics at the contextual level describe how supportive or detrimental the communities where people live and work might be to their health and access to health services. Relevant measures include educational level, ethnic

# FIGURE 1.1. A BEHAVIORAL MODEL OF HEALTH SERVICES USE INCLUDING CONTEXTUAL AND INDIVIDUAL CHARACTERISTICS.

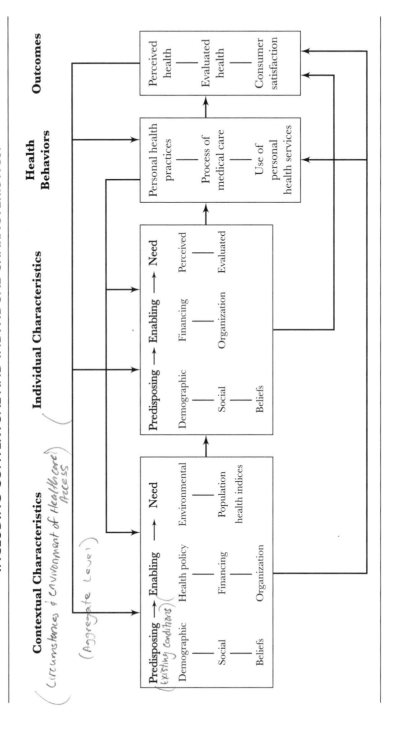

and racial composition, proportion of recent immigrants, employment level, and crime rate.

Beliefs refer to underlying community or organizational values and cultural norms and prevailing political perspectives regarding how health services should be organized, financed, and made accessible to the population.[6]

***Contextual Enabling Characteristics.*** Health policies are authoritative decisions made pertaining to health or influencing the pursuit of health.[7] They can be public policies made in the legislative, executive, or judicial branch of government, at all levels from local to national. They can also be policies made in the private sector by such decision makers as executives of managed care organizations concerning product lines, pricing, or marketing, or by accrediting agencies such as the Joint Commission on Accreditation of Health Care Organizations (JCAHO) or quality assessment organizations such as the National Committee for Quality Assurance (NCQA).

Financing characteristics are described by an array of contextual measures that suggest resources potentially available to pay for health services, including per capita community income, and wealth. Other financial characteristics are incentives to purchase or provide services, such as rate of health insurance coverage, relative price of medical care and other goods and services, and method of compensating providers. Also included here are per capita expenditures for health services.

Organization at the contextual level includes the amount and distribution of health services facilities and personnel as well as how they are structured to offer services. Structure includes supply of services in the community, such as the ratios of physicians and hospital beds to population. Structure also includes how medical care is organized in a particular institution or delivery system where people receive care, as with office hours and location of service, provider mix, utilization and quality control oversight, and outreach and education programs.

***Contextual Need Characteristics.*** Environmental need characteristics include health-related measures of the physical environment, among them the quality of housing, water, and air (for example, residing in a county that met national ambient air quality standards throughout the year).[8] Other measures suggesting how healthy the environment might be are injury or death rate (such as rate of occupational injury and disease and related deaths) as well as death rates from motor vehicle injuries, homicides, and firearms.

Population health indices are more general indicators of community health that may or may not be associated with the physical environment. These indices include general and condition-specific rates of mortality (for example, infant mortality; age-adjusted mortality; and mortality rates for heart disease, cancer, stroke, HIV); morbidity (incidence of preventable childhood communicable diseases and AIDS, and prevalence of cancer, hypertension, and untreated dental caries); and disability (disability days due to acute conditions and limitation of activity due to chronic conditions).

The arrows in Figure 1.1 leading from the contextual characteristics indicate that they can influence health behaviors and outcomes in multiple ways. They can work through individual characteristics, as when increased generosity of a state Medicaid program leads to previously uninsured low-income children being covered by health insurance and subsequent increase in their use of health services. Contextual characteristics can also influence health behaviors and outcomes directly, over and above their influence through individual characteristics, as when presence of community health clinics in a metropolitan statistical area leads to increased use of primary care services by low-income persons independent of personal income or other individual characteristics. Understanding the nature of contextual influences on access to care presents many analytic challenges,[9] but it may permit important new insights into how to improve access to care.

***Individual Predisposing Characteristics.*** Demographic factors such as age and gender of the individual represent biological imperatives suggesting the likelihood that people will need health services.[10] Social factors determine the status of a person in the community as well as his or her ability to cope with presenting problems and command resources to deal with those problems. Traditional measures include an individual's education, occupation, and ethnicity. Expanded measures might include people's social network and social interactions that can facilitate or impede access to services.[11] Health beliefs are attitudes, values, and knowledge people have about health and health services that can influence their subsequent perception of need and use of health services.

***Individual Enabling Characteristics.*** Financing of health services for the individual involves the income and wealth available to the individual to pay for services. Financing also includes the effective price of health care to the patient, determined by having insurance and cost-sharing requirements.

Organization of health services for the individual describes whether or not the individual has a regular source of care and the nature of that source (private doctor, community clinic, emergency room). It also includes means of transportation and reported travel time to and waiting time for care.

***Individual Need Characteristics.*** Perceived need is how people view their own general health and functional state. Also included here is how they experience and emotionally respond to symptoms of illness, pain, and worry about their health condition. Perceptions about the importance and magnitude of a health problem or symptom lead to a decision to seek medical care (or not to do so). Perceived need is largely a social phenomenon that, when appropriately modeled, should itself be largely explainable by social characteristics (such as ethnicity or education) and health beliefs (health attitudes, knowledge about health care, and so on).

Evaluated need represents professional judgment and objective measurement about a patient's physical status and need for medical care (blood pressure readings, temperature, and blood cell count, as well as diagnoses and prognoses for particular conditions the patient experiences). Of course, evaluated need is not simply, or even primarily, a valid and reliable measure from biological science. It also has a social component and varies with the changing state of the art and science of medicine, clinical guidelines and protocols, and prevailing practice patterns, as well as the training and competency of the professional expert doing the assessment.

Logical expectations of the model are that perceived need helps us better understand the care-seeking process and adherence to a medical regimen, while evaluated need is more closely related to the kind and amount of treatment that is given after a patient has presented to a medical care provider.

***Health Behaviors.***  Personal health practices are behaviors on the part of the individual that influence health status. They include diet and nutrition, exercise, stress reduction, alcohol and tobacco use, self-care, and adherence to medical regimens. The process of medical care is the behavior of providers interacting with patients in the process of care delivery.[12] General process measures might relate to patient counseling and education, test ordering, prescribing patterns, and quality of provider-patient communication. Process measures might also describe the specifics of caregiving for particular conditions, such as whether a provider checks a CD4 cell count in a person with HIV disease or reviews the patient's record of home glucose monitoring in a diabetic.

Use of personal health services is the essential component of health behaviors in a comprehensive model of access to care. The purpose of the original behavioral model was to predict health services use, measured rather broadly as units of physician ambulatory care, hospital inpatient services, and dental care visits. We hypothesized that predisposing, enabling, and need factors would have differential ability to explain use depending on what type of service was examined.[13] Hospital services used in response to more serious problems and conditions would be primarily explained by need and demographic characteristics, while dental services (considered more discretionary) would more likely be explained by social conditions, health beliefs, and enabling resources.

We expected all the components of the model to explain ambulatory physician use because the conditions stimulating care seeking would generally be viewed as less serious and demanding than those resulting in inpatient care but more serious than those leading to dental care. More specific measures of health services use are now being employed to describe a particular medical condition or type of service or practitioner, or they are linked in an episode of illness to examine continuity of care.[14] For example, a longitudinal study of rheumatoid arthritis measures patient visits to various types of providers, treatment used, level of patient compliance with treatment, and associated changes in functional status and pain over time. Although specific measures are, in many ways, likely to be more informative, the more global ones (number of physician visits, self-rated general health status) still have a role to play. Global measures are used to assess the overall effects of health policy changes over time.

***Outcomes.*** One kind of result or outcome of health behavior and contextual and individual characteristics is an individual's or patient's perceived health status. This depends on many factors in addition to use of personal health services, including all of the contextual factors as well as an individual's demographic and social characteristics, health beliefs, and personal health practices. Perceived health status indicates the extent to which a person can live a functional, comfortable, and pain-free existence. Measures include reports of general perceived health status, activities of daily living, and disability.

Evaluated health status is dependent on the judgment of the professional, on the basis of established clinical standards and state-of-the-art practices. Measures include tests of patient physiology and function as well as diagnosis and prognosis regarding their condition. Outcome measures of perceived and evaluated heath may appear suspiciously like perceived and evaluated need measures. Indeed, they are. The ultimate outcome validation of improved access is to reduce individual needs previously measured and evaluated.

Consumer satisfaction is how individuals feel about the health care they receive. It can be judged by patient ratings of waiting time, travel time, communication with providers, and technical care received. From a health plan perspective, an ultimate outcome measure of patient satisfaction in this era of managed care might be whether or not enrollees choose to switch plans.[15]

Central to the model shown in Figure 1.1 is feedback, depicted by the arrows from outcomes to health behaviors, individual characteristics, and contextual characteristics. Feedback allows insights about how access might come to be improved. For example, outcomes might influence contextual characteristics, as illustrated by Karen Davis, president of the Commonwealth Foundation.[16] Davis noted that the continued failure of our health services system to provide access to care, particularly for vulnerable populations, as well as the generally low level of satisfaction of the public with the health services system lead her to conclude that our health care system needs to be fundamentally changed. Such conclusions, drawn by enough influential people, as well as dissatisfaction on the part of the public might ultimately lead to health policy changes in the country and subsequent reforms in financing and organizing health services with the intent to improve access to care. These health policy reforms would represent a major contextual change in the American health care delivery system.

Feedback, of course, can occur at the community or institutional level as well as at the national level. Certainly there are expectations that feedback to health care institutions from JCAHO or NCQA might result in contextual changes in the institutions' organization and processes of care for their patients.

## Defining and Improving Dimensions of Access to Care

Access to medical care is a relatively complex multidimensional phenomenon. Over several decades, the behavioral model has been used as a tool to help define and differentiate these dimensions.[17] In this section, we review dimensions of access and suggest how access can be improved through health policy and delivery system intervention (see Figure 1.2).

*Potential Access.* Potential access is measured by the enabling variables of the behavioral model at both the contextual (health policy, financing) and individual (regular source of care, health insurance, income) levels. More enabling resources constitute the means for use and increase the likelihood that it will take place.

*Realized Access.* Realized access is the actual use of services. Realized access indicators include utilization of physician, hospital, dental and other health services. Historically, the United States experienced improving trends in access as measured by an increasing health services utilization rate. Access to health services was considered an end goal of policy change. Progressive policies designed to increase access were implemented in the 1950s and 1960s to increase the number of physicians, augment hospital beds in rural communities, and create Medicare and Medicaid. Potential access measures (regular source of care, health insurance) were used as indicators of greater access. Realized access measures (utilization of hospital and physician services) were employed to monitor and evaluate policies designed to influence health services use.

The U.S. health care system evolved from decision making grounded in altruism through increasing access and supply of resources to a position of caution and financial prudence.[18] The predominant focus on increasing medical care utiliza-

## FIGURE 1.2. THE POLICY PURPOSES OF ACCESS MEASURES.

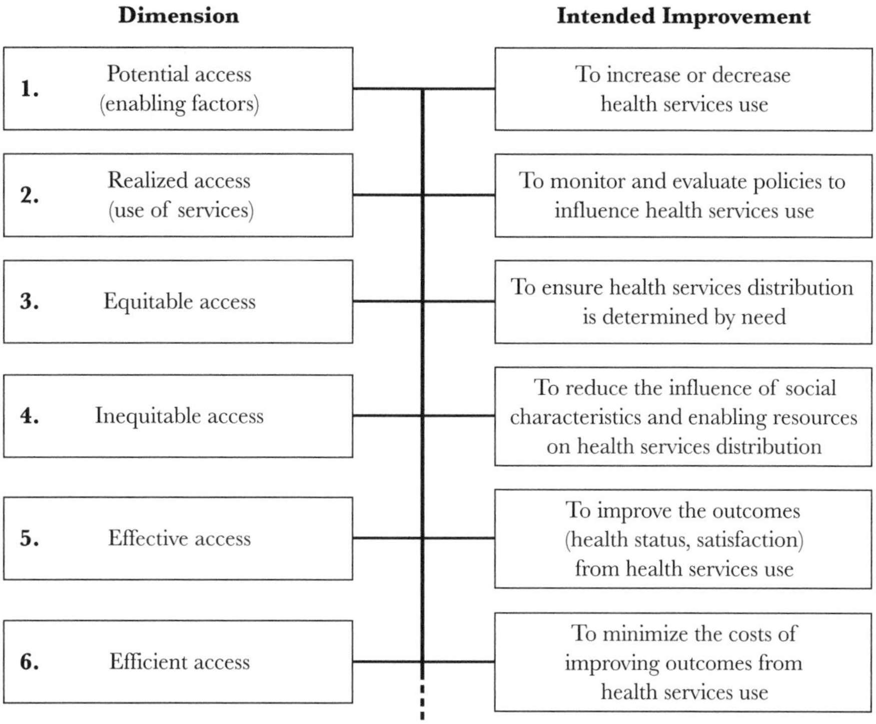

| Dimension | Intended Improvement |
|---|---|
| **1.** Potential access (enabling factors) | To increase or decrease health services use |
| **2.** Realized access (use of services) | To monitor and evaluate policies to influence health services use |
| **3.** Equitable access | To ensure health services distribution is determined by need |
| **4.** Inequitable access | To reduce the influence of social characteristics and enabling resources on health services distribution |
| **5.** Effective access | To improve the outcomes (health status, satisfaction) from health services use |
| **6.** Efficient access | To minimize the costs of improving outcomes from health services use |

tion shifted in the 1970s to concern for health care cost containment and creation of mechanisms to limit access to health care. Examples of policies designed to limit access are coinsurance, deductibles, utilization review, and the genesis of managed care. In the 1980s and early 1990s, in competing with fee-for-service organizations, managed care enjoyed double-digit growth in profit margins.[19] However, over time its growth slowed, and managed care organizations came under considerable scrutiny regarding whether they limited needed services for their enrollees.

This managed care backlash led to a downward trend in health maintenance organization (HMO) enrollment in the mid-1990s through 2000; however, during the same time period Medicaid managed care continued to expand rapidly.[20] In response to the managed care backlash and escalating health care costs, the major commercial health plans turned from capitation and utilization review to high co-payments, shifting costs to consumers, tied networks with variable co-insurance, and medical management programs focusing on high-cost patients.[21] Plans continue to experiment with new provider networks, payment systems, and referral practices designed to lower costs while improving service delivery, which has been a challenging proposition for the industry.[22]

Another incremental health policy reform initiative, the Medicare prescription drug benefit, for years has been at the forefront of congressional debate. Pharmaceuticals are a major out-of-pocket expense and threaten the financial security of lower-income beneficiaries. Policy makers grappled with deciding who should bear these costs and whether subsidies could be extended to assist lower-income beneficiaries.[23] These issues are discussed in some detail in Chapter Twenty, on Medicare reform.

Among commercial plans, 64 percent of prescription drug benefits offered through employers used tiered co-payment systems in 2004, up from 28 percent in 2000.[24] Under these arrangements, employees paid lower co-pays for generic drugs and higher fees for branded drugs, which encouraged use of less costly generic drugs. However, cost sharing for prescription drugs has the potential for reducing utilization and health status of seniors,[25] and high out-of-pocket expenditures for prescription drugs have been associated with adverse health outcomes.[26] Other methods used by companies to control utilization and costs include shifting costs to employees, disease management programs, providing incentives to doctors who meet treatment guidelines, and reducing workers' co-pay if they go to doctors with the best track record in efficiency (best result for the best price).[27]

*Equitable Access.* Equitable (as well as inequitable) access is defined according to which determinants (age, ethnicity, insurance status, symptoms) of realized access are dominant in predicting utilization. Equity is in the eye of the beholder. Value judgments about which components of the model should explain utilization in an equitable health care system are crucial to the definition. Traditionally, equitable access has been defined as occurring when demographic variables (age and gender), and especially need variables, account for most of the variance in utilization.[28]

*Inequitable Access.* Inequitable access occurs when social characteristics and enabling resources such as ethnicity or income determine who gets medical care. The social justice movement, dominant in the 1960s and early 1970s with the passage of Medicare and Medicaid, sought to ensure that health services distribution was determined by need and to reduce the influence of social characteristics and enabling resources on health services distribution.

Equity of access to medical care is the value judgment that the system is deemed fair or equitable if need-based criteria (rather than enabling resources such as insurance coverage or income) are the main determinants of whether or not—or how much—care is sought. Subgroup disparities in use of health services (say, according to race or ethnicity, or health insurance coverage) would be mini-

mized in a fair and equitable system, while underlying need for preventive or ill-
ness-related health care would be the principal factor determining utilization.

   Policies to improve social justice include the health disparities initiatives, State
Children's Health Insurance Program (SCHIP), the Federal Safety Net Initiative,
and recruiting more minorities to the health professions. The landmark 2003 report by the Institute of Medicine (IOM), *Unequal Treatment,* revealed that even if
insurance status and income are controlled for, blacks and Hispanic Americans
have poorer health outcomes.[29] Forty years after civil rights legislation was enacted
in the mid-1960s, racial inequities in health and healthcare persist that are due to
socioeconomic status, racial segregation, and inequities in access to quality medical care.[30] Policy levers have been proposed to address health disparities, such as
the central role of the Centers for Medicare and Medicaid Services (CMS) in overseeing quality of care through measurement and certification, adherence to the
HHS Office of Minority Health (OMH) national standards for cultural competence in health care, and creating a state minority health policy report card.[31] For
more in-depth analysis of health disparities and policy implications, see Chapters
Two, Three, and Four.

   A $48 billion federal action in the form of SCHIP stimulated virtually every
state to expand coverage for low-income children.[32] Prior to the enactment of
SCHIP, little progress had been made in more than fifteen years to reduce the population of uninsured children.[33] Attracting children into these programs depended
on ease of enrollment, cost-sharing requirements, whether programs were pack-
aged in such a way to reduce stigma, the effectiveness of outreach efforts, and overcoming administrative and nonfinancial barriers.[34] But is SCHIP an effective and
efficient policy intervention for improving health care access for children's safety-
net resources?[35] Several evaluation studies have demonstrated that SCHIP was associated with improved access, continuity, and quality of care, and a greater
proportion of care delivered within the regular source of medical and dental care.[36]

   Additionally, parents reported that having health insurance for children reduced family stress, enabled the children to obtain the care they needed, and eased
family burdens, producing an overall positive impact for children and their families.[37] In sharp contrast to state initiatives to extend public insurance for children,
there has been virtually no change in the generosity of public programs for adults
nationally, although public coverage has improved in some states (among them
Arizona, Tennessee, and Vermont) and declined in others (California and New
York as examples).[38]

   Other policies promoting social justice have been created to support safety-
net providers who care for uninsured and underinsured persons.[39] The institutional safety-net system consists of a patchwork of community clinics, hospitals,
and other programs whose nature varies dramatically across the country, many

funded by the Health Resources and Services Administration (HRSA). However, financing for safety-net institutions has always been tenuous and subject to changing politics, available resources, and public policies.[40]

In 2002, the Bush administration launched a five-year initiative to expand the health center system by adding twelve hundred new and expanded health center sites and increasing the number of patients served from 10.3 million in 2001 to an estimated 16 million by 2006.[41]

HRSA manages the consolidated health center program, funding a national network of more than thirty-seven hundred organizations, which include community health centers, migrant health centers, health care for the homeless, school-based health centers, and public housing primary care centers. HRSA's seven strategic goals are to improve access, health outcomes, and quality; reduce disparities; improve public health systems and emergency response; and achieve excellence in management practice.[42]

Other examples of policy and programmatic efforts to improve social justice are initiatives to recruit more underrepresented minorities (URM) to the health professions. Research has shown that URM health professionals are culturally competent and more willing to provide care to underserved populations. One such initiative was funded by the Robert Wood Johnson Foundation and the California Endowment, furnishing a combined $25 million to sponsor the Dental Pipeline, Profession, and Practice Program in fifteen accredited dental schools in the United States.[43] The Pipeline initiative was developed to help address the critical shortage of oral health care for underserved populations. The Pipeline program objectives are to (1) increase recruitment and retention of underrepresented minority and low-income students; (2) revise didactic and clinical curricula to support community-based educational programs; and (3) establish community-based clinical education programs that give dental students and residents sixty days of experience in this patient care environment. Critical outcomes of the Pipeline initiative are the practice settings selected by recent graduates and the percentage of underserved populations these entry-level dentists expect to serve in their practice.

***Effective Access.*** The cost-containment movement became more sophisticated in the late 1980s and 1990s. The next generation of health services research transitioned to measuring the impact of health services utilization on health outcomes. Accordingly, the IOM Committee on Monitoring Access to Medical Care defined *access* as timely use of personal health services to achieve the best possible health outcomes.[44] This definition relies on use of health services and health outcomes as a yardstick for judging whether access has been achieved. The resulting measures are referred to as effective access.

Measures of effectiveness examine the relative impact of health services utilization within the context of other predisposing, enabling, need, and health-behavior variables. Predisposing variables, such as age, gender, and social support variables, can influence the patient's health status following treatment. Access to personal enabling resources (health insurance, income, regular source of care) can result in expeditious medical treatment with highly trained practitioners using state-of-the-art medical technology. Conversely, lack of enabling resources can lead to delay in seeking medical advice or episodic, fragmented treatment with a potential negative impact on health outcomes and satisfaction with medical care.

Researchers conducting effectiveness and outcomes research have developed strategies for risk adjustment to control for the effects of medical need (severity of illness, number of symptoms, and comorbidities) before intervention.[45] Personal health practices (diet, exercise, stress management) and compliance with medical regimens prior and subsequent to treatment can also influence health outcomes. Analytical models used to determine the effect of alternative medical treatments on health outcomes must consider the influence of these varying personal and behavioral factors, as well as contextual differences in health care delivery systems and external environment.

***Efficient Access.*** Most recently, concerns about cost containment have been combined with those directed to improving health outcomes. The results are measures of efficient access. They are similar to measures of effective access with the added emphasis on assessing resources used to influence outcome.

Improvement is attained by promoting health outcomes while minimizing the resources required to attain improved outcomes. Aday and colleagues describe efficiency as producing the combination of goods and services with the highest attainable total value, given limited resources and technology.[46] Efficiency is an attempt to quantify the cost-effectiveness or cost benefit of health services to determine the extent to which finite private, public, or personal resources should be invested in ensuring access to those procedures.[47]

An example of policy and programmatic change to improve efficient access is the Government Performance and Results Act mandated by Congress in 1993. The purpose of the legislation was to improve efficiency and accountability for the federal dollars spent on health care. In response, HRSA created the Office of Performance Review (OPR) in 2002. The community health center cottage industry of the past is transforming into a network of professionally managed organizations. OPR's core functions are to collaboratively conduct performance reviews with HRSA funded organizations, track regional and state trends, provide policy and grantee feedback to HRSA, and offer technical assistance on performance measurement and improvement. HRSA is moving toward increased use of common, structured, and standardized data strategies to carry out an effective system of performance measurement. The performance measures, defined as outcomes and effort to produce outcomes, are designed to create a culture and technology for efficiently using federal dollars to improve access for underserved populations.[48]

Part of a larger trend in the health care industry today, performance measurement and improvement is being promoted by organizations such as the Institute for Healthcare Improvement (IHI) and the National Center for Healthcare Leadership (NCHL).[49]

## Trends in Access to Care

In this section, trends in access are examined according to several dimensions of access. We consider changes over time in potential access (health insurance coverage), realized access (use of hospital, physician, and dental services), and equitable access (health insurance and health services use according to income and race). We also examine some key research findings concerning effective and efficient access.

### Potential Access (Enabling Health Insurance)

Table 1.1 reports a critical potential access measure: health care coverage for persons under sixty-five years of age from 1984 to 2002. The uninsured proportion of the population increased from 14 to 17 percent in that time period. Medicaid coverage actually increased (from 7 to 12 percent), but the overall decline in coverage resulted from a drop in the proportion covered by private insurance, from 77 to 70 percent.

The proportion of population eighteen to forty-four who were uninsured increased during the 1980s and 1990s, reaching 23 percent in 2002. The proportion covered by private insurance decreased for every age group between 1984 and 2002. Between 1984 and 2002, the proportion of all children covered under Medicaid increased from 12 to 25 percent. This increase reflected the expanded Medicaid income eligibility enacted by Congress in the mid-1980s and SCHIP, first implemented in the late 1990s (see Chapter Two).

The results overall leave little doubt that a decline in potential access has occurred for the U.S. adult population since the early 1980s because of diminution in private health insurance coverage.

### Realized Access (Utilization Over Time)

Table 1.2 presents a historical perspective of personal health care use for the U.S. population from 1928–1931 to 2002. It presents trend data on realized access for three types of service: those in response to serious illness (hospital admissions), ser-

## TABLE 1.1. HEALTH INSURANCE COVERAGE FOR PERSONS UNDER SIXTY-FIVE, BY AGE, RACE AND ETHNICITY, AND POVERTY LEVEL.

*Percentage of Population*

| | Private Insurance[e] | | | | Medicaid[e] | | | | Not Covered[e] | | | |
|---|---|---|---|---|---|---|---|---|---|---|---|---|
| | 1984 | 1995 | 1999 | 2002 | 1984[f] | 1995[f] | 1999[g] | 2002[g] | 1984 | 1995 | 1999 | 2002 |
| **Age** | | | | | | | | | | | | |
| Under 18 | 73 | 65 | 69 | 64 | 12 | 21 | 18 | 25 | 14 | 13 | 12 | 11 |
| 18–44 | 77 | 77 | 72 | 69 | 5 | 8 | 6 | 7 | 17 | 20 | 21 | 23 |
| 45–64 | 83 | 80 | 79 | 77 | 3 | 6 | 4 | 5 | 10 | 11 | 12 | 13 |
| **Race and ethnicity[a]** | | | | | | | | | | | | |
| White, non-Hispanic[c] | 82 | 79 | 80 | 78 | 5 | 9 | 7 | 9 | 13 | 15 | 15 | 15 |
| Black, non-Hispanic[c] | 59 | 55 | 58 | 56 | 19 | 26 | 19 | 21 | 20 | 18 | 19 | 19 |
| Hispanic, Mexican[b] | 55 | 44 | 48 | 44 | 11 | 19 | 12 | 18 | 33 | 36 | 38 | 37 |
| Hispanic, Puerto Rican[b] | 51 | 49 | 51 | 51 | 29 | 31 | 27 | 28 | 18 | 18 | 20 | 19 |
| Hispanic, Cuban[b] | 72 | 63 | 71 | 62 | 5 | 14 | 8 | 15 | 22 | 22 | 20 | 21 |
| Asian[c] | 71 | 68 | 73 | 71 | 9 | 11 | 8 | 10 | 18 | 18 | 16 | 17 |
| **Percent of poverty level[a,d]** | | | | | | | | | | | | |
| Below 100 percent | 33 | 23 | 26 | 27 | 31 | 45 | 35 | 39 | 35 | 32 | 36 | 31 |
| 100–149 percent | 62 | 48 | 43 | 39 | 7 | 18 | 17 | 25 | 27 | 32 | 35 | 33 |
| 150–199 percent | 78 | 65 | 59 | 57 | 3 | 8 | 10 | 15 | 17 | 24 | 27 | 26 |
| 200 percent or more | 92 | 88 | 87 | 84 | 1 | 2 | 2 | 3 | 6 | 9 | 9 | 11 |
| Total[a] | 77 | 71 | 73 | 70 | 7 | 11 | 9 | 12 | 14 | 16 | 16 | 17 |

*Notes:*

[a] Age adjusted to year 2000 U.S. Standard populations.

[b] Persons of Hispanic origin may be white, black, or Asian or Pacific Islander.

[c] Includes persons of Hispanic and non-Hispanic origin.

[d] Poverty level is based on family income and family size, using Bureau of the Census poverty thresholds.

[e] The sum of percentages for private insurance, Medicaid, and not-covered may not sum to 100 percent because other types of health insurance (Medicare, military) do not appear in the table and because persons with private insurance as well as Medicaid are counted in both columns.

[f] Includes other public assistance.

[g] Includes state sponsored plans and State Children's Health Insurance Program (SCHIP).

*Source:* National Center for Health Statistics. Health United States, 2004. Hyattsville, Md.: National Center for Health Statistics, 2004, pp. 345, 348, 350.

vices for a combination of primary and secondary care (physician visits), and services for conditions that are rarely life threatening and generally considered discretionary but still have an important bearing on people's functional status and quality of life (dental visits).

### TABLE 1.2. PERSONAL HEALTH CARE USE BY INCOME.

|  | 1928–31[a] | 1952–53[a] | 1963–64[a] | 1974[a] | 1997[b] | 2002[b] |
|---|---|---|---|---|---|---|
| Hospital admissions (per 100 persons per year) |  |  |  |  |  |  |
| Low-income[c] | 6 | 12 | 14 | 19 | 19 | 16 |
| Middle-income[d] | 6 | 12 | 14 | 14 | 12 | 12 |
| High-income[e] | 8 | 11 | 11 | 11 | 8 | 8 |
| Total | 6 | 12 | 13 | 14 | 12 | 12 |
| Physician visits[g] |  |  |  |  |  |  |
| Low-income[c] | 2.2 | 3.7 | 4.3 | 5.3 | 19% | 18% |
| Middle-income[d] | 2.5 | 3.8 | 4.5 | 4.8 | 15% | 15% |
| High-income[e] | 4.3 | 6.5 | 5.1 | 4.9 | 13% | 12% |
| Total | 2.6 | 4.2 | 4.5 | 4.9 | 14% | 13% |
| Percentage seeing a dentist (within one year)[f] |  |  |  |  |  |  |
| Low-income[c] | 10 | 17 | 21 | 35 | 48 | 48 |
| Middle-income[d] | 20 | 33 | 36 | 48 | 51 | 52 |
| High-income[e] | 46 | 56 | 58 | 64 | 73 | 71 |
| Total | 21 | 34 | 38 | 49 | 65 | 65 |

*Notes:*
[a]Various national surveys reported in Andersen, R., and Anderson, O. "Trends in the Use of Health Services." In H. E. Freeman, S. Levine, and L. G. Reeder (eds.), *Handbook of Medical Sociology* (3rd ed.). Upper Saddle River, N.J.: Prentice Hall, 1979, pp. 374, 378, 379.

[b]National Center for Health Statistics. *Health United States,* 2004. Hyattsville, Md.: National Center for Health Statistics, 2004, pp. 289, 247, 265.

[c]Lowest 15–27 percent of family income distribution for 1928–1931, 1952–53, 1963–64, 1974. Below poverty for 1997, 2002.

[d]Middle 51–73 percent of family income distribution for 1928–1931, 1952–53, 1963–64, 1974. 100 percent to <200 percent of poverty threshold for 1997, 2002.

[e]Highest 12–32 percent of family income distribution for 1928–1931, 1952–53, 1963–64, 1974. 200 percent or greater of the poverty threshold for 1997, 2002.

[f]Estimates only for persons two years of age and older, 1997, 2002.

[g]Mean number of physician visits per person per year for 1928–1931, 1952–53, 1963–64, 1974. Percent of population with ten or more visits per year for 1997, 2002.

The hospital admission rate for the U.S. population doubled between 1928 and 1931 (six admissions per one hundred persons per year) and the early 1950s (twelve admissions). A rising standard of living, the advent of voluntary health insurance, the increasing legitimacy of the modern hospital as a place to deliver babies and treat acute illness, and the requirements necessary for developing sophisticated medical technology all contributed to expanded use of the acute care hospital. Hospital admissions further increased in the 1960s and early 1970s (reaching fourteen admissions per hundred persons per year in 1974), reflecting continued growth in medical technology, private health insurance, and the advent of Medicare coverage for the elderly and Medicaid coverage for the low-income population in 1965.

However, beginning in the mid-1970s use of the acute care hospital began to decline, dropping to twelve admissions per hundred population by 2002. There was also a substantial decrease in average length of stay per admission during this period, from 7.5 days in 1980 to 6.5 days in 1990 and 4.9 days in 2002.[50] Those declines accompanied increasing an effort to contain health care costs by shifting care from the more expensive inpatient setting to less expensive outpatient settings, a shift from fee-for-service to prospective payments by Medicare, reduced coverage and benefits with increasing co-insurance and deductibles for health insurance, and a shift in certain medical technology and styles of practice that meant reduced reliance on the inpatient settings.

Contributing to the decline of inpatient volume since 1980 has been the significant growth of managed care. (See Chapter Nineteen, on managed care, by Kominski and Melnick.) This growth of managed care with its emphasis on utilization review and cost containment contributed to reduction in hospital admissions and the length of hospital stays.

Physician visits (Table 1.2), like inpatient services, increased substantially from 1928 to 1931 (2.6 visits per person per year) to the early 1950s (4.2 visits), for many of the same reasons hospital admissions were increasing in this period. However, unlike hospital admissions the number of physician visits continued to increase, reaching 4.9 visits in 1974 and 5.8 in 1996.[51] By 2002, 13 percent of the population had 10 or more physician visits per year. In part, the continued growth of managed care, with its relative deemphasis of the inpatient setting and greater focus on outpatient settings, may account for the divergence in trends of these basic realized access measures.

Trends in dental visits (Table 1.2) for the total U.S. population paralleled those for physician visits. Twenty-one percent of the population visited a dentist in 1928–1931, and the proportion increased consistently, reaching one-half of the population in 1974. Further increases in the last three decades resulted in 65 percent of the population visiting a dentist in 2002.

### Equitable Access (Health Insurance and Use According to Income and Race)

Combined with Tables 1.1 and 1.2, Table 1.3 presents health insurance coverage and personal health care use by race and income for the U.S. population for selected years. Recall that we have suggested "equitable access" is indicated by similar levels of insurance coverage and use by various income and ethnic groups. "Inequitable access" is indicated by discrepancies in coverage and use for these groups.

### TABLE 1.3. PERSONAL HEALTH CARE USE BY RACE OR ETHNICITY.

|  | 1964[a] | 1981–1983[b,c] | 1997[d,i] | 2002[d,i] |
|---|---|---|---|---|
| Hospital admissions (per 100 persons per year) | | | | |
| White[f] | 11 | 12 | 10 | 10 |
| Black[e,g] | 8 | 14 | 13 | 12 |
| Hispanic[h] | — | — | 11 | 10 |
| Total | 11 | 12 | 10 | 12 |
| Percentage seeing a physician (within one year) | | | | |
| White[f] | 68 | 76 | 84 | 84 |
| Black[e,g] | 58 | 75 | 83 | 85 |
| Hispanic[h] | 58 | 75 | 75 | 74 |
| Total | 61 | 76 | 84 | 84 |
| Percentage seeing a dentist (within one year)[f] | | | | |
| White[f] | 45 | 57 | 67 | 67 |
| Black[e,g] | 22 | 39 | 57 | 55 |
| Hispanic[h] | — | 42 | 53 | 53 |
| Total | 43 | 54 | 65 | 65 |

*Notes:*

[a] National Center for Health Statistics. *Health United States, 1993.* Hyattsville, Md.: National Center for Health Statistics, 1994, pp. 174, 179, 180.

[b] For hospital admissions and percentage seeing a doctor: National Center for Health Statistics. *Health United States, 1988.* Hyattsville, Md.: National Center for Health Statistics, 1989, pp. 107, 111.

[c] For percentage seeing a dentist: National Center for Health Statistics. *Health United States, 1999.* Hyattsville, Md.: National Center for Health Statistics, 1999, p. 242.

[d] National Center for Health Statistics. *Health United States, 2004.* Hyattsville, Md.: National Center for Health Statistics, 2004, pp. 289, 247, 265.

[e] 1964 includes all other races.

[f] 1964 includes white Hispanics.

[g] 1964 includes black Hispanics.

[h] Persons of Hispanic origin may be of any race.

[i] For percentage seeing a dentist, includes only persons two years of age and older.

*Health Insurance.* Table 1.1 suggests considerable inequity in insurance coverage in 1980 continuing to the present time. Minorities and low-income people are generally least likely to have private health insurance. However, there are striking differences among minority groups regarding private health insurance coverage in 2002. Blacks (56 percent), Mexicans (44 percent), and Puerto Ricans (51 percent) are far below the national average (70 percent), but Cubans (62 percent) are somewhat closer and Asians (71 percent) essentially equal the national average. Medicaid compensates for some of this inequity but still left an especially high proportion of Mexicans (37 percent) and the lowest-income groups (below 150 percent of federal poverty guidelines, 31–33 percent) uninsured in 2002.

The trends in Table 1.1 suggest a somewhat mixed picture as to whether inequity in health insurance coverage is increasing over time. Between 1984 and 2002 coverage through private health insurance declined while the proportion covered by Medicaid increased for white non-Hispanics and most minority groups. The decrease in private insurance coverage tended to be offset by an increase in Medicaid so that the proportion left uninsured, for both whites and minorities, was about the same in 2002 as 1984—except for Mexicans, for whom the uninsured proportion increased from 33 to 37 percent over this eighteen-year period, indicating greater inequity. One reason for the rise in number of uninsured among Mexicans is their relatively high immigration rate into the United States during this same period. Recent immigrants are less likely to have health insurance coverage.

Trends in insurance coverage according to income level since 1984 generally suggest increased inequity (Table 1.1). Between 1984 and 2002, private health insurance coverage of low-income groups declined considerably (with the greatest decline, from 62 to 39 percent, for those with incomes of 100–149 percent of poverty). There was also a decline for the highest-income group over this period, but it was much less (from 92 to 84 percent) as a large majority of the highest-income group retained private health insurance coverage. Increasing Medicaid coverage compensated for decline in private insurance coverage for the lowest-income group so that the proportion uninsured was similar in 1984 (34 percent) and 2002 (31 percent). This was not the case for the lower-income groups above poverty, for whom the proportion of uninsured rose considerably—from 27 to 33 percent for those at 100–149 percent of poverty and from 17 to 26 percent for those at 150–199 percent of poverty. Consequently, it appears that inequity in insurance coverage has been increasing for these lower-income groups above poverty.

*Hospital Admissions.* Tables 1.2 and 1.3 suggest greater equity according to income and race for hospital admissions since use by low-income and minority groups compared to the rest of the population has grown consistently over the past seventy years.

However, such a general conclusion about improvement in equity needs to be qualified in important ways. First, the relative needs of the low-income and minority populations for acute hospital care are often much greater. Also, higher use of inpatient hospital care suggests that limited access to preventive and primary services at an earlier time might increase subsequent need for inpatient hospital services for serious acute and uncontrolled chronic disease problems (see Chapter Two, by Yancey, Bastani, and Glenn, on health disparities; and Chapter Three, by Morales and Ortega, on health care disparities).

In 1928–1931 the highest-income group had the highest admission rate (Table 1.2). By the 1950s, the rate equalized. In subsequent years, rate by income diverged, with the lowest-income group increasing relative to those with higher incomes so that by 2002 the lowest income had a rate (sixteen per hundred) twice that of the highest-income group (eight per hundred). Does this indicate that inequity exists in favor of the low-income group? Probably not. Studies taking into account the need for medical care suggest that greater use among low-income persons can be largely accounted for by their higher rates of disease and disability.[52]

The hospital admission rate in 1964 for whites (eleven per hundred) was still considerably higher than that for blacks (eight per hundred; Table 1.3). However, by the 1980s the rate for blacks exceeded that for whites, and the higher rate for blacks continued through the 1990s. The higher hospital admission rate for blacks, similar to that for low-income people, can be largely accounted for by greater level of medical need.[53] Unlike the case with blacks, the admission rate for most Hispanics only now approaches the rate for non-Hispanic whites. For the period 1992–1995, the age-adjusted proportion of the population with one or more hospital stays within a year was 6.1 percent for Mexicans and 6.3 percent for Cubans, compared to 6.5 percent for non-Hispanic whites. Among major Hispanic groups, only the percent for Puerto Ricans (8.4) exceeded the non-Hispanic white rate.[54] However, as shown in Table 1.3 by 2002 the admission rate was similar for Hispanics and White non-Hispanics (10 admissions per 100 persons per year).

***Physician Visits.*** The trends in Tables 1.2 and 1.3 also suggest increasing equity for physician visits according to income level and ethnicity. In 1928–1931, the lowest-income group averaged only one-half as many visits to the doctor (2.2 visits) as the highest-income group (4.3 visits; Table 1.2). Over time, the gap narrowed. By 1974, the lowest-income group was actually visiting a physician more than the higher-income groups, and the difference increased in the 1980s and 1990s. Again, research suggests that the apparent excess for the low-income population can be accounted for by their greater level of medical need.[55]

Similar trends have taken place among the black population (Table 1.3), but parity with the white population in the proportion seeing a doctor did not take place until the early 1980s, and the proportion seeing a doctor has remained about the same for blacks and whites in 2002. The average number of physician contacts per year for most Hispanic groups (Mexican, 5.1; Cuban, 4.5) remained considerably below the figures for blacks (6.2) and non-Hispanic whites (6.3) during the years 1992–1995. As with hospital inpatient services, the rate of use of physician visits for Puerto Ricans for physician contacts (6.4) exceeded that for other Hispanic groups.[56]

In 2002 (Table 1.3), 74 percent of all Hispanics had a physician visit within a year, compared to 84 percent for non-Hispanic Whites and 85 percent for blacks.

***Dental Visits.*** Tables 1.2 and 1.3 tell a story of major inequity according to income and race in dental visits that existed in 1928–1931 and continued into the first decade of this century. The proportion seeing a dentist has increased considerably for all income and racial groups. Still, by 2002 only 48 percent of the low-income group saw a dentist, compared to 71 percent of those in the highest-income group (Table 1.2). Further, 55 percent and 53 percent of blacks and Hispanics respectively saw a dentist, compared to 67 percent of whites (Table 1.3).

## Effective Access

The effectiveness-and-outcomes movement initiated in the late 1980s was in response to several major developments converging on the national scene.[57] The Health Care Financing Administration (HCFA) proposed a research program called the Effectiveness Initiative, stimulated by its need to (1) ensure quality of care for thirty million Medicare beneficiaries, (2) determine which medical practices worked best, and (3) aid policy makers in allocating Medicare resources. At about the same time, an Outcomes Research Program was authorized by Congress, largely inspired by the work of John Wennberg and associates in small-area variations in utilization and outcomes of medical interventions. A third major development stimulating the effectiveness movement stemmed from efforts led by Robert Brook and associates to determine whether medical interventions within the normal practice setting were being used appropriately. Within the same time period, the Agency for Health Care Policy and Research (AHCPR, renamed the Agency for Healthcare Research and Quality, AHRQ) was created, with responsibility for overseeing development of medical practice guidelines—practical application of the outcomes-and-effectiveness research movement.

Prior to the Effectiveness Initiative, research findings were hampered by weak study designs (that is, observational and cross-sectional) that were incapable of determining the clear direction of effects and their potential causality.[58] Most studies used mortality as the outcome variable, which was shown to be more sensitive to environmental and socioeconomic factors than medical care utilization.[59] Moreover, the appropriate risk adjustments were usually not available in mortality data sets.

The Medical Outcomes Study (MOS) was undertaken in response to these methodological limitations. The MOS sampled physicians and patients from various health care settings—traditional indemnity (fee-for-service, FFS) plans, independent practice associations (IPA), or HMOs—to investigate the relationships among structure, process, and medical outcomes. Specifically, the MOS was designed to (1) determine whether variation in medical outcomes was explained by differences in the system of care (structure and process) and medical specialty; and (2) develop instruments to assess and monitor medical outcomes (clinical endpoints, functioning, perceived general health status and well-being, and satisfaction with treatment).[60] Ultimately, research results demonstrated that multiple factors—(patient mix, medical specialty and system of care, influence patient outcomes, and—when patient and physician characteristics are controlled—quality indicators of primary care) vary across systems of care.[61]

Now almost two decades later, outcomes research has led to advances such as development of outcome measures for clinical research and practice, insights into current practice and practice variation, refinement and clarification of clinical hypotheses, new expectations for clinical care, and an explosion of interest in outcomes and effectiveness research.[62] However, the expectation that outcomes research would be readily translated into practice has not been realized. It is now understood that effectiveness is strongly influenced by contextual and environmental factors and that evidence should guide not only clinical decision making (evidence-based medicine) but also decision making about the administrative and organizational aspects of care related to access, quality, and outcomes ("evidence-based management").

"Evidence-based medicine" and evidence-based management have emerged from the effectiveness movement. Evidence-based medicine (EBM) synthesizes research results from multiple clinical trials to help clinicians make judicious use of the best scientific evidence for patient care decisions. EBM has been defined as an "effective series of mechanisms not only for improving health quality, but also for reducing medical errors precipitated in part by clinical practice variation."[63] These variations translate into sizeable disparity in the quality and safety of medical care and ultimately result in poor outcomes and associated health disparities.

In the late 1990s, AHRQ conceived the Evidence-Based Practice Center Program, designed to encourage private organizations (health plans and professional societies) to improve practice through clinical guidelines, quality initiatives, and coverage decisions.[64] Centers produced evidence reports and technology assessments, and a National Guideline Clearinghouse was created.[65] By the end of the 1990s, it was widely accepted that guidelines should be based on evidence, and that consensus-based methods were acceptable only if there was insufficient evidence to support an evidence-based approach.[66]

Evidence-based management, on the other hand, has enjoyed less investment in research on managerial practice and few randomized experimental trials to furnish the evidence.[67] Implementation of research knowledge in the practice setting has been even slower in health care management than in medicine to be implemented in the practice setting.[68] In fact, most of the innovation today is occurring within academic-practitioner collaboratives executed in the delivery system setting, where researchers collaborate with practitioners to measure and improve clinical or organizational performance, for example, through the IHI disease collaboratives, or employing a balanced scorecard approach such as that used by the NCHL Leadership Excellence Networks. Moving at a slower pace, evidence-based management is progressing nonetheless in response to growing concern that leaders and managers in large health systems are making strategic decisions based on evidence that is not systematically gathered or assessed.[69]

The demand for health services organizations to demonstrate their effectiveness in providing quality patient services will continue to grow. Federal and state governments, managed care organizations, JCAHO, and businesses and insurers purchasing and paying for medical services have all insisted on greater accountability.[70] Evidence-based medicine and evidence-based management are two complementary approaches for achieving more effective outcomes in the health services industry.

## Efficient Access

Efficiency studies have been conducted at the contextual level (national health care systems and health plans) and the individual level (consumer behavior). At the macroeconomic level, comprehensive data available on major, industrialized countries have been used to compare health services utilization, health resources and expenditures, and health outcomes. For example, the Organization for Economic Cooperation and Development (OECD) study comparing per capita health care expenditures in major industrialized countries found that the United States spent about 40 percent more than Canada and almost three times more than the countries with the lowest expenditures. The large expenditure gap for the United States was not offset by health outcome advantages, which raised concerns that resources were being misallocated to services with low benefit relative to cost.[71]

Efficiency analyses conducted at the level of the health plan have been used to compare traditional indemnity plans with FFS providers to HMOs.[72] Other efficiency studies have concentrated on the size and personnel mix of physician practices and other medical care delivery settings.[73] Results from these efficiency studies can be used for making managed care contract specifications to ensure that services are accessible, efficient, and effective. Efficiency analyses focusing on consumers and providers have investigated the effects of cost sharing on health services utilization to determine optimal combinations of cost sharing and managed care.[74] In summary, efficiency analysis is conducted at multiple levels (international comparative, health plan, delivery system, provider, consumer) to assess the relative cost for improving health outcomes.

## Conclusion

Is access improving or declining in the United States? for whom? and according to what measures? Although we have documented continuing increases in some realized access measures, notably physician and dental visits, inpatient hospital use has been declining for twenty-five years. However, the declining hospital use rate reflects, in part, the shift to outpatient services and greater emphasis on primary care, possibly reducing the need for acute inpatient services. A key potential access measure, health insurance, reveals that although a growing number of people are being covered by Medicaid, there has been a decline in the number covered by private insurance in the last twenty years and an overall increase in the proportion without any health insurance coverage.

Low-income and black populations appear to have achieved equity of access according to gross measures of hospital and physician utilization (not adjusting for their greater need for medical care) but continue to lag considerably in receipt of dental care.

Equity has certainly not been achieved regarding health insurance coverage; the proportion of uninsured is 50 percent higher for blacks and more than twice as high for Hispanics and the low-income population, compared to the uninsured rate for whites. Further, numerous investigations have noted great inequity in access for low-income and minority populations regarding not having a regular source of care; not getting preventive care; delay in obtaining needed care; and higher rates of morbidity, hospitalization, and mortality that could have been avoided with appropriate access to care. Many of these documented discrepancies are rising over time.[75] Improving access to care can be greatly facilitated by a new generation of access models and indicators, which should stress the importance of contextual as well as individual characteristics in promoting policies to improve access for defined populations.[76] They should focus on the extent to which medical care contributes to people's health. Access measures should be developed specifically for particular vulnerable population groups. These measures are especially important because of the cross-cutting needs of many of the vulnerable groups: persons with

HIV/AIDS, substance abusers, migrants, homeless people, people with disabilities, and those suffering from family violence.[77] Improving equity, effectiveness, and efficiency should be the guiding norms for research on access.[78]

# Notes

1. Phillips, K. A., Morrison, K. R., Andersen, R., and Aday, L. A. "Understanding the Context of Health Care Utilization: Assessing Environmental and Provider-Related Variables in the Behavioral Model of Utilization." *Health Services Research*, 1998, *33*, 571–596; and Litaker, D., Koroukian, S. M., and Love, T. E. "Context and Healthcare Access: Looking Beyond the Individual." *Medical Care*, 2005, *43*, 531–540.

2. Davidson, P. L., Andersen, R. M., Wyn, R., and Brown, E. R. "A Framework for Evaluating Safety-Net and Other Community-Level Factors on Access for Low-Income Populations." *Inquiry*, 2004, *41*, 21–38; and Robert, S. A. "Socioeconomic Position and Health: The Independent Contribution of Community Socioeconomic Context." *Annual Review of Sociology*, 1999, *25*, 489–516.

3. Andersen, R. M. *A Behavioral Model of Families' Use of Health Services.* Research Series no. 25. Chicago: Center for Health Administration Studies, University of Chicago, 1968; and Andersen, R. M. "Revisiting the Behavioral Model and Access to Medical Care: Does It Matter?" *Journal of Health and Social Behavior*, 1995, *36*, 1–10.

4. Donabedian, A. *Exploration in Quality Assessment and Monitoring. Vol. 1: The Definition of Quality and Approaches to Its Assessment.* Ann Arbor, Mich.: Health Administration Press, 1980.

5. Bindman, A. B., and Gold, M. R. (eds.). "Measuring Access Through Population-Based Surveys in a Managed Care Environment: A Special Supplement to HSR." *Health Services Research*, 1998, *33*, 611–766.

6. Andersen, R. M., Smedby, B,, and Anderson, O. W. *Medical Care Use in Sweden and the United States—A Comparative Analysis of Systems and Behavior.* Research Series no. 27. Chicago: Center for Health Administration Studies, University of Chicago, 1970; Andersen, R. M., Anderson, O. W., and Smedby, B. "Perceptions of the Response to Symptoms of Illness in Sweden and the United States." *Medical Care*, Jan.-Feb. 1968, *6*(1), 18–30; Andersen, R. M., and Smedby, B. "Changes in Response to Symptoms of Illness in the United States and Sweden." *Inquiry*, June, 1975, *12*(2), 116–127. Reprinted in G. K. Chacko (ed.), *Health Handbook, 1976: An International Reference on Care and Cure.* Amsterdam: North Holland, 1976.

7. Longest, B. B., Jr. *Health Policymaking in the United States.* (2nd ed.) Chicago: Health Administration Press, 1998.

8. National Center for Health Statistics. *Health, United States, 1999, with Health and Aging Chart Book.* Hyattsville, Md.: National Center for Health Statistics, 1999.

9. Robert (1999); and Snijders, T.A.B., and Bosker, R. J. *Multilevel Analysis: An Introduction to Basic and Advanced Multilevel Modeling.* Thousand Oaks, Calif.: Sage, 1999.

10. Hulka, B. S., and Wheat, J. R. "Patterns of Utilization: The Patient Perspective." *Medical Care*, 1985, *23*, 438–460.

11. Bass, D. M., and Noelker, L. S. "The Influence of Family Caregivers on Elders' Use of In-Home Services: An Expanded Conceptual Framework." *Journal of Health and Social Behavior*, 1987, *28*, 184–196; Guendelman, S. "Health Care Users Residing on the Mexican Border: What Factors Determine Choice of the U.S. or Mexican Health System?" *Medical*

*Care*, 1985, *23*, 438–460; and Portes, A., Kyle, D., Eaton, W. W. "Mental Illness and Help-Seeking Behavior Among Mariel Cuban and Haitian Refugees in South Florida." *Journal of Health and Social Behavior*, 1993, *33*, 283–298; Pescosolido, B. A., Wright, E. R., Alegria, M., and Vera, M. "Social Networks and Patterns of Use Among the Poor with Mental Health Problems in Puerto Rico." *Medical Care*, 1998, *36*, 1057–1072; and Heck, K. E., and Parker, J. D. "Family Structure, Socioeconomic Status and Access to Health Care for Children." *Health Services Research*, 2002, *37*, 173–186.

12. Donabedian (1980).
13. Andersen (1968).
14. Andersen (1995).
15. Cunningham, P. J., and Kohn, L. "Health Plan Switching: Choice or Circumstance?" *Health Affairs*, 2000, *19*, 158–164.
16. Davis, K. Baxter Allegiance Foundation Prize for Health Services Research, acceptance speech, June 24, 2000, Los Angeles. New York: Commonwealth Fund, 2000.
17. Andersen, R, and Davidson, P. "Measuring Access and Trends." In R. Andersen, T. Rice, and G. Kominski (eds.) *Changing the U.S. Health Care System* (1st ed.). San Francisco: Jossey-Bass, 1996.,
18. McManus, S. M., and Pohl, C. M. "Ethics and Financing: Overview of the U.S. Health Care System." *Journal of Health and Human Resources Administration*, 1994, *16*(3), 332–349.
19. Kenkel, P. J. "HMO Profit Outlook Begins to Brighten." *Modern Healthcare*, 1989, *19*, 98; Larkin, H. "Law and Money Spur HMO Profit Status Changes." *Hospitals*, 1989, *63*, 68–69; Coyne, J. S., and Meadows, D. M. "California HMOs May Provide National Forecast." *Healthcare Financial Management*, 1991, *45*, 36–39.
20. Marquis, M. S., Rogowski, J. A., and Escarce, J. J. "The Managed Care Backlash: Did Consumers Vote with Their Feet." *Inquiry*, 2004–05, *41*(4), 376–390. Gluck, M. E. "A Medicare Prescription Drug Benefit." *Medicare Brief*, 1999, *1*, 1–13; Mechanic, D. "The Rise and Fall of Managed Care." *Journal of Health Social Behavior*, 2004, *45*, Suppl., 76–86.
21. Robinson, J. C. "Reinvention of Health Insurance in the Consumer Era." *Journal of the American Medical Association*, 2004, *291*(15), 1880–1886.
22. Mays, G. P., Claxton, G., and White, J. "Marketwatch: Managed Care Rebound? Recent Changes in Health Plans' Cost Containment Strategies." *Health Affairs*, 2004, July–Dec.; Suppl. Web Exclusives: W4-427-36; Draper, D. A., and Claxton, G. "Managed Care Redux: Health Plans Shift Responsibilities to Consumers." Issue Brief, Center for Studying Health System Change, 2004, *79*, 1–4; Mays, G. P., Hurley, R. E., and Grossman, J. M. "An Empty Tool Box? Changes in Health Plans' Approaches for Managing Costs and Care." *Health Services Research*, 2003; *38* (1, Pt. 2), 375–393.
23. Etheredge, L. "Purchasing Medicare Prescription Drug Benefits, a New Proposal." *Health Affairs*, 1999, *18*(4), 7–19.
24. Barrett, A., and Arndt, M. "Health Costs: Good News at Last." *Business Week*, May 30, 2005, pp. 28–31.
25. Barrett and Arndt (2005); Rice, T., and Matsuoka, K. Y. "The Impact of Cost-Sharing on Appropriate Utilization and Health Status: A Review of the Literature on Seniors." *Medical Care Research Review*, 2004, *61*(4), 415–452.
26. Heisler, M., and others., "The Health Effects of Restricting Prescription Medication Use Because of Cost." *Medical Care*, 2004, *42*(7), 626–634.
27. Barrett and Arndt (2005).
28. Andersen, R. M., Kravits, J., and Anderson, O. *Equity in Health Services: Empirical Analysis in Social Policy.* Boston: Ballinger, 1975.

29. Institute of Medicine (IOM). *Unequal Treatment: Confronting Racial and Ethnic Disparities in Health Care.* Washington, D.C.: National Academies Press, 2003; Lavizzo-Mourey, R., Richardson, W. C., Ross, R. K., and Rowe, J. W. "A Tale of Two Cities." *Health Affairs,* 2005, *24* (2), 313–315.

30. Smith, D. B. "Racial and Ethnic Health Disparities and the Unfinished Civil Rights Agenda." *Health Affairs,* 2005, *24*(2), 317–324.

31. Lurie, N., Jung, M., and Lavizzo-Mourey, R. "Disparities and Quality Improvement: Federal Policy Levers." *Health Affairs,* 2005, *24*(2), 354–364; Eichner, J., and Vladeck, B. C. "Medicare as a Catalyst for Reducing Health Disparities." *Health Affairs,* 2005, *24* (2), 365–375; Moy, E., Dayton, E., and Clancy, C. M. "Compiling the Evidence: The National Healthcare Disparities Reports." *Health Affairs,* 2005, *24* (2), 376–387; Trivedi, A. N., and others. "Creating a State Health Policy Report Card." *Health Affairs,* 2005, *24*(2), 388–396.

32. Alpha Center. "State of the States." Prepared for State Coverage Initiatives, Robert Wood Johnson Foundation, Jan. 2000.

33. Newacheck, P. W., and others. "Adolescent Health Insurance Coverage: Recent Changes and Access to Care." *Pediatrics,* 1999, *104,* 195–202.

34. Reschovsky, J. D., and Cunningham, P. J. "CHIPing away at the Problem of Uninsured Children: Why Children Lack Health Insurance and Implications for the New State Children's Health Insurance Program." Center for Studying Health System Change. n.d. [http://www.hschange.com/researcher/rr2_toc.html]; Reschovsky, J. D., and Cunningham, P. J. "CHIPing Away at the Problem of Uninsured Children." Issue Brief. Center for Studying Health System Change, 1998, 14, 1–7.; Newacheck, P. W., Hung, Y. Y., Park, M. J., Brindis, C. D., Irwin, C. E. "Disparities in Adolescent Health and Health Care: Does Socioeconomic Status Matter?" *Health Services Research,* 2003, *38*(5), 1235–1252.

35. Long, S. H., and Marquis, M. S. "Geographic Variation in Physician Visits for Uninsured Children: The Role of the Safety Net." *Journal of the American Medical Association,* 1999, *281,* 2035–2040.

36. Lave, C. R., and others. "Impact of a Children's Health Insurance Program on Newly Enrolled Children." *Journal of the American Medical Association,* 1998, *279,* 1820–1825; Szilagyi, P. G., and others. "Improved Access and Quality of Care After Enrollment in the New York State Children's Health Insurance Program (SCHIP)." *Pediatrics,* 2004, *113*(5), 395–404.

37. Lave, and others (1998); Damiano, P. C., Willard, J. C., Momany, E. T., and Chowdhury, J. "The Impact of the Iowa S-SCHIP program on Access, Health Status, and the Family Environment." Ambulatory Pediatrics, 2003, *3*(5), 263–269.

38. Gilmer, T., Kronick, R., and Rice, T. "Children Welcome, Adults Need Not Apply: Changes in Public Program Enrollment Across States over Time." *Medical Care Research and Review,* 2005, *62*(1), 56–78.

39. Institute of Medicine. *America's Health Care Safety Net: Intact But Endangered.* Washington, D.C.: National Academy of Science, 2000.

40. Fishman, L. E., and Bentley, J. D. "The Evolution of Support for Safety-Net Hospitals." *Health Affairs,* 1997, *16,* 30–47; Gaskin, D. J., and Hadley, J. "Identify Urban Safety Net Hospitals and the Populations They Serve." (Abstract.) *Abstract Book, Association for Health Services Research,* 1997, *14,* 62–63.

41. Health Resources and Services Administration, HRSA. News Release, June 1, 2005, "HHS Awards 86 Grants Worth More Than $30 Million to Expand Health Center Services and Strengthen America's Health Care Safety Net." HRSA Press Office [www.hhs.gov/news/press/2005pres/20050601.html].

42. Health Resources and Services Administration, HRSA 2005. [http://www.hrsa.gov/performancereview/protocol.htm] (last accessed June 30, 2005).

43. Bailit, H., Formicola, A., Herbert. K,, and Stavisky, J. "The Origins and Design of the Pipeline Program." *Journal of Dental Education*, 2005, *69*(2), 232–238; Andersen, R. M., and others "Pipeline, Profession, and Practice Program: Evaluating Change in Dental Education." *Journal of Dental Education*, 2005, *69*(2), 239–248.

44. Institute of Medicine (U.S.), Committee on Monitoring Access to Personal Health Care Services. *Access to Health Care in America.* (M. Millman, ed.). Washington, D.C.: National Academy Press, 1993.

45. Iezzoni, L. *Risk Adjustment for Measuring Healthcare Outcomes* (3rd ed.). Chicago: Health Administration Press, 2003.

46. Aday, L. A., Begley, C. E., Lairson, D. R., and Slater, C. H. *Evaluating the Health Care System: Effectiveness, Efficiency, and Equity* (2nd ed.). Ann Arbor, Mich.: Health Administration Press, 1998.

47. Aday, L. A. "Access to What and Why? Towards a New Generation of Access Indicators." Proceedings of the Public Health Conference on Records and Statistics, DHHS Pub. No. 94214. Washington, D.C.: U.S. Government Printing Office, 1993.

48. Davidson, P. L. *Performance Measurement and Improvement: The Future for HRSA-funded Health Centers.* Manuscript in preparation, Oct. 2005.

49. Institute for Healthcare Improvement (IHI) [http://www.ihi.org/ihi]; National Center for Healthcare Leadership (NCHL) [http://www.nchl.org].

50. National Center for Health Statistics. *Health United States, 2004.* Hyattsville, Md.: National Center for Health Statistics, 2004.

51. National Center for Health Statistics (1999), p. 229.

52. Davis, K., and Rowland, D. "Uninsured and Underserved: Inequities in Health Care in the United States." *Milbank Quarterly*, 1983, *61*, 149–176.

53. Manton, K., Patrick, C., and Johnson, K. "Health Differentials Between Blacks and Whites: Recent Trends in Mortality and Morbidity." *Milbank Quarterly*, 1987, *65* (supp. 1), 129–199.

54. Hajat, A., Lucas, J. B., and Kington, R. "Health Outcomes Among Hispanic Subgroups: United States, 1992–95." Advance Data from Vital and Health Statistics, no. 310. Hyattsville, Md.: National Center for Health Statistics, 2000.

55. Davis and Rowland (1983).

56. Hajat, Lucas, and Kington. (2000).

57. Heithoff, K. A., and Lohr, K. N. (eds.). *Effectiveness and Outcomes in Health Care.* Washington, D.C.: National Academy Press, 1993.

58. Aday, Begley, Lairson, and Slater (1998).

59. Martini, C., Allen, J. B., Davidson, J., and Backett, E. M. "Health Indexes Sensitive to Medical Care Variation." *International Journal of Health Services*, 1977, *7*, 293–309.

60. Tarlov, A., and others. "The Medical Outcomes Study: An Application of Methods for Monitoring the Results of Medical Care." *Journal of the American Medical Association*, 1989, *262*, 925–930; Ware, J. E. "Measuring Patient Function and Well-Being: Some Lessons from the Medical Outcomes Study." In Heithoff and Lohr (1993); Kravitz, R. L., and others. "Differences in the Mix of Patients Among Medical Specialties and Systems of Care: Results from the Medical Outcomes Study." *Journal of the American Medical Association*, 1992, *267*, 1617–1623.

61. Kravitz and others (1992); Greenfield, S., and others. "Variations in Resource Utilization Among Medical Specialties and Systems of Care: Results from the Medical Outcomes

Study." *Journal of the American Medical Association*, 1992, *267*, 1624–1630; Safran, D. G., Tarlov, A. R., and Rogers, W. H. "Primary Care Performance in Fee-for-Service and Prepaid Health Care Systems: Results from the Medical Outcomes Study." *Journal of the American Medical Association*, 1994, *271*, 1579–1586.

62. Stryer, D. B., Siegel, J. E., Rodgers, A. B. "Outcomes Research: Priorities for an Evolving Field." *Medical Care*, 2004, *42*(4 suppl), III-1–5.

63. Eddy, D. M. "Evidence-Based Medicine: A Unified Approach." *Health Affairs*, 2005, *24* (1), 8–17.

64. Iglehart, J. K. "The New Imperative: Producing Better Evidence." *Health Affairs*, 2005, *24* (1), 7.

65. Eddy (2005).

66. Eddy (2005).

67. Kovner, A. R., Elton, J. J., and Billings, J. "Transforming Health Management: An Evidence-Based Approach." *Frontiers of Health Services Management*, 2000, *16*(4), 3–24.

68. Rundall, T. G. "Refocusing Future Faculty on Evidence-Based Health Services Management Research." *Journal of Health Administration Education*, Fall 2003, *20*(4), 263–273.

69. Kovner, and others (2000).

70. White, A. W., and Wager, K. A. "The Outcomes Movement and the Role of Health Information Managers." *Topics in Health Information Management*, May 1998, *18*, 1–2.

71. Aday, Begley, Lairson, and Slater (1998).

72. Aday, Begley, Lairson, and Slater (1998); Manning, W. A., Liebowitz, A., and Goldberg, G. A. "A Controlled Trial of the Effect of a Prepaid Group Practice on Use of Services." *New England Journal of Medicine*, 1984, *310*, 1505–1510.

73. Reinhardt, U. "A Production Function for Physician Services." *Review of Economics and Statistics*, 1972, *54*, 55–66; Smith, K. R., Miller, M., and Golladay, F. L. "An Analysis of the Optimal Use of Inputs in the Production of Medical Services." *Journal of Human Resources*, 1972, *7*, 208–255; Brown, D. M. "Do Physicians Underutilize Aides?" *Journal of Human Resources*, 1988, *23*, 342–355; and Rohrer, J. E., and Rohland, B. M. "Oversight of Managed Care for Behavioral Sciences." *Journal of Public Health Management and Practice*, 1998, *4*, 96–100.

74. Shapiro, M. F., Ware, J. E., and Sherbourne, C. D. "Effects of Cost Sharing on Seeking Care for Serious and Minor Symptoms: Results of a Randomized Controlled Trial." *Annals of Internal Medicine*, 1986, *104*, 246–251; Rohrer and Rohland (1998).

75. Institute of Medicine (1993); Institute of Medicine (2003); and Moy, E., Dayton, E., and Clancy, C. M. (2005).

76. Bindman and Gold (1998); Docteur, E. R., Colby, D. C., and Gold, M. "Shifting the Paradigm: Monitoring Access in Medicare Managed Care." *Health Care Financing Review*, 1996, *17*, 5–21.

77. Aday, L. A. *At Risk in America: The Health and Health Care Needs of Vulnerable Populations in the United States.* San Francisco: Jossey-Bass, 1993.

78. Aday, Begley, Lairson, and Slater (1998).

CHAPTER TWO

# ETHNIC DISPARITIES IN HEALTH STATUS

Antronette K. Yancey
Roshan Bastani
Beth A. Glenn

During the past one hundred years, dramatic gains have been made in the overall health of the U.S. population. One common, albeit gross, indicator of the general health of a population is life expectancy, which increased by thirty years during the twentieth century.[1] Because of the adverse social conditions attendant to slavery, Reconstruction, and the Jim Crow legislation of that era, it is understandable that the life expectancy of blacks lagged substantially behind that of whites in 1900. It is unconscionable that, although the gap has narrowed in some areas, ethnic disparities in health status that existed at the turn of the twentieth century persist as we enter the twenty-first century.

There is ample evidence that ethnic minorities experience higher rates of morbidity and mortality across many disease states.[2] Historically, the ideals of social justice and equality have served as the impetus for eliminating health disparities.[3] Although these factors remain compelling, the growing diversification of the U.S. population is an additional rationale for eliminating inequity. Figure 2.1 presents data on the ethnic distribution of the U.S. population in 2000 and projections for 2100. According to the 2000 census, slightly more than 70 percent of the population was white, with the remaining 30 percent made up of ethnic minorities (less than 5 percent Asian, more than 10 percent African American, more than 10 percent Latino/Latina). Ethnic minorities are projected to constitute more than 50 percent of the total population by 2060, with the largest growth expected to occur among Latinos and Asians. In addition, the relative youth of

## FIGURE 2.1. U.S. POPULATION (2000 CENSUS) AND PROJECTIONS FOR 2100.

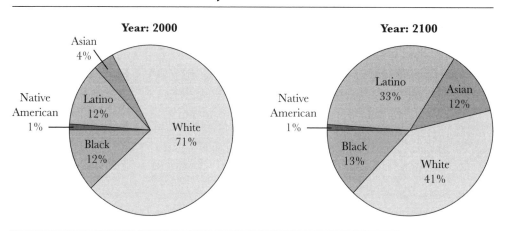

ethnic minority populations currently will magnify existing disparities in the future, as the average age of the entire population advances, particularly among minority groups. Therefore today, and increasingly in the future, the overall health and economic well-being of the U.S. population can be maintained and enhanced only by addressing ethnic disparities in health status and their determinants.

Because the disease burden over the past century has shifted from communicable to chronic diseases, inequality in chronic disease burden represents one of the most critical areas of health disparities today. Chronic diseases account for more than 75 percent of health care expenditures and deaths annually.[4] This is in contrast to the early 1900s, when chronic disease accounted for less than one-quarter of all deaths.[5] Despite steady improvement in the health of all Americans, ethnic minorities continue to experience poorer health status, especially with regard to chronic disease. In fact, the current obesity epidemic threatens to end the steady rise in overall life expectancy of the past two centuries and contributes disproportionately to chronic disease disparities. Therefore this chapter describes current health status disparities, reviews the potential determinants of observed disparities, and outlines future directions for policy and practice, with specific emphasis on the contribution of chronic disease.

## Epidemiology of Health Disparities

In this section, we review the evidence related to ethnic disparities in major health indicators.

## Life Expectancy

Life expectancy is one of the summary statistics most commonly used to describe the health of a population. During the past century, we have seen a dramatic increase in life expectancy, from less than forty-seven years in the early 1900s to more than seventy-seven by the year 2002.[6] Although increased life expectancy has been observed for all ethnic groups, ethnic disparities in life expectancy remain fairly constant. Figure 2.2 shows the average life expectancy by ethnicity and gender according to population-based data from 1999.[7] Within each ethnic group, women have a higher life expectancy than men. However, substantial differences are found among ethnic groups regardless of gender. The longest average life expectancy is seen among Asian women (86.5 years) and the shortest among American Indian and Alaska Native men (67.6), a difference of more than eighteen years. In general, Asians have the longest life expectancy of any ethnic group, followed by Latinos, whites, African Americans, and American Indians.

## Major Causes of Mortality

Although life expectancy provides global information about disparities, it does not inform us about the underlying causes. Table 2.1 shows the top ten causes of mortality for all adults living in the United States in 2002, the relative rank of each cause within ethnic groups, and age-adjusted death rate. For the overall population, chronic diseases comprise six of the top ten causes of death. Heart disease

### FIGURE 2.2. LIFE EXPECTANCY BY ETHNICITY AND GENDER.

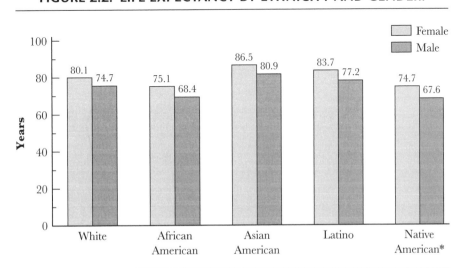

## TABLE 2.1. LEADING CAUSES OF DEATH, BY ETHNICITY, 2002.

| Causes of Death | White | | | African American | | | American Indian and Alaska Native | | | Asian American and Pacific Islander | | | Latino | | |
|---|---|---|---|---|---|---|---|---|---|---|---|---|---|---|---|
| | Rank | Percentage | Death Rate | Rank | Percentage | Death Rate | Rank | Percentage | Death Rate | Rank | Percentage | Death Rate | Rank | Percentage | Death Rate |
| Heart disease | 1 | 28.9 | 236.7 | 1 | 26.8 | 308.4 | 1 | 19.9 | 157.4 | 2 | 26 | 134.6 | 1 | 23.8 | 180.5 |
| All cancers | 2 | 22.9 | 191.7 | 2 | 21.6 | 238.8 | 2 | 17.5 | 125.4 | 1 | 26.1 | 113.6 | 2 | 19.8 | 128.4 |
| Cerebrovascular diseases | 3 | 6.6 | 54.2 | 3 | 6.5 | 76.3 | 5 | 4.6 | 37.5 | 3 | 9.2 | 47.7 | 4 | 5.5 | 41.3 |
| Chronic lower respiratory diseases | 4 | 5.5 | 45.4 | 8 | 2.7 | 31.2 | 7 | 3.6 | 30.1 | 7 | 3 | 15.8 | 8 | 2.6 | 20.6 |
| Unintentional injuries | 5 | 4.3 | 37.5 | 5 | 4.3 | 36.9 | 3 | 12 | 53.8 | 4 | 3.5 | 17.9 | 3 | 8.6 | 30.7 |
| Diabetes mellitus | 6 | 2.8 | 23.1 | 4 | 4.4 | 49.5 | 4 | 6 | 43.2 | 5 | 3.1 | 17.4 | 5 | 5 | 35.6 |
| Influenza and pneumonia | 7 | 2.8 | 22.6 | | | | 9 | 2.4 | 20.4 | 6 | 3 | 17.5 | 9 | 2.4 | 19.2 |
| Alzheimer's disease | 8 | 2.6 | — | | | | | | | | | | | | |
| Non-malignant kidney diseases | 9 | 1.6 | — | 9 | 2.6 | — | | | | 9 | 1.7 | — | | | |
| Septicemia | | | | 10 | 2.1 | — | | | | 10 | 1.1 | — | | | |
| Suicide | 10 | 1.4 | 12 | | | | 8 | 2.6 | 10.2 | 8 | 1.7 | 5.4 | | | |
| Homicide | | | | 6 | 2.9 | 21 | 10 | 2.2 | 8.4 | | | | 7 | 2.7 | 7.3 |
| HIV/AIDS disease | | | | 7 | 2.7 | 22.5 | | | | | | | 6 | 2.9 | 5.8 |
| Chronic liver disease | | | | | | | 6 | 4.4 | 22.8 | | | | | | |
| Certain conditions originating in the perinatal period | | | | | | | | | | | | | 10 | 2.1 | — |

Source: National Center for Health Statistics (U.S.). Health, United States, 2004. Atlanta: Centers for Disease Control and Prevention, 2004.

ranks number one for all ethnic groups except Asian Americans. However, the mortality rate from heart disease is not equal among the groups. African Americans rank highest, followed by whites, Latinos, American Indians, and Asian Americans. Cancer is the second leading cause of death for all groups except Asian Americans, for whom it ranks first. Cancer mortality rate is highest among African Americans, followed by whites, Latinos, American Indians, and Asian Americans and Pacific Islanders. The death rate for the most common cancers (breast, lung, prostate, colorectal) varies by ethnicity in a pattern similar to overall cancer mortality. African Americans and whites are most likely to die of these cancers, followed by Latinos and Asian Americans and Pacific Islanders. However, for some less common cancers, such as stomach and liver, Asian Americans and Latinos have the highest observed death rate. Cerebrovascular diseases constitute the third leading cause of death overall. African Americans are most likely to die of cerebrovascular disease, followed by whites, Asian Americans and Pacific Islanders, Latinos, and American Indians. The death rate for chronic lower respiratory disease, the fourth leading cause overall, is highest among whites and lowest among Asian Americans and Pacific Islanders. Unintentional injuries are the fifth leading cause of death overall but third for American Indians and Latinos. American Indians have a substantially higher frequency of death from unintentional injury than all other groups. Several causes of death, although not among the top ten for the overall population or whites, pose a significant health risk to ethnic minorities. For example, African Americans, Latinos, and American Indians have substantially higher death rates from homicide than whites and Asian Americans. Similarly, HIV/AIDS ranks higher among African Americans and Latinos than for the other ethnic groups.

## Years of Potential Life Lost

Examining the years of potential life lost from specific causes of death is another way of assessing health status. Figure 2.3 presents data regarding the years of potential life lost for all ethnic groups 2000.[8] YPLL-75, or the years of potential life lost before age seventy-five, indicates the average per 100,000 persons, assuming that each person would otherwise live to age seventy-five. Similar to the pattern observed for life expectancy, significant health disparities remain, despite improvement in this health indicator across all ethnic groups during the past twenty years. Across all causes of death, African Americans have the highest average YPLL, followed by American Indians and Alaskan Natives, whites, Latinos, and Asian Americans and Pacific Islanders. The YPLL for African Americans is more than three times that of Asian Americans and Pacific Islanders, and nearly twice as high as the YPLL for whites. The two largest contributors to the disproportionately high YPLL rate among African Americans are cancer (17.8 percent of

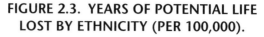

## FIGURE 2.3. YEARS OF POTENTIAL LIFE LOST BY ETHNICITY (PER 100,000).

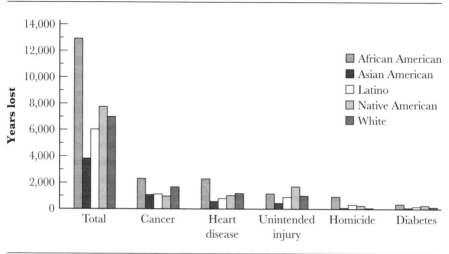

all YPLL) and heart disease (17.6 percent). Among American Indians and Alaskan Natives, the most important contributors to YPLL are unintentional injury (21.9 percent) and heart disease (13.3 percent). For whites, cancer (24 percent) and heart disease (16.9 percent) account for the highest proportion of YPLL. Cancer is the most important contributor to YPLL among Latinos, accounting for 18 percent of all YPLL, followed by unintentional injury (15.2 percent).

## Morbidity

It is important to examine morbidity, in addition to mortality, as an indicator of health status. This indicator incorporates the observation that some common diseases markedly impairing quality of life often do not result in shortened life span or in death. Arthritis and rheumatism are a common cause of disability in the United States, accounting for 17 percent of cases of disability among individuals fifteen years or older.[9] The second most common cause of disability is back or spinal problems (13.5 percent). It should be noted that neither disability appears as a common cause of death. Five of the remaining leading causes of disability can be considered chronic diseases: heart problems (11.1 percent), lung or respiratory problems (6.8 percent), hypertension (5.1 percent), diabetes (3.9 percent), and stroke (2.5 percent).

Another method of assessing ethnic differences in disability is to calculate the disability-free life expectancy or to assess the limitation of activity that is due to chronic conditions. Disability-free life expectancy is the percentage of the life span an individual can expect to live free of major disability. Whites and Asian Americans and Pacific Islanders enjoy the longest life expectancy free of disability (82 percent), followed by Latinos (78 percent), African Americans (74 percent), and American Indians and Alaskan Natives (69 percent). Figure 2.4 presents data regarding limitation of activity caused by chronic conditions, by ethnicity.[10] Approximately 25 percent of American Indians and Alaskan Natives report experiencing a limitation in instrumental activities of daily living (IADL), or activities related to independent living such as preparing meals, managing money, personal shopping, and housework. African Americans have the second highest rate, with 18 percent reporting such limitation. More than 13 percent of Latinos report an IADL limitation. Asian Americans and whites have the lowest rate of limitation in IADL (fewer than 12 percent). Of note, this indicator is one of the few that finds Latinos to have slightly poorer health than whites.

## Epidemiology of Health Disparities: Summary

Across all the indicators of health status mentioned here, African Americans are the most disadvantaged. This is a reflection of four centuries of exploitation and oppression—forced immigration, enslavement, and brutal subjugation during the majority of their tenure in the United States. The advances of the civil rights movement, heralding greater (but far from equal) educational, housing, and employment opportunities, encompass less than 10 percent of their history in this

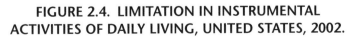

**FIGURE 2.4. LIMITATION IN INSTRUMENTAL ACTIVITIES OF DAILY LIVING, UNITED STATES, 2002.**

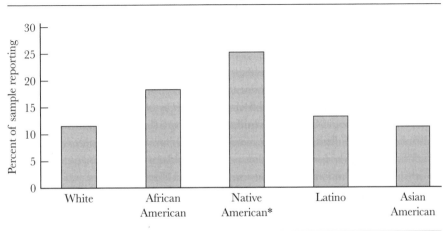

country. They experience the highest mortality rates for heart disease, cancer, type 2 diabetes mellitus, and cerebrovascular disease. In addition, homicide and HIV/AIDS emerge as leading causes of death among African Americans, but not for the overall population. Other significant health issues that affect African Americans in particular are high incidence rates of obesity, infant and maternal mortality, and smoking among middle-aged men. Infant mortality is a particularly critical health concern for African Americans. In 2002, the African American infant mortality rate (13.9 infant deaths per thousand live births) was more than two times the rate for Latinos, whites, and Asian Americans and Pacific Islanders (each fewer than 6 per thousand live births),[11] and the gap has widened appreciably during the past two decades.[12] Although the infant mortality rate decreases with higher education, the rate for African Americans exceeds that for all other ethnic groups at every level of education.[13] The African American infant mortality rate for women with the highest level of education is higher than that for women with the lowest level of education from other ethnic groups.

Latinos as a group have lower mortality rates from most of the leading causes of death. This is despite the fact that they exhibit many of the socioeconomic characteristics consistently associated with poor health status, such as lower income and level of education. This phenomenon has been labeled the "Latino or Hispanic Paradox,"[14] and it is far more pronounced for mortality than morbidity statistics (for example, type 2 diabetes mellitus). Several hypotheses have been advanced to explain this paradox, although the root causes remain unknown. Among the explanations for the paradox are lack of reliable data, the possibility that many older Latinos return to their native country when they become ill or are close to death, difference in risk factors for the major causes of death, cultural factors, and the suggestion that migration to the United States occurs principally among the healthiest individuals from the home country. It is also important to note that data on Latinos are often aggregated across a diverse group of people of differing nationalities, ethnicities, and races as well as varying migration history (which may mask disparities among subgroups). For example, although Latinos experience a lower death rate from all cancers combined as well as for the most common cancers (lung, colon, prostate), they have higher incidence rates of stomach, liver, gallbladder, and cervical cancer than whites and the general population.[15] Finally, Latinos are the fasting-growing population in the United States, amplifying the importance of more fully understanding the health of this group. Recent data on the effect of acculturation on health status among Latinos indicate that health status declines with increasing acculturation,[16] as is seen for example in the rise of obesity and type 2 diabetes mellitus in this group.[17]

In terms of overall mortality, the rate for American Indians is lower than for African Americans but higher than for whites, Latinos, and Asian Americans.[18]

However, they are the most disadvantaged with respect to disability-free life expectancy, and the second most disadvantaged when health status is measured by potential years of life lost. Research on the health of American Indians and Alaskan Natives has been hampered by lack of data. When data are collected on race and ethnicity, American Indians and Alaskan Natives are often coded as "other" and combined with other groups. Even when studies specifically recruit samples of American Indians, as in the Behavioral Risk Factor Surveillance System, small sample size can make a population estimate unreliable and unstable, and the methods used to collect data (such as telephone interviews) often fail to reach a representative sample of this small and unique population.[19] The health of American Indians was negatively affected originally when European settlers brought diseases that were previously unknown to native populations. Since that time, American Indians have endured substantial hardship and oppression, negatively affecting their health status. Three of the top ten health threats for American Indians are not among the top ten for the total U.S. population: chronic liver disease (sixth), suicide (eighth), and homicide (tenth). In addition, unintentional injury ranks third as a cause of death in this group.[20] Alcohol abuse is considered a key underlying cause for the higher mortality from these four causes of death. Data from the Behavioral Risk Factor Surveillance System found that binge drinking (consuming five or more drinks on one occasion in the past month) among American Indians or Alaskan Natives was quite prevalent. The rate within the American Indian and Alaskan Native sample was 18.9 percent, compared to 14.3 percent for whites, 8.7 percent for African Americans, 16.2 percent for Latinos, and 6.7 percent for Asians.[21] Type 2 diabetes mellitus also ranks relatively high as a cause of death within this ethnic group (third) compared to the overall population (sixth), and it is pervasive among such tribes as the Pima and Zuni.[22]

The Asian American and Pacific Islander population has been referred to as the "model minority," given their wealth and better health status as reflected in a variety of indicators. However, there are a number of critical issues to consider in understanding the health of this population. As with Latinos, immigration may select for the healthiest individuals. The category Asian American and Pacific Islander encompasses an extraordinarily diverse group of people originating from many countries with widely varying socioeconomic characteristics, immigration history, culture, and social standing in the United States. Unfortunately, the majority of research studies to date have collapsed all individuals of Asian descent into one category. This aggregation masks considerable subgroup differences for general indicators such as mortality as well as for incidence of particular diseases. For example, Asian Indian women have the highest life expectancy (88.1 years), whereas Pacific Islander men have a life expectancy among the lowest at 70.5 years.[23] Vietnamese have the highest mortality rates for cervix and liver cancers while the Japanese have the lowest.[24] In addition, as among all immigrant groups, increasing acculturation is often linked to diminished health status.[25] Asian Americans as a group present a unique opportunity to examine the effect of acculturation by examining the incidence of certain conditions across groups with more recent immigration history (for example, Koreans) compared to those who have lived in the United States for many generations (Japanese). An illustration of this effect can be found in recent data showing that although Japanese women residing in Japan have one of the lowest rates of breast cancer in the world, Japanese women residing in Los Angeles County have overtaken white women with respect to breast cancer incidence.[26]

## Factors Underlying Chronic Disease-Related Disparities

Paralleling our focus on the major disease states compromising health in describing the epidemiology of ethnic disparities in health status, in this section we emphasize the underlying factors responsible for the majority of morbidity, disability, and mortality. McGinnis and Foege's classic article[27] identified the *actual* causes of more than 80 percent of "preventable" mortality as diet, physical inactivity, tobacco, and alcohol. Thus we highlight these behavioral risk factors in presenting the underlying contributors to a broad spectrum of health status disparities. It is important to keep in mind that the actual cause of more than half of all deaths is not known, and thus identified determinants or risk factors generally explain only a modest amount of the variance in most disease processes.

Of the many theoretical models of determinants of health, we have elected to use the Evans-Stoddart model to depict the broad categories of variables contributing to health (see Figure 2.5) and as an organizing framework for our discussion of those most closely linked to disparities.[28] We have selected several categories of determinants to be highlighted in detail, on the basis of the malleability of the determinant and the availability of data.

Specifically, we discuss behavioral, socioeconomic, and physical and social environmental factors that influence individual response, focusing especially on current areas of scientific investigation in public health. Although we recognize that behavioral and biological responses often overlap, we focus on the behavioral variables. The genetic contribution to observed racial and ethnic variation in health is considered minor, and consequently is not examined here. Race and ethnicity are essentially a sociocultural and ideological construct, as reflected in the considerable genetic variation within racial groups and relatively little consistent between-group variation (consider the general failure of efforts to link racial phenotypes to biological typologies).[29] Disparities in health care access and utilization

## FIGURE 2.5. THEORETICAL FRAMEWORK.

**Determinants of Health (Evans-Stoddart Model)**

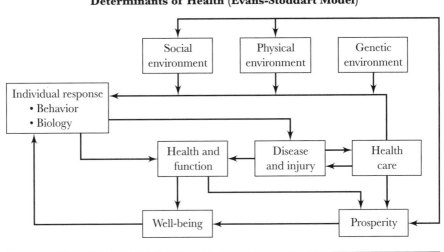

are also associated with health disparities but are not discussed in this chapter; they are the subject of Chapter Three, by Morales and Ortega.

## Behavioral Risk Factors

Individual behaviors are the final common pathway through which genetic, economic, physical, and social environmental factors influence health. They are symptomatic of the major contributors to health disparities to be discussed later. Public health surveillance of these behaviors or conditions allows quantification of adverse exposure and disease as a bellwether of future disease incidence, providing an opportunity for targeted intervention.

Obesity is increasingly recognized as a major driver of chronic disease disparities.[30] Rates of being overweight and of obesity (defined as a body mass index [BMI] at or greater than 25 kg/m$^2$ and 30 kg/m$^2$, respectively) are increasing across the population but even more rapidly in certain ethnic groups: including African Americans, Latinos, American Indians, and Pacific Islanders.[31] Physical inactivity and poor dietary quality—the antecedents of obesity—are commensurately more common in ethnic minority groups in general except Asian Americans, though certain healthful dietary components are more often consumed in these groups (legumes among African Americans and Latinos, fruits and vegetables among Latinos).[32] Asian Americans as a group have lower incidence of being overweight or obese.[33] However, the negative health effects of being overweight begin to occur at a lower BMI among Asian Americans compared to individuals of other ethnicities. Lower socioeconomic status is associated with obesity, but higher socioeconomic status is less protective against obesity for African Americans than for Latinos and whites.[34]

Tobacco use varies in form and prevalence among ethnic groups. Twenty-two percent of American adults are currently smokers, 25.2 percent of men and 20 percent of women.[35] The overall rate of tobacco use among African Americans is similar to the overall population (22.4 percent). However, among African American women it is 18.7 percent, slightly lower than the national average for women.[36] Compared to whites, African Americans tend to start smoking at a later age and are more inclined to attempt to quit smoking but less likely to succeed. The later age at initiation of smoking among African American women is reflected in a lower relative risk of obstructive lung disease compared to white women.[37] The smoking rate among Latinos (16.7 percent) is lower than for the general population and is especially low among Latinas (10.8 percent).[38] American Indian and Alaskan natives have the highest tobacco use of all ethnic groups at 40.8 percent overall, equal among men and women. A higher proportion of American Indian and American Indian tobacco users use smokeless tobacco products compared to the general population. Asian Americans and Pacific Islanders smoke at the lowest rate (13.3 percent overall), although it has been observed that use for Asians varies widely among Asian subgroups and between genders, and it may increase with acculturation. Tobacco consumption among adolescents from all ethnic minority groups appears to be on the rise.

Alcohol use patterns also vary considerably across ethnic groups. In general, men have a higher rate of alcohol use and heavy drinking than women. Whites have more alcohol use across all age groups; however, problem-related drinking and the negative consequences of alcohol are more prevalent among African Americans, American Indians and Alaskan Natives, and Latinos than whites. Several studies have found that American Indians and Latinos of Mexican origin may be particularly likely to be dependent on alcohol.[39] Alcohol use among Asians, although lower than for other ethnic groups, has been found to vary widely within ethnic groups and a higher rate is seen among U.S.-born people than in immigrant populations.

Ethnic disparities in health status have traditionally been ascribed to poor health behaviors, primarily those described here, and to limited access to health care. It has become increasingly clear, however, that individual-level behavioral variables are closely linked with environmental-level variables that govern the ease or difficulty of access to healthy or unhealthy options and choices. These environmental exposures are further examined in the later discussion of socioeconomic, physical, and social environmental influences.

## Socioeconomic Status

Poverty is the most powerful determinant of health,[40] with African Americans and Latinos substantially overrepresented among households in poverty.[41] Children of color are even more impoverished—for example, in Los Angeles County 21 percent of Asian Americans and Pacific Islanders, 37 percent of African Americans, and 46 percent of Latino children live at or below the poverty level, compared with 9 percent of whites.[42]

However, higher income inequality, rather than absolute deprivation, may also have an adverse influence on health.[43] Several theories have been advanced to explain the relationship between income inequality and adverse health outcomes.[44] The psychosocial pathway theory postulates that inequality affects health through individual perceptions of low position in the social hierarchy, which in turn can have an effect on biological response (for instance, blood pressure) or maladaptive behavior (smoking, homicide). The material deprivation pathway theory proposes that inequality affects health through an accumulation of negative exposures and lack of resources held by individuals at the bottom of a social hierarchy. There is evidence that income inequality is growing in the United States, with the income of the upper 1 percent of the population growing 139 percent between 1979 and 2001 to more than $700,000, while the income of the middle fifth rose by just 17 percent (to $43,700) and the income of the poorest fifth rose only 9 percent.[45]

Researchers often use singular indicators of SES such as income, education, or occupational attainment interchangeably. However, the interaction among these indicators may differ by ethnic group. For example, formal education does not have the same socioeconomic return for blacks as for whites.[46] At the same level of education, research has found, whites have higher income and occupational attainment as compared to blacks. Furthermore, there is evidence to indicate that, at an individual level, increasing SES does not have the same benefits on the health of blacks compared to whites.[47] Data indicate that even at a higher level of education, blacks experience poorer physical health outcomes such as increased infant mortality compared to whites.[48]

Finally, community-level socioeconomic measures have not been adequately captured in most analyses examining the effect of SES on health. Research has shown that socioeconomic characteristics of the neighborhood in which an individual lives (average income, percentage of unemployment) predict morbidity and mortality above and beyond individual characteristics.[49] Ethnic minorities are significantly more likely to live in disadvantaged or resource-poor communities relative to whites. A study by Jargowsky[50] found that though only 6 percent of poor whites lived in a high-poverty area in 1990, 34 percent of poor blacks and 22 percent of poor Latinos lived in such areas. A recent analysis of a fairly socioeconomically homogeneous multiethnic sample controlled for twelve community-level variables (among them robbery arrests and income inequality). However, disparities persisted in coronary heart disease risk, obesity, and hypertension among black women compared to white women.[51] Pathways by which these community-level variables influence health are elaborated later in this section.

## Physical Environmental Influences

Many tobacco control efforts implemented over the past two decades have focused on creating changes in the physical environment. The success of these efforts in reducing smoking speaks to the powerful influence of the physical environment on health behaviors. Some of the most effective tobacco control efforts have included federal laws prohibiting tobacco sales to minors, state smoking bans in public places, and federal and state policies that encourage a smoke-free workplace among grant recipients. Although many policies and laws have been enacted, adherence to and enforcement of these controls is lower in communities of color. In addition, the shift in focus of tobacco marketing to the developing world, where few such controls have been implemented, results in the addiction of many Asian American and Latino men who later immigrate to the United States.

Researchers are now beginning to elucidate the link between ecological factors, such as access to high-quality or poor-quality food, and the onset of such conditions as cardiovascular disease and diabetes.[52] Studies show that minority neighborhoods have fewer supermarkets and fewer high-quality food options.[53] Other studies demonstrate that African American neighborhoods have a disproportionate number of fast food restaurants.[54] In addition, diners in lower-income, minority neighborhoods have fewer healthy options available to them in restaurants, in both food selection and preparation.[55] These areas have been termed "food deserts" by English researchers.[56] Numerous studies demonstrate that regular consumption of fast food can lead to higher BMI, contributing to obesity and related illnesses.[57] Recent studies also link periodic food insecurity to overconsumption, obesity, and poor mental health.[58]

Product consumption preferences and purchasing behaviors are also influenced by commercial advertising, marketing, and promotion. There is increasing evidence of concentrated media marketing and advertising of a range of commercial products targeted to specific ethnic groups that may contribute to health risk behavior disparities, especially tobacco, alcohol, and nutrient-poor food consumption.[59] Severely constraining billboard and television advertising and counteradvertising campaigns (adolescent-targeted social marketing to counter the claims of tobacco industry advertising) are credited with contributing to decreased tobacco use. However, the decrease in, for example, tobacco billboard advertising has been accompanied by more advertising of other unhealthy products. For example, billboards in predominantly African American and Latino neighborhoods in Chicago were found to advertise alcohol five times as frequently as those in predominantly white areas.[60] Similarly, fewer advertisements for healthier food and beverage products are found in magazines and television shows targeting African Americans compared to those targeting "general audiences," and a significantly greater number of advertisements for unhealthy products.[61] In addition, Lewis and her colleagues[62] have recently identified substantially more point-of-sale advertising and promotions, with many more for unhealthy than healthy foods, in restaurants in lower-income African American and Latino communities in Los Angeles County than in its more affluent white communities. This commercial marketing is also likely to influence physical activity and sedentary behavior patterns (automobile and other private transportation usage, audiovisual electronic media consumption), and work is beginning in this area to elucidate these relationships.

Though less studied than its influence on nutritional intake, the influence of physical surroundings on physical activity patterns has recently received much attention. Lower-income and minority neighborhoods have fewer recreational facilities, private or community gardens, less safety (perceived and actual), insufficient lighting, and urban design with few concessions to pedestrians.[63] Interestingly, the major difference is that lower-income neighborhoods have fewer free recreational facilities (such as parks) compared to higher-income neighborhoods, although no differences are observed for frequency of paid usage facilities (such as gyms). In addition to these environmental stressors or disincentives (which also include noise, traffic congestion, and information overload), environmental psychologists point to neighborhood disorder (less "defensible space," incivility) exerting a negative influence on physical activity and restorative features such as foliage, water, and spatial vistas that reduce stress positively influencing physical activity.[64]

Health-compromising physical characteristics of workplace and residential environments are well characterized elsewhere and are only summarized here. Workplace and residential environmental characteristics have been found to influence multiple health outcomes, in particular intentional and unintentional injury, disability, chronic disease morbidity, and mortality. Potential exposures occurring in these environments include noise, toxic chemical or biological hazards (tobacco smoke, lead, asbestos, dioxin, tuberculosis, vehicle emissions), hazardous equipment, hazardous natural elements (ionizing and nonionizing radiation, heights, bodies of water, heat), poor ergonomic design of equipment, lack of adherence to safety protocols or safety equipment usage, traffic hazards, poorly maintained streets and sidewalks, and firearms. People of ethnic minority background are more likely to work and live in an environment that can have a detrimental effect on health.

## Social Environmental Influences

As has been illustrated here, socioeconomic position explains many, but not all, of the ethnic differences in health status. For example, 1979–1989 life-expectancy differentials between white men earning less than $10,000 and those earning more than $25,000 were less than those for black men in similar economic circumstances (-6.6 years vs. -7.4 years, respectively).[65] This might be interpreted to indicate that poverty exerts a greater negative influence on mortality among blacks than whites. Recent evidence points to additional explanations for the more adverse effect of poverty on the health of people of color:

- Cumulative effects of prolonged exposure to individual stressors
- Long-term effects of an early childhood or prenatal environment of deprivation[66]
- Reaction to macrosocial factors. In today's world, social comparisons extend beyond what was formerly possible only at the neighborhood level. Marketing by mass media to children and adolescents fosters a desire for goods and services (enjoyed by affluent whites) that are beyond the means of working and middle-class families.

Racial and ethnic discrimination is the primary social environmental influence cited, given that negative attitudes toward individuals from ethnic minority groups are still commonplace[67]; racism may also interact with other forms of discrimination, based on gender, sexual orientation, disability, or age.[68] Social experiences are translated and transformed into biological responses ("embodied"), enhancing or eroding health.[69] Thus social disparities mediate gene expression, which is the greater contributor to health disparities than gene frequency (genotype).[70] A full explication of this topic is beyond the scope of this chapter. Here we briefly summarize the major issues attendant to investigation of the association between discrimination and health outcomes.

Epidemiological investigation of the health effects of discrimination has used three main approaches[71]:

1. *Indirect, individual-level,* inferring discrimination when established risk factors do not fully explain ethnic differences in health outcomes; for example, formal education does not produce the same returns in improved health for blacks as whites, similar to its lesser return in wealth and income.[72]
2. *Direct, individual-level,* examining association between self-reported discrimination and particular individual health outcomes (blood pressure, peptic ulcer disease).
3. *Institutional, population-level,* examining association between group-level measures of discrimination and population health outcomes.

The major mediators of the relationship between discrimination and health are:[73] economic and social deprivation (for instance, diminished access to goods and services, substandard education, poor health care); exposure to hazardous physical, chemical, and biological agents (lead-based paint, parasites); socially inflicted trauma (mental, physical, or sexual abuse or neglect); and targeted marketing of legal and illegal health-compromising substances (tobacco, energy-dense but nutrient-poor foods). These mediators exert their influence through psychological and physiological responses to perceived or internalized discrimination among those discriminated against, and individual and institutional policies and practices by those perpetrating discrimination that produce socioeconomic disadvantage or personal injury. One common example of the latter is work-related stress. Relegation to a position not commensurate with one's talents, or to certain types of lower-status job, increases the likelihood of an individual being subjected to high psychological demands with little decisional latitude or control or social support, an independent contributor to coronary heart disease risk.[74] Another example is reflected in the political expedience of the generalized stigmatization of people of Middle Eastern and South Asian descent following the 2001 terrorist attacks in the United States carried out by Islamic radicals—presenting an interesting parallel to the stigmatization of Asians following the Japanese attack on Pearl Harbor.

## Factors and Influences: Summary

Socioeconomic status (SES) is a major contributor to ethnic disparities in health. In fact, ethnicity is frequently a proxy for SES in public health research and surveillance, because the dramatic skew in the income distribution of African Americans and Latinos compared to whites and acculturated subgroups of Asian Americans precludes appropriate SES matching. Lower SES is responsible for increased exposure to many of the physical and sociocultural environmental conditions contributing to health risk behaviors and compromising health status, among them long-term effects of the early childhood or prenatal environment.

However, income inequality may also be an important contributor to poorer health, and economic indicators demonstrate that the gap between rich and poor is increasing dramatically while opportunities for upward social mobility are declining.[75] This disproportionately disadvantages ethnic minority populations and likely contributes to ethnic health disparities. In addition to absolute or relative economic deprivation, recent evidence suggests that the health of ethnic minorities may be negatively affected by macrosocial factors such as the mass media's promotion of social comparisons beyond what can be observed at the neighborhood level.

Racial and ethnic discrimination is the primary social environmental contributor to health disparities, exerting both acute or immediate effects (anger, hostility) and cumulative effects of prolonged exposure to individual stressors. Discrimination also influences the physical environment, through institutional policies and practices on the part of those perpetrating discrimination that produce socioeconomic disadvantage or personal injury.

## Future Directions and Policy Implications

Population demographic shifts, including both aging and ethnic diversification, will further increase attention to and need for programmatic and policy intervention to eliminate health disparities. In particular, as the obesity epidemic strains the health care system and otherwise increases societal economic burden, there is clearly a need for a shift in health policy focus, and ultimately the health services funding focus, from treatment to disease prevention and health promotion. The increasing contribution of obesity-related disparities to overall health disparities and burden of disease will also drive this necessary shift; a range of sectors must engage in structural and systemic change to stem the epidemic.

The paucity of data, from public health practice surveillance, observational epidemiological research, and in particular policy and programmatic intervention evaluation or research, constitutes a major concern in this or any discussion of disparities. Our ability to identify, understand, and monitor progress in addressing disparities is severely limited by the underrepresentation of people of ethnic minority and low-income backgrounds in surveillance and research.[76] In both surveillance and research, data must be disaggregated and sufficiently "local" (beyond city or county to zip code and census tract, to really reach communities or neighborhoods) if we are to accurately capture and monitor disparities and assess and refine intervention efforts.

The existence of positive ethnic disparities (rate of disease and risk behavior in ethnic minority populations lower than for whites) or attenuation of disparities in relation to the severity of socioeconomic disadvantage is noteworthy. A number of sociocultural protective factors create resilience and mitigate the effects of adversity. Such factors within the Mexican and Central American Latino communities may include the effect of strong identification with the culture of origin on healthy food choices,[77] and family and neighborhood cohesion creating optimal birth outcomes.[78] The lower level of nonmalignant lung disease among African American women and lower smoking rate among African American adolescents may reflect a protective response to discrimination manifested in active resistance to tobacco company exploitation of the black community, as in organizing to prevent introduction of the Uptown cigarette brand. Having role models and mentors has been associated with such positive outcomes as ethnic identity, academic achievement, physical activity, and self-esteem in adolescence.[79] Also, a lower level of overweight self-perception may protect against eating disorders, poor body image, and sedentary behavior in Latinos, Pacific Islanders, and African Americans.[80] The sociocultural environment may in fact be as important as the physical environment in supporting physical activity participation,[81] as reflected in the comparable physical activity of Pacific Islanders and whites.[82] The fact that, for example, dancing or movement to music is normative throughout adulthood in African American, Latino, and other communities of color along with their collectivist rather than individualist values are cultural assets that may increase receptivity to intervention approaches reintegrating brief bouts of physical activity into organizational (that is, workplace) routines.[83]

In addition, the relative health advantages observed for Asian Americans and Latinos are likely to dissipate over time, given the negative effect of acculturation on health status. Also, the health indicators that show the greatest benefit for Latinos and Asian Americans—life expectancy and death rate—do not yet reflect significant changes in risk factor status occurring over the past ten years. For example, among immigrants obesity and tobacco use, poorer dietary quality, and lower level of physical activity have been correlated with increased length of stay in the United States.[84] "Softer" measures, such as self-reported disability and lower perceived health status, are already more common in these groups than among whites, a harbinger of excess future disease and death.

For all these reasons, health services policy and health care organizations must extend beyond their accustomed boundaries of medical care delivery to address the physical, social, and economic environmental conditions undergirding health disparities. Changes in the health care system will have a diminishing influence on the health status of the population without immediate, careful, and considerable attention to eliminating health disparities.

# Notes

1. National Center for Health Statistics (U.S.). *Health, United States, 2004.* Atlanta: Centers for Disease Control and Prevention, 2004.
2. Lavizzo-Mourey, R., and others. "A Tale of Two Cities." *Health Affairs,* 2005, *24*(2), 313–315; Satcher, D., and others. "What If We Were Equal? A Comparison of the Black-White Mortality Gap in 1960 and 2000." *Health Affairs,* 2005, *24*(2), 459–464; Smith, D. B. "Racial and Ethnic Health Disparities and the Unfinished Civil Rights Agenda." *Health Affairs,* 2005, *24*(2), 317–324.
3. Smith, J. P. "Healthy Bodies and Thick Wallets: The Dual Relation Between Health and Economic Status." *Journal of Economic Perspectives,* 1999, *13*(2), 144–166.
4. Centers for Disease Control and Prevention (U.S.), and National Center for Chronic Disease Prevention and Health Promotion (U.S.). *Chronic Disease Overview.* [http://www.cdc.gov/nccdphp/overview.htm, June, 2005].

5. Population Reference Bureau. *Major Causes of Death in the United States and Peru.* [http://www. prb.org/content/navigationmenu/prb/educators/human_population/health2, June 2001].

6. National Center for Health Statistics (2004).

7. *Methodology and Assumptions for the Population Projections of the United States*: 1999–2100 [microform]. Washington, D.C.: Population Projections Program, Population Division, U.S. Census Bureau, Department of Commerce, 2000; *Regional Differences in Indian Health 1998–99.* Washington, D.C.: Indian Health Service, U.S. Dept. of Health and Human Services, 2001.

8. National Center for Health Statistics (2004).

9. "Prevalence of Disabilities and Associated Health Conditions—United States, 1991–1992." *Morbidity and Mortality Weekly Report*, 1994, *43*(40), 730–731, 737–739.

10. National Center for Health Statistics (2004).

11. National Center for Health Statistics (2004).

12. Frisbie, W. P., and others. "The Increasing Racial Disparity in Infant Mortality: Respiratory Distress Syndrome and Other Causes." *Demography*, 2004, *41*(4), 773–800.

13. Lu, M. C., and Halfon, N. "Racial and Ethnic Disparities in Birth Outcomes: A Life-Course Perspective." *Maternal and Child Health Journal*, 2003, *7*(1), 13–30.

14. Hayes-Bautista, D. E., and others. "An Anomaly Within the Latino Epidemiological Paradox: The Latino Adolescent Male Mortality Peak." *Archives of Pediatrics and Adolescent Medicine*, 2002, *156*(5), 480–484.

15. American Cancer Society. *Cancer Facts & Figures for Hispanics/Latinos 2003–2005.* [http:// www.cancer.org/downloads/STT/CPED2003PWSecured.pdf]. Atlanta: American Cancer Society, 2003.

16. Balcazar, H., Peterson, G., and Cobas, J. A. "Acculturation and Health-Related Risk Behaviors Among Mexican American Pregnant Youth." *American Journal of Health Behavior*, 1996, *20*(6), 433–435; Guendelman, S., and Abrams, B. "Dietary Intake Among Mexican-American Women: Generational Differences and a Comparison with White Non-Hispanic Women." *American Journal of Public Health*, 1995, *85*(1), 20–25.

17. Smith, S. C., Jr., and others. "Discovering the Full Spectrum of Cardiovascular Disease: Minority Health Summit 2003—Report of the Obesity, Metabolic Syndrome, and Hypertension Writing Group." *Circulation*, 2005, *111*(10), 134–139.

18. National Center for Health Statistics (2004).

19. Denny, C. H., Holtzman, D., and Cobb, N. "Surveillance for Health Behaviors of American Indians and Alaska Natives. Findings from the Behavioral Risk Factor Surveillance System, 1997–2000." *Morbidity and Mortality Weekly Report, Surveillance Summary*, 2003, *52*(7), 1–13.

20. National Center for Health Statistics (2004).

21. Bolen, J. C., and others. "State-Specific Prevalence of Selected Health Behaviors, by Race and Ethnicity—Behavioral Risk Factor Surveillance System, 1997." *Morbidity and Mortality Weekly Report Surveillance Summary*, 2000, *49*(2), 1–60.

22. Ritenbaugh, C., and Goodby, C. S. "Beyond the Thrifty Gene: Metabolic Implications of Prehistoric Migration into the New World." *Medical Anthropology*, 1989, *11*(3), 227–236.

23. Johnson, H. P., and Hayes, J. M. "The Demographics of Mortality in California: Population Trends and Profiles." *California Counts*, 2004, *5*(4).

24. Glanz, K. *Cancer in Women of Color Monograph.* Bethesda, Md.: National Cancer Institute, Department of Health and Human Services, 2003.

25. Deapen, D., and others. "Rapidly Rising Breast Cancer Incidence Rates Among Asian-American Women." *International Journal of Cancer*, 2002, *99*(5), 747–750; Gomez, S. L., and others. "Immigration and Acculturation in Relation to Health and Health-Related Risk

Factors Among Specific Asian Subgroups in a Health Maintenance Organization." *American Journal of Public Health*, 2004, *94*(11), 1977–1984.

26. Deapen and others (2002).

27. McGinnis, J. M., and Foege, W. H. "Actual Causes of Death in the United States." *Journal of the American Medical Association*, 1993, *270*(18), 2207–2212.

28. Evans, R. G., and Stoddart, G. L. "Producing Health, Consuming Health Care." In R. G. Evans, M. L. Barer, and T. R. Marmor (eds.), *Why Are Some People Healthy and Others Not?: The Determinants of Health of Populations.* New York: A. de Gruyter, 1994.

29. Mays, V. M., and others. "Classification of Race and Ethnicity: Implications for Public Health." *Annual Review of Public Health*, 2003, *24*, 83–110; Wilkinson, D. Y., and King, G. "Conceptual and Methodological Issues in the Use of Race as a Variable: Policy Implications." *Milbank Quarterly*, 1987, *65* Suppl. 1, 56–71.

30. Smith, Jr., and others (2005); Yancey, A. K., and others. "Discovering the Full Spectrum of Cardiovascular Disease: Minority Health Summit 2003—Report of the Advocacy Writing Group." *Circulation*, 2005, *111*(10), 140–149; Swinburn, B., Gill, T., and Kumanyika, S. "Obesity Prevention: A Proposed Framework for Translating Evidence into Action." *Obesity Review*, 2005, *6*(1), 23–33.

31. U.S. Department of Health and Human Services. "The Surgeon General's Call to Action to Prevent and Decrease Overweight and Obesity." Washington, D.C.: Office of the Surgeon General, Public Health Service, U.S. Department of Health and Human Services, 2001.

32. Bermudez, O. I., and others. "Hispanic and Non-Hispanic White Elders from Massachusetts Have Different Patterns of Carotenoid Intake and Plasma Concentrations." *Journal of Nutrition*, 2005, *135*(6), 1496–1502; Lucas, J. W., Schiller, J. S., and Benson, V. "Summary Health Statistics for U.S. Adults: National Health Interview Survey, 2001." *Vital Health Statistics*, 2004, *10*(218), 1–134; Smit, E., and others. "Estimates of Animal and Plant Protein Intake in U.S. Adults: Results from the Third National Health and Nutrition Examination Survey, 1988–1991." *Journal of the American Dietary Association*, 1999, *99*(7), 813–820; Popkin, B. M., Siega-Riz, A. M., and Haines, P. S. "A Comparison of Dietary Trends Among Racial and Socioeconomic Groups in the United States." *New England Journal of Medicine*, 1996, *335*(10), 716–720.

33. Smith, Jr., and others (2005).

34. Williams, D. R. "Racial/Ethnic Variations in Women's Health: The Social Embeddedness of Health." *American Journal of Public Health*, 2002, *92*(4), 588–597.

35. Centers for Disease Control and Prevention (U.S.), and National Center for Chronic Disease Prevention and Health Promotion (U.S.). *Chronic Disease Overview.* [http://www.cdc.gov/nccdphp/overview.htm], June 2005.

36. Centers for Disease Control and Prevention and National Center for Chronic Disease Prevention and Health Promotion (2005).

37. Williams (2002).

38. Centers for Disease Control and Prevention and National Center for Chronic Disease Prevention and Health Promotion (2005).

39. *National Household Survey on Drug Abuse: 1991–93.* Rockville, Md.: National Institute on Drug Abuse, Division of Epidemiology and Statistical Analysis; Alcohol, Drug Abuse, and Mental Health Administration, Public Health Service, U.S. Department of Health and Human Services, 1994;:*Results from the 2003 National Survey on Drug Use and Health: National Findings.* Rockville, Md.: National Institute on Drug Abuse Division of Epidemiology and Statistical

Analysis; Alcohol, Drug Abuse, and Mental Health Administration, Public Health Service, U.S. Department of Health and Human Services , 2004.

40. Lynch, J. W., Kaplan, G. A., and Shema, S. J. "Cumulative Impact of Sustained Economic Hardship on Physical, Cognitive, Psychological, and Social Functioning." *New England Journal of Medicine*, 1997, *337*(26), 1889–1895.

41. Robert, S. A., and House, J. S. "Socioeconomic Inequalities in Health: Integrating Individual-, Community-, and Societal-Level Theory and Research." In G. L. Albrecht, R. Fitzpatrick, and S. Scrimshaw, (eds.) *Handbook of Social Studies in Health and Medicine*. Thousand Oaks, Calif.: Sage, 2000.

42. "Public Health. Los Angeles County Department of Health Services." [http://www.lapublichealth.org]. Los Angeles: County Department of Health Services, 2005.

43. Lynch, Kaplan, and Shema (1997); Kawachi, I. "Income Inequality and Health." In L. F. Berkman and I. Kawachi (eds.), *Social Epidemiology*. New York: Oxford University Press, 2000; Kaplan, G. A., and others. "Inequality in Income and Mortality in the United States: Analysis of Mortality and Potential Pathways." *British Medical Journal*, 1996, *312*(7037), 999–1003.

44. Lynch, J. W., and others. "Income Inequality and Mortality: Importance to Health of Individual Income, Psychosocial Environment, or Material Conditions." *British Medical Journal*, 2000, *320*(7243), 1200–1204.

45. Scott, J., and Leonhardt, D. "Shadowy Lines That Still Divide." *New York Times*, May 15, 2005, p. A-1.

46. Lillie-Blanton, M., and Laveist, T. "Race/Ethnicity, the Social Environment, and Health." *Social Science Medicine*, 1996, *43*(1), 83–91.

47. Anderson, N. B., and Armstead, C. A. "Toward Understanding the Association of Socioeconomic Status and Health: A New Challenge for the Biopsychosocial Approach." *Psychosomatic Medicine*, 1995, *57*(3), 213–225.

48. Williams, D. R., and Collins, C. "U.S. Socioeconomic and Racial Differentials in Health: Patterns and Explanations." *Annual Review of Sociology*, 1995, *21*, 349–386.

49. Diez-Roux, A. V., and others. "Neighborhood Environments and Coronary Heart Disease: A Multilevel Analysis." *American Journal of Epidemiology*, 1997, *146*(1), 48–63; Haan, M., Kaplan, G. A., and Camacho, T. "Poverty and Health. Prospective Evidence from the Alameda County Study." *American Journal of Epidemiology*, 1987, *125*(6), 989–998.

50. Jargowsky, P. A. *Poverty and Place: Ghettos, Barrios, and the American City*. New York: Russell Sage Foundation, 1997.

51. Finkelstein, E. A., and others. "Racial/Ethnic Disparities in Coronary Heart Disease Risk Factors Among WISEWOMAN Enrollees." *Journal of Women's Health*, 2004, *13*(5), 503–518.

52. Hill, J. O., and Peters, J. C. "Environmental Contributions to the Obesity Epidemic." *Science*, 1998, *280*(5368), 1371–1374; Stokols, D. "Establishing and Maintaining Healthy Environments: Toward a Social Ecology of Health Promotion." *American Psychologist*, 1992, *47*(1), 6–22.

53. Sloane, D. C., and others. "Improving the Nutritional Resource Environment for Healthy Living Through Community-Based Participatory Research." *Journal of General Internal Medicine*, 2003, *18*(7), 568–575; Morland, K., and others. "Neighborhood Characteristics Associated with the Location of Food Stores and Food Service Places." *American Journal of Preventive Medicine*, 2002, *22*(1), 23–29.

54. Block, J. P., Scribner, R. A., and DeSalvo, K. B. "Poverty, Race, and Fast Food: A Geographical Analysis." *Journal of General Internal Medicine*, 2002, *17* (Suppl. 1), 151.

55. Lewis, L. B., and others. "African Americans' Access to Healthy Food Options in South Los Angeles Restaurants." *American Journal of Public Health*, 2005, *95*(4), 668–673.

56. Whelan, A., and others. "Life in a Food Desert." *Urban Studies*, 2002, *39*, 2083–2100; Wrigley, N., Warm, D., and Margetts, B. "Deprivation, Diet, and Food-Retail Access: Findings from the Leeds 'Food Deserts' Study." *Environment and Planning*, 2003, *35*, 151–188.

57. Thompson, O. M., and others. "Food Purchased away from Home as a Predictor of Change in BMI Z-score Among Girls." *International Journal of Obesity Related Metabolic Disorders*, 2004, *28*(2), 282–289; French, S. A., Story, M., and Jeffery, R. W. "Environmental Influences on Eating and Physical Activity." *Annual Review of Public Health*, 2001, *22*, 309–335.

58. Heflin, C. M., Siefert, K., and Williams, D. R. "Food Insufficiency and Women's Mental Health: Findings from a 3-Year Panel of Welfare Recipients." *Social Science Medicine*, 2005, *61*(9), 1971–1982.

59. French, Story, and Jeffery (2001); Wakefield, M., and others. "Role of the Media in Influencing Trajectories of Youth Smoking." *Addiction*, 2003, *98* Suppl. 1, 79–103; Hackbarth, D. P., Silvestri, B., and Cosper, W. "Tobacco and Alcohol Billboards in 50 Chicago Neighborhoods: Market Segmentation to Sell Dangerous Products to the Poor." *Journal of Public Health Policy*, 1995, *16*(2), 213–230; Parloff, R. "Is Fat the Next Tobacco?" *Fortune*, 2003, *147*(2), 50–54.

60. Hackbarth, Silvestri, and Cosper (1995).

61. Pratt, C. A., and Pratt, C. B. "Comparative Content Analysis of Food and Nutrition Advertisements in *Ebony*, *Essence*, and *Ladies' Home Journal*." *Journal of Nutrition Education*, 1995, *27*(1), 128–133; Tirodkar, M. A., and Jain, A. "Food Messages on African American Television Shows." *American Journal of Public Health*, 2003, *93*(3), 439–441.

62. Lewis and others (2005).

63. Booth, K. M., Pinkston, M. M., and Poston, W. S. "Obesity and the Built Environment." *Journal of the American Dietetic Association*, 2005, *105*(5 Suppl. 1), 110–117; Estabrooks, P. A., Lee, R. E., and Gyurcsik, N. C. "Resources for Physical Activity Participation: Does Availability and Accessibility Differ by Neighborhood Socioeconomic Status?" *Annals of Behavioral Medicine*, 2003, *25*(2), 100–104; Powell, L. M., Slater, S., and Chaloupka, F. J. "The Relationship Between Community Physical Activity Settings and Race, Ethnicity, and SES." *Evidence-Based Preventive Medicine*, 2004, *1*(2), 135–144; Humpel, N., Owen, N., and Leslie, E. "Environmental Factors Associated with Adults' Participation in Physical Activity: A Review." *American Journal of Preventive Medicine*, 2002, *22*(3), 188–199.

64. King, A. C., and others. "Theoretical Approaches to the Promotion of Physical Activity: Forging a Transdisciplinary Paradigm." *American Journal of Preventive Medicine*, 2002, *23*(2 Suppl.),15–25.

65. Population Reference Bureau (2001).

66. Population Reference Bureau (2001); Halfon, N., and Hochstein, M. "Life Course Health Development: An Integrated Framework for Developing Health, Policy, and Research." *Milbank Quarterly*, 2002, *80*(3), 433–479, iii.

67. Williams, D. R., and Jackson, P. B. "Social Sources of Racial Disparities in Health." *Health Affairs*, 2005, *24*(2), 325–334; Williams, D. R. "Race, Socioeconomic Status, and Health: The Added Effects of Racism and Discrimination." *Annals of the New York Academy of Science*, 1999, *896*, 173–188.

68. Fiscella, K., and Williams, D. R. "Health Disparities Based on Socioeconomic Inequities: Implications for Urban Health Care." *Academy of Medicine*, 2004, *79*(12), 1139–1147; Cochran, S. D., Mays, V. M., and Sullivan, J. G. "Prevalence of Mental Disorders, Psychological Distress, and Mental Health Services Use Among Lesbian, Gay, and Bisexual Adults in the United States." *Journal of Consulting and Clinical Psychology*, 2003, *71*(1),53–61.

69. Krieger, N. "Embodiment: A Conceptual Glossary for Epidemiology." *Journal of Epidemiological Community Health*, 2005, *59*(5), 350–355.

70. Krieger, N. "Stormy Weather: Race, Gene Expression, and the Science of Health Disparities." *American Journal of Public Health*, 2005, *95*(12), 2155–2160.

71. Krieger, N. "Discrimination and Health." In L. F. Berkman and I. Kawachi (eds.), *Social Epidemiology*. New York: Oxford University Press, 2000.

72. Robert and House (2000).

73. Fiscella and Williams (2004); Krieger, N. "Discrimination and Health." In L. F. Berkman and I. Kawachi (eds.). *Social Epidemiology*. New York: Oxford University Press, 2000; Patrick, D. L., and Wickizer, T. M. "Community and Health." In B. C. Amick (ed.), *Society and Health*. New York: Oxford University Press, 1995.

74. Theorell, T. "Working Conditions and Health." In L. F. Berkman and I. Kawachi (eds.), *Social Epidemiology*. New York: Oxford University Press, 2000.

75. Scott and Leonhardt (2005).

76. Yancey, A. K., and others. "Population-Based Interventions Engaging Communities of Color in Healthy Eating and Active Living: A Review." *Preventing Chronic Disease*, 2004, *1*(1), 1–18; Yancey, A. K., Ortega, A. N., and Kumanyika, S. K. "Effective Recruitment and Retention of Minority Research Participants." *Annual Review of Public Health*, 2006, *27*, 1–28.

77. Smith, W. E., Day, R. S., and Brown, L. B. "Heritage Retention and Bean Intake Correlates to Dietary Fiber Intakes in Hispanic Mothers—Que Sabrosa Vida." *Journal of the American Dietary Association*, 2005, *105*(3), 404–411; discussion 411–412.

78. Lara, M., and others. "Acculturation and Latino Health in the United States: A Review of the Literature and Its Sociopolitical Context." *Annual Review of Public Health*, 2005, *26*, 367–397.

79. DuBois, D. L., and Silverthorn, N. "Natural Mentoring Relationships and Adolescent Health: Evidence from a National Study." *American Journal of Public Health*, 2005, *95*(3), 518–524; Yancey, A. K., Siegel, J. M., and McDaniel, K. L. "Role Models, Ethnic Identity, and Health-Risk Behaviors in Urban Adolescents." *Archives of Pediatrics and Adolescent Medicine*, 2002, *156*(1), 55–61; Beier, S. R., and others. "The Potential Role of an Adult Mentor in Influencing High-Risk Behaviors in Adolescents." *Archives of Pediatrics and Adolescent Medicine*, 2000, *154*(4), 327–331.

80. Morrison, T. G., Kalin, R., and Morrison, M. A. "Body-Image Evaluation and Body-Image Investment Among Adolescents: A Test of Sociocultural and Social Comparison Theories." *Adolescence*, 2004, *39*(155), 571–592; Muris, P., and others. "Biological, Psychological, and Sociocultural Correlates of Body Change Strategies and Eating Problems in Adolescent Boys and Girls." *Eating Behaviors*, 2005, *6*(1), 11–22; Yancey, A. K., and others. "Ethnic and Gender Differences in Overweight Self-Perception: Relationship to Sedentariness." *Obesity Research*, 2006, *14*, 980–988.

81. Stahl, T., and others. "The Importance of the Social Environment for Physically Active Lifestyle—Results from an International Study." *Social Science and Medicine*, 2001, *52*(1), 1–10.

82. Lucas, Schiller, and Benson (2004).

83. Yancey, A. K., Ory, M. G., and Davis, S. M. "Dissemination of Physical Activity Promotion Interventions in Underserved Populations." *American Journal of Preventive Medicine*, forthcoming.

84. Kaplan, M. S., and others. "The Association Between Length of Residence and Obesity Among Hispanic Immigrants." *American Journal of Preventive Medicine*, 2004; *27*(4), 323–326.

CHAPTER THREE

# DISPARITIES IN HEALTH CARE

Leo S. Morales
Alexander N. Ortega

Racial and ethnic disparities in health care pervade the American health care system. Several reviews of the scientific literature document the existence of racial and ethnic disparities in the processes and outcomes of care for a variety of diseases and clinical conditions, including cardiovascular disease, cancer, HIV/AIDS, and other chronic conditions as well as in delivery of preventive services.[1] Similarly, a recently published national report on health care disparities that draws on multiple data sources finds that blacks, Hispanics, Asians, and American Indians and Native Alaskans were more likely than whites to receive lower-quality care across a range of quality-of-care indicators.[2]

The Institute of Medicine's report on the quality of health care in the United States identifies six aims for improving performance of the health care system: safety, effectiveness, patient-centeredness, timeliness, efficiency, and equity.[3] Equity, as defined by the IOM, is the delivery of health services of equal quality to all individuals regardless of such personal characteristics as gender, socioeconomic status, geographic location, and race or ethnicity. Thus the existence of disparities in care represents a failure of the American health care system and signals the need for attention and reform.

Addressing racial and ethnic disparities in care is of growing importance because the population of the United States is more diverse than ever. Between 2000 and 2050 the Hispanic population is expected to increase as a percentage of the U.S. population from 13 to 24 percent, the Asian population is expected to grow from 4 to 8 percent, and the black population is expected to grow from 13 to 15 percent. Over the same period, the non-Hispanic white population is expected to decrease as a percentage of the U.S. population from 69 percent to 50 percent. If racial and ethnic minorities continue to receive lower-quality care than the majority population, a substantial portion of the U.S. population will have suboptimal health status, which will in turn affect labor market productivity and national health care spending.[4]

We begin this chapter by defining our view of disparities in care. Next, we review some of the historical factors that have contribute to the patterns of disparities we observe today. In the following sections we summarize some of the evidence documenting racial and ethnic disparities in the treatment of some diseases. In the final sections of the chapter, we summarize a number of ongoing initiatives to reduce disparities in care.

# Definition of Disparity in Health Care

A distinction can be made between disparity in health and disparity in health care. The former refers to racial and ethnic differences in morbidity and mortality and is influenced by a variety of factors (social, environmental, behavioral, biological), only one of which is health care. With recent advances in human genomics, much more attention is being given to the genetic basis for racial and ethnic disparities in health.[5] Disparities in health per se are discussed in a separate chapter in this volume. In this chapter, we focus on disparities in health care.

Various perspectives on disparities in health care have been adopted by researchers over time. Some have viewed all differences in health care between racial and ethnic groups as constituting disparities. From this point of view, differences in the use of services are viewed as disparities regardless of coexistent differences in access to care, insurance coverage, personal preferences, clinical need, or clinical appropriateness. It has been suggested that in some cases lower use of services may constitute an advantage, in particular where overuse is thought to lead to excess morbidity or mortality.

Others have taken a narrower perspective, defining disparity as a difference in care not accounted for by a difference in access to care, personal preference, clinical need, or clinical appropriateness (see Figure 3.1). In this narrower view, two groups of factors are identified as responsible for disparities in care. The first is system-level factors such as the structure of health care systems and the legal and regulatory environment in which those systems operate. These may include structural factors such as underfunding of hospitals that predominantly serve minority patients or organizational characteristics such as inadequate workforce diversity or

## FIGURE 3.1. INSTITUTE OF MEDICINE MODEL OF DISPARITIES IN HEALTH CARE.

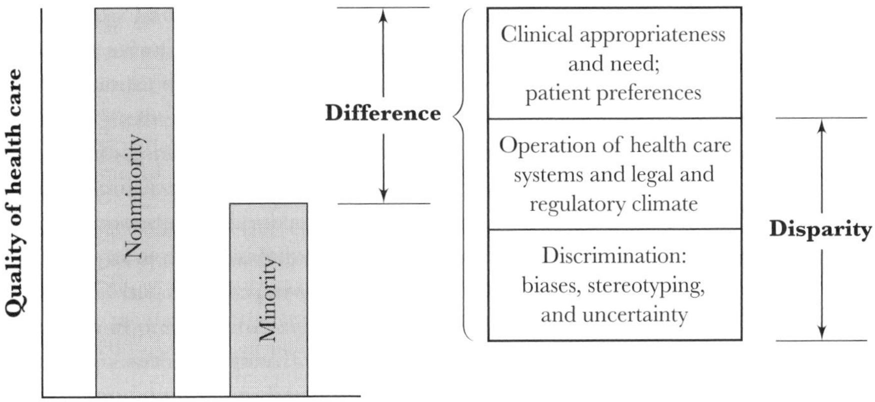

Source: Institute of Medicine (IOM), *Unequal Treatment: Confronting Racial and Ethnic Disparities in Health Care,* Washington, D.C.: National Academies Press, 2003.

the absence of policy and procedures that promote culturally competent care. The second group of factors is discrimination at the patient-provider level, whether it takes the form of bigotry and prejudice or unconscious stereotyping.

The broader perspective of disparities in care is often taken by analysts because of data limitations. Few datasets include information on quality of care, race and ethnicity, or patient needs. It is also true that few datasets can differentiate between the effects of structural or legal and regulatory factors on the one hand and discrimination on the other. As we show in the following sections, the literature tends to support the view that all three sets of factors are operating to produce disparities in care.

# Historical Overview of Disparities in Medical Care

The Tuskegee Syphilis Study, a forty-year study by the U.S. Public Health Service of untreated syphilis in black men from Alabama, is typically cited as a central reason many black Americans do not participate in medical studies or seek needed health care, but the legacy of distrust of and mistreatment by the medical establishment toward minorities predates the Tuskegee study.[6] Minorities in the United States, in particular African Americans and Mexican Americans (the largest subgroup of Latinos), have a long history of segregation in medical care and of receiving poor-quality care.[7] Inequity in medical care began with racial segregation and slavery in American history. Slaves were able to obtain care only in slave hospitals, which were typically staffed by other slaves, slave owners, and their family members.[8] After emancipation, the federal government set up more than ninety hospitals for the emancipated slaves, but only one remained as of the end of the 1800s: Howard University Medical Center.[9] In segregated America, no one took responsibility for the delivery of care for African Americans. Through considerable struggle, black medical professionals began taking charge of care for black Americans. But this transformation was difficult; in the early 1900s blacks were restricted from mainstream professional medical societies, as well as most medical schools.[10] In fact, in 1900 only seven medical schools were training blacks at all.[11] In the late 1800s, black physicians led efforts to establish black hospitals, starting with the Provident Medical Center in Chicago.[12] For both African Americans and Mexican Americans, public health and other medical societies did not begin taking responsibility for their health until they were deemed a threat to the health of whites;[13] thus the type of care delivered was generally in the form of hygiene control and treatment of infectious diseases.

## Factors Related to Disparities Among African Americans

African Americans in the United States experience on average excess morbidity and mortality across a range of chronic and infectious diseases compared with non-Latino whites. Researchers have identified a variety of risk factors that contribute to these disparities (recall Chapter Two) For example, African Americans in the United States are disproportionately represented among the poor and people who live in the inner city. Socioeconomic status and race are associated with a slew of disease risk factors, among them access to primary health care, behaviors (diet, smoking, physical activity), access to resources and social capital, and environmental and psychosocial stressors. Minority and low-income populations are also less likely to receive effective public health and prevention messages that could help prevent disease.

Studies have found that African Americans are less likely to have private insurance and more likely to be publicly insured, underinsured, or uninsured than whites.[14] This is an important risk factor because insurance coverage is related to access to primary care, continuity of care, site of care, and the type and quality of care received, where publicly and uninsured patients often receive less care and poorer quality. Site of care is also important; some studies assert that, for example, patients in community health clinics are less likely to receive high-quality care because such clinics tend to be understaffed and poorly resourced and cannot deliver highly effective care across a range of illnesses and health problems.

Some argue that racial disparities in medical treatment are rooted in discrimination on the part of providers and health care systems, while others disagree and posit that there is insufficient empirical evidence to support that the disparities are due to conscious or subconscious discrimination.[15] Nonetheless, there is abundant evidence to note that disparities in health care are persistent, are deeply seated, and exist across many medical disciplines, practices, and populations (children, adults, elderly). Most researchers would agree that disparities in treatment are a result of myriad factors including patient preferences and behaviors, provider constraints and practices, and system or institutional policies (see Figure 3.2).

***Patient Factors.*** Many patient-related factors are associated with access to and use of health care. Some of these factors are more salient to African American patients than nonminority patients. Patient perception of health status and views of specific diseases and the patient's ability to accept and cope with illness are all associated with health care use. Psychosocial constructs such as readiness for change, perceived self-efficacy, self-reliance, and fatalism are all related to individual decision making.[16] Patient trust, level of comfort with medical providers, and satisfaction with care are all important factors for health care entry and retention.[17]

***Provider Factors.*** A number of African Americans in the United States come from disadvantaged communities and households. High-income, well-educated, and empowered patients are able to demand, expect, and obtain high-quality health care and have positive health outcomes. These expectations come, in part, from having the resources, privileges, opportunities, state of mind, and prestige that advantaged individuals may expect.[18] The medical establishment remains dominated by white, upper-class, and middle-class men; accordingly, there exists

## FIGURE 3.2. FACTORS RELATED TO HEALTH CARE USE AND THEIR SYNERGIES.

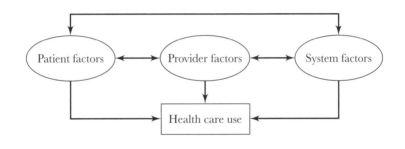

considerable discordance between patient and provider demographics. It is reasonable to believe that most providers feel more comfortable communicating with patients who share similar demographics and background. Researchers have asserted that how providers communicate and understand their patients is likely to influence the effectiveness and continuity of care. If the provider stereotypes or misunderstands the patients, then clinical decision making may be compromised. For instance, Schulman and colleagues,[19] who reported on a sample of more than seven hundred physicians who were surveyed to determine recommendations for managing chest pain during videotaped, scripted interviews, found that black women were less likely to be referred for cardiac catheterization than white men. This study suggested that race and gender play significant and synergistic roles in how providers manage their patients.

Provider communication is associated with patient satisfaction, adherence to recommendations, and health outcomes,[20] which may have consequential effects on the type of service sought (emergency versus primary care). Providers who communicate effectively with their patients and are sensitive to process tend to have patients who are satisfied and understand their health issues; even more important, they are more likely to follow through with treatment and continue to seek primary care services.[21] It is important to note that for low-income minority populations communication is mostly directed by medical providers, so examination of process needs to concentrate not only on patients but also on physicians. This also extends to the communication of office staff, nurses, and physician assistants.

In pediatrics, it has been observed that minority children tend to receive poor-quality care, which is usually delivered in a busy community-based ambulatory care center or a hospital-based clinic.[22] Underuse of clinical practice guidelines (CPG) among providers of minority and low-income patients has also been observed. A national study of pediatricians showed that participants reported using ten CPGs for asthma.[23] The study reported that CPG use was more common among pediatricians who practiced in an HMO. Surveyed pediatricians said they were more likely to use CPGs if they were easy-to-follow, feasible, logical, and evidence-based.

*System Factors.* System factors have also been implicated in health care disparities. For instance, it is important that systems promote and foster cultural competency not only for providers but also for office and administrative staff. A report by the Association for Clinicians for the Underserved entitled "Assessment of Childhood Asthma Management and Care in Region III's Indigent and Minority Populations"[24] detailed the major system barriers reported by fifty-one pediatric clinicians. The report was the result of an Office of Disease Prevention and Health Promotion (ODPHP) inquiry into the increased morbidity and mortality rates for asthmatic children that persist despite acceptance of "excellent" evidence-based clinical practice guidelines. Of eight challenges identified, three predominated: (1) resources not available onsite to provide evidence-based care, (2) reimbursement practices, and (3) uncoordinated medical homes (primary care sites) that do not deliver effective asthma education materials. The clinicians reported resource deficits impede patient access to specialty care, trained case management educators, home health services, pharmaceuticals, and equipment. Poor coordination of services, as a result of the failure of the community-based system of care to serve as the "medical home" for underserved populations, and the lack of culturally appropriate patient and family education materials sensitive to the literacy, language, and cultural diversity of the populations served were major issues.

## Factors Related to Disparities Among Latinos

Latinos make up a diverse group of people who come from differing national origins and who have various histories and political ties with the United States. Much like other ethnic groups in the United States, Latinos have a range of immigration and migration patterns. For instance, many Latinos in the Southwest have a family history that can be traced in the region well before the colonization of the American Southwest following the Treaty of Guadalupe Hildalgo. Puerto Ricans have a history in the United States that goes back to the Jones Act in 1917 (almost twenty years after the Treaty of Paris ended the Spanish-American War), stipulating that Puerto Rico was a U.S. territory whose inhabitants were entitled to U.S. citizenship. Other Latino groups from the Americas and the Caribbean have an immigration history that is sometimes tied with refugee status, as with the Cubans who sought refuge in the United States after the Bay of Pigs fiasco.

Given the changing demographics of the United States, the significance of Latino health and health care access and use can be expected to increase. According to recent U.S. census data,[25] Latinos make up approximately 13 percent of the total population. Within the Latino population, those of Mexican and Puerto Rican descent make up the two largest groups, accounting for 58.5 percent and 9.6 percent, respectively, of the entire U.S. Latino population (not including the 3.5 million U.S. citizens in Puerto Rico). Latinos also make up the largest minority group of children and adolescents. Census[26] data show Latinos numbering 16 percent (11.6 million) of the U.S. population under the age of eighteen.

Studies document that Latinos tend to have worse access to health care, worse morbidity as a result of lack of care or treatment, and poorer quality of care than nonminorities. Many factors have been implicated in disparities in access to and quality of care for Latinos. For instance, studies have reported that Latinos, compared with nonminorities, have a low rate of insurance coverage, usually as a result of noncitizen status or low-wage or migrant employment; have worse geographic access to care, usually because of migration or living in a farm area; and receive low-quality care, usually because of language discordance between them and their medical providers. Disparities in insurance and access differ, however, with the group. For instance, Puerto Ricans born on the island are citizens by birth, facilitating circular migration and enabling them to qualify for certain federal and state health programs (Medicaid, S-CHIP, and Medicare).

If insured, Latinos have a high presence in public insurance programs,[27] mainly Medicaid. Medicaid is characterized by higher per capita resource constraints and stricter limits or covered services, variables that relate to poor access and quality of care. Low Medicaid capitation payments have been linked to restricted provider networks for health care organizations enrolling minority beneficiaries,[28] thus limiting the pool of available providers.

For Spanish-speaking populations in the United States, the language barrier can affect the quality of care through poor communication exchanged with physicians. As a result, there can be deficient transfer of important information such as details of disease, consequences of treatment or lack of treatment, and medication regimens, all of which can lead to ineffective disease management or prevention. Many Latinos delay seeking care until their condition is severe. Delay coupled with the need for effective medical interpreters and providers make Latinos more vulnerable and potentially more expensive to treat and more complicated to manage than other ethnic groups who speak English well.[29]

## Scientific Evidence of Disparities in Health Care

In the following six sections, we review some of the evidence supporting the existence of disparities in health care. Because the literature on disparities in care is extensive, spanning several decades, we selected six condition-specific areas of research for our review: cardiovascular disease, cancer, renal disease and transplantation, HIV/AIDS, asthma, and mental health. These areas were selected for a variety of reasons. Cardiovascular disease, cancer, renal disease and transplantation, and HIV-AIDS were selected because they are among the most studied areas of racial and ethnic disparities in care. Asthma was selected because African Americans and some Hispanic subgroups (Puerto Ricans, for instance) are disproportionately affected. Finally, because the other areas included in this review focus on physical domains of health status, we elected to include mental health.

### Cardiovascular Disease

Coronary artery disease (CAD) and acute myocardial infarction (AMI) are the most analyzed topics among studies of racial and ethnic disparities in care. Although blood pressure and cholesterol screening are generally common for both blacks and whites, one study using seven federal datasets found that hospitalization rates for hypertension, angina, and congestive heart failure were higher for blacks than whites across almost all age groups—suggesting that screening is insufficient to prevent heart disease in blacks.[30]

Studies of racial and ethnic disparities in cardiovascular disease have become increasingly sophisticated in their control and adjustment for confounders.[31] An examination of their results indicates that, barring a few exceptions (usually because samples were small), African Americans with CAD or AMI are significantly less likely to receive appropriate cardiac procedures or therapies than whites.[32]

African Americans are less likely than whites to be catheterized; when it is done, they are 20–50 percent less likely to undergo a revascularization procedure. They are also less likely to receive beta blockers, thrombolytic drugs, or aspirin when indicated.[33] There are similar, though less consistent, findings for Hispanics.[34] In one study of AMIs based on the Corpus Christi heart study, Mexican Americans were 40 percent less likely to receive thrombolytic therapy than comparable whites.[35] In a Veterans Administration study, Hispanics were 70 percent less likely than whites to receive thrombolytic therapy. These results held in both teaching and nonteaching hospitals after controlling for age, sex, disease severity, symptom expression, comorbidity, health insurance or payor, and physician specialty.[36]

A significantly lower rate of coronary artery bypass graft surgery (CABG) among African Americans were found in a large study at Duke Medical Center. Included among those who did not receive treatment were patients at highest risk, who would have been expected to have the highest benefit. In the same study, the five-year mortality rate was significantly higher for blacks than for whites.[37] A study of revascularization procedures at major medical centers in New York State found that rates for angioplasty and CABG among African Americans were lower than those for comparable whites. This study examined patients who had been categorized by widely accepted criteria as "inappropriate," "appropriate," or "necessary" for revascularization. For those for whom revascularization was classified as necessary, African Americans were 37 percent less likely to undergo angioplasty or CABG compared to whites.[38] No difference was found between Hispanics and whites in the same category. In another study, blacks were less likely than whites to undergo cardiac catheterization and revascularization, less likely to be given newer antiplatelet agents during hospitalization, and less likely to receive lipid-lowering agents and smoking cessation counseling at time of hospital discharge.[39]

The role of race in clinical decision making regarding cardiovascular disease has also been investigated. In one study where a committee of cardiologists and cardiothoracic surgeons made decisions about CABG versus angioplasty for 938 patients after catheterization—decisions based only on a presentation by a cardiology fellow, and thus effectively blinded to the patient's race—the rate of revascularization was similar for blacks and whites, though blacks were more likely to receive angioplasty and whites more likely to receive CABG.[40] A study that included Medicare patients treated for myocardial infarction in 4,609 hospitals found that on average blacks were treated at "hospitals with lower-quality medical treatment but higher-quality surgical treatment." Nevertheless "blacks received fewer surgical treatments than whites admitted to the same hospital."[41] A study that examined six-month outcomes among patients who underwent diagnostic cardiac catheterization found that blacks, compared to whites, had significantly higher incidence of angina and worse outcomes in five of eight functional status domains after adjustment for baseline characteristics. This study found that a lower rate of revascularization for blacks appeared to be responsible for the outcome differences.

## Cancer

Studies of racial and ethnic disparities in cancer incidence and prevalence, screening, stage at diagnosis, as well as treatment and survival have been attributed to a range of factors, among them differences in tumor biology, genetics, cultural differences and folk beliefs, socioeconomic status, problems of access to continuity of care, physician practice style and communication with patients, and interaction among all of these factors.[42] Racial bias is used less often to explain disparities, though some studies have found an unexplained effect of race after accounting for other variables.[43]

Whereas black and Hispanic females have a lower incidence of breast cancer compared to whites, they also tend to present to their doctors with more advanced disease and thus have poorer prognosis and shorter survival time compared to whites.[44] Differences in prognosis and survival time among white, African American, and Hispanic women were found by early studies to be attributable almost entirely to racial and ethnic differences in socioeconomic status,[45] though biological factors and cultural beliefs were also suggested as factors. Data from National Health Interview Surveys reported similarly on having a screening mammogram among black, Hispanic, and white women in 1990.[46] Mammography and Pap smear rates differed, though, among ethnic subgroups (Colombian, Dominican, Ecuadorian, Puerto Rican, Caribbean, Haitian, and U.S.-born black women).[47]

Racial variation in diagnosis was found in some studies. One of them found that older black women were consistently less likely than comparable white women to receive a mammogram, perhaps because physicians were unable or unwilling to spend the additional time necessary to educate black women about the importance of the procedure.[48] Suggested explanations for a finding that indicated African American, Hispanic, and Asian women had less timely follow-ups than whites after an abnormal finding on a screening mammogram included patient preferences, insurance coverage, and discriminatory practices among providers.[49] A more recent study indicates that there is significant variation in mammography screening within racial and ethnic groups, with immigrants having a substantially lower mammography rate than nonimmigrants within the same racial and ethnic group, and that limitations in the national survey databases lead to overestimation of mammogram use, particularly for low-income racial and ethnic minorities due to higher survey nonresponse in these groups.[50]

Variation in treatment was also found in some studies, though not all. One study found that black patients received "significantly different care" than whites for four out of ten treatment procedures for breast cancer, although they were not the most clinically important.[51] Shavers and Brown found that, after controlling for clinical factors, black women are less likely than white women to receive breast conserving surgery (BCS) and radiation. After undergoing BCS, black women and women from other racial and ethnic minority groups are less likely than whites to have radiation therapy.[52] In addition, black women also receive lower chemotherapy dosage than white women.[53] Other studies found similar rates and types of treatment among African American, Hispanic, and white women.[54]

Similar patterns according to race and ethnicity were found for men and women with colorectal cancer. In one study, blacks were treated less aggressively than whites with similar disease, even after adjusting for insurance coverage, hospital type, and comorbidities. The authors were unable to determine if the differences were attributable to social, cultural, or economic differences. In contrast, no differences were found in treatment or survival in a study in the free-care VA system[55] or in the equal-access Department of Defense health care system.[56] A study of elderly Tennesseans enrolled in both Medicaid and Medicare found no significant difference in overall outcomes for black and white patients, though blacks were less likely to have surgery.[57]

A notable difference was found for early stage nonsmall-cell lung cancer. After controlling for variables, researchers found that blacks were only about half as likely as whites to undergo surgery that can substantially increase the likelihood of surviving for five years or longer. This difference was suggested as attributable to either patient preference or physician's decision.[58]

## Renal Disease and Transplantation

African Americans and Native Americans have the highest incidence of risk of illness and death from end-stage renal disease (ESRD) among minorities. Among Native Americans, for example, the rate is four times that for whites. This is due to more hypertension, diabetes, and sickle cell disease among blacks, diabetes among Native Americans, and less access to or use of early primary care intervention for both groups. The two main treatments for ESRD are dialysis and renal transplantation. Although ESRD treatment is specifically supported by a Medicare program, kidney transplantation varies by race.

One study found that time from renal failure to transplantation, time from renal failure to wait listing, and time from wait listing to transplantation were all longer for blacks than for whites, Asian Americans, and Native Americans.[59] Another study, using a telephone survey of a representative national sample of ESRD patients, found that within the first year on dialysis 30 percent of white respondents but only 13.5 percent of black respondents were placed on a waiting list, and three times as many whites as blacks received a kidney.[60] Additionally, a cohort study of more than forty-one thousand ESRD patients on the waiting lists of all 238 renal transplant centers in the United Network for Organ Sharing from 1994 to 1996 showed that blacks, Hispanics, and Asians, patients of any race or ethnicity who were less well educated, and those with limited financial resources were much less likely to receive a transplant.[61] Another study reported that even though American Indians were more likely than whites to be identified as potential transplant candidates and referred to a transplant center, and there were no significant differences for the same between Hispanics and whites, both American Indians and Hispanics were less likely to be placed on a waiting list and were much less likely than whites to undergo renal transplantation.[62]

Reasons for these differences are debated and may involve numerous factors. One study attributed 60 percent of the difference in rate of waiting list entry for blacks and whites, and about half of the difference in transplantation rate, to race-related differences in socioeconomic status, biologic factors associated with the complicated immunologic problems of donor-recipient matching by human leukocyte antigens, disease severity and the presence of contraindications, and patient preferences or choices.[63] Yet another study found that differences in socioeconomic status were only a minor contributor.[64]

Many studies showed that African American patient preferences, including refusal of and disinterest in transplantation, is an important contributing factor.[65] A large sample of ESRD patients in four regions of the United States showed that black patients were less likely than whites to want a transplant.[66] A larger difference was apparent in the rate at which blacks and whites were fully informed of the options and referred for evaluation of a transplant. A study that examined physicians' beliefs about racial differences in referral for renal transplantation related that whereas physicians did not view patient-physician communication and trust as important reasons for racial differences in care, black patients were less likely than white patients to report receiving some or a lot of information about transplantation (55 percent versus 74 percent).[67] Another study found that one of the contributors associated with black disinterest in transplantation was fatalism, based on lifelong experience of perceived racial discrimination.[68]

## HIV/AIDS

Over the past two decades, infection with HIV and progression to AIDS have disproportionately affected African Americans and Hispanics. For example, in 2002 HIV/AIDS was the sixth leading cause of death among African Americans and tenth leading cause of death among Hispanic males, whereas it did not place among the ten leading causes of death for white males.[69] Relatively few studies have examined racial variation in diagnosis or treatment. Evidence from those that have examined these differences indicate that African Americans and Hispanics are less likely than whites to receive various medications or to undergo some diagnostic procedures, though they vary by source of care.[70] A study of the relative risk of six-year mortality among ethnic groups found Hispanics to have a significantly shorter median of survival (15.5 months) than whites (23.8 months) and blacks (35.1 months).[71] One study found that blacks and Latinos, compared to whites, had an inferior pattern of care in many measures that examined service and medication utilization.[72] Another study showed that blacks (and to a lesser degree Hispanics) were less likely to undergo bronchoscopy and tended to receive less timely administration of prophylaxis against opportunistic infection in many hospitals, but these disparities did not exist in the free-care VA hospital system.[73]

Among gay and bisexual men with HIV, another study found that whites were about 60 percent more likely than blacks to be taking antiretroviral drugs, after adjusting for access to care and insurance status.[74] Among patients appearing at a teaching hospital for treatment, blacks were found to be 40 percent less likely than whites to have previously received antiretroviral drugs or prophylaxis against opportunistic infection, regardless of income and insurance status.[75] Possible reasons for the difference were misconceptions about HIV/AIDS among blacks, distrust of health authorities, and "prescribing habits" of providers.

Additionally, many studies have found difficulty in physician-patient communication in HIV/AIDS cases, particularly in discussing decisions about end-of-life care and resuscitation[76] and when there was racial or ethnic discordance between patient and physician. One study found that physicians at a teaching hospital were more comfortable discussing the results of clinical trials with white patients than racial and ethnic minorities.[77] Patient mistrust and conspiracy beliefs are also a factor. One study found that 27 percent of 520 black adults in ten randomly selected census tracts agreed with the statement "HIV/AIDS is a man-made virus that the federal government made to kill and wipe out black people," and an additional 23 percent were undecided.[78]

Suggesting that more information beyond risk behavior and partner type distinctions are needed to understand racial and ethnic disparities in HIV risk, one study concluded that blacks and Latinos had a higher prevalence of HIV compared to whites even though whites most frequently reported potentially risky sex and drug-using behaviors.[79] This multisite venue-based survey of fifteen-to-twenty-two-year-old males found black and multiethnic black men experienced nine times, and Latinos about twice, the fully adjusted odds of infection compared to whites.[80]

## Asthma

Asthma is a major health problem across many socioeconomic and racial and ethnic categories. However, blacks and Latinos, especially Puerto Ricans, share a disproportionate burden from asthma.[81] Asthma is the most common chronic condition afflicting children in the United States. Among children, blacks and Latinos have worse morbidity and blacks have more mortality due to asthma than all other racial or ethnic groups of children.[82] The asthma death rate among U.S. blacks is approximately three times more than for whites.[83] Between the ages of five and thirty-four (when asthma is easier to distinguish from other causes of ventilatory impairment), blacks experience an asthma mortality rate approximately three to five times higher than that of whites.[84] Multiple risk factors have been implicated for asthma morbidity and mortality for minorities: tobacco smoke exposure, obesity, air pollution, house dust mite allergen, cockroaches, and cat hair.[85] An elevated level of severe asthma and related hospitalization among inner-city minority children is associated with features of health care and treatment, such as inadequate use of long-term controller steroid medications and overuse of quick-acting reliever drugs such as albuterol.[86] Researchers have observed that poor asthma management and control among racial and ethnic minorities is associated with a slew of factors, including poor provider-patient communication, deficient access to and use of high-quality and effective primary care, poor perceived patient and family efficacy to manage asthma, and perceived inadequate treatment efficacy by patients and their families.[87]

Studies have reported that mismanagement of asthma for minority children is partly attributable to such provider factors as inadequate knowledge or use of national asthma clinical guidelines.[88] Evidence shows that Latino children are less likely than white children to be prescribed inhaled corticosteroids and other maintenance medications, regardless of insurance coverage, severity of asthma, and other determinants such as site of care or primary care contacts.[89] One study of children in three managed care organizations found a difference in dispensing of controller agents but similar rates of prescription,[90] and in a separate study the same group of researchers found that medication was prescribed less to Latinos in five health care organizations in Massachusetts.[91] The researchers reported that reduced use of corticosteroids and controller medication by minorities may have been due to a combination of lower adherence and prescription by physicians compared to whites. Minority children with asthma are also less likely than white children to receive preventive therapy or obtain equipment that helps them manage their asthma.[92]

## Mental Health

Improving mental health services access and utilization has been a top health policy priority in the United States. The attention to mental health care comes from increasing awareness that many people who meet diagnostic criteria for mental illness do not seek or obtain needed care. Several studies have demonstrated that minorities, particularly blacks and Latinos, are less likely to use mental health services than whites. In the U.S. Surgeon General's Supplement *Mental Health: Culture, Race, and Ethnicity*, it is noted that ethnic and racial minorities have less access to mental health care than whites, and that they are less likely to receive needed care and stay in care.[93] The disparities in mental health care use seem to persist even after accounting for variation in psychopathology across groups.[94]

The reasons minorities underuse mental health services are multifactorial. Considerable attention in mental health services research has focused on the role of payment and insurance. Many people in the United States lack sufficient insurance coverage to cover mental health; many health plans also limit the number of visits people may have over time. Further, some plans require costly copay or do not allow people to go out of plan to find a suitable provider. Other barriers include lack of access to providers who speak the same language, especially for low-acculturated Latinos.[95] There are also accessibility factors, such as location and awareness of available services.

Growing awareness of other factors that might account for disparity in mental health service use that go beyond payment mechanisms has been occurring in the literature. For example, researchers are focusing on factors such as health beliefs, knowledge of mental health problems, and coping mechanisms such as self-reliance and social networks.[96] For example, two reports of island Puerto Ricans demonstrated a high level of psychiatric disorder but also high denial and self-reliance.[97] Denial can be a maladaptive coping strategy, especially if it results in little or no usage of needed mental health care. The extent to which denial is more or less prevalent in minority populations relative to nonminority populations is unknown. For Latinos, some researchers have focused on the role of families and social networks in both protecting members from morbidity and being part of the pathway to mental health care.[98] Other factors that have been examined as potential determinants of mental health care disparities for all minorities include stigma, discrimination, and racism.[99]

## Reducing Disparities in Care

In response to the ever-growing body of literature documenting the existence of racial and ethnic disparities in care, there have been and continue to be numerous efforts to address racial and ethnic disparities in care. Examples of these efforts exist in the public and private sectors of U.S. society. In the public sector, for example, the Department of Health and Human Services has convened a council on disparities. This group assembles leaders across HHS under the assistant secretary for health to coordinate and maximize the effectiveness of the many federal efforts to eliminate disparities and to identify and evaluate new opportunities for eliminating disparities.

Directed by the congress, the Agency for Healthcare Research and Quality has begun producing a yearly National Healthcare Disparities Report (www. qualitytools.ahrq.gov/disparitiesreport), documenting variations in quality of care by racial and ethnic groups. This reports draws on data from numerous national surveys, including the Medical Expenditure Panel Survey, the National Health Interview Survey, the National Immunization Survey, the National Ambulatory Care Survey, and many others. The purpose of this report is to illuminate areas of greatest need and track reduction in disparities over time.

In the private sector, the National Business Group on Health, a Washington D.C.-based private nonprofit organization representing more than two hundred large employers, health care companies, benefits consultants, and vendors, has developed an employer toolkit for reducing disparities (www.businessgrouphealth.org). This toolkit is designed to give employers information and practical strategies to assess and reduce racial and ethnic health disparities within their workforce. It includes various summary papers covering topics such as making the business case for reducing disparities; it offers employee surveys that employers can use to assess and monitor disparities directly.

In a public-private effort, AHRQ and the Robert Wood Johnson Foundation have launched a national health plan learning cooperative to reduce disparities and improve health. This effort includes ten of America's foremost health plans: Aetna, Anthem, Cigna, Harvard Pilgrim, HealthPartners, Highmark, Kaiser Permanente, Molina, UnitedHealth Group, and WellPoint. This group plans to collect health care quality data by racial and ethnic group and develop interventions to reduce disparities in the treatment of diabetes and other chronic conditions. Lessons learned by the participating plans in the collaborative will be shared with the greater health care community.

To address language barriers faced by Spanish-speaking patients, the Robert Wood Johnson Foundation has also funded Hablamos Juntos, a four-year $10 million effort to improve patient-provider communication (www.hablamosjuntos.org). This project has funded ten sites to develop new (and improve existing) language interpretation programs, upgrade signage for non-English speaking patients, and enhance Spanish-translated health information materials, targeting regions of the United States that have seen rapid growth in the number of Hispanics over the last decade. Funded sites include many new destinations for Hispanic immigrants, notably Washington State, Alabama, Rhode Island, Nebraska, South Carolina, Tennessee, and Pennsylvania, as well as more established destinations such as California, Texas, and Virginia.

Various other efforts are in place to help address disparities. The National Committee for Quality Assurance, the largest accreditor of private health plans in the United States, is in the process of developing measures of quality to monitor racial and ethnic disparities in managed care settings (www.ncqa.org). Once developed, these measures will be integrated into NCQA's Health Plan Employer Data and Information Set (HEDIS) measurement set. Although not yet used for accreditation, NCQA HEDIS measures have been applied to report racial and ethnic disparities in care. For example, according to four HEDIS measures collected by Medicare health plans, blacks were less likely than whites to receive breast cancer screening, eye examinations for patients with diabetes, beta-blocker medication after myocardial infarction, and follow-up after hospitalization for mental illness.[100] The Joint Commission on Accreditation of Healthcare Organizations is also in the process of developing and incorporating new measures for hospital accreditation that focus on racial and ethnic disparities in care (www.jcaho.org). Like NCQA, JCAHO accredits health care organizations, focusing on hospitals rather than health (www.jcaho.org).

# Summary

It is evident from the medical and public health literatures that disparities in health care are prevalent, with racial and ethnic minorities receiving lower-quality care in a variety of health care settings and across a range of medical conditions. A number of factors account for disparities in care, among them legal and structural factors as well as patient and provider factors. From a historical perspective, these findings are not surprising; racial and ethnic minorities have experienced discrimination and segregation in health care settings since the founding of the United States. Although efforts to address racial and ethnic disparities in care are multiple and ongoing, if not overcome minority patients can be expected to continue to have suboptimal health status, which will in turn affect labor market productivity and national health care spending. With the growing size of minority populations in the United States, addressing disparities in care is a paramount health policy issue.

# Notes

1. Geiger, H. J. "Racial and Ethnic Disparities in Diagnosis and Treatment: A Review of the Evidence and a Consideration of Causes." In B. D. Smedley, A. Y. Stith, and A. R. Nelson (eds.), *Unequal Treatment: Confronting Racial and Ethnic Disparities in Health Care.* Washington D.C.: National Academies Press, 2003.
2. Department of Health and Human Services (DHHS). *2004 National Healthcare Disparities Report.* Rockville, Md.: Agency for Healthcare Research and Quality, U.S. Department of Health and Human Services, 2004.
3. Institute of Medicine (IOM). *Crossing the Quality Chasm.* Washington, D.C.: National Academies Press, 2001.
4. Bound, J., Waidmann, T., Schoenbaum, M., and Bingenheimer, J. B. "The Labor Market Consequences of Race Differences in Health." *Milbank Quarterly,* 2003, *81*(3), 441–473.
5. Fine, M. J., Ibrahim, S. A., and Thomas, S. B. "The Role of Race and Genetics in Health Disparities Research." *American Journal of Public Health,* Dec. 2005, *95*(12), 2125–2128.
6. Gamble, V. N. "Under the Shadow of Tuskegee: African Americans and Health Care." *American Journal of Public Health,* 1997, *87,* 1773–1778.
7. Abel, E. K. "'Only the Best Class of Immigration': Public Health Policy Toward Mexicans and Filipinos in Los Angeles, 1910–1940." *American Journal of Public Health,* 2004, *94,* 932–939; Gamble, V. N. *Making a Place for Ourselves: The Black Hospital Movement, 1920–1945.* New York: Oxford University Press, 1995.
8. Gamble (1995); Smith, D. B. *Health Care Divided.* Ann Arbor: University of Michigan Press, 1999.
9. Smith (1999).
10. Gamble (1995); Smith (1999).
11. Smith (1999).
12. Gamble, V. N. "The Provident Hospital Project: An Experiment in Race Relations and Medical Education." *Bulletin of the History of Medicine,* 1991, *65,* 457–475.
13. Abel (2004); Gamble (1995).
14. Kaiser Commission on Medicaid and the Uninsured. *Health Insurance Coverage in America.* Washington, D.C.: Kaiser Family Foundation, 2004.
15. Epstein, R. A. "Disparities and Discrimination in Health Care Coverage: A Critique of the Institute of Medicine Study." *Perspectives in Biology and Medicine,* 2005, *48*(1 Suppl.), S26–41.
16. Lewis, R. K., and Green, B. L. "Assessing the Health Attitudes, Beliefs, and Behaviors of African Americans Attending Church: A Comparison from Two Communities." *Journal of Community Health,* 2000, *25,* 211–224; Lorig, K. R., Ritter, P. L., and Gonzalez, V. M. "Hispanic Chronic Disease Self-Management: A Randomized Community-Based Out-

come Trial." *Nursing Research*, 2003, *52*, 361–369; Ortega, A. N., and Alegría, M. "Self-Reliance, Mental Health Need, and the Use of Mental Healthcare Among Island Puerto Ricans." *Mental Health Services Research*, 2002, *4*, 131–140; Wolff, M., and others. "Cancer Prevention in Underserved African American Communities: Barriers and Effective Strategies—A Review of the Literature." *Wisconsin Medical Journal*, 2003, *102*, 36–40.

17. Sheppard, V. B., Zambrana, R. E., and O'Malley, A. S. "Providing Health Care to Low-Income Women: A Matter of Trust." *Family Practice*, 2004, *21*, 484–491; Shi, L., and Stevens, G. D. "Disparities in Access to Care and Satisfaction Among U.S. Children: The Roles of Race/Ethnicity and Poverty Status." *Public Health Reports*, 2005, *120*, 431–441.

18. Gornick, M. E. *Vulnerable Populations and Medicare Services.* New York: Century Foundation Press, 2000.

19. Schulman, K. A., and others. "The Effect of Race and Sex on Physicians' Recommendations for Cardiac Catheterization." *New England Journal of Medicine*, 1999, *340*, 618–626.

20. Bartlett, E. E., and others. "The Effects of Physician Communication Skills on Patient Satisfaction, Recall, and Adherence." *Journal of Chronic Diseases*, 1984, *37*, 755–764; Ong, L. M., and others. "Doctor-Patient Communication: A Review of the Literature." *Social Science and Medicine*, 1995, *40*, 903–918; Stewart, M. "What Is a Successful Doctor-Patient Interview? A Study of Interactions and Outcomes." *Social Science and Medicine*, 1984, *19*, 167–175.

21. Saha, S., and others. "Patient-Physician Racial Concordance and the Perceived Quality and Use of Health Care." *Archives of Internal Medicine*, 1999, *159*, 997–1004.

22. Shi, L. "Type of Health Insurance and the Quality of Primary Care Experience." *American Journal of Public Health,* 2000, *90*(12), 1848–1855.

23. Flores, G., and others. "Pediatricians' Attitudes, Beliefs, and Practices Regarding Clinical Practice Guidelines: A National Survey." *Pediatrics*, 2000, *105*, 496–501.

24. Association of Clinicians for the Underserved. *Assessment of Childhood Asthma Management and Care in Region III's Indigent and Minority Populations: A Final Report.* (PSC no. 99T101465). Kenbridge, Va.: Clinical Regional Advisory Network-Region 3, 2000.

25. U.S. Census Bureau. *Census Bureau Releases Population Estimates by Age, Sex, Race and Hispanic Origin* (CB03–16). [http://www.census.gov/Press-Release/www/2003/cb03–16.html] (accessed on Dec. 15, 2005).

26. U.S. Census Bureau. *Current Population Survey. Population by Sex, Age, Hispanic Origin, and Race: March 2000.* [http://www.census.gov/population/socdemo/hispanic/p20–535/tab01–1.txt] (accessed Jan. 6, 2006).

27. Institute of Medicine (IOM). *Unequal Treatment: Confronting Racial and Ethnic Disparities in Health Care.* Washington, D.C.: National Academies Press, 2003.

28. Tai-Seale, M., Freund, D., and LoSasso, A. "Racial Disparities in Service Use Among Medicaid Beneficiaries After Mandatory Enrollment in Managed Care: A Difference-in-Differences Approach." *Inquiry*, 2001, *38*, 49–59.

29. IOM (2003).

30. Holmes, J. S., Arispe, I. E., Moy, E. "Heart Disease and Prevention: Race and Age Differences in Heart Disease Prevention, Treatment and Mortality." In Moy, E. (ed.), "Health Care Quality and Disparities: Lessons from the First National Reports." *Medical Care*, 2005, *43*,(3 Suppl.), I33-I41.

31. Geiger (2003).

32. Maynard, C., and others. "Blacks in the Coronary Artery Surgery Study: Risk Factors and Coronary Artery Disease." *Circulation*, 1986, *74*, 64–71; Hannan, E. L., and others. "Interracial Access to Selected Cardiac Procedures for Patients Hospitalized with Coronary Artery Disease in New York State." *Medical Care*, 1991, *29*, 430–441; Udyvarhelyi, I. S., and

others. "Acute Myocardial Infarction in the Medicare Population. Process of Care and Clinical Outcomes." *Journal of the American Medical Association*, 1992, *268*, 2530–2536; Ayanian, J. Z., and others. "Racial Differences in the Use of Revascularization Procedures After Coronary Angiography." *Journal of the American Medical Association*, 1993, *269*, 2642–2646; Franks, A. L., and others. "Racial Differences in the Use of Invasive Coronary Procedures After Acute Myocardial Infarction in Medicare Beneficiaries." *Ethnicity and Disease*, 1993, *3*, 213–220; Whittle, J., and others. "Racial Differences in the Use of Invasive Cardiac Procedures in the Department of Veterans Affairs Medical System." *New England Journal of Medicine*, 1993, *329*, 621–627; Peterson, E. D., and others. "Racial Variation in Cardiac Procedure Use and Survival Following Acute Myocardial Infarction in the Department of Veterans Affairs." *Journal of the American Medical Association*, 1994, *271*, 1175–1180; Giles, W. H., and others. "Race and Sex Differences in Rates of Invasive Cardiac Procedures in U.S. Hospitals. Data from the National Hospital Discharge Survey." *Archives of Internal Medicine*, 1995, *155*, 318–324; Carlisle, D. M., Leake, B., and Shapiro, M. F. "Racial and Ethnic Differences in the Use of Invasive Cardiac Procedures Among Cardiac Patients in Los Angeles County, 1986 Through 1988." *American Journal of Public Health*, 1995, *85*, 352–356; Stone, P. H., and others. "Influence of Race, Sex, and Age on Management of Unstable Angina and Non-Q-wave Myocardial Infarction: The TIMI III Registry." *Journal of the American Medical Association*, 1996, *275*, 1104–1112; Gornick, M. E., Eggers, P. W., and Reilly, T. W. "Effects of Race and Income on Mortality and Use of Services Among Medicare Beneficiaries." *New England Journal of Medicine*, 1996, *335*, 791–799; Sedlis, S. P., and others. "Racial Differences in Performance of Invasive Cardiac Procedures in a Department of Veterans Affairs Medical Center." *Journal of Clinical Epidemiology*, 1997, *50*, 899–901; Weitzman, S., and others. "Gender, Racial, and Geographic Differences in the Performance of Cardiac Diagnostic and Therapeutic Procedures for Hospitalized Acute Myocardial Infarction in Four States." *American Journal of Cardiology*, 1997, *79*, 722–726; Peterson, E. D., and others. "Racial Variation in the Use of Coronary Revascularization Procedures: Are the Differences Real? Do They Matter?" *New England Journal of Medicine*, 1997, *336*, 480–486; Hannan, E. L., and others. "Access to Coronary Artery Bypass Surgery by Race/Ethnicity and Gender Among Patients Who Are Appropriate for Surgery." *Social Science and Medicine*, 1999, *50*, 813–828; Canto, J. G., and others. "Relation of Race and Sex to the Use of Reperfusion Therapy in Medicare Beneficiaries with Acute Myocardial Infarction." *New England Journal of Medicine*, 2000, *342*(15), 1094–1100.

33. Geiger (2003).
34. Goff, D. C., and others. "A Population-Based Assessment of the Use and Effectiveness of Thrombolytic Therapy: The Corpus Christi Heart Project." *Annals of Epidemiology*, 1995, *5*, 171–178; Mickelson, J. K., Blum, C. M., and Geraci, J. M. "Acute Myocardial Infarction: Clinical Characteristics, Management and Outcome in a Metropolitan VA Medical Center Teaching Hospital." *Journal of the American College of Cardiology*, 1997, *29*: 915–925; Canto, J. G., and others. "Presenting Characteristics, Treatment Patterns, and Clinical Outcomes of Non-Black Minorities in the National Registry of Myocardial Infarction 2." *New England Journal of Medicine*, 1998, *82*(9), 1013–1018; Hannan and others (1999).
35. Goff (1995).
36. Geiger (2003).
37. Peterson and others (1997).
38. Hannan, E. L., Kilburn, H. Jr, O'Donnell, J. F., Lukacik, G., and Shields, E. P. "Interracial Access to Selected Cardiac Procedures for Patients Hospitalized with Coronary Artery Disease in New York State." *Medical Care*, 1991, *29*(5), 430–441.

39. Sonel, A. F., and others. "Racial Variations in Treatment and Outcomes of Black and White Patients with High-Risk Non-ST-Elevation Acute Coronary Syndromes: Insights from CRUSADE." *Circulation*, 2005, *111*(10), 1225–1232.

40. Okelo, S., and others. "Race and the Decision to Refer for Coronary Revascularization. The Effect of Physician Awareness of Patient Ethnicity." *Journal of the American College of Cardiology.* 2001, *38*, 698–704.

41. Barnato, A., and others. "Hospital-Level Racial Disparities in Acute Myocardial Infarction Treatment and Outcomes." *Medical Care*, 2005, *43*(4), 308–319.

42. Geiger (2003).

43. Eley, J. W., and others. "Racial Differences in Survival from Breast Cancer. Results of the National Cancer Institute Black/White Cancer Survival Study." *Journal of the American Medical Association*, 1994, *272*, 947–954.

44. Shinagawa, S. M. "The Excess Burden of Breast Carcinoma in Minority and Medically Underserved Communities: Application, Research, and Redressing Institutional Racism." *Cancer*, Mar. 1, 2000, *88*(5 Suppl), 1217–1223; IOM (2003).

45. Dayal, H., Power, R. N., and Chen, C. "Race and Socioeconomic Status in Survival from Breast Cancer." *Journal of Chronic Diseases*, 1982, *35*, 675–683; Bassett, M. T., and Krieger, N. "Social Class and Black-White Differences in Cancer Survival." *American Journal of Public Health*, 1986, *76*, 1400–1403.

46. Breen, N., and Kessler, L. "Changes in the Use of Screening Mammography: Evidence from the 1987 and 1990 National Health Interview Surveys." *American Journal of Public Health*, 1994, *84*, 62–67.

47. Mandelblatt, J. S., and others. "Breast and Cervical Cancer Screening Among Multiethnic Women: Role of Age, Health, and Source of Care." *Preventive Medicine*, 1999, *28*, 418–425; O'Malley, A. S., and others. "Continuity of Care and the Use of Breast and Cervical Cancer Screening Services in a Multiethnic Community." *Archives of Internal Medicine*, 1997, 157, 1462–1470.

48. Burns, R. B., and others. "Black Women Receive Less Mammography Even with Similar Use of Primary Care." *Annals of Internal Medicine*, 1996, *125*, 173–182.

49. Chang, S. W., and others "Racial Differences in Timeliness of Follow-up After Abnormal Screening Mammography." *Cancer*, 1996, *78*, 1395–1402.

50. Peek, M. E., and Han, J. H. "Disparities in Screening Mammography: Current Status, Interventions, and Implications." *Journal of General Internal Medicine*, 2004, *19*, 184–194.

51. Diehr, P., and others. "Treatment Modality and Quality Differences for Black and White Breast Cancer Patients Treated in Community Hospitals." *Medical Care*, 1989, *27*, 942–954.

52. Shavers, V. L., and Brown, M. L. "Racial and Ethnic Disparities in Receipt of Cancer Treatment." *Journal of the National Cancer Institute*, 2002, *94*, 334–357; Mandelblatt, J. S., and others. "Variations in Breast Carcinoma Treatment in Older Medicare Beneficiaries: Is It Black or White?" *Cancer*, 2002, *95*(7), 1401–1414.

53. Griggs, J. J., and others. "Racial Disparity in the Dose and Dose Intensity of Breast Cancer Adjuvant Chemotherapy." *Breast Cancer Research and Treatment*, 2003, *81*, 21–31.

54. Farrow, D. C., Hunt, W. C., and Samet, J. M. "Geographic Variation in the Treatment of Localized Breast Cancer." *New England Journal of Medicine*, 1992, *326*, 1097–1101; Satariano, E. R., Swanson, G. M., and Moll, P. P. "Nonclinical Factors Associated with Surgery Received for Treatment of Early-Stage Breast Cancer." *American Journal of Public Health*. 1992, *82*, 195–198.

55. Dominitz, J. A., Samsa, G. P., Landsman, P., and Provenzale, D. "Race, Treatment and Survival Among Colorectal Carcinoma Patients in an Equal-Access Medical System." *Cancer*, 1998, *82*, 2312–2320.

56. Optenberg, S. A., and others. "Race, Treatment and Long-Term Survival from Prostate Cancer in an Equal-Access Medical Care Delivery System." *Journal of the American Medical Association*, 1995, *274*, 1599–1605.

57. Rogers, S. O., Ray, W. A., and Smalley, W. E. "A Population-Based Study of Survival Among Elderly Persons Diagnosed with Colorectal Cancer: Does Race Matter If All Are Insured?" *Cancer Causes Control*, 2004, *15*(2), 193–199.

58. Bach, P. B., Cramer, L. D., Warren, J. L., and Begg, C. B. "Racial Differences in the Treatment of Early-Stage L Cancer." *New England Journal of Medicine*, 1999, *341*, 1198–1205.

59. Eggers, P. W. "Racial Differences in Access to Kidney Transplantation." *Healthcare Financing Review*, 1995; *17*, 89–103.

60. Ozminkowski, R. J., White, A. J., Hassol, A., and Murphy, M. "Minimizing Racial Disparity Regarding Receipt of a Cadaver Kidney Transplant." *American Journal of Kidney Diseases*, 1997, 30, 856–858.

61. Kasiske, B. L., London, W., and Ellison, M. D. "Race and Socioeconomic Factors Influencing Early Placement on the Kidney Transplant Waiting List." *Journal of the American Society of Nephrology*, 1998, *9*, 2141–2147.

62. Sequist, T. D., and others. "Access to Renal Transplantation Among American Indians and Hispanics." *American Journal of Kidney Diseases*, 2004, *44*(2), 344–352.

63. Ozminkowski, White, Hassol, and Murphy (1997).

64. Byrne, C., Nedelman, J., and Luke, R. G. "Race, Socioeconomic Status, and the Development of End-Stage Renal Disease." *American Journal of Kidney Diseases*, 1994, *23*, 16–22.

65. Geiger (2003).

66. Ayanian, J. Z., Cleary, P. D., Weissman, J. S., and Epstein, A. M. "The Effect of Patients' Preferences on Racial Differences in Access to Renal Transplantation." *New England Journal of Medicine*, 1999, *341*, 1661–1669.

67. Ayanian, J. Z., and others. "Physicians' Beliefs About Racial Differences in Referral for Renal Transplantation." *American Journal of Kidney Diseases*, 2004, *43*(2), 350–357.

68. Klassen, A. C., and others. "The Relationship Between Patients' Perspective on Disadvantage and Discrimination and Listing for Kidney Transplantation." *American Journal of Public Health*, 2002, *92*(5), 811–817.

69. National Center for Health Statistics (NCHS). *Health, United States, 2005, with Chartbook on Trends in the Health of Americans.* Hyattsville, Md.: National Center for Health Statistics, 2005.

70. Geiger (2003).

71. Cunningham, W. E., and others. "Ethnic and Racial Differences in Long-Term Survival from Hospitalization for HIV Infection." *Journal of Health Care for the Poor and Underserved*, 2000, *11*(2), 163–178.

72. Shapiro, M. F., and others. "Variations in the Care of HIV-Infected Adults in the United States." *Journal of the American Medical Association*, 1999, *281*(24), 2305–2315.

73. Bennett, C. L., and others. "Racial Differences Among Hospitalized Patients with Pneumocystis Carinii Pneumonia in Chicago, New York, Los Angeles, Miami and Raleigh-Durham." *Archives of Internal Medicine*, 1995, *155*, 1586–1592.

74. Graham, N.M.H., and others. "Access to Therapy in the Multicenter AIDS Cohort Study." *Journal of Clinical Epidemiology*, 1994, *27*, 1003–1012.

75. Moore, R. D., Stanton, D., Gopalan, R., and Chaisson, R. E. "Racial Differences in the Use of Drug Therapy for HIV Disease in an Urban Community." *New England Journal of Medicine*, 1994, *330*(11), 763–768.

76. Haas, J., and others. "Discussion of Preferences for Life-Sustaining Care by Persons with AIDS: Predictors of Failure in Patient-Physician Communication." *Archives of Internal Medicine*, 1993, *153*, 1241–1248.

77. Stone, V. E., Mauch, M. Y., and Steger, K. A. "Provider Attitudes Regarding Participation of Women and Persons of Color in AIDS Clinical Trials." *Journal of Acquired Immune Deficiency Syndromes Human Retrovirology,* Nov. 1, 1998, *19*(3), 245–253.

78. Klonoff, E. A., and Landrine, H. "Do Blacks Believe That HIV/AIDS Is a Government Conspiracy Against Them?" *Preventive Medicine,* 1999, *28*(5), 451–457.

79. Harawa, N. T., and others. "Associations of Race/Ethnicity with HIV Prevalence and HIV-Related Behaviors Among Young Men Who Have Sex with Men in 7 Urban Centers in the United States." *Journal of Acquired Immune Deficiency Syndrome,* 2004, *15*(35), 526–536.

80. Harawa and others (2004).

81. Centers for Disease Control and Prevention (CDC). "Self-Reported Asthma Prevalence and Control Among Adults—United States, 2001." *Morbidity and Mortality Weekly Report,* 2003, *52,* 381–384.

82. CDC (2003).

83. CDC (2003).

84. Marder, D., and others. "Effect of Racial and Socioeconomic Factors on Asthma Mortality in Chicago." *Chest,* 1992, *101*(6 Suppl.), 426S-429S; Weiss, K. B., Gergen, P. J., and Crain, E. F. "Inner-City Asthma: The Epidemiology of an Emerging U.S. Public Health Concern." *Chest,* 1992, *101*(6 Suppl.), 362S-367S.

85. Gilliland, F. D., and others. "Maternal Smoking During Pregnancy, Environmental Tobacco Smoke Exposure and Childhood Lung Function." *Thorax,* 2000, 55, 271–276; Luder, E., Melnik, T. A., and DiMaio, M. "Association of Being Overweight with Greater Asthma Symptoms in Inner City Black and Hispanic Children." *Journal of Pediatrics,* 1998, *132,* 699–703; Pearce, N., Beasley, R., Burgess, C., and Crane, J. *Asthma Epidemiology: Principles and Methods.* New York: Oxford University Press, 1998.

86. Ortega, A. N., and Calderon, J. G. "Pediatric Asthma Among Minority Children." *Current Opinion in Pediatrics,* 2000, *12,* 579–583.

87. Ortega and Calderon (2000).

88. Bender, B., and others. "Measurement of Children's Asthma Medication Adherence by Self Report, Mother Report, Canister Weight, and Doser CT." *Annals of Allergy, Asthma, and Immunology,* 2000, *85,* 416–421; Rand, C. S., and others. "Adherence with Therapy and Access to Care: The Relationship to Excess Asthma Morbidity Among African-American Children." *Pediatric Asthma and Immunology,* 1994, *8,* 179–184; Flores and others (2000).

89. Kozyrskyj, A. L., Mustard, C. A., Cheang, M. S., and Simons, E. R. "Income-Based Drug Benefit Policy: Impact on Receipt of Inhaled Corticosteroid Prescriptions by Manitoba Children with Asthma." *Canadian Medical Association Journal,* 2001, *165,* 897–902; Ortega, A. N., and others. "Use of Health Services by Insurance Status Among Children with Asthma." *Medical Care,* 2001, *39,* 1065–1074; Ortega, A. N., and others. "Impact of Site of Care, Race, and Hispanic Ethnicity on Medication Use for Childhood Asthma." *Pediatrics,* 2002, *109*(1). [http://www.pediatrics.org/cgi/content/full/109/1/e1]; Finkelstein, J. A., and others. "Underuse of Controller Medications Among Medicaid-Insured Children with Asthma." *Archives of Pediatrics and Adolescent Medicine,* 2002, *156,* 562–567; Lieu, T. A., and others. "Racial/Ethnic Variation in Asthma Status and Management Practices Among Children in Managed Medicaid." *Pediatrics,* 2002, *109,* 857–865; Halterman, J. S., and others. "Inadequate Therapy for Asthma Among Children in the United States." *Pediatrics,* 2000, *105*(1 Pt. 3), 272–276.

90. Finkelstein, J. A., and others. "Self-Reported Physician Practices for Children with Asthma: Are National Guidelines Followed?" *Pediatrics,* 2000, *106,* 886–896.

91. Finkelstein, J. A., and others. "Quality of Care for Preschool Children with Asthma: The Role of Social Factors and Practice Setting." *Pediatrics,* 1995, *95,* 389–394.

92. Finkelstein and others (1995).
93. Department of Health and Human Services (DHHS). *Mental Health: Culture, Race, and Ethnicity—A Supplement to Mental Health: A Report of the Surgeon General.* Rockville, Md.: Center for Mental Health Services, Substance Abuse and Mental Health Services Administration, DHHS, 2001.
94. Alegría, M., and others. "Changes in Access to Mental Health Care Among the Poor and Non-Poor: Results from the Health Care Reform in Puerto Rico." *American Journal of Public Health*, 2001, *91*, 1431–1434; Vega, W. A., and Alegría, M. "Latino Mental Health and Treatment in the United States." In M. Aguirre-Molina, C. W. Molina, and R. E. Zambrana (eds.), *Health Issues in the Latino Community.* San Francisco: Jossey-Bass, 2001.
95. Zambrana, R. E., and others. "The Relationship Between Psychosocial Status of Immigrant Latino Mothers and Use of Emergency Pediatric Services." *Health and Social Work*, 1994, *19*, 93–102; Miranda, M. R., and others. "Mexican American Dropouts in Psychological Therapy as Related to Level of Acculturation." In M. R. Miranda (ed.), *Psychotherapy with the Spanish-Speaking: Issues in Research and Service Delivery.* (Monograph no. 3.) Los Angeles: Spanish-Speaking Mental Health Research Center, University of California, 1976.
96. Ortega, A. N., and Alegría, M. "Denial and Its Association with Mental Health Care Use: A Study of Island Puerto Ricans." *Journal of Behavior and Health Services Research*, 2005, *32*, 320–331; Pescosolido, B. A., and others. "Social Networks and Patterns of Use Among the Poor with Mental Health Problems in Puerto Rico." *Medical Care*, 1998, *36*, 1057–1072; Ortega and Alegría (2002).
97. Ortega and Alegría (2005, 2002).
98. Pescosolido (1998); Rogler, L. H., and Cortes, D. E. "Help-Seeking Pathways: A Unifying Concept in Mental Health Care." *American Journal of Psychiatry*, 1993, *150*, 554–561.
99. Ginzberg, E. "Access to Health Care for Hispanics." *Journal of the American Medical Association*, *1991*, *265*(2), 238–247; De la Rosa, M. "Health Care Needs of Hispanic Americans and the Responsiveness of the Health Care System." *Health and Social Work*, 1989, *14*, 104–113; Giachello, A. L. "Hispanics and Health Care." In P. S. Cafferty, S. J. Pastora, and W. C. McCready (eds.), *Hispanics in the United States: A New Social Agenda.* New Brunswick. N.J.: Transaction Books, 1988; Sue, S. "Community Mental Health Services to Minority Groups: Some Optimism, Some Pessimism." *American Psychologist*, 1977, *32*(8), 616–624.
100. Schneider, E. C., Zaslavsky, A. M., and Epstein, A. M. "Racial Disparities in the Quality of Care for Enrollees in Medicare Managed Care." *Journal of the American Medical Association*, 2002, *287*(10), 1288–1294.

CHAPTER FOUR

# PUBLIC POLICIES TO EXTEND HEALTH CARE COVERAGE

E. Richard Brown
with Shana Alex Lavarreda

The United States remains alone among the economically developed countries in not providing health care coverage to its entire population. In 2004, nearly forty-six million Americans were uninsured—people who have no private or public health insurance of any kind.[1]

This chapter examines the origins and status of the American system of health care coverage and the options available to extend coverage to the uninsured. First, it describes the current state of health insurance coverage, with an examination of historical trends and the public policies that have shaped the current system. The chapter concludes with a review of the major policy options to extend coverage to the remaining uninsured population.

Why is health insurance coverage important? It is the principal financial means by which people can obtain health care services. The importance of health insurance coverage has been shown in cross-sectional surveys that compare the access of insured and uninsured people, and in panel or longitudinal studies that examine over time the effects of losing or gaining health insurance on access and health status.[2]

The United States has repeatedly toyed with major reforms to establish a universal social insurance program to extend health care coverage to the entire population. Each time it has failed to come to grips with this issue or has adopted partial reform. After these repeated failures to enact comprehensive reform, and despite the partial solutions that have been adopted, the problems of lack of coverage remain a continuing challenge to the U.S. health system and the nation's political institutions.

## The Uninsured

The large and growing number of Americans who have no health care coverage continues to be one of the most compelling—and intractable—policy and political issues in the United States. In 1984, an estimated thirty million Americans, 14.3 percent of the nonelderly population, were uninsured at any point in time (Table 4.1). By 1995, a year after the end of the most extensive effort to enact universal coverage, the uninsured rate reached 15.9 percent. It rose in 1997 to 17.4 percent, dipped during the economic boom from 1998 to 2001, and rose again with the economic decline, reaching 17.2 percent in 2003 and declining again in 2004.[3]

By 2004, an estimated 45.8 million persons were uninsured, including eight million children under age eighteen and thirty-seven million adults ages eighteen to sixty-four.[4] About 297,000 persons age sixty-five or over (just 0.8 percent of all persons in this age group) were completely uninsured in 2004; nearly all the elderly

**TABLE 4.1. PERCENTAGE OF NONELDERLY POPULATION WHO ARE UNINSURED, AGES 0–64, UNITED STATES, SELECTED YEARS.**

| Year | Percentage of Persons Age 0–64 |
|------|-------------------------------|
| 1984 | 14.3 |
| 1995 | 15.9 |
| 1997 | 17.4 |
| 1998 | 16.5 |
| 1999 | 16.0 |
| 2000 | 16.8 |
| 2001 | 16.2 |
| 2002 | 16.5 |
| 2003 | 17.2 |
| 2004 | 16.6 |

*Sources:* National Health Interview Survey. 1984 and 1995 data from *Health, United States, 2004.* Hyattsville, Md.: National Center for Health Statistics, 2004; 1997–2004 data from Cohen, R. A., and Martinez, M. E. *Health Insurance Coverage: Estimates from the National Health Interview Survey, 2004.* Hyattsville, Md.: National Center for Health Statistics, 2005.

receive at least Medicare coverage and most have some other coverage that reduces Medicare's cost sharing (deductibles and co-insurance) and covers some services that are not Medicare benefits. Because the uninsured population includes so few elderly persons, most analysts of this problem focus on the nonelderly population.

More than eight in ten (83 percent) of the nonelderly uninsured are working adults and their children. Half (49 percent) of the uninsured are in a family headed by at least one employee who works full-time all year, and another 14 percent are in a family of full-time employees who work less than a full year (Figure 4.1). The self-employed and their children account for 8 percent of the uninsured, twice their proportion of the nonelderly population.[5]

Three-fourths of the uninsured have low or moderate family income. More than half (55 percent) have income below 200 percent of the federal poverty level (that is, less than about $38,600 for a family of four in 2004), and another fifth (18 percent) have moderate family income (between 200 percent and 299 percent of the poverty level; Figure 4.2). The low and moderate incomes of the uninsured mean that efforts to extend coverage to them require considerable financial assistance to make it affordable, assistance that can come only from employers or government. Although 53 percent of the entire nonelderly population have a family

## FIGURE 4.1. FAMILY WORK STATUS OF UNINSURED NONELDERLY PERSONS, UNITED STATES, 2003.

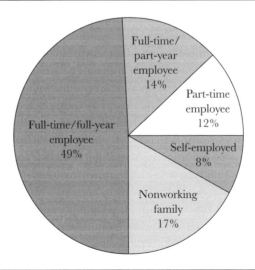

*Source:* Analysis of March 2004 Current Population Survey by UCLA Center for Health Policy Research.

### FIGURE 4.2. FAMILY INCOME OF UNINSURED NONELDERLY PERSONS, UNITED STATES, 2003.

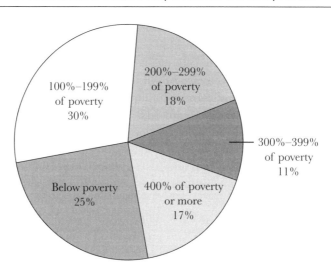

*Note:* Total family income relative to the federal poverty level.

*Source:* Analysis of March 2004 Current Population Survey by UCLA Center for Health Policy Research.

income at least three times the poverty level (about $58,000 for a family of four), only about one in four (28 percent) of the uninsured have a family income that high. It is unlikely that any of the uninsured below this level could afford a significant share of the costs of family coverage, although those with income above 400 percent of poverty could help pay for their health insurance.

Because of their predominance in the population, half of the uninsured are non-Latino whites, but ethnic minorities have a disproportionately high uninsured rate. More than one out of three nonelderly Latinos (35 percent), one in five African Americans (21 percent), and one in five Asian Americans and Pacific Islanders (20 percent) are uninsured, compared to 13 percent of non-Latino whites.[6]

Twelve states have an uninsured rate of 20 percent or more of their nonelderly population, while seven states have below 12 percent. Differences across states are driven mainly by state variations in employment-based health insurance, which itself is explained by differences in labor market characteristics (such as firm size, industry, and unionization). But state differences are also influenced by the generosity of each state's eligibility policies for Medicaid and other public health care insurance programs.[7]

## Employer-Sponsored Private Health Insurance Coverage

In 2003, 63 percent of the nonelderly obtained private health insurance through their own employment or that of a family member (Figure 4.3). Another 4 percent purchased private health insurance on their own through the nongroup market. Among all nonelderly persons with any private health insurance, more than 90 percent obtained it through employment. How did employment-based health insurance gain such a dominant position in the United States, despite the absence of any nationwide requirement that employers provide their workers with coverage?

From World War II through the mid-1970s, private health insurance covered a growing proportion of the American population. World War II generated several conditions that encouraged expansion of private health insurance. Cost-plus government war contracts reimbursed many employers for all their labor costs, reducing their opposition to giving workers increased compensation. Federal wage-and-price controls exempted employee benefits, giving employers an opportunity to increase workers' noncash compensation in response to demands from labor unions in a very tight labor market and a war-focused economy. Federal tax

### FIGURE 4.3. HEALTH INSURANCE COVERAGE OF NONELDERLY PERSONS BY SOURCE OF COVERAGE, UNITED STATES, 2003.

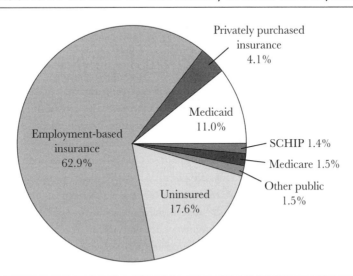

*Source:* Analysis of March 2004 Current Population Survey by UCLA Center for Health Policy Research.

policies allowed employers to deduct premiums for health plans from business revenues and allowed employees to deduct employer-paid health insurance premiums from taxable earnings, affording significant tax advantages. By 1945, enrollment in hospital insurance plans had spread to 24 percent of the population, up from 10 percent in 1940. After the war, commercial insurance companies, following the early leadership of not-for-profit Blue Cross plans, pushed into the employer-sponsored health insurance market. By 1950, private hospital insurance covered 51 percent of the population; by 1962, about 70 percent of the entire population had hospital benefits and 65 percent were covered for physicians' surgical services.[8]

Private health insurance was popular among consumers of health services because it spread the risk of expensive medical conditions across a large population base, reducing the threat of personal bankruptcy in the event of serious health problems and making health services financially more accessible to the covered population. It was also popular among hospitals, physicians, and other health care providers because it created a stable base of revenues that reduced their risk of bankruptcy during recession and permitted them to expand and introduce new technologies during good years. Expansion of private health insurance coverage was the financial foundation for the rapid growth of medical care, including escalating investments in medical technology, hospitals, and specialty care.

The large proportion of the uninsured who are in working families—83 percent—underscores the less-than-universal character of employment-based health insurance. Employment-based health insurance peaked in the mid-1970s and has ebbed and flowed since that time, especially with each expansion and contraction of the economy. This dynamic is illustrated by changes in job-based insurance coverage following the recession of the early 1990s. The proportion of the nonelderly population with job-based coverage rose from 63 percent in 1994 (as the country was just beginning to emerge from recession) to 67 percent in 2001 (as the economy boomed), and it fell back to 63 percent in 2003.[9]

The lack of health insurance coverage among the working population is primarily the result of many workers having little or no access to such coverage. Many employers do not offer health benefits, some workers are not eligible for benefits when they are offered, and some workers who are offered and eligible for health benefits do not accept them. The proportion of employers who offer health benefits to at least some of their workers (the "offer rate") has fluctuated slightly with economic booms and declines, rising to a peak of 69 percent of all firms in 2000, including virtually all firms with two hundred or more workers and two-thirds of smaller firms. But even with the economic recovery beginning in 2002, the proportion of smaller firms that offer health benefits declined every year through 2005, driven by the growing costs of health insurance and by economic pressure to cut labor costs.[10]

There is some evidence of a decline in eligibility for health benefits (the "eligibility rate") among employees who work less than full-time, full-year and a decline among full-time, full-year employees in acceptance of health insurance when it is offered and they are eligible (the "take-up rate"). The eligibility rules are set by employers and are usually related to the number of hours worked per week, duration of employment with the firm, and some other factors. Workers may affect their own eligibility if they have the ability to work more or fewer hours. Between 1987 and 1996, the take-up rate declined significantly among young workers, Hispanic workers, those with low educational attainment, and those with low wages.[11] Eligibility and take-up rates have changed little since then, increasing slightly during the economic boom of the late 1990s and more recently declining among small firms.

Nevertheless, concern is mounting that the recent decline in employment-based insurance reflects a fundamental flaw in the current U.S. health care system. The rising costs of health insurance are the product in part of uncontrolled growth in health care costs and spending. The rising cost of health care is driving down the prevalence of job-based insurance, particularly comprehensive insurance, as these cost increases push employers to shift costs to their workers and then workers respond by dropping their coverage because the cost of health insurance has risen far faster than workers' earnings.[12]

The probability that a worker is offered health benefits, in general, depends on the labor market in which the worker is competing for a job. Firms are much less likely to offer health benefits if they are small, pay lower wages, do not offer other benefits (such as paid vacation and sick leave), have no union workers, have high workforce turnover, and have more part-time workers. They also are less likely to offer health benefits if their workers are disproportionately Latino, younger, less educated, or female—in large part because such workers are more likely to be employed in these low-wage sectors of the economy.[13] Because these groups have no subsidy from their employer or the government, their low-to-moderate income makes private purchase of health insurance unaffordable.

Thus, private health insurance has not served all sectors of American society. The elderly and the poor were effectively priced out of the market for private coverage even in its period of rapid growth during the 1950s and early 1960s. In 1958, although 86 percent of the upper-income third of all American families had some type of private health insurance, only 42 percent of the lower-income third had any coverage at all. Like the lower working class and the poor, the elderly were unable to obtain adequate private hospitalization coverage at a price they could afford. In 1958, only 43 percent of those age sixty-five and over had insurance for hospital care, compared to at least two-thirds of the nonelderly population.[14] Although private health insurance dramatically reduced disparities in the use of health services related to income for the population with coverage, it remained for Medicare and Medicaid to significantly improve access for the elderly and the poor.

## Medicare, Medicaid, and SCHIP

By 1960, political pressures to enact public programs to provide for the poor, especially the low-income elderly, had become irresistible. The Kerr-Mills Act, enacted in that year, offered generous matching federal grants to states to encourage them to develop medical care programs for the elderly poor and the nonelderly disabled and blind. But the program was implemented unevenly by the states, with the bulk of the federal funds going to a handful of states that developed comprehensive programs. Senior citizen groups and the nation's major labor unions were not assuaged by this public assistance program; they continued to demand health insurance under Social Security, not a welfare program.[15]

The November 1964 election gave the Democrats a landslide victory (the most lopsided popular vote in the twentieth century) and President Lyndon Johnson both a clear mandate for his Great Society reforms and a Democratic Congress (two-thirds in both houses) to enact them. The next year, Congress established Medicare, a social insurance program for hospital care and voluntary insurance for physician services for the elderly, and Medicaid, a public assistance program for poor people who meet "categorical" requirements. Medicare was a landmark in American health care reform because, as a contributory program that afforded entitlement to health benefits without a means test, it was the first successful enactment of social insurance for health services. Medicaid was also important because of its broad potential scope of benefits and population coverage, despite its public assistance (or welfare) character resting on means testing.

### Medicare: Improving Access for the Elderly

Medicare has extended coverage to virtually all the elderly and to many blind and long-term-disabled nonelderly persons for a significant portion of their medical expenses. It is the largest source of public financing for health care services in the United States. People age sixty-five and over with social security benefits are automatically entitled to receive Medicare Part A (coverage for hospital services) and to enroll in Medicare Part B (coverage for physician and other services). Part A is a mandatory program financed by a special social security tax paid by all workers and deposited in the Medicare Trust Fund, while Part B is a voluntary plan funded by beneficiary premium payments and contributions from the U.S. Treasury. In 2003, Medicare covered forty-one million beneficiaries (thirty-five million aged and six million disabled enrollees), at a cost of $271 billion.[16]

Medicare is a social insurance program. This is a very important characteristic. Like Social Security, Medicare Part A is a contributory program, which means that everyone who works contributes to it through a tax on earnings. Medicare is also an entitlement program, which means that everyone is eligible for Medicare on reaching age sixty-five or, if younger, meeting a stringent disability test. It is not a means-tested welfare program; this distinction will become clear as we discuss Medicaid.

Medicare quickly improved access to medical services, especially hospital care, for the elderly and disabled. But even under Medicare—an entitlement program with uniform benefits and standards—beneficiary access problems remain. In the program's first few years, more affluent elderly beneficiaries received more physician and hospital services than did the lower-income elderly. Similarly, white Anglo beneficiaries received more health services than did African American beneficiaries. Over time, however, both income and racial differentials were reduced. Recent studies have found that the vast majority of Medicare beneficiaries report no access problems, but some groups do encounter serious barriers. About one in seven Medicare beneficiaries do not have a usual source of care or have not seen a physician for a medical problem that warranted medical attention. Studies that examine access to specific procedures consistently find differences by race in the rate of selected diagnostic and treatment procedures performed. African American beneficiaries are less likely than Anglo beneficiaries to receive a variety of high-technology procedures.[17]

Despite Medicare's impact in improving access to care of elderly and disabled beneficiaries, the program's cost-sharing provisions for covered services posed financial barriers for many. Premium costs for Medicare Part B, deductibles, and co-insurance impose out-of-pocket expenses on the beneficiary. In addition, physicians can bill beneficiaries for more than Medicare's allowed fee (called "balance billing"), although the Omnibus Budget Reconciliation Act of 1989 limited these extra fees to no more than 15 percent of the Medicare payment rate. Nearly nine in ten beneficiaries purchase supplemental "Medigap" coverage to offset deductibles and co-insurance as well as cover some additional services; many individually purchase private supplemental insurance or receive it through a current or former employer. An estimated 17 percent of Medicare beneficiaries also qualify for financial assistance and supplemental benefits under their state Medicaid programs because their income is very low.[18]

Many Medicare beneficiaries obtained their supplemental coverage through managed care plans (HMOs), called "Medicare+Choice" in recent years but now called "Medicare Advantage." Medicare+Choice plans were especially attractive because they covered services (in particular prescription drugs) that the basic Medicare program did not. They also covered preventive health services such as screening mammograms and Pap tests, which were not covered by Medicare until 1991.

In 2005, 13 percent of Medicare beneficiaries were enrolled in a managed care plan, ranging from less than 1 percent in seventeen states to more than 20 percent in six states. Many private plans, unhappy with the amount of money they were getting per enrollee, withdrew from the program, reducing the number of Medicare managed care plans from a high of 346 in 1998 to 179 in 2005. Payments to Medicare HMOs were raised by the Congress and President Bush to attract such plans back into serving Medicare beneficiaries. As a result of increased payment to Medicare HMOs, they now receive more on average than the program would have spent if those enrollees had remained in the fee-for-service Medicare program—8.4 percent more in 2004, according to a study by the Commonwealth Fund.[19]

There have been additional problems with the Medicare managed care program. Termination of service by Medicare plans increases difficulty for beneficiaries in getting and paying for care, often forcing them to pay a higher premium, increasing their out-of-pocket cost for services, and requiring them to change health care providers. In addition, there was high turnover among Medicare+Choice primary care providers in many states, forcing elderly and disabled beneficiaries to change health care providers. Overall, after controlling for beneficiary characteristics, enrollees in Medicare+Choice plans were more likely to receive key preventive services and reported fewer problems with paperwork, information, and customer service, but those in the traditional Medicare fee-for-service program reported better overall access to and experiences with care.[20]

During its first four decades, Medicare's lack of coverage for several key benefits limited its effectiveness for many types of health service, particularly for lower-income beneficiaries. One notable absence of coverage is for long-term care services. Medicare restricts coverage for nursing home stays and home health visits to posthospital use of limited duration, imposing hardship on the elderly who must use extensive personal resources to pay for care. If they become poor or impoverished because of medical expenses, they may apply to Medicaid, which has become the nation's largest payer for long-term care.

Perhaps foremost among Medicare's gaps was the lack of coverage for prescription drugs. This problem grew over time for the elderly and others who on average use more medication than younger groups do. Out-of-pocket costs for prescription drugs took an ever-increasing share of seniors' income as a growing number of drugs were prescribed for more conditions and as the high prices charged by pharmaceutical manufacturers pushed up prescription drug expenditures. A growing demand to cover prescription drugs under Medicare eventually generated enough political support to push the Congress to enact a coverage program. The Medicare Prescription Drug, Improvement, and Modernization Act of 2003 (MMA) established a new and complex prescription drug benefit beginning in 2006 (the prescription drug benefit is described in Chapter Twenty), bringing expected relief to many elderly persons with high expenses. President George W. Bush and the Republican majority in Congress created the prescription drug benefit as a private program, except in areas where private plans were very limited, overcoming objections by Democratic congressional leaders who argued for having the program run by the federal Medicare program. The MMA, for the first time in Medicare's four decades, will require beneficiaries to choose among private drug plans, with a complex set of rules and options that may well test the viability of such privatization strategies in the Medicare program.

## Medicaid: Improving Access for the Poor

Medicaid was enacted in 1965 to offer coverage to poor persons who were eligible for federally supported, state-run welfare programs. These welfare programs give cash assistance to families with dependent children (formerly Aid to Families with Dependent Children, or AFDC) and to the disabled, the blind, and the elderly (those receiving Supplemental Security Income/State Supplemental Payment program income). Through this latter component, Medicaid assists elderly Medicare beneficiaries who could not afford the required cost sharing for Medicare or supplemental insurance. Medicaid is administered by the states under federal guidelines that require minimum standards for eligibility, benefits, and (in some cases) provider payments. Funding is shared between the federal government and the states, with the federal share (called the Federal Medical Assistance Percentage, or FMAP) ranging from 50 percent up to 77 percent.

In 2002, Medicaid covered nearly fifty million persons at a cost of $213.5 billion. Half of Medicaid beneficiaries are low-income children, about a quarter are low-income women, and the remaining quarter are low-income disabled and elderly persons. Medicaid spending is tilted toward the elderly (who in 2002 accounted for 9 percent of all recipients and averaged about $10,965 per person) and toward the disabled (who made up 16 percent of recipients and averaged about $10,455 per person, compared to children, who constitute 50 percent of all Medicaid recipients and average about $1,305 per child).[21]

There is substantial evidence that Medicaid is responsible for a significant increase in use of health services among low-income persons. In 1964, two years before the Medicaid program began operation, poor people averaged 4.3 doctor visits per year, compared to 4.6 visits for the nonpoor. By the mid-1970s, when nearly all states were operating Medicaid programs, poor adults averaged more physician visits than nonpoor adults, and the gap between poor and nonpoor children had been reduced (though not eliminated). However, use of a greater volume of services by the poor may not necessarily indicate complete equity in access because of the poorer health status of many low-income people.[22]

Medicaid's positive effect on the utilization rate of low-income people is, of course, limited to those who are eligible for the program. Numerous studies have found that Medicaid beneficiaries, in contrast to uninsured low-income persons, use health services at a rate comparable to that of higher-income people, after adjusting for differences in health status. Among the poor and near-poor who are sick or in poor health, those uninsured during the entire year use far fewer medical services than those who have Medicaid for even part of the year.[23]

Studies have found that loss of Medicaid coverage has an adverse impact on the health status of low-income people, especially among persons with chronic illness. Loss of Medicaid has a serious adverse impact on access to health services and on the health status of anyone with a chronic illness such as diabetes or high blood pressure.[24]

Despite its important contributions, Medicaid's ability to improve access to medical care for the nation's low-income population has been hampered by several factors. State-level discretion in the Medicaid program has resulted in great variation across states in the population covered and the benefits provided. Federal guidelines define mandatory eligible populations and covered benefits, but they allow states considerable latitude beyond this floor. States vary markedly in their Medicaid income eligibility level for a family, which ranges from one state with income eligibility below 50 percent of the federal poverty level for parents of eligible Medicaid children to eleven states with income eligibility at or above 200 percent. States also differ in the benefits covered in the Medicaid program. Each state defines its own package of benefits beyond the mandatory services defined by federal Medicaid law. For example, coverage for such essential services as prescription drugs, physical therapy, occupational therapy, respiratory care services, and corrective eyeglasses are all optional. The reimbursement level for Medicaid also varies considerably across states, contributing to differences by state in the rate of physician participation.[25]

Medicaid's limitations in covering the poor were exacerbated by budget cuts during the Reagan administration and ratcheting down by states of income limits for AFDC eligibility. As a result, Medicaid enrollees as a proportion of all poor persons declined from 51 percent in 1981 to 45 percent in 1982. Beginning in the mid-1980s, however, Congress enacted a series of expansions in Medicaid income

eligibility in order to extend Medicaid's beneficial effects to more low-income pregnant women and their children. Although only 51 percent of poor children were
on Medicaid in 1985, 60 percent were covered by Medicaid in 1994, an important reversal of the trend of a decade earlier.[26]

Most of this increase was aimed at ensuring financial access to pregnant
women to enable them to obtain prenatal care early in pregnancy in order to improve birth outcomes and the health of infants of Medicaid-eligible pregnant
women. Congress required states to cover pregnant women up to 133 percent of
the poverty level and encouraged states to voluntarily expand coverage up to 185
percent of poverty. This extension of Medicaid to a population well above the income eligibility for cash public assistance programs partially severed the historic
link between Medicaid and welfare. In addition, Congress required states to increase fees for obstetric care to attract an adequate number of providers, and it
appropriated other funds for enhanced perinatal care. By 2002, thirty-four states
had expanded coverage of pregnant women beyond the federally mandated level,
all fifty states had streamlined the eligibility process at least to some extent, and
forty-four states offered Medicaid reimbursement for enhanced prenatal services.
More than one-third of all births in the United States (37 percent) now are paid
for by Medicaid, while other programs fund improvement in the supply and accessibility of prenatal care services and nutritional and other supports for mothers and young children.[27]

The Medicaid program's improvements in eligibility for pregnant women to
meet specific public health goals is a valuable example of how public policy may
be used directly to improve access. The findings regarding the effects Medicaid
expansion has on use of prenatal care and birth outcomes vary. Some studies show
improvement in access to care and birth outcomes, while others do not. These
findings suggest that there are multiple components to providing prenatal care
that include, but go beyond, improving financial access: outreach and educational
programs, case management, and supply of providers.[28]

The expansion of Medicaid coverage appeared to come to a halt with enactment and implementation of the Personal Responsibility and Work Opportunity Reconciliation Act of 1996, better known as welfare reform. Nationally,
Medicaid coverage fell from 12.5 percent of the nonelderly population overall in
1994 to 10.4 percent in 1998, but it fell even more sharply among nonworking
families, from 52.8 percent in 1994 to 40.8 percent in 1998.[29] As the economy
continued to improve, some families and individuals who formerly relied on Medicaid might have obtained low-wage jobs that permitted some access to health
benefits, or earned more money that enabled them to pay the employee's share
of premiums. However, many of these newly employed workers and their families found themselves in low-wage jobs without health benefits and joined the ranks

of the uninsured. Although welfare reform promises public assistance recipients that they will receive transitional Medicaid coverage for at least a year when they leave public assistance, both advocates and analysts argue that this policy is inadequately implemented.[30]

Finally, many noncitizen families refrained from applying for Medicaid. Welfare reform legislation together with the Illegal Immigration Reform and Immigrant Responsibility Act of 1996 restricted all noncitizens' eligibility for Medicaid and greatly broadened application of a "public charge" classification for those who used any public benefits. Noncitizen parents feared being labeled a public charge if they enrolled themselves or their children (even children who were born in the United States and thus are citizens) in a means-tested program. They were concerned that the classification would be used against them if they tried to renew their visas, return to the United States from abroad, or apply for citizenship.[31] This problem was ameliorated by policies issued in May 1999 by the Immigration and Naturalization Service (now called the U.S. Citizenship and Immigration Services), specifying that noncitizens will not be classified as a public charge if they or their children enroll in Medicaid, unless they receive long-term care under Medicaid.

One important characteristic of the Medicaid program is its origin as a public assistance program. Welfare programs, even federally supported ones such as Medicaid, tend to be administered by the states, albeit under some federal regulation. Unlike Medicare, which is administered as a social insurance program by the federal government and includes the same eligibility and benefits throughout the country, the Medicaid program is administered by the states. Medicaid is in reality fifty-one programs, with variations in eligibility and benefits across all fifty states and the District of Columbia.

Many of the problems associated with Medicaid are the legacy of its welfare-based origin. Welfare programs tend to rely on stigmatizing means tests, usually conducted in welfare offices.[32] It is noteworthy that there is no stigma attached to Medicare, which is viewed as a universal entitlement, a social contract between the nation's young and old generations. Nor is there stigma associated with the tax exemption of employer-paid health insurance for largely middle- and upper-income workers, which cost the federal government about $188.5 billion in 2004—a health insurance subsidy program that no one calls welfare.[33] Despite Medicaid's welfare origins, expansion of eligibility in the 1980s to low-income pregnant women and children at a higher income level—nearly twice the poverty level for pregnant women and infants—loosened the connection with welfare and created the logic for 1990s policies that went further.

A second important characteristic of Medicaid is that it is an entitlement program. Anyone who meets Medicaid's eligibility requirements is entitled to receive its benefits. Expenditures for these benefits generate a cost to the state and draw the specified federal matching payment. In this way, Medicaid differs from block grant programs, in which the federal government gives the states a maximum allocation, such that once a state has expended its allocation, any additional services for eligible persons become the fiscal responsibility of the state alone. This characteristic has been the nub of major conflict between liberals and conservatives, with liberals defending Medicaid as an entitlement and conservatives often proposing to turn it into a block grant—as they tried unsuccessfully to do in 1996, when welfare reform ended entitlement of poor children and families to cash assistance. President Bush has also proposed turning Medicaid at least partly into a block grant program, indicating that this issue remains alive and may yet alter the fundamental character of Medicaid.

***Expanding Medicaid Eligibility.*** With the failure to enact national health care reform, many states looked to Medicaid, among other approaches, to extend coverage to their uninsured residents. Numerous states have expanded or otherwise modified their Medicaid programs with the aid of a waiver under sections 1115 and 1915(b) and (c) of the Social Security Act. These waivers, which must be granted by the federal Health Care Financing Administration, permit states to modify eligibility, payment methods, and other characteristics in their Medicaid programs. These waivers permit states to require Medicaid beneficiaries to enroll in a managed care plan, on the expectation that managed care enables the state to slow the growth of its Medicaid expenditures and, in some cases, improve access to health services. Most of the recent waivers also extend coverage to the working poor and their families, who were not previously eligible for Medicaid, promising to use at least some of the expected savings from managed care to expand coverage to low-income uninsured persons.[34] By 2004, 60.7 percent of all Medicaid beneficiaries were enrolled in managed care, up from 9.5 percent in 1991.[35]

By the end of 2004, twenty states had comprehensive health care reform Medicaid waivers, most to expand enrollment to optional populations.[36] Tennessee undertook the most ambitious expansion as it replaced its fee-for-service Medicaid program with TennCare, a fully capitated managed care program. By the end of 1999, TennCare had enrolled more than 1.3 million Medicaid beneficiaries in managed care, including more than 506,000 who did not fit traditional Medicaid eligibility. Altogether, by 2004, sixteen waiver states covered 1.4 million persons who would not have been eligible without the waiver.[37]

States can also cover parents of children who are income-eligible for Medicaid, under the new section 1931 of the Social Security Act (added as part of welfare reform in 1996), which allows states considerable flexibility in setting Medicaid income eligibility for families. By 2002, however, only twenty-seven states had used either section 1931 or an 1115 waiver to cover parents to at least 100 percent of the poverty level.[38] Other states remain well below that level.

However, by 2004 budget pressures at the state level had put a halt to many planned expansions. States found themselves unable to fund the programs for which they had been granted federal waivers. Tennessee modified its TennCare waiver to allow for *dis*enrollment of 323,000 adults in optional populations from their program because of budgetary constraints. This drastic move, which generated a great deal of opposition within the state, signified the immense fiscal pressure states face with their Medicaid budgets. During an economic recession, state revenues decrease but applications for state programs increase. Between 2000 and 2003, total costs for Medicaid jumped by one-third to $276 billion, with much of this cost borne by states that are required by law to balance their annual budgets while facing huge tax revenue shortfalls and deficits.

During this same period, rapidly increasing health care costs pushed up both private insurance premiums and public programs costs. In fact, both Medicaid premiums and spending per enrollee had much lower rates of increase than those of private insurers. States used a variety of mechanisms, including volume purchasing and direct controls over reimbursement, to control Medicaid cost increases before turning to restrictions on eligibility, enrollment, and benefits.[39]

Medicaid managed care has a mixed record. On some measures, such as having a regular provider and receiving preventive health care services, Medicaid managed care beneficiaries appear to be doing better than their fee-for-service counterparts, but managed care enrollees are more likely to report not getting needed care and more dissatisfaction with some aspects of their care. There is, however, a growing body of evidence that, overall, managed care plans offer Medicaid beneficiaries access to health services that is at least as good as in the fee-for-service Medicaid program and quality of care that is equal to or better than care in the fee-for-service program.[40] Nevertheless, there is little evidence that managed care reduces Medicaid costs, in part because most Medicaid managed care enrollees have not been the higher-cost disabled or elderly for whom substantial savings might be realized, and in part because Medicaid expenditures per beneficiary were already ratcheted down to an extremely low level in many states.

## The State Children's Health Insurance Program (SCHIP)

With the collapse in 1994 of efforts to cover the entire population, many health care reform advocates joined with children's advocacy groups to expand coverage for children. They focused a great deal of attention on the fact that there were then more than eleven million uninsured children eighteen or younger in the United States, many of whom had low family incomes that were nonetheless above their state's often less-than-generous Medicaid income eligibility level. Children are an appealing group to cover, both because there is wide political support for public programs that benefit children and because insuring children costs much less than insuring adults.

In 1997, Congress enacted the State Children's Health Insurance Program (SCHIP), offering funds to states to expand health insurance coverage to uninsured, low-income, and moderate-income children. Although liberals and conservatives fought over whether to make SCHIP an entitlement that expanded Medicaid or a block grant that established a separate program that relies on private insurance, in the end Congress compromised on a generous block grant that could be used by the states to do either or both.

SCHIP was generous in two ways. First, it enabled states to set the income eligibility level up to 200 percent of the federal poverty level (in 2003, up to $24,240 for a family of two or $30,520 for a family of three) or even higher. Second, it gives states more generous matching funds than under Medicaid—30 percent higher than the state's federal Medicaid match, up to 85 percent of a state's expenditures. This was an incentive to induce states to implement the program quickly and vigorously. SCHIP implementation began slowly, falling short of early enrollment goals, but it has picked up speed since 2000 and significantly helped slow the growth in the uninsured population. By 2003, four million children nationwide were enrolled in SCHIP.[41]

Early examinations indicated that most of the program's enrollment came from children who were previously insured through private coverage, not uninsured children as intended. However, as states' SCHIP programs matured and outreach efforts intensified, more and more children who previously had no insurance enrolled in the program.[42] Among children with chronic health conditions (such as asthma), SCHIP has achieved significant success in reducing the uninsured rate.[43] Early research showed that access to quality health care received by SCHIP enrollees was dramatically higher than when they were uninsured.[44]

As SCHIP enrollments expanded, these state programs faced the same budgetary pressures as did Medicaid. Although some states were able to continue expanding their SCHIP programs throughout the recession from 2000 to 2003, twenty-three restricted enrollment and retention. Eight states imposed an explicit enrollment freeze, while the rest rolled back application simplifications in order to reduce enrollment indirectly. By July 2004, twenty-two states had imposed additional co-payments on SCHIP enrollees to decrease state expenditures.[45]

In spite of these cutbacks, the SCHIP program is a successful model for modern expansion of public coverage. Together with Medicaid, SCHIP expanded eligibility for and enrollment in public health insurance programs for children whose low- and moderate-income families did not have access to affordable employment-based

insurance. Between the Medicaid and SCHIP public programs and private employment-based coverage, the United States is clearly moving—albeit haltingly
and with some steps backward—toward a policy of offering affordable health care
coverage to all children.

# Reforms to Expand Private Coverage

In addition to expanding the population groups covered through Medicaid and
SCHIP, states have also experimented with an array of reforms aimed at expanding private coverage to the uninsured population. The collapse of national
health care reform efforts has increased pressure to implement state solutions,
rather than national ones, to rising health care costs and access problems. However, states vary in their political and economic capacity to effectively implement
reforms, and they also lack the legislative authority to enact reforms that would
achieve universal coverage.

The main approaches that states and the federal government have pursued
to expand private coverage of the uninsured include reform of insurance laws to
increase affordability or access to coverage, creation of purchasing alliances or cooperatives, and in a few states passage of legislation mandating coverage. To varying degrees, these approaches build on the existing employment-based insurance
system, strengthening the connection between coverage and work.

## Small Group and Individual Health Insurance Reform

Compared to larger groups, small groups and individuals face higher premiums
for health insurance as a result of higher marketing and administrative costs and
more difficulty in managing risk in this market. Consequently, they also face such
problems as frequent jumps in premiums, frequent changes in insurance carriers,
and medical underwriting (that is, basing premiums on the particular group's expected use of health services).[46]

Furthermore, groups or individuals considered at highest risk were often unable to obtain any coverage. The Consolidated Omnibus Budget Reconciliation
Act of 1985 (COBRA), for example, addressed this problem by requiring employers and insurers to allow employees who lost or changed their employment to
keep their health insurance if they pay 102 percent of the full premium. Although
this provision is useful to higher-risk persons who are very concerned about being
without coverage, it does not help those who cannot afford the full cost of their
health plan—the situation facing the great majority of the uninsured, and especially those who have become unemployed.

The Health Insurance Portability and Accountability Act (HIPAA) of 1996 required states to reform their individual and small-group health insurance markets. It guaranteed that individuals could buy health insurance without exclusion for a preexisting condition if they (1) have been covered by an employer-sponsored health plan for at least eighteen months, (2) exhaust any continuation of their employer's health benefits available through COBRA, (3) are not eligible for any other public or private health insurance, and (4) were uninsured no longer than two months. HIPAA also limited insurers' ability to exclude preexisting conditions and prohibited them from defining pregnancy as a preexisting condition. It prohibited employers from charging employees higher premiums according to health status or other factors related to potential usage, and it required insurers to guarantee issuance and renewal of health insurance for small employers (those with two to fifty employees). HIPAA also gradually raised the tax deductibility for health insurance purchased by self-employed persons from 30 percent in 1996 to 100 percent by the year 2003.

What HIPAA did not do was limit the amount an insurer could charge for coverage that it guaranteed. As a result, HIPAA-protected coverage is often unaffordable to individuals who need it, resulting in a negligible impact on the uninsured population. Moreover, since almost all states had already enacted some type of small-group and individual market insurance reforms,[47] HIPAA served to bring all the states up to a uniform national standard, rather than dramatically change the accessibility and affordability of coverage. In sum, reforms that extend guaranteed coverage to small groups and individuals help regulate the market, but they have limited impact in expanding coverage unless they are accompanied by some form of subsidy.

## Purchasing Groups

Unlike high-risk pools that offer private health insurance to individuals, purchasing groups target small businesses. These organizations are designed to increase small firms' purchasing power in the private health insurance market and lower their administrative costs related to arranging for coverage of their workers. Eight out of ten (79 percent of) small firms that do not offer health benefits cite the high cost of coverage as a "very important" reason they do not do so, far ahead of any other reason.[48] State-sponsored cooperatives enable small businesses to pool the risk of insurance coverage, thus lowering premium costs and improving their bargaining power in the health insurance market. National estimates from the 1997 Robert Wood Johnson Foundation Employer Health Insurance Survey suggest that about one-quarter of all businesses participate in a purchasing pool and that smaller businesses are more likely to participate. The survey also found that pools modestly increased the availability of employee choice among plans and promoted information for employees about plan quality, but pooling did not increase the accessibility or affordability of insurance for employers.[49]

## Employer Mandates

The reforms of the private health insurance market that have been discussed so far were intended to make coverage available to employers or individuals whose high risk or small size make it difficult to find coverage at rates available to other employers or individuals. Such reforms may help small firms reduce their disadvantage in the health insurance market relative to larger firms. But they do not make health insurance more affordable for employers of low-wage workers, for whom the still-high cost of health insurance would substantially increase their labor costs relative to other employers in their industry who do not offer health benefits. Nor do these reforms make health insurance premiums more affordable for the moderate- and low-income working individuals and families who make up the majority of the uninsured.

To make health insurance more affordable to the uninsured population—as well as to stabilize the employment-based system for financing health insurance—there has been considerable national and state interest in requiring employers to help pay for coverage for their employees. Despite the apparent value of an employer mandate, only Hawaii has implemented this reform. The ability of states to adopt employer mandates has been thwarted by the federal Employee Retirement Income Security Act (ERISA), which exempts self-insured businesses from state insurance regulations and taxes, although it does not bar states from regulating health insurance coverage that employers purchase for their employees.[50] Nationally, just over half (54 percent) of all medium and large firms self-insure (that is, assume all or part of the financial risk of coverage), greatly limiting states' authority over the employer group insurance market.[51] Hawaii is the only state that received a congressional exemption from ERISA for its employer mandate because Hawaii enacted its mandate legislation in 1974, before ERISA itself was enacted.

Both ERISA and the political and economic opposition by business groups to employer mandates led a few other states that in the late 1980s planned to enact mandate policies to abandon their efforts or place on hold implementation of the mandate, but in 2003 California enacted SB 2, a "pay or play" law that mandated employers with fifty or more workers to provide health benefits or pay into a state-administered fund that would furnish private health insurance for eligible workers and their families. Employer mandates have been vehemently opposed by employers, especially through interest groups representing small business and large low-wage employers. California's attempt to implement its pay-or-play legislation was thwarted by a referendum initiative that won very narrowly in November 2004 (49.2% in favor and 50.8% against), repealing SB 2. Inclusion of a provision that employers help pay for their workers' health insurance coverage also generated one of the most aggressive and effective lobbying campaigns against President Clinton's health care reform proposal—perhaps constituting the crushing blow.

# Frustrations on the Road to Universal Coverage

For at least the last half century, many Americans have found the concept of government health insurance an appealing way to cover the population. Funded by taxes and administered as a universal national program by the federal government, or by a combination of federal and state governments, such a social insurance program would pay physicians, hospitals, and other health care providers, eliminating the need for private health insurance. Since 1965, Medicare has made available virtually universal coverage for the elderly, but throughout much of the twentieth century repeated efforts to enact a universal system for the entire population have consistently foundered.

## Social Insurance: The Elusive Option

Social insurance systems have many advantages. Canada's single-payer system, a social insurance program that received a great deal of attention in the United States in the late 1980s and early 1990s, has been an efficient means of extending universal coverage with comprehensive health benefits.

The Canadian system has many advantages that attracted Americans at the beginning of the 1990s. Canada's provincial-run national program features universal coverage, very good access to primary care, patients' freedom to choose their own physicians, a superior record of controlling expenditures for physicians and hospitals, lower administrative costs, lower out-of-pocket costs for patients, and less restricted clinical autonomy for physicians.[52] However, steady reduction in federal support for the provincial programs, from 50 percent in 1971 to just 23 percent in 1997, exacerbated by the ever-rising cost of new medical technologies, has led to lower per capita spending, a shortage of medical personnel and facilities, and increased waiting time for specialty care and surgery. The decline in federal support and its sequelae yielded a dramatic decline in popular satisfaction with the system, with the proportion of the public saying "On the whole the system works pretty well, and only minor changes are needed to make it work better" falling from 56 percent in 1988 to just 20 percent in 1998. Growing dissatisfaction, though rooted in funding constraints, has created fertile ground for arguments by market-oriented policy makers that Canada should allow employers and individuals to supplement government-funded health care with private insurance and services, which is otherwise restricted. Nevertheless, Canada's public system retains strong popular support, even as conservative and liberal political leaders ramp up a national debate.[53]

Despite the advantages of social insurance and at least nominal support among the American public, social insurance proposals have not fared well in the United States since the enactment of Medicare. Although the single-payer proposals[54] introduced into Congress in the health care reform effort of the early 1990s received substantial support from some unions and consumer-based organizations, they could not overcome the powerful opposition of an array of interest groups representing health care providers, insurers, and business. In November 1994, California voters rejected (by a 73-27 margin) a Canadian-style single-payer ballot initiative that was opposed by a very well-funded campaign.

Given the particular political system of the United States, universal coverage reforms of all kinds are likely to continue to face stiff opposition, despite their demonstrated need. Adding to the difficulties, people with differing political viewpoints who agree on the need for universal coverage can disagree sharply on the means by which to achieve that end. Those who believe in market-based reforms tend to favor using federal tax credits for individual purchase of health insurance, thereby subsidizing consumer purchase.

However, research has shown that this alone would have little effect on reducing the number of uninsured nationwide. Most of the uninsured are in middle-income or low-income tax brackets, paying already low or, for those with very low earnings, no income tax. The savings from a tax credit would likely be just 3-6 percent of the actual cost of the premium required for purchasing health insurance.[55] Additionally, tax credits cost the government much more per dollar value of insurance provided ($2.36 to $12.98) than expanding public programs would ($1.17 to $1.33).[56] Finally, the Congressional Budget Office noted that tax credits would likely subsidize individuals who already have insurance and hurt those who would lose their insurance as employers dropped their offered coverage because of the federal government subsidy. This would result in very few of the uninsured gaining coverage.[57]

A growing number of states have taken it on themselves to expand public programs such as the Medicaid and SCHIP expansions discussed earlier in this chapter. Along with those programs, states (and in some cases counties) have developed their own insurance programs to fill in the gaps left between Medicaid and those who earn enough to either get coverage through their employer or buy it on their own. Maine launched Dirigo Health in June 2003 as a broad strategy to improve the state's health care system, which included universal access to health coverage. The state government entered into a public-private partnership with Blue Shield of Maine and Anthem Blue Cross to provide coverage, as well as mandating that employers offer coverage to their employees. However, funding streams and cost issues remained under discussion by an internal task force, as of September 2005.[58]

California also enacted an employer mandate in 2003, which was repealed a year later, as discussed earlier. Other efforts to expand coverage at the state level range from proposals for mandates on individuals to buy coverage to proposals for universal coverage of children, building on the relatively successful expansions of Medicaid and SCHIP. In 2006 Massachusetts enacted an individual mandate, with promised subsidies, and in 2005 Illinois enacted a program to offer some form of coverage, private or public, to all children.

## Political Barriers to Universal Coverage Reform

There are many barriers to adopting policy options that would lead to universal coverage. The effort at health care reform in the early 1990s started out with massive public support, but many forces combined to sap the political momentum for change. As we entered the 1990s, nine out of ten Americans, driven by fear of losing health insurance coverage and being unable to afford the rising cost of care, told pollsters that they believed the nation's health care system needed fundamental change or complete rebuilding.[59] The same proportion of chief executive officers of Fortune 500 corporations, whose attention was focused on their rising health benefit costs, supported fundamental change or complete rebuilding of the nation's health care system.[60] Three-fourths of these corporate executives said the problems could not be solved by companies working on their own and that government must play a bigger role. The leaders of four major national business organizations jointly appealed to the Congress to "do something" about health care costs.[61]

This impressive support for comprehensive reform dissipated rapidly as opposition interest groups eroded public support and threw their impressive weight against congressional efforts to find a consensus.[62] The Clinton administration created a cumbersome policy process to develop and promote its health care proposal, and (unlike reform opponents) the administration waged a feckless public campaign that did not mobilize grassroots support. Popular support for any specific proposal began to decline. Waning prospects for health care reform encouraged major employers to turn from policy change to other options to lower their own costs, including encouraging or forcing their employees into managed care and limiting their own costs by providing employees with a fixed contribution for health benefits.

As managed care plans tightly controlled utilization, they created a backlash in the late 1990s that, combined with extraordinary economic growth and a tight labor market, encouraged employers to seek looser arrangements for care.[63] Many employers and their employees turned increasingly to preferred provider organizations, but the PPOs in part fueled a rapid increase in health care spending, sending health insurance premiums up by double digits every year from 2001 to 2004, with no signs of relief on the horizon.[64] Increasingly, conservative political and business leaders became advocates for "consumer-directed health plans," which are designed to make patients and families more conscious of each dollar spent on health care by making them more directly responsible for the financial consequences of their health care utilization.

President Bush and many business groups soon went further, making high-deductible heath plans into their primary cost-control strategy.[65] These plans replace comprehensive health insurance with catastrophic coverage plans, often paired with "health savings accounts." In a high-deductible heath plan, the average annual deductible for an individual is $2,790 and the average share-of-cost for covered benefits is $2,857—a total of more than $5,600 in financial exposure—after paying premiums that average $1,204 for a twenty-year-old to $3,306 for a fifty-five-year-old. Family coverage imposes even more potential liability, totaling $10,593 in deductibles and out-of-pocket costs, plus premiums averaging $2,772 for a family with a twenty-year-old primary subscriber to $5,518 for a family with a fifty-five-year-old primary subscriber. High-deductible health plans have experienced rapid growth, as the number of covered lives more than doubled to one million between September 2004 and March 2005, according to America's Health Insurance Plans, the industry's trade association.[66]

There is substantial evidence that a large number of Americans are already underinsured. An estimated one-fourth to one-half of all personal bankruptcies in the United States are due to medical care costs. Between two-thirds and four-fifths of all these individuals had health insurance at the time they incurred their expenses, although people with medical insurance were more likely than those without it to have suffered a recent lapse in coverage.[67] Problems paying for medical care go well beyond the more than six hundred thousand medical care debt-related bankruptcies in 2002, the majority of them affecting people with health insurance.

There is growing evidence that many families with medical bills find it increasingly difficult to pay for them. One national survey estimated that nearly twenty million families experienced problems paying the bills they got for medical care, leading nearly two-thirds of them to report difficulty paying for other basic necessities such as rent, mortgage payments, transportation, and food.[68]

Underlying this successful frustration of health care reform efforts is (in addition to other factors discussed previously) the nation's political system itself. Compared to all parliamentary democracies that have developed a national health insurance system, the U.S. political system, institutions, and culture pose significant challenges to enacting major reforms.[69]

In the United States, political power is dispersed—divided between the executive (the government), the legislative body, and the judiciary—rather than concentrated, making it more difficult for the government to push through controversial reforms. In parliamentary democracies, the government represents a majority party or coalition in the parliament, creating a greater concentration of political power and fewer opportunities for blocking legislation that the government supports.

In the United States, the government (headed by the president or a governor) gains office through a winner-take-all election that reduces the opportunity for third parties to influence policy; this is quite a different situation from parliamentary systems. The winner-take-all provision encourages parties to "market" themselves to the broadest part of the electorate and discourages formation of political parties with a coherent policy or political commitment that is considered binding on a candidate elected in the party's name.

These systemic conditions make U.S. political parties weak institutions. They are organized as a loose coalition and more focused on fundraising than on policy guidance. The weakness of political parties opens a wide door to interest group influence in the policy process. The influence of interest groups has been greatly enhanced by the growing dominance of expensive television advertising in political campaigns and the dependence of parties and candidates on large donations from interest groups, corporations, and individuals with resources to give.[70] Thus a political party that "controls" the White House and the Congress—as the Democrats did in 1993 and 1994—lacks coherence and a means of enforcing its policy platform. In a parliamentary democracy, parties have more political coherence and more leverage over legislators elected on the party slate.

Compounding the weakness of parties, labor unions in the United States historically have played a more modest political role than they do in other industrial democracies. In most parliamentary democracies, the power of the labor-controlled party, generally representing working families and individuals, was a critical factor in enacting national health insurance. In the United States, throughout the twentieth century and at the beginning of the current century, labor tied itself to the Democratic Party, which it influences but does not control. In contrast to labor's relatively weak role, business-oriented interest groups in the United States assert a broad and powerful influence and have repeatedly undermined or vetoed efforts to enact national health insurance.

Finally, the United States has an ingrained political culture that supports weak government, a tradition that goes back to the very founding of the country. The United States has never developed either a strong civil service or a tradition of people looking to government to solve social problems—a different set of popular expectations than prevail in a number of other democracies.

There are additional political and economic barriers for states that try to tackle these problems outside a national framework. ERISA limits states' ability to regulate employer health and welfare benefit programs. Limited state fiscal resources create competition among constituencies and interest groups, especially when the state's fiscal condition is tight—and state residents who lack health insurance coverage tend not to be among the more influential political groups. Elected officials fear raising taxes, which would be needed to fund a health insurance subsidy, because higher taxes may encourage some businesses to move to other states or countries, and a vote for higher taxes certainly would be a weapon in a challenger's hands at the next election. Finally, many elected officials worry that generous public subsidies for health insurance coverage will attract a lot of low-income people to move to the state.

## In the Twenty-First Century: Important Roles for Research and Policy

The new century brought no signs of improvement in our system of providing and paying for health care coverage. If anything, health insurance coverage appears to be continuing its long and bumpy slide. Employer-funded health insurance seems to respond to changes in the economy but otherwise shows little evidence of expansion to uninsured working families. Changes in the labor market—the decline in manufacturing, the increase in low-wage service-sector jobs, and the increasing use of temporary and part-time employment arrangements—as well as the decline in real (inflation-adjusted) income among working families and individuals have, over time, eroded the foundation of the nation's voluntary private health insurance system. Many employers are raising employee contributions for health benefits, especially for family coverage, which makes the employee contribution increasingly unaffordable for low-wage workers and contributes to growing the ranks of the uninsured. In the long run, these structural changes are likely to undermine our reliance on private employment-based health insurance.

Compounding this diminishing private insurance coverage, recent declines in Medicaid coverage have offset the small gains in private insurance that resulted from improved employment in the strong economy. The growing number and proportion of the population who are completely uninsured places enormous burdens on those individuals and families; they must cope with reduced access and increased personal expense. But this problem also burdens others who help pay for whatever health services the uninsured receive; this includes employers and employees, who pay for private health insurance; and state and local taxpayers, who bear the financial burden of public hospitals and clinics for the medically indigent.

SCHIP and other modest public-sector incremental reforms help states address these problems. Taken together, SCHIP and Medicaid supply expanded federal and state resources to cover uninsured working families and (with ingenuity) individuals. The critical question is whether there is sufficient political will to maximize the use of these resources and extend affordable coverage to the entire population for good access to quality health care.

Despite the many political challenges, there is support for government to expand and strengthen health insurance coverage. Americans express strong support for universal coverage, although support for any particular approach is thin. In an election-focused public opinion poll in 2000, seven in ten adults said the federal government should help increase the number of Americans covered by health insurance, but only 38 percent were willing to pay additional taxes for a major government program to cover all of the uninsured.[71] Nevertheless, administration and congressional proposals to use federal funds to expand coverage receive broad support, and a number of states (including some with Republican governors, such as Wisconsin and Massachusetts) have taken significant steps to cover their uninsured residents. The path to universal coverage in the United States may well be through federal support and incentives to states to develop their own strategies to cover their entire population.[72] It almost certainly will require a strong grassroots campaign by a broad coalition that favors it, including senior citizens groups, consumer organizations, women's organizations, people of color, and labor unions, which have recently been undergoing a revitalization and resurgence.

Health services research continues to be important to help policy makers and the public understand the impact of these trends. Health services research has played an important role in identifying gaps in insurance coverage, monitoring the effects of those gaps, and modeling the impact of reform options on coverage and costs. The devolution of responsibility for funding and oversight of publicly financed programs enhances the importance of state- and local-level studies. In addition, studies of the effects of devolution and related policy changes on low-income populations and ethnic and racial minorities—especially studies that examine differences across states and local areas—are particularly important.

Studies of the effect of the type of insurance plan on access and on the process and quality of care become increasingly important as managed care and market-based prices dominate the health care field. The shift of both public and private purchasers to managed care exposes the gaps in knowledge as to which aspects of managed care promote effective use of services and which impede appropriate use.[73]

Policy intervention is needed to shore up growing gaps in coverage. Health services research is needed to inform policy analyses and development. Whether solutions are developed at the state level or the federal, through private-sector insurance and financing or through public programs and taxes, with social insurance programs such as Medicare or means-tested programs such as Medicaid and SCHIP, the United States cannot escape the need for fundamental reforms that extend coverage to its entire population.

# Notes

1. Walt, C. D., Proctor, B. D., and Lee, C. H. *Income, Poverty, and Health Insurance Coverage in the United States, 2004.* Washington, D.C.: U.S. Census Bureau, 2005.
2. Aday, L., Andersen, R., and Fleming, G. V. *Health Care in the U.S.: Equitable for Whom?* Thousand Oaks, Calif.: Sage, 1980; Aday, L., and others. *Evaluating the Health Care System: Effectiveness, Efficiency and Equity* (2nd ed.). Chicago: Health Administration Press, 1998; Marquis, M. S., and Long, S. H. "Reconsidering the Effect of Medicaid on Health Care Services Use." *Health Services Research*, 1996, *30*, 791–808; Lurie, N., and others. "Termination of Medi-Cal Benefits: A Follow-up Study One Year Later." *New England Journal of Medicine*, 1986, *314*, 1266–1268.
3. Measurement differences (between surveys in questions asked, and changes in questions over time within the same repeated survey,) make it difficult to track rates over the years. The data reported here are from a series of surveys that were conducted by the same federal agency (the Agency for Healthcare Research and Quality, which operated under a series of names during this period), the National Health Interview Survey, conducted annually by the National Center for Health Statistics, and that used generally similar methodologies over the years, thus increasing the comparability of the estimates during this twenty-year period. These estimates differ somewhat from those derived from the U.S. Census Bureau's Current Population Survey (CPS).
4. Walt, Proctor, and Lee (2005). Estimates in this paragraph are from the March 2004 Current Population Survey, conducted by the U.S. Census Bureau, analyzed by the UCLA Center for Health Policy Research.
5. Author's analysis of March 2004 Current Population Survey.
6. Author's analysis of March 2004 Current Population Survey.
7. Analysis of March 2004 Current Population Survey. See also Shen, Y.-C., and Zuckerman, S., "Why Is There State Variation in Employer-Sponsored Insurance?" *Health Affairs*, 2003, *22*(1), 241–251.
8. Mueller, M. S. "Private Health Insurance in 1973: A Review of Coverage, Enrollment, and Financial Experience." *Social Security Bulletin*, Feb. 1975, *38*, 21–40; Mueller, M. S. "Private Health Insurance in 1975: A Review of Coverage, Enrollment, and Financial Experience." *Social Security Bulletin*, June 1977, *40*, 3–21; Cambridge Research Institute. *Trends Affecting the U.S. Health Care System.* Washington, D.C.: Health Resources Administration, 1976.
9. Author's analysis of March 1995, 2001, and 2004 Current Population Survey by the UCLA Center for Health Policy Research.
10. Gabel, J., and others. "Health Benefits in 2005: Premium Increases Slow Down, Coverage Continues to Ebb." *Health Affairs*, 2005, *24*(3), 1273–1280; and Kaiser Family Foundation and Health Research and Educational Trust. *Employer Health Benefits, 2005 Annual Survey.* Menlo Park, Calif.: Henry J. Kaiser Family Foundation, 2004. See also Fronstin, P., Herman, R., and Greenwald, M., "Small Employers and Health Benefits: Findings from the

2002 Small Employer Health Benefits Survey." *EBRI Issue Brief,* 2003, *253,* 1–21; and Collins, S. R., Schoen, C., Doty, M. M., and Holmgren, A. L. "Job-Based Health Insurance in the Balance: Employer Views of Coverage in the Workplace." *Commonwealth Fund Issue Brief,* Mar. 2004.

11. Estimates for some years vary, depending on the data source. The estimates in this paragraph are from Cooper, P. F., and Steinberg Schone, B. "More Offers, Fewer Takers for Employment-Based Health Insurance: 1987 and 1996." *Health Affairs,* 1997, *16*(6), 142–149. See also Rice, T., and others. *Trends in Job-Based Health Insurance Coverage.* Los Angeles: UCLA Center for Health Policy Research, 1998; and Farber, H. S., and Levy, H. "Recent Trends in Employment-Sponsored Health Insurance Coverage: Are Bad Jobs Getting Worse?" (Working paper.) Princeton University Industrial Relations Section, July 1998; and analyses of February 1995, 1997, 1999, and 2001 Current Population Survey by the UCLA Center for Health Policy Research.

12. Gilmer, T., and Kronick, R., "It's the Premiums, Stupid: Projections of the Uninsured Through 2013." *Health Affairs,* Apr. 5, 2005 (e-pub). See also Fronstin, P. "The Erosion of Employment-Based Health Insurance: Costs, Structural and Non-Structural Changes in the Economy." Paper presented at annual meeting of the American Public Health Association, Nov. 1997; and U.S. General Accounting Office. *Employment-Based Health Insurance: Costs Increase and Family Coverage Decreases.* (GAO/HEHS-97–35.) Washington, D.C.: U.S. General Accounting Office, Feb. 1997; Kronick, R., and Gilmer, T. "Explaining the Decline in Health Insurance Coverage, 1979–1995." Unpublished paper, Oct. 1997.

13. *Employer Health Benefits. 1999 Annual Survey.* Menlo Park, Calif.: Kaiser Family Foundation, and Health Research and Educational Trust, Oct. 1999; and Fronstin, Herman, and Greenwald (2003), and author's analysis of February 1999 Current Population Survey.

14. Somers, H. W., and Somers, A. R. *Doctors, Patients and Health Insurance.* Washington, D.C.: Brookings Institution, 1961.

15. Marmor, T. R. *The Politics of Medicare.* Chicago: Aldine, 1970; Starr, P. *The Social Transformation of American Medicine.* New York: Basic Books, 1982.

16. "Brief Summaries of Medicare and Medicaid." Baltimore, Md.: Centers for Medicare and Medicaid Services (CMS), November 5, 2005 [http://www.cms.hhs.gov/MedicareProgram RatesStats/downloads/MedicareMedicaidSummaries2005.pdf] (accessed Aug. 27, 2006); "Medicare Enrollees, Selected Years." CMS, [http://www.cms.hhs.gov/researchers/ pubs/datacompendium /2003/03pg30.pdf] (accessed Sept. 21, 2005); "Program Benefit Payments, Selected Fiscal Years." CMS, [http://www.cms.hhs.gov/ researchers/pubs/data compendium/2003/03pg3.pdf] (accessed Sept. 21, 2005).

17. Mitchell, J. B., and Khandker, R. K. "Black-White Treatment Differences in Acute Myocardial Infarction." *Health Care Financing Review,* 1995, *17,* 61–70; Davis, K. "Equal Treatment and Unequal Benefits: The Medicare Program." *Milbank Memorial Fund Quarterly/Health and Society,* 1975, *53,* 449–488; Long, S. H., and Settle, R. F. "Medicare and the Disadvantaged Elderly: Objectives and Outcomes." *Milbank Memorial Fund Quarterly/Health and Society,* 1984, *62,* 609–656; Link, C. R., Long, S. H., and Settle, R. F. "Equity and the Utilization of Health Services by the Medicare Elderly." *Journal of Human Resources,* 1982, *17,* 195–212; Physician Payment Review Commission (PPRC). *Annual Report to Congress, 1994.* Washington, D.C.: Physician Payment Review Commission, 1994; Wenneker, M. B., and Epstein, A. M. "Racial Inequalities in the Use of Procedures for Patients with Ischemic Heart Disease in Massachusetts." *Journal of the American Medical Association,* 1989, *261,* 253–257; McBean, A. M., and Gornick, M. "Differences by Race in the Rates of Procedures Performed in Hospitals for

Medicare Beneficiaries." *Health Care Financing Review,* 1994, *15,* 77–90; Ayanian, J. Z., and others. "Acute Myocardial Infarction: Process of Care and Clinical Outcomes." *Journal of the American Medical Association,* 1993, *269,* 2642–2646.

18. Cubanski, J., and others. *Medicare Chartbook* (3rd ed.). Kaiser Family Foundation, Summer 2005. [www.kff.org] (accessed Sept. 21, 2005).

19. Cubanski and others (2005), p. 29; Biles, B., Nichols, L., and Cooper, B. "The Cost of Privatization: Extra Payments to Medicare Advantage Plans." (Issue brief.) New York: Commonwealth Fund, 2004.

20. Cubanski and others (2005), p. 29; Biles, B., Dallek, G., and Nicholas, L. H., "Medicare Advantage: Déjà Vu All over Again?" *Health Affairs,* Dec., 2004, *15,* W4586-W4597; Booske, B. C., Lynch, J., and Riley, G. "Impact of Medicare Managed Care Market Withdrawal on Beneficiaries." *Health Care Financing Review,* 2002, *24*(1), 95–115; Landon, B. E., and others. "Comparison of Performance of Traditional Medicare vs. Medicare Managed Care." *Journal of the American Medical Association,* 2004, *291*(14), 1744–1752.

21. "Brief Summaries of Medicare and Medicaid" CMS (2005).

22. Health Resources Administration (HRA). *Health of the Disadvantaged. Chart Book II.* DHHS pub. no. (HRA) 80–633. Washington, D.C.: U.S. Government Printing Office, Sept. 1980; Aday, L., and Andersen, R. "Equity of Access to Medical Care: A Conceptual and Empirical Overview." In *Securing Access to Health Care: The Ethical Implications of Differences in the Availability of Health Services.* Washington, D.C.: President's Commission for the Study of Ethical Problems in Medicine and Biomedical and Behavioral Research, 1983.

23. Berk, M. L., Schur, C. L., and Cantor, J. C. "Ability to Obtain Health Care: Recent Estimates from the Robert Wood Johnson Foundation National Access to Care Survey." *Health Affairs,* Fall 1995, *14*(3), 139–146; Schoen, C., and others. "Insurance Matters for Low Income Adults: Results from a Five State Survey." *Health Affairs,* 1997, *16*(5), 163–171; Millman, M. (ed.). *Access to Health Care in America.* Washington, D.C.: National Academy Press, Institute of Medicine, 1993; Newacheck, P. "Access to Ambulatory Care for Poor Persons." *Health Services Research,* 1988, *23,* 401–419; Wilensky, G. R., and Berk, M. L. "Health Care, the Poor, and the Role of Medicaid." *Health Affairs,* 1982, *1,* 93–100; Kasper, J. D. "Health Status and Utilization: Differences by Medicaid Coverage and Income." *Health Care Financing Review,* Summer 1986, *7,* 1–17; Freeman, H. E., and Corey, C. R. "Insurance Status and Access to Health Services Among Poor Persons." *Health Services Research,* 1993, *28*(5), 531–541; Nelson, K. M., and others. "The Association Between Health Insurance Coverage and Diabetes Care: Data from the 2000 Behavioral Risk Factor Surveillance System." *Health Services Research,* 2005, *40*(2), 361–372; Almeida, R. A., Dubay, L. C., and Ko, G. "Access to Care and Use of Health Services by Low-income Women." *Health Care Finance Review,* Summer 2001, *22*(4), 27–47; Simpson, L., and others. "Health Care for Children and Youth in the United States: Annual Report on Patterns of Coverage, Utilization, Quality, and Expenditures by Income." *Ambulatory Pediatrics,* 2005, *5*(1), 6–44.

24. Lurie, N., Ward, N. B., Shapiro, M. F., and Brook, R. H. "Termination from Medi-Cal: Does It Affect Health?" *New England Journal of Medicine,* 1984, *311,* 480–484; Lurie, N., and others. "Termination of Medi-Cal Benefits: A Follow-up Study One Year Later." *New England Journal of Medicine,* 1986, *314,* 1266–1268.

25. Eligibility information from NGA Center for Best Practices. "MCH Update 2002: State Health Coverage for Low-Income Pregnant Women, Children, and Parents." June 2003; benefits information from Kaiser Commission on Medicaid and the Uninsured. "Medicaid: An Overview of Spending on 'Mandatory' vs. 'Optional' Populations and Services."

June 2005; other information from Centers for Medicare and Medicaid Services. "Medicaid At-a-Glance 2003." [http://www.cms.hhs.gov/states/maaghm.asp] (accessed July 26, 2005).

26. Rowland, D., Lyons, B., and Edwards, J. "Medicaid: Health Care for the Poor in the Reagan Era." *Annual Review of Public Health*, 1988, *9*, 427–450; Rosenbaum, S., and Darnell, J. *Medicaid Section 1115 Demonstration Waivers: Approved and Proposed Activities as of November 1994.* Washington, D.C.: Kaiser Commission on the Future of Medicaid, 1994.

27. NGA Center for Best Practices. "MCH Update 2002." June 2003.

28. Loranger, L., and Lipson, D. *The Medicaid Expansions for Pregnant Women and Children.* Washington, D.C.: Alpha Center, 1995; Ray, W. A., Mitchel, E. F. Jr., and Piper, J. M. "Effect of Medicaid Expansions on Preterm Birth." *American Journal of Preventive Medicine*, 1997, *13*(4), 292–297; Dubay, L., and others. "Changes in Prenatal Care Timing and Low Birth Weight by Race and Socioeconomic Status: Implications for the Medicaid Expansions for the Medicaid Expansions for Pregnant Women." *Health Services Research*, 2001, *36*(2), 373–398; Guillory, V. J., and others. "Prenatal Care and Infant Birth Outcomes Among Medicaid Recipients." *Journal of Health Care for the Poor and Underserved*, 2003, *14*(2), 272–289; Hessol, N. A., Vittinghoff, E., and Fuentes-Afflick, E. "Reduced Risk of Inadequate Prenatal Care in the Era After Medicaid Expansions in California." *Medical Care*, 2004, *42*(5), 416–422; and Kaestner, R., Dubay, L., and Kenney, G. "Managed Care and Infant Health: An Evaluation of Medicaid in the U.S." *Social Science and Medicine*, 2005, *60*, 1815–1833.

29. Author's analysis of March 1995 and 1999 Current Population Survey data.

30. Krebs-Carter, M., and Holahan, J. "State Strategies for Covering Uninsured Adults." (Discussion paper.) Washington, D.C.: Urban Institute, Feb. 2000; Holl, J. L., Slack, K. S., and Stevens, A. B. "Welfare Reform and Health Insurance: Consequences for Parents." *American Journal of Public Health*, 2005, *95*(2), 279–285.

31. Perry, M. J., Stark, E., and Valdez, R. B. *Barriers to Medi-Cal Enrollment and Ideas for Improving Enrollment: Findings from Eight Focus Groups in California with Parents of Potentially Eligible Children.* Menlo Park, Calif.: Henry J. Kaiser Family Foundation, 1998.

32. For evidence of Medicaid's stigmatizing welfare image, see Perry, Stark, and Valdez (1998).

33. Sheils, J., and Haught, R. "The Cost of Tax-Exempt Health Benefits in 2004." *Health Affairs*, Feb. 25, 2004 Web Exclusive, W4-106–W4-112 [http://content.healthaffairs.org/cgi/content/full/hlthaff.w4.106v1/DC1].

34. Kronick, R., and Gilmer, T. "Insuring Low-Income Adults: Does Public Coverage Crowd out Private?" *Health Affairs*, 2002, *21*(1), 225–239; Dubay, L., and Kenney, G. "Expanding Public Health Insurance to Parents: Effects on Children's Coverage Under Medicaid." *Health Services Research*, 2003, *38*(5), 1283–1301; and Busch, S. H., and Duchovny, N. "Family Coverage Expansions: Impact on Insurance Coverage and Health Care Utilization of Parents." *Journal of Health Economics*, 2005, *24*, 876–890.

35. "Medicaid Managed Care Enrollment as of June 30, 2004." Fact Sheet. Centers for Medicare and Medicaid Services. [http://www.cms.hhs.gov/medicaid/managedcare/mcsten04.pdf] (accessed July 27, 2005).

36. "State Waiver Programs and Demonstrations." Center for Medicare and Medicaid Services. [http://www.cms.hhs.gov/medicaid/waivers/waivermap.asp] (accessed July 27, 2005); "States with Comprehensive Health Care Reform Demonstrations." Dec. 31, 2004. Washington, D.C.: CMS Website.

37. CMS. "State Waiver Programs and Demonstrations." Website, 2005.

38. Kaiser Commission on Medicaid and the Uninsured. "Medicaid Enrollment and Spending Trends." Fact Sheet, June 2005.

39. Kaiser Commission on Medicaid and the Uninsured (2005).

40. Rosenbaum, Shin, Markus, and Darnell (2000); Kaiser Commission on the Future of Medicaid. *Medicaid and Managed Care: Lessons from the Literature.* Menlo Park, Calif.: Henry J. Kaiser Family Foundation, 1995; General Accounting Office. *Medicaid: States Turn to Managed Care to Improve Access and Control Costs.* (GAO/HRD-93–46.) Washington, D.C.: U.S. General Accounting Office, Mar. 1993; Coughlin, T. A., and Long, S. K. "Effects of Medicaid Managed Care on Adults." *Medical Care,* 2000, *38*(4), 433–446; Landon, B. E., and others. "The Evolution of Quality Management in State Medicaid Agencies: A National Survey of States with Comprehensive Managed Care Programs." *Joint Commission Journal on Quality Improvement,* 2002, *28*(2), 72–82; Garrett, B., Davidoff, A. J., and Yemane, A. "Effects of Medicaid Managed Care Programs on Health Services Access and Use." *Health Services Research,* 2003, *38*(2), 575–594; and Garrett, B., and Zuckerman, S. "National Estimates of the Effects of Mandatory Medicaid Managed Care Programs on Health Care Access and Use, 1997–1999." *Medical Care,* 2005, *43*(7), 649–657.

41. Kaiser Commission on Medicaid and the Uninsured. "Enrolling Uninsured Low-Income Children in Medicaid and SCHIP." Fact Sheet, Mar. 2005.

42. Cunningham, P. J., Hadley, J., and Reschovsky, J. "The Effects of SCHIP on Children's Health Insurance Coverage: Early Evidence from the Community Tracking Survey." *Medical Care Research and Review,* 2002, *59*(4), 359–383; and Lo Sasso, A. T., and Buchmueller, T. C. "The Effect of the State Children's Health Insurance Program on Health Insurance Coverage." *Journal of Health Economics,* 2004, *23,* 1059–1082.

43. Davidoff, A., Kenney, G., and Dubay, L. "Effects of the State Children's Health Insurance Program Expansions on Children with Chronic Health Conditions." *Pediatrics,* 2005, *116*(1), 34–42.

44. Kempe, A., and others. "Changes in Access, Utilization, and Quality of Care After Enrollment into a State Child Health Insurance Plan." *Pediatrics,* 2005, *115*(2), 364–371.

45. Ross, D. C., and Cox, L. "Beneath the Surface: Barriers Threaten to Slow Progress on Expanding Health Coverage of Children and Families." Kaiser Commission on Medicaid and the Uninsured, publication no. 7191, Oct. 2004.

46. Thorpe, K. "Expanding Employment-Based Health Insurance: Is Small Group Reform the Answer?" *Inquiry,* 1992, *29,* 128–136; Jensen, G. A. and Morrisey, M. A. "Small Group Reform and Insurance Provision by Small Firms, 1989–1995." *Inquiry,* 1999, *36*(2), 176–187; and Davidoff, A., Blumberg, L., and Nichols, L. "State Health Insurance Market Reforms and Access to Insurance for High-Risk Employees." *Journal of Health Economics,* 2005, *24*(4), 725–750.

47. Riley, T. "State Health Reform and the Role of 1115 Waivers." *Health Care Financing Review,* 1995, *16,* 139–149.

48. *Employer Health Benefits. 2004 Annual Survey,* Menlo Park, Calif.: Kaiser Family Foundation, and Health Research and Educational Trust, Sept. 2004. See also Small Business Administration. *The State of Small Business: A Report of the President.* Washington, D.C.: U.S. Government Printing Office, 1987.

49. Long, S. H., and Marquis, S. M. "Pooled Purchasing: Who Are the Players?" *Health Affairs,* July–Aug. 1999, *18,* 105–111.

50. Butler, P. *ERISA Preemption Primer.* Washington, D.C.: Alpha Center, and National Academy for State Health Policy, 2000. See also Butler, P. *ERISA Implications for SB 2.* Oakland, Calif.: California HealthCare Foundation, Mar. 2004.

51. *Employer Health Benefits 2004.*

52. Fuchs, V. R., and Hahn, J. S. "How Does Canada Do It? A Comparison of Expenditures for Physicians' Services in the United States and Canada." *New England Journal of Medicine,* 1990, *323,* 884–890; Evans, R. G., and others. "Controlling Health Expenditures: the Canadian Reality." *New England Journal of Medicine,* 1989, *320,* 571–577; U.S. Congressional Budget Office. "Single-Payer and All-Payer Health Insurance Systems Using Medicare's Payment Rates." CBO Staff Memorandum. Washington, D.C.: U.S. Congressional Budget Office, Apr. 1993; Woolhandler, S., and Himmelstein, D. U. "The Deteriorating Administrative Efficiency of the U.S. Health Care System." *New England Journal of Medicine,* 1991, *324,* 1253–1258; General Accounting Office. *Canadian Health Insurance: Lessons for the United States.* (GAO/HRD-91-90.) Washington, D.C.: U.S. Government Accounting Office, June 1991; Hayes, G. J., Hayes, C., and Dykstra, T. "Physicians Who Have Practiced in Both the U.S. and Canada Compare Systems." *American Journal of Public Health,* 1993, *83,* 1544–1548; Evans, R. G. "Going for the Gold: The Redistributive Agenda Behind Market-Based Health Care Reform." *Journal of Health Politics, Policy, and Law,* 1997, *22,* 427–466; Evans, R. G., and Roos, N. P. "What Is Right About the Canadian Health Care System?" *Milbank Quarterly,* 1999, *77,* 393–399; Commission on the Future of Health Care in Canada. *Building Values: The Future of Health Care in Canada—Final Report.* Ottawa: Commission on the Future of Health Care in Canada, Nov. 2002; Deber, R. B. "Health Care Reform: Lessons from Canada." *American Journal of Public Health,* 2003, *93,* 20–24.

53. Iglehart, J. K. "Revisiting the Canadian Health Care System." *New England Journal of Medicine,* 2000, *342,* 2007–2012; Donelan, K., and others. "The Cost of Health System Change: Public Discontent in Five Nations." *Health Affairs,* May-June 1999, *18,* 206–216.

54. Bills introduced into the U.S. Senate by Paul Wellstone and into the House of Representatives by Jim McDermott and John Conyers to create a Canadian-style single-payer system, and the bill introduced into the House of Representatives by Pete Stark to make Medicare universally available.

55. Glied, S., and Remler, D. K. "The Effect of Health Savings Accounts on Health Insurance Coverage." (Issue Brief.) Commonwealth Fund, Apr. 2005.

56. Gruber, J. "Tax Policy for Health Insurance." *NBER Working Paper Series,* Working Paper 10977. National Bureau of Economic Research, Dec. 2004.

57. "Budget Options, February 2005." Washington, D.C.: Congressional Budget Office, 2005; "How Many People Lack Health Insurance and for How Long?" Washington, D.C.: Congressional Budget Office, May 2003.

58. "Payers, State Officials Disagree over Funding for Maine's DirigoChoice Program." Kaiser Daily Health Policy Report. [www.kaisernetwork.org] (accessed Sept. 2, 2005); [www.dirigohealth.maine.gov] (accessed Sept. 2, 2005); "Massachusetts Officials Announce New Regulations for 'Free-Care' Program." Kaiser Daily Health Policy Report. [www.kaisernetwork.org] (accessed Aug. 4, 2005).

59. Blendon, R. J., and Taylor, H. "Views on Health Care: Public Opinion in Three Nations." *Health Affairs,* Spring 1989, *8,* 149–157.

60. Cantor, J. C., and others. "Business Leaders' Views on American Health Care." *Health Affairs,* 1991, *10,* 98–105.

61. Rosenblatt, R. A. "Business Groups Plead for Health-Care Support." *Los Angeles Times,* Nov. 16, 1989, p. A20.

62. West, M. W., Heith, D., and Goodwin, C. "Harry and Louise Go to Washington: Political Advertising and Health Care Reform." *Journal of Health Politics, Policy, and Law,* 1996, *21,* 35–68; Podhorzer, M. "Unhealthy Money: Health Reform and the 1994 Elections." *International*

*Journal of Health Services*, 1995, *25*, 393–401; and *Well-Healed: Inside Lobbying for Health Care Reform*. Washington, D.C.: Center for Public Integrity, 1994.

63. Mechanic, D. "The Rise and Fall of Managed Care." *Journal of Health and Social Behavior*, 2004, *45*(Suppl.), 76–86; and Marquis, M. S., Rogowski, J. A., and Escarce, J. J. "The Managed Care Backlash: Did Consumers Vote with Their Feet?" *Inquiry*, 2004–05, *41*(4), 376–390.

64. *Employer Health Benefits 2004 Annual Survey*. Kaiser Family Foundation and Health Research and Educational Trust, Sept. 2004.

65. Robinson, J. C. "Reinvention of Health Insurance in the Consumer Era." *Journal of the American Medical Association*, 2004, *291*(15), 1880–1886; Draper, D. A., and Claxton, G. "Managed Care Redux: Health Plans Shift Responsibilities to Consumers." (Issue brief.) Center for Studying Health System Change, Mar. 2004; Davis, K. "Will Consumer-Directed Health Care Improve System Performance?" *Health Services Research*, 2004, *39*(4, part II), 1219–1233.

66. "Number of HSA Plans Exceeded One Million in March 2005." Washington, D.C.: America's Health Insurance Plans, Mar. 2005.

67. Levitt, J. C. "Transfer of Financial Risk and Alternative Financing Solutions." *Journal of Health Care Finance*, 2004, *30*(4), 21–32; Jacoby M., Sullivan T., and Warren E. "Medical Problems and Bankruptcy Filings." *Norton's Bankruptcy Adviser*, May 2000, 1, 2, 10; Himmelstein, D. U., Warren, E., Thorne, D., and Woolhandler, S. "Illness and Injury as Contributors to Bankruptcy." *Health Affairs*, Feb. 2, 2005 [e-pub, ahead of print].

68. May, J. H., and Cunningham, P. J., "Tough Trade-Offs: Medical Bills, Family Finances and Access to Care." Issue brief no. 85, Center for Studying Health System Change, June 2004. See also Costello, D. "At What Cost?" *Los Angeles Times*, Apr. 4, 2005.

69. See Weissert, C. S., and Weissert, W. G. *Governing Health: The Politics of Health Policy*. Baltimore, Md.: Johns Hopkins University Press, 1996; Skocpol, T. *Boomerang: Clinton's Health Security Effort and the Turn Against Government in U.S. Politics*. New York: Norton, 1996; Morone, J. A. *The Democratic Wish: Popular Participation and the Limits of American Government*. New York: Basic Books, 1990; Navarro, V. "Why Some Countries Have National Health Insurance, Others Have National Health Services, and the U.S. Has Neither." *Social Science and Medicine*, 1989 *28*, 887–898; Rothman, D. J. "A Century of Failure: Health Care Reform in America." *Journal of Health Politics*, Policy, and Law, 1993, *18*, 271–286.

70. Corrado, A., and others (eds.). *Campaign Finance Reform: A Sourcebook*. Washington, D.C.: Brookings Institution, 1997.

71. Morin, R., and Broder, D. S. "A Health Care Muddle." *Washington Post*, July 28, 2000, p. A01; McGregor, D. "Deciphering the Polls on the Health Issue." *Congressional Quarterly Weekly Report*, 1994, *52*, 1846; Blendon, R. J., and Brodie, M. "Public Opinion and Health Policy." In T. J. Litman and L. S. Robins (eds.), *Health Politics and Policy* (3rd ed.). Albany, N.Y.: Delmar, 1997.

72. See "The Health Security for All Americans Act" (S. 2888, 106th Congress) by Sen. Paul Wellstone (D-Minn.).

73. Bindman, A. B., and Gold, M. R. (eds.). "Measuring Access to Care Through Population-Based Surveys in a Managed Care Environment." *Health Services Research*, 1998, *33*(3, part 2), 611–766.

PART TWO

COSTS OF HEALTH CARE

CHAPTER FIVE

# MEASURING HEALTH CARE COSTS AND TRENDS

## Thomas H. Rice

In 2006, U.S. health care expenditures are expected to eclipse the $2 trillion mark. It is difficult to fathom such a large number. To put it in perspective, suppose you lined up a trillion dollar bills end to end. They would stretch all the way to the sun—and back to earth![1]

This chapter focuses on how these health care expenditures are measured and then discusses the trends. It concludes with a discussion of whether health care cost control is even necessary, as a bridge to the following chapter, where particular strategies are evaluated. Although data and measurement may seem a bit pedestrian to the analyst interested in proceeding quickly to policy issues, this is an unfortunate viewpoint. Accurate data on national health care spending are necessary in order to enact appropriate health policy reforms. (A blunter reason for accurate data that may ring true to the policy analyst comes from computer programming: "garbage in, garbage out.") Once these tools are in hand, Chapter Six can analyze alternative methods of containing health care expenditures.

## Measuring Health Care Expenditures

As just noted, understanding measurement is essential if one is to fully appreciate many issues that are currently in the forefront of health policy. To give one example, debate continues about whether the United States—a country that relies more heavily than others on markets in its health care system—has been as successful as other countries in controlling health expenditures. Resolution of this ostensibly straightforward issue would yield insight as to the potential savings or losses, if any, that might accrue if the United States adopted some aspects of other countries' organization and financing systems. But to ascertain an accurate answer to this question, it is necessary to understand how health expenditures are compiled in various countries as well as how they *can* be compared.[2] This section of the chapter discusses a number of key issues concerning measurement of health care expenditures.

## Expenditures Versus Costs

Most policy discussions employ the term *costs* rather than expenditures; indeed, the next chapter also adopts this convenience. It is important to understand that the two concepts are hardly the same.

Expenditures, of course, mean how much is spent on a particular thing. As discussed in Chapter Four, in a fee-for-service system expenditures are simply the product of unit prices and the quantity of goods or services purchased. Total expenditures can then be broken down in a number of ways, such as by type of service (for example, hospital expenditures, physician expenditures) or by payer source (private insurers, Medicare, out-of-pocket).

In contrast, costs apply to the production process. Specifically, the term refers to the value of resources used in producing a good or service. There are two distinct definitions of cost: accounting and economic. The accounting definition includes only the value of the resources used in production (that is, labor and capital). The difference between the sales revenue from a good or service and the accounting cost is defined as net revenue or profit.

This differs from the economic definition of cost. To an economist, the term includes not only the value of resources expended in the production process but in addition a "normal" return on investment.[3] Using their definition, economists predict that in a competitive market profit levels are near zero—that is, a typically efficient producer garners only a normal rate of return on investment. The persistence of an economic profit level far above zero over a long period of time may indicate the existence of "market failure," which in turn might call for government policy intervention.

Accounting and economic profits are therefore related to each other. The latter is approximately equal to the former minus a normal rate of return on investment.[4] But both definitions of *cost* differ from the definition of *expenditure*. The distinction is shown in Figure 5.1; for simplicity, we use the economic definition of *cost* and compare that to the definition of *expenditure*. In the figure, the horizontal axis shows the quantity of a particular good or service; the vertical axis, sales prices

### FIGURE 5.1. DISTINCTION BETWEEN
### ACCOUNTING AND ECONOMIC PROFITS.

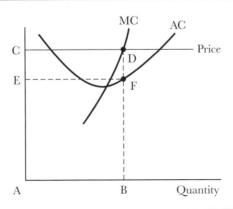

and production costs. MC refers to marginal costs—the cost of producing the last unit of output. AC is average cost of output, and Price is the selling price. Both of the cost curves include a normal rate of return on investment.

Health care *expenditures* are equal to the rectangle ABCD, which is simply the selling price multiplied by the quantity sold, AB. In contrast, economic *costs* are shown by a smaller rectangle, ABEF; this is average costs (AE) multiplied by the quantity sold (AB). In this example, expenditure exceeds cost by the rectangle CDEF. This implies that excess profits are being obtained by firms in the industry. Other firms therefore may be stimulated to enter the market to reap these profits, which in turn may drive down price and restore profit to a normal level. If this does not occur, then some form of government intervention may be necessary to correct market failure.

With these distinctions in mind, we can address the question of whether we should spend most of our effort analyzing health care cost or expenditure. Although both are useful, it turns out to be considerably easier to conduct analyses of the entire health care system using the concept of expenditure. This is because it is extremely difficult to obtain reliable data on cost; private firms are rarely expected to report their internal cost data to any sort of governmental body. One exception is Medicare hospital costs, because such data are collected by the federal government. But for other sectors—physician care, pharmaceuticals, and the like (and for services that are covered by private insurers rather than Medicare and Medicaid)—reliable data on costs are exceedingly difficult to obtain. The remainder of this chapter, then, focuses on measurement and trends in health care expenditure rather than cost. First, however, we discuss measuring changes in unit price.

## Measuring Health Care Prices

The most common measure of health care prices in the United States is the medical care component of the Consumer Price Index (CPI). The CPI, which is published monthly by the Bureau of Labor Statistics, gives information on the change in prices charged to urban consumers for a variety of consumer goods and consumers.[5]

To obtain the index, the CPI begins with a common "market basket" of goods and services. The monthly price data are obtained from urban localities that represent about 80 percent of the U.S. population. To form the index, each item in the market basket is given a weight representing its relative importance in the spending patterns of urban consumers. An index is then formed that compares the change in prices in a current time period to a base period (usually 1982–1984) whose index value is set to a value of 100. For example, in 2003 the medical care component of the CPI had a value of 297.1, which means that medical care prices were nearly three times what they were during the base period.

As shown later in this chapter when trends are presented, the medical care component of the CPI is further subdivided into several categories, making it possible to monitor inflation in various health-related markets. The two main subcategories are medical care services and medical care commodities. Within services, there are separate indices constructed for physicians' services, dental services, eye care, other medical professionals, hospital rooms, other inpatient services, and hospital outpatient services. Within commodities, separate indices exist for prescription drugs, over-the-counter drugs and medical supplies, internal and respiratory over-the-counter drugs, and medical equipment and supplies.

There are a number of limitations to the CPI.[6] First, and perhaps most important, the CPI measures change in price, not in expenditure. It does not take into account change in the quantity of services provided, only the price.

Second, the CPI measures changes in prices, not price levels. The index cannot be used to compare difference in health care prices among parts of the country. Suppose, for example, that in 2003 the medical component of the CPI was 304 in New York City, and 290 in Los Angeles. All that one could say is that prices rose faster in New York than Los Angeles since the base year in which the index was set to 100. It cannot be concluded that health care prices necessarily are lower in Los Angeles than New York.

Third, the CPI measures the price charged, not the price received by a producer. This is a critical distinction because of the prevalence of discounts offered by providers to managed care plans such as preferred provider organizations (PPOs). In some competitive parts of the country, such as California, providers' list or billed charges are illusory; almost no one pays them. However, these prices are exactly what is measured by the CPI. What this means is that the CPI might overstate the amount of medical care inflation in certain parts of the country because over time the true price of care has deviated further below the billed charge.

Fourth, the CPI measures changes in price for a fixed market basket of consumer goods. In fact, the entire notion of the CPI is based on the existence of such an apples-to-apples comparison. By using a standard market basket of goods, it is possible to determine how price alone has changed. But this also leads to two difficulties. First, people do change their consumption habits over time, so the market basket being measured by the CPI may become increasingly irrelevant. The Bureau of Labor Statistics (BLS), the federal agency responsible for the index, is dealing with this problem by updating the composition of the market basket more frequently than it did previously. The second difficulty is that the CPI does not take into account change in the quality of goods and services produced—although again, BLS is currently grappling with this problem. To illustrate this issue, note that an increase in per diem hospital charges over the last twenty years is likely to be exaggerated by the CPI. Over this period, hospital rooms have become much more expensive not only from inflation but also because of enhancements in the type of services and facilities available to the hospital patient. In theory, the CPI should hold these changes constant and look only at price inflation of hospital care of a given quality. This has not been the practice, however.

Fifth, the CPI measures only changes in consumers' expenditures (premiums plus out-of-pocket payments). If, as in the case of hospital care, a majority of expenditures are not paid out of pocket, then the index does not capture the majority of underlying inflation. This could bias the index figures because there has been a gradual movement away from out-of-pocket expenditure toward more employer and government payment, which is not included in the CPI.[7] (We may now be witnessing a reversal of this trend with increased patient cost sharing as part of many job-based health insurance plans, but at the time of writing the aggregate data are not clear on this point.)

These caveats are not meant as criticism; any differently configured index would raise a host of other problems. Rather, the limitations of the CPI must simply be understood when using the index.

## Measuring Expenditures

This section examines U.S. expenditures and international comparisons.

***U.S. Expenditures.*** There are many sources of data on U.S. health expenditure; space does not permit separate discussion of each. Rather, we focus on the primary source: the national health accounts produced by the Office of the Actuary of the Centers for Medicare and Medicaid Services (CMS), which is housed in the U.S. Department of Health and Human Services. Trends in these data are presented later in the chapter.

Data on U.S. national health expenditures are published regularly—usually annually—in journals such as *Health Affairs* and the *Health Care Financing Review.*[8] The data for one year can be viewed best as a matrix. Each row of the matrix represents the group that spends the money, whereas each column indicates the provider of services that receives the funds. (An example is presented later in the chapter, as Table 5.5.) A cell in the matrix therefore represents how much a particular payer (for example, a private insurer) spends on a specific service (say, hospital care). Because these same data are compiled annually, by comparing the matrices of several years one can calculate the rate of change in expenditure in various components of the health care sector.

In viewing the matrix, one might think that the data come from a single, consistent source. They do not. Literally dozens of sources are used to piece the matrices together. Some of the data are collected relatively systematically, but others are not. For example, data from the Medicare program are systemically collected by CMS through the Medicare Statistical System (MSS). One file in the MSS, the hospital insurance claims file, contains information on each beneficiary's spending for Part A (hospital) services, while the supplementary Medicare insurance file includes similar data for Part B (primarily physician) services. Although somewhat more unwieldy, Medicaid data are also collected from the states in a consistent format by HCFA.

But because there are no national data collection requirements for private insurers, other aspects of the matrices have to be pieced together from multiple data sources. Some are more systematic than others. Hospital expenditures, for example, largely come from a single source: the American Hospital Association's annual survey of hospitals. But out-of-pocket expenditures come from any number of sources: a consumer expenditures survey, conducted by the Bureau of Labor Statistics; periodic surveys of nursing homes, conducted by the National Center for Health Statistics; surveys about home health care, conducted by the Visiting Nurse Association; physician and dentist surveys, conducted by the American Medical Association and the American Dental Association; data about outpatient clinic services, collected by the Bureau of the Census; and information about Community Health Centers, collected by the Health Resources and Services Administration. As discussed at the end of the chapter, the lack of a consistent data source makes it difficult to successfully administer certain types of health care reform, particularly regulatory ones such as national expenditure targets.

Over the years, there have been various revisions to the national health accounts. The most noteworthy ones, which applied to the estimates beginning in 1988, employed new data sources and produced a higher level of detail.[9]

There are, nevertheless, a number of problems, most of which are caused by the lack of source data:

- The accounts are unable to distinguish between some inpatient and outpatient expenditures (for example, salaried physician care counted as hospital rather than physician expenditure).
- Premium expenditures by consumers (Medicare Part B payments, private insurance premiums) are included as payment made by insurers rather than as out-of-pocket expenditure by consumers.
- Some capital expenditures are double-counted.

These and other issues, as well as recommendations for improving the accounts, have been discussed in a report published by a technical advisory panel.[10]

***International Comparisons.*** The primary source of data on international health care spending for more than two dozen developed (and some developing) countries is collected by the Organization for Economic Cooperation and Development (OECD), which is based in Paris. These data are published in periodic articles in the journal *Health Affairs* and also appear in the annual government publication *Health United States.*[11] Data from the OECD database are presented later in the chapter.

The previous discussion about U.S. health expenditures focused on the lack of a consistent data source. As can be imagined, the problem of lacking consistent data is even greater when one compares data from two dozen countries. Those who compile the OECD data have attempted to make them reliable by disseminating definitions of key terms as well as common accounting principles to all member countries. Nevertheless, one must use a great deal of caution in employing the data because of differences in definition, source of data, and variation in accuracy among the countries.

Among the areas of particular concern:

- How countries distinguish between health and social services. Some, for example, may classify certain domiciliary care to the elderly as health, while others might not.
- How countries distinguish between hospital and long-term care. In some countries the distinction between the two is much finer than in the United States, with more long-term care being provided in hospitals.
- Accurate conversion of numerous currencies to a common unit. This is typically done through purchasing power parities (PPPs), which take into account buying power in different countries. For this reason, it is probably safer to rely

on figures pertaining to the proportion of a country's national income devoted to health than to an absolute monetary amount.

• Underreporting of certain categories of expenditure by some countries, which is due in part to data limitations.

Two of the researchers involved in the initial efforts to compile the OECD data, Schieber and Poullier, have responded to various criticisms of the data by noting that "these data have the advantage of being based on an internationally accepted functional classification; receiving direct comment and input from the statistical offices of the countries; and having methodology, sources, and underlying assumptions widely disseminated."[12]

## Trends in Health Care Expenditure

This section is divided into three parts: trends in prices, U.S. expenditures, and international expenditures.

### U.S. Prices

Table 5.1 presents the values for the major components of the CPI from 1980 to 2003, while Table 5.2 shows the corresponding annual rates of change. Tables 5.3 and 5.4 present similar data for some of the items that make up the medical care component of the CPI.

### TABLE 5.1. CONSUMER PRICE INDEX FOR ALL ITEMS: UNITED STATES, SELECTED YEARS, 1980–2003.

| Year | All Items | Medical Care | Food | Apparel | Housing | Energy |
|------|-----------|--------------|------|---------|---------|--------|
| | | | *Consumer Price Index* | | | |
| 1980 | 82.4 | 74.9 | 86.8 | 90.9 | 81.1 | 86.0 |
| 1990 | 130.7 | 162.8 | 132.4 | 124.1 | 128.5 | 102.1 |
| 1995 | 152.4 | 220.5 | 148.4 | 132.0 | 148.5 | 105.2 |
| 2000 | 172.2 | 260.8 | 167.8 | 129.6 | 169.6 | 124.6 |
| 2001 | 177.1 | 272.8 | 173.1 | 127.3 | 176.4 | 129.3 |
| 2002 | 179.9 | 285.6 | 176.2 | 124.0 | 180.3 | 121.7 |
| 2003 | 184.0 | 297.1 | 180.0 | 120.9 | 184.8 | 136.5 |

*Note:* 1982–1984 = 100.

*Source:* U.S. Department of Health and Human Services, Public Health Service, Health United States, 2004, p. 327. [http://www.cdc.gov/nchs/hus.htm].

## TABLE 5.2. ANNUAL CHANGE IN CONSUMER PRICE INDEX FOR ALL ITEMS: UNITED STATES, SELECTED YEARS, 1980–2003.

| Year | All Items | Medical Care | Food | Apparel | Housing | Energy |
|------|-----------|--------------|------|---------|---------|--------|
| | *Average Annual Percentage Change* | | | | | |
| 1980–1990 | 4.7 | 8.1 | 4.3 | 3.2 | 4.7 | 1.7 |
| 1990–1995 | 3.1 | 6.3 | 2.3 | 1.2 | 2.9 | 0.6 |
| 1995–2000 | 2.5 | 3.4 | 2.5 | −0.4 | 2.7 | 3.4 |
| 2000–01 | 2.8 | 4.6 | 3.2 | −1.8 | 4.0 | 3.8 |
| 2001–02 | 1.6 | 4.7 | 1.8 | −2.6 | 2.2 | −5.9 |
| 2002–03 | 2.3 | 4.0 | 2.2 | −2.5 | 2.5 | 12.2 |

*Note:* 1982–1984 = 100.

*Source:* U.S. Department of Health and Human Services, Public Health Service, Health United States, 2004, p. 327. [http://www.cdc.gov/nchs/hus.htm].

Beginning with Tables 5.1 and 5.2, we see that since 1980 medical care prices have grown far faster than other prices in the U.S. economy. Between 1980 and 2003, they rose fourfold, whereas the index as a whole increased only 2.3 times, and the other components listed grew even less. The pattern is most pronounced in the early years; between 1980 and 1990 medical prices rose by an average of 8.1 percent annually, compared to 4.7 percent for the CPI as a whole. Since then, price increases have lessened somewhat, although still usually double those of the other sectors of the economy.

Tables 5.3 and 5.4 show the patterns within the medical care sector. The largest growth rate was for hospital, which increased by a factor of 5.7 from 1980 to 2003. As mentioned earlier, however, one should be skeptical about this number because the CPI does not do a good job of accounting for the changing nature of the hospital product. What is most noteworthy is that after relatively low inflation in the middle to late 1990s, there has been a resurgence in most medical price increases, although not as great as in the 1980s.

## U.S. Expenditures

Table 5.5 presents 2002 data on U.S. health expenditures from the national health accounts. The rows give information on the source of funds, while the columns indicate the provider of services receiving the funds. Some noteworthy aspects of the data:

## TABLE 5.3. CONSUMER PRICE INDEX FOR
## ALL ITEMS AND FOR MEDICAL CARE COMPONENTS:
## UNITED STATES, SELECTED YEARS, 1980–2003.

|  | 1980 | 1990 | 1995 | 2000 | 2001 | 2002 | 2003 |
|---|---|---|---|---|---|---|---|
|  | *Consumer Price Index* | | | | | | |
| CPI, all items | 82.4 | 130.7 | 152.4 | 172.2 | 177.1 | 179.9 | 184.0 |
| Less medical care | 82.8 | 128.8 | 148.6 | 167.3 | 171.9 | 174.3 | 178.1 |
| CPI, all services | 77.9 | 139.2 | 168.7 | 195.3 | 203.4 | 209.8 | 216.5 |
| All medical care | 74.9 | 162.8 | 220.5 | 260.8 | 272.8 | 285.6 | 297.1 |
| Medical care services | 74.8 | 162.7 | 224.2 | 266.0 | 278.8 | 292.9 | 306.0 |
| Professional medical services | 77.9 | 156.1 | 201.0 | 237.7 | 246.5 | 253.9 | 261.2 |
| Physician services | 76.5 | 160.8 | 208.8 | 244.7 | 253.6 | 260.6 | 267.7 |
| Dental services | 78.9 | 155.8 | 206.8 | 258.5 | 269.0 | 281.0 | 292.5 |
| Eye care | — | 117.3 | 137.0 | 149.7 | 154.5 | 155.5 | 155.9 |
| Services by other medical professionals | — | 120.2 | 143.9 | 161.9 | 167.3 | 171.8 | 177.1 |
| Hospital and related services | 69.2 | 178.0 | 257.8 | 317.3 | 338.3 | 367.8 | 394.8 |
| Medical care commodities | 75.4 | 163.4 | 204.5 | 238.1 | 247.6 | 256.4 | 262.8 |
| Prescription drugs and medical supplies | 72.5 | 181.7 | 235.0 | 285.4 | 300.9 | 316.5 | 326.3 |
| Nonprescription drugs and medical supplies | — | 120.6 | 140.5 | 149.5 | 150.6 | 150.4 | 152.0 |

*Source:* U.S. Department of Health and Human Services, Public Health Service, *Health United States 2004,* p. 327. [http://www.cdc.gov/nchs/hus.htm].

- Government expenditures account for 44 percent of total health expenditures, 76 percent of which are federal. Government pays far more of the bill for hospital care (59 percent) than for physician services (34 percent).
- Although out-of-pocket costs make up on average 16 percent of total expenditures, this figure varies tremendously by type of service. It ranges from only 3 percent for hospital care to 25 percent for nursing home care, 36 percent for other personal care, and 30 percent for prescription drugs.
- Private insurance pays a substantial proportion (more than 30 percent) of expenditure for hospital, physician, and prescription drugs but only 7.5 percent for nursing home care.

### TABLE 5.4. AVERAGE ANNUAL CHANGE IN CONSUMER PRICE INDEX FOR ALL ITEMS AND FOR MEDICAL CARE COMPONENTS, UNITED STATES, SELECTED YEARS, 1980–2003.

| | 1980–90 | 1990–95 | 1995–2000 | 2000–01 | 2001–02 | 2002–03 |
|---|---|---|---|---|---|---|
| CPI, all items | 4.7 | 3.1 | 2.5 | 2.8 | 1.6 | 2.3 |
| Less medical care | 4.5 | 2.9 | 2.4 | 2.7 | 1.4 | 2.2 |
| CPI, all services | 6.0 | 3.9 | 3.0 | 4.1 | 3.1 | 3.2 |
| All medical care | 8.1 | 6.3 | 3.4 | 4.6 | 4.7 | 4.0 |
| Medical care services | 8.1 | 6.6 | 3.5 | 4.8 | 5.1 | 4.5 |
| Professional medical services | 7.2 | 5.2 | 3.4 | 3.7 | 3.0 | 2.9 |
|   Physicians services | 7.7 | 5.4 | 3.2 | 3.6 | 2.8 | 2.7 |
|   Dental services | 7.0 | 5.8 | 4.6 | 4.1 | 4.5 | 4.1 |
|   Eye care | — | 3.2 | 1.8 | 3.2 | 0.6 | 0.3 |
|   Services by other medical professionals | — | 3.7 | 2.4 | 3.3 | 2.7 | 3.1 |
|   Hospital and related services | 9.9 | 7.7 | 4.2 | 6.6 | 8.7 | 7.3 |
| Medical care commodities | 8.0 | 4.6 | 3.1 | 4.0 | 3.6 | 2.5 |
|   Prescription drugs and medical supplies | 9.6 | 5.3 | 4.0 | 5.4 | 5.2 | 3.1 |
|   Nonprescription drugs and medical supplies | — | 3.1 | 1.2 | 0.7 | −0.1 | 1.1 |

*Source:* U.S. Department of Health and Human Services, Public Health Service, *Health United States, 2004,* p. 327. [http://www.cdc.gov/nchs/hus.htm].

Table 5.6 shows annual rate of change in U.S. health expenditures, by type of service, between 1980 and 2003. Expenditure growth has slowed since 1990, but it is still far higher than in the rest of the economy. There has also been a resurgence of growth during the 2000s. In examining types of service, note that the most important trend is the tremendous growth in spending on pharmaceuticals, which has hovered around 15 percent per year since 1995. This far exceeds all other service types, which have grown in the single digits.

Analysts have not only studied past trends in expenditures; they have also used simulation models to project what expenditures will be in future years. One recent

## TABLE 5.5. PERSONAL HEALTH CARE EXPENDITURES, BY TYPE OF EXPENDITURE AND SELECTED SOURCES OF PAYMENT, 2002.

| Source of Payment | Total | Hospital Care | Physician Service | Prescription Drug | Nursing Home Care | Other Personal Care |
|---|---|---|---|---|---|---|
| | | | *Amount in Billions* | | | |
| Personal health care expenditures | 1340.2 | 486.5 | 339.5 | 162.4 | 103.2 | 248.6 |
| | | | Percentage of Total | | | |
| Out-of-pocket payments | 15.9 | 3.0 | 10.1 | 29.9 | 25.1 | 35.8 |
| Private health insurance | 35.8 | 33.9 | 49.1 | 47.8 | 7.5 | 25.0 |
| Other private funds | 4.2 | 4.2 | 6.9 | NA | 3.4 | 3.5 |
| Government | 44.2 | 58.9 | 33.8 | 22.3 | 64.0 | 35.6 |
|   Medicaid | 18.7 | 17.1 | 7.2 | 17.5 | 49.3 | 18.3 |
|   Medicare | 20.0 | 30.7 | 20.3 | 1.6 | 12.5 | 10.2 |

*Source:* U.S. Department of Health and Human Services, Public Health Service, *Health United States, 2004,* pp. 330–331.

## TABLE 5.6. ANNUAL CHANGE IN PERSONAL HEALTH CARE EXPENDITURES BY TYPE OF SERVICE, UNITED STATES, 1980–2002.

| Year | All Expenditures | Hospital | Physician | Nursing Home | Prescription Drug | Other Personal Care |
|---|---|---|---|---|---|---|
| | | *Average Annual Percentage Change* | | | | |
| 1980–1990 | 11.0 | 96.0 | 12.8 | 11.5 | 12.9 | 11.1 |
| 1990–1995 | 7.2 | 6.2 | 7.0 | 7.2 | 8.6 | 9.6 |
| 1995–2000 | 5.5 | 3.8 | 4.2 | 4.7 | 14.9 | 5.4 |
| 2000–01 | 8.5 | 7.5 | 8.5 | 5.7 | 15.9 | 7.2 |
| 2001–02 | 8.8 | 9.5 | 7.7 | 4.1 | 15.3 | 7.2 |

*Source:* U.S. Department of Health and Human Services, Public Health Service, *Health United States 2004,* pp. 330–331. [http://www.cdc.gov/nchs/hus.htm].

set of projects was computed by the Centers for Medicare and Medicaid Services.[13] It concluded that the proportion of gross national project accounted for by health expenditures will increase from 15.4 percent in 2004 to 18.7 percent in 2014.

In considering these figures, one should keep in mind that such projections often turn out to be quite off the mark. For example, in a report published in 1992, the Congressional Budget Office estimated that health expenditures would consume about 18 percent of GDP by the year 2000.[14] The more likely figure was 13.3 percent.

Needless to say, accurately projecting health spending is difficult at best. One problem is that, over time, the estimates can become increasingly farfetched. An analysis of these issues was conducted by Warshawsky, who concluded that "even the most conservative projections, which assume either robust economic growth, improved demographic trends, or some moderation in health care price inflation, foresee the health care sector consuming more than a quarter of national output by [the year] 2065. If, on the other hand, current relative price trends continue, economic growth remains anemic, demographic trends continue or worsen, or the health care sector becomes a major user of capital, [simulation models] predict that health care expenditures will comprise between a third to a half of national output."[15]

Aside from a number of technical assumptions, the problem with believing these projections is that they assume, on some level at least, continuation of current expenditure trends. This is unlikely to be the case as health care further crowds out other public and private expenditures. Nevertheless, the increasing ability of new medical technologies and soon, perhaps genetic therapies, to improve people's health, coupled with the inability of the U.S. Congress to approve health care reform containing strong cost control measures, lends credence to the belief that health expenditures will continue growing rapidly in the years to come.

### International Expenditures

Table 5.7 shows total health expenditures as a percentage of GDP in OECD countries over the period 1980–2001. The 2001 figure for the U.S., 14.1 percent, is almost one-third higher than for any other country; only Germany and Switzerland also exceeded the 10 percent mark. Not shown in the table are per capita expenditures expressed in dollars. In 2001, the U.S. figure was about $5,021, a full 51 percent higher than the next (for Switzerland).[16]

## The Need for Timely and Complete Data Systems

An important issue facing the United States is availability of accurate and timely data on national health care utilization rates and expenditures. The United States does not have a system in place that allows it to compute expenditures for the

## TABLE 5.7. HEALTH EXPENDITURES AS A PERCENTAGE OF GROSS DOMESTIC PRODUCT: SELECTED COUNTRIES AND YEARS, 1980–2001.

| Country | 1980 | 1990 | 1995 | 2001 |
|---|---|---|---|---|
| Australia | 7.0 | 7.8 | 8.2 | 9.2 |
| Austria | 7.6 | 7.1 | 8.2 | 7.7 |
| Belgium | 6.4 | 7.4 | 8.6 | 9.0 |
| Canada | 7.1 | 9.0 | 9.2 | 9.7 |
| Denmark | 9.1 | 8.5 | 8.2 | 8.6 |
| Finland | 6.4 | 7.8 | 7.5 | 7.0 |
| France | NA | 8.6 | 9.5 | 9.5 |
| Germany | 8.7 | 8.5 | 10.6 | 10.7 |
| Greece | 6.6 | 7.4 | 9.6 | 9.4 |
| Iceland | 6.2 | 8.0 | 8.4 | 9.2 |
| Ireland | 8.4 | 6.1 | 6.8 | 6.5 |
| Italy | NA | 8.0 | 7.4 | 8.4 |
| Japan | 6.4 | 5.9 | 6.8 | 8.0 |
| Luxembourg | 5.9 | 6.1 | 6.4 | NA |
| Netherlands | 7.5 | 8.0 | 8.4 | 8.9 |
| New Zealand | 5.9 | 6.9 | 7.2 | 8.1 |
| Norway | 6.9 | 7.7 | 7.9 | 8.0 |
| Portugal | 5.6 | 6.2 | 8.3 | 9.2 |
| Spain | 5.4 | 6.7 | 7.6 | 7.5 |
| Sweden | 8.8 | 8.2 | 8.1 | 8.7 |
| Switzerland | 7.6 | 8.5 | 10.0 | 11.1 |
| United Kingdom | 5.6 | 6.0 | 7.0 | 7.6 |
| United States | 8.8 | 12.0 | 13.4 | 14.1 |

*Source:* U.S. Department of Health and Human Services, Public Health Service, *Health United States, 2004,* p. 325. [http://www.cdc.gov/nchs/hus.htm].

entire health care sector in a consistent and timely fashion. Such a data set would be extremely beneficial, and perhaps even essential, for enacting certain types of health care reform, particularly those that are regulatory in nature.

The problem, in a nutshell, is this: the U.S. government does not require private insurers to collect and release data on expenditures. Such data, if available in a consistent format, would increase the country's flexibility in adopting various types of reform.

One of the reforms discussed in the next chapter that are designed to control health care costs is use of expenditure targets, which applies to a fee-for-service system. Under such a system, unit prices are adjusted annually if utilization is above or below a designated target. To implement such a system requires timely data on health expenditures on a subnational (statewide) basis for all payers. (The current dearth of statewide data is one important impediment to enacting major health care reform.) Current data systems, however, do not support such a system, largely because private insurers and health plans are not required to compile aggregate utilization and expenditure information.

## Is Cost Control Even Necessary?

This chapter has discussed how health care costs are measured and has shown recent levels and trends. The next chapter considers various methods of controlling these costs. Before doing so, one must ask a natural question: if it is even necessary to control national health expenditures.

The question is not a trivial one. If people wish to spend more on health care, and consequently less on other things, why should they be stopped—particularly when it seems increasingly clear that certain new medical devices, products, and procedures can improve the quality and length of life?

It turns out that there are several reasons cost control is important and likely to be in the forefront of health policy for years to come. First, there are significant opportunity costs associated with additional spending. A dollar spent on health cannot be spent on such other things as education, housing, or consumer goods. Cost control continues to be a major issue simply because it is imprudent to waste money in the face of so many strong consumer desires and societal needs.

Second, there are various ways in which the health care market is imperfect, which fact may lead to more spending than is desirable. Unlike other goods and services, health care services are often well insured, which insulates consumers from facing their true cost (that is, resource value). In addition, because consumer information is often poor, people may demand medical goods and services in part because of strong advertising, or because they are "induced" to do so by providers who have a pecuniary incentive to increase demand.

Third, government now pays for almost half of U.S. health care spending. With recent government deficits, the future of social programs is worrisome. Medicare faces the prospect of more recipients and fewer contributors as the baby boom generation retires; problems for Medicaid are close at hand, with nearly all states engaged in significant eligibility, benefit, or reimbursement cuts.

Finally, one of the major reasons that the number of uninsured persons continues to rise in the United States is health care costs. Although more employers are offering insurance than in the past, fewer workers are purchasing it because they cannot afford the premiums.[17] This trend is likely to accelerate if health care costs continue to grow at a pace far outstripping the rest of the economy. In summary, then, there are compelling reasons to believe not only that health care costs will remain a central policy interest but also that their control is in the national interest.

# Notes

1. A dollar bill is roughly six inches, or half a foot, long. Lining up two trillion of them would stretch one trillion feet, or more than twice the ninety-three million miles between the earth and the sun. Expenditure projections are from Heffler, S., and others. "U.S. Health Spending Projections for 2004–2014." *Health Affairs* (Web exclusive), Feb. 23, 2005, W5-74–W5-85.

2. A tremendous amount of effort has gone into compiling accurate health expenditure figures across countries. For a presentation of the most recent estimates by the Organization for Economic Cooperation and Development (OECD), which has sponsored much of this work, see Reinhardt, U. E., Hussey, P. S., and Anderson, G. F. "U.S. Health Care Spending in an International Context." *Health Affairs,* May–June 2004, *23*(3), 10–25.

3. Miller, R. L., and Meiners, R. E. *Intermediate Microeconomics.* New York: McGraw-Hill, 1986.

4. There are other distinctions in how economists and accountants define cost. Specifically, economic profits equal an organization's cash flow minus a normal rate of return on investment. Further discussion of this issue can be found in textbooks on corporate finance.

5. For more information on the index, see the U.S. Department of Labor's Consumer Price Index Website [http://www.bls.gov/cpi/].

6. Feldstein, P. *Health Care Economics* (6th ed.). Clifton Park, N.Y.: Thomson Delmar Learning, 2004.

7. Feldstein (2004).

8. At the time of writing, the most recent version was Strunk, B. C., Ginsburg, P. B., and Cookson, J. P. "Tracking Health Care Costs: Declining Growth Trend Pauses in 2004." *Health Affairs* (Web exclusive), June 21, 2005, W5-286–W5-295.

9. Office of National Cost Estimates. "Revisions of the National Health Accounts and Methodology." *Health Care Financing Review,* Summer 1990, *11,* 42–54.

10. Haber, S. G., and Newhouse, J. P. "Recent Revisions to and Recommendations for National Health Expenditures Accounting." *Health Care Financing Review,* Fall 1991, *13,* 111–116.

11. For the most recent article, see Reinhardt, Hussey, and Anderson (2004).

12. Schieber, G. J., and Poullier, J. "International Health Spending: Issues and Trends." *Health Affairs,* Spring 1991, *10,* 106–116.

13. Heffler, S., and others (2005).

14. Congressional Budget Office. *Projections of National Health Expenditures.* Washington, D.C.: Congressional Budget Office, Oct. 1992.

15. Warshawsky, M. J. "Projections of Health Care Expenditures as a Share of the Gross Domestic Product: Actuarial and Macroeconomic Approaches." *Health Services Research,* Aug. 1994, *29,* 293–313.

16. U.S. Department of Health and Human Services, Public Health Services. *Health United States, 2004.* [http://www.cdc.gov/nchs/hus.htm].

17. Gabel, J., and others. "Health Benefits in 2004: Four Years of Double-Digit Premium Increases Take Their Toll on Coverage." *Health Affairs,* Sept.–Oct. 2004, *23*(5), 200–209.

CHAPTER SIX

# CONTAINING HEALTH CARE COSTS

Thomas H. Rice
Gerald F. Kominski

Since publication of the two previous editions of this book in 1996 and 2001, much has changed in the area of cost (that is, expenditure) containment. During the 1980s, per capita health care expenditures grew by almost 10 percent per year. The first half of the 1990s saw a reduction to 6.2 percent per year, and the period from 1995 to 1999 to the historically low level of 4.5 percent per year. Since then, expenditures have begun to climb again, rising at more than 7 percent per year between 1999 and 2002.[1] At the time of this writing, they show little sign of receding.

When the 2001 edition was published, we did not know whether health care expenditure increases had peaked. There was some reason to believe this to be the case, given recent cost-containment successes of HMOs. That edition of the book was written just before the so-called managed care backlash was unleashed in full force—one of the reasons for the upsurge in spending. Not surprisingly, then, historical predictions about future costs have been notoriously unreliable. Studies published in the beginning of the 1990s predicted that U.S. health expenditures would consume 18 percent of national income by the year 2000. When that year arrived, they were only 13.3;[2] since that time they have risen considerably, to 15.3 percent in 2003. Some analysts are again projecting large increases, to almost 19 percent by 2014.[3] History has taught us to view these projections skeptically, but it still behooves us to understand the factors responsible for rising costs and how these increases can be stemmed.

Why have we seen expenditure increases go back and forth? Although analysts disagree about the exact reasons for the reduction in the 1990s, most would argue that it related to the growth of managed care, particularly HMOs. By moving largely from a fee-for-service system to a capitated-based one (at least for those under age sixty-five), all parties have less economic incentive to increase service volume. Furthermore, many would argue that competition between health care plans set in motion strong forces to keep premiums, and hence total expenditures, lower than they would be otherwise.

So why are they rising again now? In addition to the managed care backlash—which led to growth in fee-for-service payment systems such as PPOs at the expense of capitated HMOs—some suggest that the main reason is the proliferation of high-tech procedures and medications, which have the potential to lengthen and improve quality of life and thus further stimulate consumer demand. Others argue that increasing reliance on private insurance and market mechanisms are—unlike the case in other industries—ineffective in the health sector because of poor consumer information and the market power held by insurers and providers.

This chapter has three purposes: to present a framework for assessing alternative cost-containment strategies, to review previous research on the success and failure of these strategies, and to suggest directions for future research that may help clarify the most effective future cost-containment options for the United States to pursue.

## Framework

Before embarking on an analysis of alternative cost-containment strategies, it is useful to construct a framework that groups together similar strategies.[4] It is possible to construct any number of frameworks. The one shown here is employed because each of the two equations relate to a major method of provider payment.[5] The first applies to the fee-for-service system, and the second to capitated systems.

(1)
$$E = \sum_{j=1}^{J} (P_j \times Q_j)$$

(2)
$$E = \sum_{j=1}^{J} (C_j \times N_j)$$

where

E = total health expenditures (or costs)

P = unit price for services

Q = quantity of services in a time period

C = cost of all services per person in a time period

N = number of persons

j = index representing each payer

Equation one states that total expenditures are equal to the product of the price of services and the quantity of services, summed over all payers. In other words, it is the sum of P times Q for Medicare, Medicaid, Blue Cross and Blue Shield, each private insurer, and so on. In contrast, equation two is oriented toward the person, not the service. In this equation, total expenditures (or costs) are simply the product of costs per person and the number of persons, again summed over all payers. Here, total expenditures would equal the number of Medicare beneficiaries multiplied by cost per beneficiary, plus the number of Blue Cross enrollees times the cost per enrollee, and so on.

The equations employ summation signs to illustrate the potential for "cost shifting." To illustrate, suppose that one payer, Medicare, successfully controls both P and Q. This clearly results in lower Medicare costs, but it does not necessarily contain systemwide health care costs. This is because hospitals and physicians might respond to Medicare's controls by trying to increase their Ps or Qs to the patients of other payers. The same thing could happen in equation two. A health plan with market clout might cut a particularly good deal with an HMO, and the HMO might respond by charging more to other insurers.

Our framework simply defines the determinants of health expenditures; what may be hidden is the fact that the success of alternative cost-containment strategies hinges on how they affect consumer and provider behavior. In equation one, for example, it might appear a reasonable strategy for controlling expenditures to lower the price of services paid to physicians. However, this would not be successful if physicians responded to these price controls by inducing their patients to obtain more services (that is, P would go down, but Q would go up).

The same is true of the capitation strategies in equation two. The most obvious approach for controlling expenditures seemingly is to control costs per person. However, if this is accomplished by paying HMOs less, they may in turn respond by seeking to enroll only the healthiest people, or by lowering the quality of care they provide.

In analyzing cost-containment strategies, then, we must be aware of the ability of providers (and others) to "game" the system to meet their own goals. Strategies that are difficult to game tend to be most successful. As an example, we argue that some hospital rate-setting programs were moderately successful in containing costs because it was difficult for hospitals to game the system by increasing admissions and length of stay. Instead, physicians rather than hospitals made these decisions, and physician payment rates were not affected by the rate-setting programs.

In contrast, certificate-of-need programs were less successful in controlling costs because hospitals were able to respond to restrictions on growth in the number of beds by purchasing more equipment and engaging in other activities that were not regulated (or that were tolerated by the regulators). Thus, in analyzing cost-containment strategies, we focus on how they influence provider and consumer behavior, which in turn strongly influences their ultimate success or failure.

Before we proceed any further, one other caveat is necessary. This chapter focuses on ways of containing costs, but it must be remembered that cost containment is not society's only goal with regard to health services; access and quality of care also matter. Consequently, if analysts find that a particular strategy is effective in controlling costs, they must also consider any spillover effects—such as decreased quality—that result. Only by considering both benefits and costs can we make the best policy decisions for reforming our health care system. In that regard, at the time of this writing there is a flurry of activity to devise "pay for performance" provider payment methods. They are designed to give providers an incentive to control costs and furnish high-quality services. This has been attempted on a limited basis, but there is currently a lack of reliable data on the most effective payment formulas or their effect on quality and costs.[6]

## Analysis of Cost-Containment Strategies

This section uses the framework just presented to review evidence regarding the cost-containment potential of various fee-for-service and capitated cost-containment strategies. Although it addresses more than a dozen such strategies, still others cannot be included because of space limitations.

Before embarking on this review, an explanation is in order. One cost containment tool could just as easily be included in the fee-for-service or capitation section: increased patient cost sharing. As will be noted, patient cost sharing requirements have been increasing rapidly, to keep utilization rates and costs down by making consumers think twice before using additional costly services. In fee-for-service, cost sharing is designed to reduce the quantity of services (Q in the first equation); under capitation arrangements, cost sharing is designed to reduce costs per person (C in the second equation). Somewhat arbitrarily, we have included it in the capitation section. One reason is the recent increases in deductible and co-payment requirements in managed care systems.

## Fee-for-Service Options

Fee-for-service options can be divided into three types, each corresponding to a term in equation one: P, Q, and E. The discussion here is divided accordingly.

*Price Options.* One type of cost-containment strategy that has been attempted at various times in the United States is controlling the unit price paid to the provider. On the hospital side, examples include state hospital rate-setting programs and use of diagnosis-related groups (DRGs). On the physician side, the Medicare and Medicaid programs have, at various times, attempted to control their costs by freezing (or even lowering) physician payments. There is also some experience in this regard from Canada. Since the early 1990s, Medicare and many Medicaid programs have adopted resource-based fee schedules, which are simply another form of price controls.

Before reviewing the available evidence, we believe it is useful to outline the overall advantages and disadvantages of price-control options. There appear to be two possible advantages. First, controlling price typically involves less administrative effort (and expense) than controlling the quantity of service. Rather than examining the appropriateness of every provider and every service, it is only necessary to ensure that payments conform to regulated amounts. Second, and related to this, price regulation tends to be less intrusive; it does not entail the type of micromanagement often encountered in the quantity-related options discussed next.

There are some disadvantages, however. First, it addresses only one component of total expenditures. As we shall see, a price-based strategy can be circumvented if providers are able to increase the quantity of service they provide. Second, these strategies can diminish the efficiency of the market. If the wrong price is chosen, the wrong quantity or mix of services may result.

Several states adopted hospital rate-setting programs in the 1970s and 1980s. These programs varied on a number of dimensions, the most important of which were whether they were voluntary or mandatory and whether they applied to some or all payers. Most (but not all) were aimed at giving hospitals an incentive to spend less by controlling hospital charges per day.

Of the twenty-five state-level programs that were in effect by the end of the 1970s, only eight were mandatory as opposed to voluntary, and only four—in Maryland, Massachusetts, New Jersey, and New York—applied to all payers.[7] In most cases, these programs established uniform payments, so that public and private insurers paid the same price for the same unit of care (for example, day of care, admission, and so on). To include Medicare in their all-payer systems, these states had to apply to the Health Care Financing Administration (HCFA, now the Centers for Medicare and Medicaid Services, or CMS) for waivers exempting them from Medicare's national payment rules. In granting these waivers, HCFA specified limits on the rate of growth in total Medicare inpatient payments, or in Medicare inpatient payments per case, under the all-payer programs.[8]

Since 1985, with the exception of Maryland these states have either lost their waivers or allowed them to expire. Ironically, one factor contributing to the financial pressure for these states to abandon waivers was the implementation of the Medicare inpatient prospective payment system (PPS) in October 1983. Because payment rates during the first three years of PPS were a blend of hospital-specific and national payment amounts, these states felt pressure from their hospital associations to abandon the waivers because hospitals could increase their Medicare revenue by joining PPS.

Most research on the subject found it was these four programs that were most effective, with savings on the order of 10–15 percent.[9] It might seem surprising that a gross strategy the likes of limiting hospital payments per day would work, but apparently it did. This is likely because of the difficulty hospitals had in gaming such a system. If a hospital wants to raise more revenue under an all-payer, mandatory rate-setting program that establishes the daily payment rate, it has two choices: increase the number of admissions, or increase length of stay. But neither option is typically available to hospitals because these decisions are made by physicians, whose fees are generally not subject to these controls. Consequently, as much as a hospital might wish to raise more revenue, it might not have the ability to do so.

Implementation of the DRG-based Medicare PPS made such gaming even more difficult (although it led to its own gaming, of course). Under the DRG system, hospitals are paid a fixed amount of money for a particular diagnosis, irrespective of how much is spent on treating a patient.[10] Hospitals therefore cannot benefit by trying to keep patients longer. Another option for garnering more revenue is to increase the number of admissions, but this has not happened, for two reasons: the physician rather than the hospital makes this decision, and hospitals found it profitable to treat patients on an outpatient basis, which is paid for separately and outside the DRG system.

There remain two other avenues for increasing revenue under DRGs: earning more from treating Medicare patients on an outpatient basis, and shifting costs to other payers. Although Medicare outpatient costs have risen rapidly, this increase has not been sufficient to cut deeply into Medicare savings.[11] Since 2000, hospital outpatient care under Medicare has been paid for using an outpatient PPS, thus further reducing revenue from outpatient care.

The same cannot be said about the shift to other payers. Over the years, researchers have found that hospitals do resort to shifting costs onto private payers. The magnitude of cost-shifting practice is shown in Table 6.1.[12] In 1990, for example, Medicare paid hospitals less than 90 percent of the costs associated with treating program patients, and Medicaid only 80 percent. In contrast, private insurers paid hospitals about 28 percent more for their patients' care than it actually cost to provide. Cost shifting has decreased substantially in the last few years, mainly because Medicare has begun to pay its share of hospital costs, and Medicaid payments have improved as well. In 2002, private insurers were paying "only" 19 percent more than their patients actually cost hospitals.

## TABLE 6.1. HOSPITAL PAYMENT-TO-COST RATIOS, 1982–2002.

| Year | Medicare | Medicaid | Private |
|------|----------|----------|---------|
| 1982 | 96.1 | 91.5 | 115.8 |
| 1986 | 101.7 | 91.8 | 116.3 |
| 1990 | 89.4 | 80.1 | 127.8 |
| 1994 | 96.9 | 93.7 | 124.4 |
| 1998 | 101.9 | 96.6 | 115.8 |
| 2002 | 97.9 | 96.1 | 119.0 |

*Source:* American Hospital Association/Lewin Group. *TrendWatch Chartbook 2004: Trends Affecting Hospitals and Health Systems.* May 2004, Table 4.4, p. 99. [http://www.ahapolicyforum.org/ahapolicyforum/trendwatch/chartbook2004.html].

Because of cost shifting, some analysts have concluded that DRGs have done little if anything to control national health care spending,[13] evidence of substantial savings in the Medicare program notwithstanding.[14] This is not necessarily an indictment of DRGs, however. If other payers were to adopt DRGs, systemwide hospital spending might be better controlled. For example, a number of state Medicaid programs have adopted payment systems based on DRGs, but most commercial insurers have not.[15]

These conclusions about the successes and failures of hospital price controls are further supported by experience with physician controls. Most studies indicate limited cost savings when physician payments are frozen or reduced, because physicians respond by providing a greater quantity of services.[16] In making its projections about physician payment costs under the new Medicare fee schedule that was implemented starting in 1992, the Congressional Budget Office concluded that for every 1 percent reduction in physician fees, the volume of services would rise by 0.56 percent.[17]

Why might these physician controls be less effective than hospital controls? It is because physicians have greater ability to game the payment system. If their payment rate drops, physicians in a fee-for-service environment can attempt to increase the volume of services (and may very well succeed). Hospitals do not tend to have this ability.

Nevertheless, physicians' ability to generate additional billing is probably limited. This is illustrated by the experience of the Canadian provinces, which have tightly controlled physician fees since the early 1970s. Although the quantity of services rose faster in Canada than in the United States over this time period, it was not nearly enough to compensate for the lower fees.[18] In a country like the United States, where there are multiple payers, an effective way for a payer to control physician spending is to pay so little to doctors that they do not want to treat such patients. This, of course, is what has happened in many state Medicaid programs. Canadian provinces do not suffer from this problem because there is only one payer; the provinces are the only game in town.

*Quantity Options.* The next group of fee-for-service cost-containment strategies are those aimed at service quantity or utilization. Examples are certificate-of-need programs, technology controls, utilization review, and practice guidelines (to name just a few). Their primary advantage over price options is that they can focus on reducing waste in the system. For example, if a particular procedure is inappropriate for a patient with a given diagnosis, quantity options can focus on the problem.

There are two disadvantages. Like the price options, they only target one component of expenditure. If providers can game utilization controls by increasing prices, then the savings from these programs are diminished. Second, the strategies are often cumbersome from an administrative standpoint, involving much bureaucracy, paperwork, and undue oversight over the practice of medicine.

The earliest examples of quantity controls were certificate-of-need (CON) programs. These programs, which became commonplace in the early 1970s, were aimed at controlling expenditures by reducing the amount of hospital resources available, both beds and equipment. Typically, hospitals needed permission for any proposed investment in excess of $100,000. A local board, called the health systems agency, ruled on a hospital's request for additional resources.

Many studies have been conducted on CON, and almost all reach the same conclusion: it did not succeed in saving money.[19] Although there was some effect on the number of hospital beds, capital equipment per bed rose even more quickly than before.[20] There are a number of reasons for this failure, but the fundamental one is that the entity making the decisions on the hospital's application (the local health systems agency, and ultimately the state) was not financially accountable for the increased cost associated with approving a hospital's request. In other words, why turn down a hospital request when the cost would be borne by such payers as Medicare, Blue Cross, or commercial insurers? On the contrary, board members would have every incentive to approve requests by their local hospital, since this would be viewed as helpful to their community and constituencies.

This is not to say that technology controls can't work; they probably can. However, they need to be implemented at a broader geographic level by an entity that is at risk for additional health care spending. The Canadian provinces give us such an example.

Despite claims to the contrary, there is no single Canadian health care system. Rather, each province has its own system, but all have to conform to various federal requirements if they are to receive federal contributions. One key point, often overlooked in the literature, is that provinces are 100 percent at risk for additional health care spending because annual federal contributions are fixed. Unlike the U.S. Medicaid program, where the federal government at least matches additional state spending, provinces do not receive an additional penny if they spend more on health care than anticipated.

Since provinces are also responsible for financing a host of other nonhealth programs, they must be judicious in allotting their tax revenues to health care. One way they do this is by controlling the diffusion of medical technology. If a hospital wants to expand or purchase equipment, it needs the province's permission, and provinces have not been eager to grant requests. The United States has far more of most technologies than Canada, measured per capita. For example, in 1999 the United States had 7.6 MRI units and 13.2 CT scanners per million people; Canada's figures were only 1.8 and 8.2, respectively.[21]

Canadians often claim that they have achieved this by regionalizing their technologies, thereby making their system more efficient. Others contend, however, that the result is rationing. Indeed, evidence from a 2002 survey of the public in five countries (Australia, Canada, New Zealand, United Kingdom, and United States) found that Canadians reported the longest waits for getting a doctor's appointment, seeing a specialist, and being admitted to a hospital. For example, 28 percent of sicker Canadians reported that a long wait for being admitted to a hospital in the past two years was a "big problem," more than double the U.S. figure of 13 percent.[22]

Up to this point, the discussion of quantity has focused not on services but on hospital beds and technologies. In the United States, however, most of the focus is aimed at particular services. This is commonly done through utilization management (UM). UM programs are normally implemented by third-party payers as a way to reduce provision of unnecessary or inappropriate services. Examples are preadmission certification of hospital stays, concurrent and retrospective review of stays, management of high-cost patients, requiring a second opinion before embarking on surgery, and profiling of physicians' practices.

There is a dearth of recent literature evaluating the impact of UM in fee-for-service settings, perhaps because more attention has been paid to capitated arrangements. This may change, however, given the recent growth of PPOs at the expense of HMOs. One recent review of the literature examined three types: utilization review, case management, and physician gate keeping. Prospective review of hospital stays was found to reduce admissions by about 10 percent, but concurrent review had little impact. Moreover, hospital outpatient utilization increased as a result, so the savings were even smaller. Studies show little impact of case management on cost control, in part because of the difficulty in coordinating the activities of a number of physicians. The literature on the cost-savings potential of physician gate keeping is too sparse for making any generalization.[23] One issue for those who are concerned about controlling future health care expenditures is that UM programs are almost universal now, meaning that we may have already gained about as much in savings as can be extracted.

The wave of the future is now on developing UM for the outpatient setting, particularly through physician profiling. However, the savings potential of these programs is still largely untested. There is strong reason to believe that UM in the outpatient setting is much more difficult to implement, because of the difficulty in knowing whether a physician who is a high spender is less efficient or more profligate, or alternatively has a more severely ill group of patients than his or her peers. Normally one tries to risk-adjust a provider's case mix, but this is difficult at the level of the individual physician, who experiences a relatively low caseload and therefore is more likely to have healthier or sicker patients as a result of random chance. The best we are likely to do—and this is now the emphasis—is to employ risk-adjustment formulas with physician groups.

The most recent UM efforts focus on developing practice guidelines. These are written protocols designed to instruct physicians on which procedures are appropriate for a patient with a particular diagnosis. The guidelines are largely being developed by researchers under the auspices of the federal Agency for Healthcare Research and Quality, although some medical specialty groups are doing so as well. One intent of the guidelines is to increase quality by reducing the amount of regional variation in health care use. It has been widely documented that parts of the country have differing surgery rates for certain procedures, and that this cannot be readily explained by variation in patient health status.[24]

Development of practice guidelines is still relatively new, so we cannot know the extent to which they might control costs. Moreover, because these programs aim far more at improving quality than cost containment, relatively little research has been conducted on the latter. There is reason to be skeptical, though. Just as practice guidelines could reduce resource use by physicians who overtreat patients by providing too many services, they could just as well increase spending by physicians who currently offer fewer services than are recommended by the guidelines. The issue, then, is whether the guidelines are likely to prescribe a quantity of service that is greater or less than what is currently being provided. Unfortunately, little recent direct evidence is available on this particular issue. Earlier, a General Accounting Office study on treatment of cancer patients gave evidence that many physicians are conducting less treatment than is suggested by the guidelines. It concluded that "20 percent of those with Hodgkin's disease, 25 percent of those with one type of lung cancer, 60 percent of those with rectum cancer, 94 percent of colon cancer patients—did not receive what [the National Cancer Institute] considers state-of-the-art treatments. This is especially troubling in that all these treatments have been proven to extend patients' survival in controlled experiments, many of which were concluded 10 or more years ago."[25]

***Expenditure Options.*** The final group of fee-for-service options are those that directly target expenditure. Some examples are Medicare's Sustainable Growth Rate (SGR) system, hospital global budgets, and national and subnational health budgeting. The overriding advantage of expenditure control is somewhat tautological; it directly aims at controlling health care expenditures. The extent to which this can succeed, however, depends in large measure on whether all health care spending is targeted, or just a component of total spending such as hospital or physician expenditures. The primary disadvantage is that implementing such controls may result in a less efficient health care system, which could reduce the quality of services.

The primary example of expenditure control in the United States was implementation of Medicare Volume Performance Standards (VPS) in the early 1990s, which was replaced by the somewhat similar SGR system, described later. The VPS system was part of the 1989 physician payment reforms adopted by Congress that also resulted in the Medicare Fee Schedule, which is based on the resource-based relative value scale (RBRVS). Congress recognized that simply redistributing physician fees to make higher payments to primary care physicians, and lower payments to specialists, though more equitable, would not by itself control burgeoning program expenditures. This was left to the VPS system.

Under the system, each year Congress set a target rate of increase in Medicare Part B physician expenditures. If actual spending exceeded the target, the next year's physician fee update was normally reduced by that amount (although Congress could do, of course, whatever it chose when the time came). Conversely, if the growth in spending was less than the target, physicians would get more. Suppose, for example, that the target for a particular year was a 10 percent increase in spending. If actual spending increased by 12 percent, the target would be exceeded. Most likely, this would be extracted the next time Congress updated Medicare physician fees. If physicians were due a 5 percent cost-of-living increase, they would likely be granted only 3 percent.

The SGR system was enacted as part of the Balanced Budget Act of 1997 and implemented in 1998. The main different between it and the VPS system was in setting the target expenditure rate of sustainable growth, which was determined by four factors: the percentage change in physician input prices, the percentage change in Part B fee-for-service enrollment, the projected change in real GDP, and the percentage change in spending for physicians' services resulting from other changes in law.[26]

The VPS and SGR systems have been criticized as being too blunt an instrument for affecting the individual physician's behavior. Because they apply nationally, individual physicians who increase their volume of services do not pay the price by experiencing a decline in fees. This happens only if all physicians behave this way. But if a physician does not increase his or her volume and other physicians do, then the first physician suffers—volume (Q) does not climb, but the fee (P) falls as a result of the behavior of other physicians. These systems therefore contain a "perverse" incentive to increase the volume of services—which is exactly what they are supposed to prevent. One way to improve the incentives is to target smaller groups of physicians, by having separate targets for each specialty, state, or state-specialty combination.[27]

The SGR system is the subject of recent intense criticism. Being anchored by a formula based, in part, on growth in the economy, it does not take into account upward trends in medical technology diffusion, which is generally acknowledged as one of the leading factors in recent health care expenditure growth. This means that the payment formula has resulted in substantial annual *reduction* in fee updates. In 2004 and 2005, they were overridden by the Congress, but this does nothing to solve the basic issue.[28] In fact, a few years earlier, in 2001, the Medicare Payment Advisory Commission (MedPAC), which advises Congress on all Medicare payment issues, recommended that the current formula be scrapped in favor of one that better recognizes the root causes of medical care inflation and adequately pays physicians for efficient provision of services to beneficiaries.[29]

To find an example of expenditure controls applied to the hospital level, we must again look to Canada. In each province, hospitals are paid an annual global budget, which is negotiated between the province and the individual hospital. If a hospital exceeds its budget, there is no guarantee that it will be compensated.

Hospital global budgets seem to work in the sense that since their inception hospital spending in Canada has risen much less quickly than in the United States. The primary way in which this has been achieved is that Canadian hospitals now have only about half as many nonphysician personnel as do their U.S. counterparts.[30] (Capital expenditures have also been controlled, but for different reasons, since they are not included in the global budgets.) One perverse effect is that Canadian hospitals seem to prefer long-staying patients who might belong in nursing homes, because these patients occupy a bed but use few other resources. Another fear is that the lack of resources is diminishing the quality of care in Canadian hospitals. What little available evidence there is indicates, however, that inpatient outcomes appear to be similar in the two countries[31] and that, with the exception of longer waits for elective services, quality and satisfaction indicators are comparable or favorable to Canada.[32]

The two aforementioned strategies—Medicare VPS and SGR and hospital global budgets—do not constitute a comprehensive cost-control policy because they are aimed at only one component of health care expenditures. A broader strategy might be to target all (or most) health expenditures at the same time, through a system of national or regional budgeting.

The typical way of controlling total expenditures in a fee-for-service system is through expenditure targets. Generally, under such a system unit prices are adjusted to ensure that targeted expenditures are met. This differs from the VPS and SGR systems in two primary ways: (1) it applies to all payers, not just to Medicare; and (2) it applies to most of the health care system, not just physician payment. Although the United States has the most experience—domestically and internationally—with using expenditure targets for paying physicians, it could nevertheless be applied to other services, such as hospitalization. In such a case, DRG payments per admission could be tied to meeting specific growth in inpatient expenditure.[33]

The advantage of such a system, of course, is that it controls expenditures directly. But there are several possible disadvantages: it might result in inefficient use of resources, it could potentially harm quality, and it requires massive amounts of timely data that currently are not being produced.

With regard to efficiency in a competitive market, in the long run price is based on the cost of producing a good or service. If the price is too high, then the incentive is to overproduce the good; if it is too low, the incentive is to underproduce. Under an expenditure target system, prices change not in response to demand and supply considerations but rather in how closely total expenditures conform to a target. The good news is that prices tend to fall when quantity is too high, so it might be argued that the system is self-correcting. The bad news is that there is no assurance that health care inputs will be used efficiently by producers if the market mechanism is circumvented. Even more troubling is the possibility that the mix of services produced is not based on what consumers would like to buy.

This touches on the second potential problem: quality. Suppose that Congress sets an austere budget level, necessitating a subsequent decline in unit prices. This may dissuade providers from delivering necessary services for fear that they will exceed the expenditure target, which in turn can result in diminished quality. Because adequate data systems do not yet exist for monitoring quality, there is a strong possibility that it will be sacrificed in favor of controlling expenditures.

Finally, there is the data problem. To make expenditure targets work in a fee-for-service system, it is necessary to have up-to-date information about the quantity of services provided to all patients. It is through this information that total expenditures are tallied and updates are made to provider prices. In the United States, however, we have no formal mechanism for obtaining timely utilization and expenditure data for privately insured patients or for publicly insured patients in managed care. It would take several years to develop such a system, but the process has not yet even started. Thus the fee-for-service method that has the greatest likelihood of controlling cost perhaps also suffers from the most shortcomings. This illustrates that there are indeed no easy answers for controlling cost under a fee-for-service system.

## Capitation Options

Equation two showed that three things are necessary to control expenditures under a capitated system: control of costs per person (C), the number of persons (N), and shifting costs between payers. This section focuses on the first component; cost shifting has already been addressed, and controlling the number of persons (say, by denying eligibility for coverage)—although clearly a cost-containment strategy—is inconsistent with the notion of equitable health care reform.

This section discusses three strategies for controlling costs under a capitated system: patient cost-sharing, HMOs, and managed competition. The treatment of the latter two is short because these strategies are dealt with in more detail in the chapter on managed care.

***Patient Cost Sharing.***  There are many ways in which insured patients can share in the cost of the services they use. There are deductibles (amount paid out of pocket before insurance benefits kick in), co-payments (fixed amount paid per covered service), and co-insurance (percentage of costs paid per service). Historically, co-payment has been the most common in capitated systems, but more recently there has been a proliferation of deductibles as well, particularly high-deductible insurance products.[34]

To illustrate these rapid increases, in point-of-service HMOs (in which enrollees can go out of network to receive care at higher fees) health plan deductibles tripled in just four years (2000–2004), from an average of $70 to $210 when using preferred providers, and they rose from $352 to $575 for nonpreferred providers. Moreover, among all firms offering prescription drug benefits that use a three-tier arrangement, co-payments for generic drugs rose 43 percent over this same four-year time period (from $7 per prescription to $10) by 62 percent (from $13 to $21) for preferred drugs, and by almost 100 percent (from $17 to $33) for nonpreferred drugs.[35]

Cost sharing is designed to make people think twice before using additional services. Nearly all research has shown that this is the case. In the most notable research endeavor on the subject, the RAND Health Insurance Experiment (HIE) conducted between 1974 and 1982, individuals who were randomly assigned to policies with zero co-insurance used substantially more services than those who had to pay out of pocket for some of their care. Specifically, it was found that people who have to pay 95 percent of charges had annual expenditures that were 28 percent less than those who paid nothing. More relevant to policy, those paying 25 percent co-insurance had expenditures 18 percent less than those with free care.[36] Subsequent studies, none of which have had the advantage of employing a true experimental design, supported the finding that patient cost sharing requirements result in a substantially lower utilization rate.[37]

The impact on this lower utilization on health status, however, is less clear. In general, the HIE found few instances (notably, high blood pressure) in which free care improved health status for the general population. It did find some significant improvements for lower-income persons in poor health. One worrisome finding in the study was that those facing higher co-payments did not cut back more on marginally effective services but rather cut their use across the board—reducing the use of care rated by experts as "highly effective" as much as care that is "less effective" or "rarely effective."[38] This implies that although potentially effective, patient cost sharing is a blunt instrument that, if used injudiciously, could impair the health of the population. It is perhaps for those reasons that most other countries have relied more on strategies targeting the suppliers than the demanders of services.

**HMOs.** Unlike its limited efforts with many so-called competitive strategies, the United States has much experience with HMOs. They have been a part of the U.S. health care system along with their cousins, point-of-service (POS) plans.[39]

HMOs are given an incentive to control costs by the fact that they are paid on a capitation basis. That is, they receive a fixed payment to provide an enrollee's care for a specific length of time, and this payment is unrelated to how much the HMO actually spends. Thus if it spends less by being more efficient (say, not hospitalizing unnecessarily), then it gets to keep more money. But how much the HMO charges in premiums is kept in check by competitive pressure; if it charges too much in premiums, fewer people are likely to enroll.

Much of the early evidence on HMOs through the 1970s focused on group- and staff-model HMOs; it indicated that they could yield substantial savings, as much as 30–40 percent over fee-for-service.[40] A savings rate on this order is now viewed as extremely optimistic. HMOs do save money, but it is difficult to know how much. On the one hand, comparison of HMOs and fee-for-service shows the savings of the former are exaggerated by the fact that, historically, HMOs have experienced favorable selection (healthier or less costly patients), although more recent evidence is pointing to the end of this trend.[41] On the other hand, HMOs probably save more than is directly attributable to them because competition between HMOs and fee-for-service plans undoubtedly results in the latter reducing their costs.

Whatever savings they generate, HMOs by themselves are probably insufficient to solve long-term problems in rising health care costs. One reason is they are subject to the same forces that raise the costs of fee-for-service medicine: overall growth in input costs and development and diffusion of expensive medical technologies. Even less evidence is available on how HMOs affect the quality of care provided. One comprehensive review of the literature found equal numbers of studies reporting better and worse quality of care in HMOs than in fee-for-service.[42]

**Managed Competition.** Analysts have recognized for years that pure competition is unlikely to work well in the health care sector. There are many reasons; two are detailed here. First, the health care market is a complicated one, with people having relatively poor information about their alternatives and the implications (for their health and their pocketbook) of making these choices. A second is biased selection; insurers may compete for the healthiest people, leaving sicker people with no source of insurance.

Advocates of managed competition believe that the marketplace can be trusted in the health care sector only if the players conform to certain rules.[43] To facilitate consumer understanding, health plans should be required to offer specific minimum benefits, or in some proposals conform to standardized benefits. The latter aids consumers in comparison shopping between alternative plans. Furthermore, certain practices on the part of insurers (such as cherry picking the healthiest people, charging unaffordably high premiums to unhealthy individuals and groups, and denying coverage for preexisting conditions) are to be prohibited. To make consumers think twice before purchasing extravagant insurance policies, employers would make a defined contribution based on the lowest-cost premium in the market. As a result, those choosing more expensive health plans would have to pay more of the premiums out of pocket, given the fixed employer premium contribution. Some proposals also tax health plans that are more expensive than the cheapest approved plan in an area. All of this is to be carried out through consortia called health insurance purchasing cooperatives (HIPCs), or health alliances.

There is no way to know whether managed competition can succeed in controlling health care costs; it has never been tried on a wide scale. Some elements of managed competition have been adopted voluntarily, however, and it is claimed that much of the success in controlling costs in the 1990s was the result of health plans and providers competing against each other.[44] It must be recognized, however, that Medicare was also successful in controlling costs over this period even outside of its HMO sector, so we are not yet in a position to draw a strong conclusion about the ability of managed competition to control costs.

# Future Research Issues in Cost Containment

Before addressing future research issues, it is necessary to ask a more basic question: Are health care costs in the United States too high? Unfortunately, it is nearly impossible to know the answer to this question. To answer it, we would have to know the benefits (tangible and intangible) that we derive from health care services, and compare them to the benefits and costs of alternative uses of our resources. Some analysts, however, have tried to answer a somewhat more limited issue: whether the increase in expenditures due to greater medical technologies is worthwhile in comparison to the medical benefits that accrue to the population. Cutler and McClellan examined the costs and benefits of medical technological changes for five medical conditions (health attacks, low-birth weight infants, depression, cataracts, and breast cancer) and concluded that the value of the first four as measured by the increase in life expectancy per dollar spent was highly cost-effective.[45]

There are, nevertheless, good reasons for ongoing research on methods to contain U.S. health care costs. First, the fact that other countries spend so much less per capita raises the possibility that there may be effective cost-control options available. Second, there is an opportunity cost; more spent on health care means less money available to spend on other societal needs. Third, and related to this, there are strong reasons to believe that the availability of new and effective medical technologies such as gene therapy will result in an even greater jump in spending. It would seem prudent that we understand what options are available to control these and other costs before health care spending absorbs even more of our national income.

If continued research on cost-containment methods is appropriate, the next question is which areas of inquiry are most fruitful. One area that spans the domestic and the international is to determine the relative contribution of price versus quantity in continued health care cost inflation. In a 2003 article that received a great deal of attention by researchers and the press ("It's the Prices, Stupid: Why the United States Is So Different from Other Countries"), the authors show that whereas utilization rates are comparable between the United States and other countries, unit prices are far higher.[46] The issue, however, is more subtle: it may be that unit prices are higher in the United States in large part as a result of more expensive inputs (for example, more technologically advanced hospitals, better-trained doctors) that can result in better-quality care. Thus a ripe area of cross-national research is what various countries are getting from their health care systems—an area of research that has begun but is still in its incipient stage.[47]

On the domestic front, there should be continued study of the effects of competition on health care costs to determine which of these approaches are most effective in controlling costs without harming quality and access. In this regard, federally sanctioned state demonstration projects are extremely desirable because they allow researchers to assess whether particular methods work on a large-scale basis. With the implementation of high-deductible Health Savings Accounts (HSAs) as part of the Medicare Modernization Act, it should be possible to assess this strategy in particular, as well as other forms of "consumer-directed" health care. In addition, research on a particular component of a competitive approach (say, a risk-adjustment formula) should continue so that the tools are available to implement selective competitive reforms if there is the political will to do so.

Regulatory approaches should be studied as well. Empirical evidence from previous and current use of price controls in the United States indicates that they are effective in controlling expenditures, improving or maintaining access, and reducing or eliminating cost shifting if applied to all payers. Nevertheless, deep distrust of increased government intervention into the health care market poses a substantial barrier to expanded use of price controls or global budgets. Thus some approaches (for instance, a single-payer system) will be difficult to test in the United States, even on a small scale. For this reason, more research on how other countries have implemented cost containment using regulatory approaches—and the effects of these approaches—is warranted.

Since the late 1980s, there has been a movement toward more funded research in the areas of medical effectiveness and clinical outcomes. Infusion of more federal monies into this branch of health services research is widely viewed as a valuable investment because of the dearth of information on which medical interventions work best. We hope, however, that this recent emphasis on outcomes research does not diminish the importance of general health services research, which seeks to address some of the larger concerns discussed in this chapter.

# Notes

1. Department of Health and Human Services, Centers for Disease Control, National Center for Health Statistics. *Health, U.S., 2004.* (Table 116.) [http://www.cdc.gov/nchs/data/hus/hus04trend.pdf#topic].

2. Congressional Budget Office. *Projections of National Health Expenditures.* Washington, D.C.: Congressional Budget Office, Oct. 1992; and Sally, T., and others. "Projections of National Health Expenditures Through the Year 2000." *Health Care Financing Review,* Fall 1991, *13,* 1–27.

3. Heffler, S., and others. "U.S. Health Spending Projections for 2004–2014." *Health Affairs,* Feb. 23, 2003 (Web exclusive), W5-74–W5-85.

4. The framework presented in this chapter is new but draws on frameworks that Rice previously published. See Rice, T. "An Evaluation of Alternative Policies for Controlling Health Care Costs." In J. A. Meyer and S. Silow-Carroll (eds.), *Building Blocks for Change: How Health Care Reform Affects Our Future.* Washington, D.C.: Economic and Social Research Institute, 1993; and Rice, T. "Containing Health Care Costs in the United States." *Medical Care Review,* Spring 1992, *49,* 19–65.

5. There is a third payment method as well: salary. In general, though, health plans do not pay salaries to providers. In cases where salary is employed, such as in group- and staff-model HMOs, health plans pay a capitation rate to physician groups, which in turn may choose to give salaries to their staff.

6. Some current efforts are described in Rosenthal, M. B., Fernandopulle, R., Song, H. R., and Landon, B. "Paying for Quality: Providers' Incentives for Quality Improvement." *Health Affairs,* 2004, *23*(2), 127–141.

7. Ashby, J. L., Jr. "The Impact of Hospital Regulatory Programs on Per Capita Costs, Utilization, and Capital Investment." *Inquiry,* Spring 1984, *21,* 45–59.

8. Davis, K., Anderson, G. F., Rowland, D., and Steinberg, E. P. *Health Care Cost Containment.* Baltimore: Johns Hopkins University Press, 1990.

9. See Robinson, J. C., and Luft, H. S. "Competition, Regulation, and Hospital Costs: 1982–1986." *Journal of the American Medical Association,* Nov. 11, 1988, *260,* 2676–681; and Thorpe, K. E. "Does All-Payer Rate Setting Work? The Case of the New York Prospective Hospital Reimbursement Methodology." *Journal of Health Politics, Policy, and Law,* 1987, *12,* 391–408.

10. So-called outlier payments are made for patients who become much more expensive than the typical patient with that diagnosis. Even with the formula, hospitals usually lose money on long-staying patients. Thus, there is little or no incentive on the part of the hospital to keep patients for a long time just so that they can reap outlier payments.

11. Chulis, G. S. "Assessing Medicare's Prospective Payment System for Hospitals." *Medical Care Review,* 1991, *48,* 167–206.

12. American Hospital Association and Lewin Group. "Chartbook 2004: Trends Affecting Hospitals and Health Systems." TrendWatch, May 2004, Table 4.4, p. 99. [http://www.ahapolicy forum.org/ahapolicyforum/trendwatch/chartbook2004.html].

13. Chulis (1991).

14. Russell, L. B., and Manning, C. L. "The Effect of Prospective Payment on Medicare Expenditures." *New England Journal of Medicine,* Feb. 16, 1989, *320,* 439–444.

15. Carter, G. M., Jacobson, P. D., Kominski, G. F., and Perry, M. J. "Use of Diagnosis-Related Groups by Non-Medicare Payers." *Health Care Financing Review,* Winter 1994, *16,* 127–158.

16. For a review of early evidence from several natural experiments, see Gabel, J., and Rice, T. "Reducing Public Expenditures for Physician Services: The Price of Paying Less." *Journal of Health Politics, Policy, and Law,* 1985, *9,* 595–609.

17. Christensen, S. "Volume Responses to Exogenous Changes in Medicare's Payment Policies." *Health Services Research,* 1992, *27,* 65–79.

18. Barer, M. L., Evans, R. G., and Labelle, R. J. "Fee Controls as Cost Controls: Tales from the Frozen North." *Milbank Quarterly,* 1988, *66,* 1–64.

19. Steinwald, B., and Sloan, F. A. "Regulatory Approaches to Hospital Cost Containment: A Synthesis of the Empirical Evidence." In M. A. Olson (ed.), *A New Approach to the Economics of Health Care.* Washington, D.C.: American Enterprise Institute for Public Policy Research, 1981.

20. Another effect was that hospitals increased purchase of equipment that cost less than the CON threshold (for instance, $100,000) and sometimes split the cost of more expensive equipment in order to circumvent the regulations.

21. Reinhardt, U. E., Hussey, P. S., and Andersen, G. F. "Cross-National Comparisons of Health Systems Using OECD Data, 1999." *Health Affairs*, 2002, *21*(1), 169–181.

22. Blendon, R. J., and others. "Common Concerns Amid Diverse Systems: Health Care Experiences in Five Countries." *Health Affairs*, 2003, *22*(3), 106–121.

23. Wickizer, T. M., and Lessler, D. "Utilization Management: Issues, Effects, and Future Prospects." *Annual Review of Public Health*, 2002, 233–254.

24. This research was originally conducted by John Wennberg and his colleagues. For a discussions of some of these issues surrounding the Medicare program, see Wennberg, J. E., Fisher, E. S., and Skinner, J. S. "Geography and the Debate over Medicare Reform." *Health Affairs*, Feb. 12, 2002 (Web exclusive), W96–W114.

25. U.S. General Accounting Office. *Cancer Treatment, 1975–1985: The Use of Breakthrough Treatments for Seven Types of Cancer.* (Pub no. PEMD-88-12BR.) Washington, D.C.: General Accounting Office, 1988.

26. Medicare Payment Advisory Commission (MEDPAC). *Report to Congress: Medicare Payment Policy.* Washington, D.C.: MEDPAC, Mar. 2000.

27. See Rice, T., and Bernstein, J. "Volume Performance Standards: Can They Control Growth in Medicare Services?" *Milbank Quarterly*, 1990, *68*, 295–319; and Marquis, M. S., and Kominski, G. F. "Alternative Volume Performance Standards for Medicare Physicians' Services." *Milbank Quarterly*, 1994, *72*, 329–357.

28. Physician Payment Review Commission. *Annual Report to Congress. Medicare Payment Policy.* Washington, D.C.: MEDPAC, Mar. 2005.

29. Physician Payment Review Commission. *Annual Report to Congress. Medicare Payment Policy.* Washington, D.C.: MEDPAC, Mar. 2001.

30. OECD Secretariat. "Health Care Expenditure and Other Data." *Health Care Financing Review*, 1989 Annual Supplement, *11*, 111–194.

31. Newhouse, J. P., Anderson, G., and Roos, L. L. "Hospital Spending in the United States and Canada: A Comparison." *Health Affairs*, 1988, *7*(5), 6–24; Detsky, A. A., Stacey, S. R., and Bombardier, C. "The Effectiveness of a Regulatory Strategy in Containing Hospital Costs: The Ontario Experience, 1967–1981." *New England Journal of Medicine*, July 1983, *309*, 151–159.

32. Blendon and others (2003).

33. Marquis, M. S., and Kominski, G. F. "Alternative Volume Performance Standards for Medicare Physicians' Services." *Milbank Quarterly*, 1994, *72*, 329–357.

34. Gabel, J., and others. "Health Benefits in 2004: Four Years of Double-Digit Premium Increases Take Their Toll on Coverage." *Health Affairs*, Sept.–Oct. 2004, *23*(5), 200–209.

35. Kaiser Family Foundation and Health Research and Educational Trust. "Employer Health Benefits: 2004 Annual Survey." (Chartpack.) Washington, D.C.: Kaiser Family Foundation, 2004.

36. Manning, W. G., and others. "Health Insurance and the Demand for Medical Care: Evidence from a Randomized Experiment." *American Economic Review*, 1987, *77*(3), 251–277.

37. Rice, T., and Morrison, K. R. "Patient Cost Sharing for Medical Services: A Review of the Literature and Implications for Health Care Reform." *Medical Care Review*, 1994, *51*(3), 235–287.

38. Lohr, K. N., and others. "Effect of Cost Sharing on Use of Medically Effective and Less Effective Care." *Medical Care,* 1986, *24* (Supplement), S31–S38.

39. Kominski, G. Commentary on Zuckerman, S., Norton, S. A., and Verrilli, D. "Price Controls and Medicare Spending: Assessing the Volume Offset Assumption." *Medical Care Research and Review,* 1998, *55*(4), 479–483.

40. Point-of-service plans are like HMOs in that the health plan receives a capitation amount for providing services. Typically, enrollees must be referred by a primary care physician before receiving hospital or specialty care. The main difference is that under POS, patients can go to providers outside of the network, but usually only by assuming a sizable co-payment (say, 40 percent of costs).

41. Schaefer, E., and Reschovsky, J. D., "Are HMO Enrollees Healthier Than Others? Results from the Community Tracking Study." *Health Affairs,* 2002, *21*(3), 249–258.

42. Miller, R. H., and Luft, H. S. "HMO Plan Performance Update: An Analysis of the Literature, 1997–2001." *Health Affairs,* 2002, *21*(4), 63–86.

43. This is the theme of the writings of Alain Enthoven. See, for example, Enthoven, A. C. "The History and Principles of Managed Competition." *Health Affairs,* 1993 Supplement, *12,* 24–48; or, more recently, Enthoven, A. C. "Employment-Based Health Insurance Is Failing. Now What?" *Health Affairs,* 2003 (Web exclusive), W3-237–W3-249.

44. Cutler, D. M., and McClellan, M. "Is Technological Change in Medicine Worth It?" *Health Affairs,* 2001, *20*(5), 11–29.

45. Strunk, B. C., Ginsburg, P. B., and Gabel, J. R. "Tracking Health Care Costs: Growth Accelerates Again in 2001." *Heath Affairs,* Sept. 25, 2002 (Web exclusive), W299–W310.

46. Anderson, G. F., Reinhardt, U. E., Hussey, P. S., and Petrosyan, V. "It's the Prices, Stupid: Why the United States Is So Different from Other Countries." *Health Affairs,* 2003, *22*(3), 89–105.

47. Most research has been done on satisfaction rates across selected countries. See, for example, Schoen, C., and others. "Primary Care and Health System Performance: Adults' Experience in Five Countries." *Health Affairs,* Oct. 28, 2004 (Web exclusive), W4-487–W4-503.

CHAPTER SEVEN

# CONTROLLING PHARMACEUTICAL PRICES AND EXPENDITURES

Stuart O. Schweitzer
William S. Comanor

Despite major changes in the U.S. health care system since the 1950s, public discourse toward the pharmaceutical industry has remained much the same: though pleased with the pharmaceutical industry's prominence and the many new drugs that promise longer and healthier lives, many Americans are outraged that drugs cost as much as they do, whether more than they used to cost or more than in other countries. The issue of pharmaceutical costs is long-standing, but many are unclear as to what "drug costs" actually means and what the underlying determinants are. The purpose of this chapter is to clarify these issues and consider some possible solutions to this problem.

Unfortunately, part of the concern over drug expenditures is misplaced by failure to recognize that drugs are an integral part of the medical care process. In many cases, drugs are a substitute for other health care inputs such as hospital stays and physician visits. H2 antagonists such as Tagamet and Zantac, for example, have practically eliminated the need for ulcer surgery, and antipsychotic drugs have substantially reduced the need for mental hospital admissions. For both of these drug classes, pharmaceutical expenditures increased after their introduction, while at the same time total medical costs due to these illnesses declined.

However, not all drugs are cost-saving substitutes. Some, like the so-called clot busters used in emergency rooms for heart-attack patients, are complements that make other services more efficient and improve outcomes. These drugs have also led to rising pharmaceutical expenditures, but few would deny their value in improving health outcomes. Drugs can be both substitutes and complements to other health care inputs.

Concern over pharmaceutical costs is further heightened by lack of clarity about the nature of the problem. Spending on any good or service is a function of both price and quantity. Is the problem of rising drug expenditures due to rising quantities of pharmaceuticals that are consumed? Or is it due to rising prices? The answers to these questions are complicated by the role played by rapid technological innovation, which leads to frequent replacement of older products by newer ones. Newer products are often more expensive than the older ones, so that expenditures may rise because of displacement, even if the prices of all drugs, new and old, as well as the number of prescriptions were to remain constant.

To understand rising drug costs, we first review trends in drug expenditures in the United States. Next we look at U.S. drug prices, considering first a series of issues that make measurement of drug prices particularly difficult. We then look at the evidence on whether U.S. drug prices are higher than those in other countries. We also examine the intertemporal relationship between price increases and quality changes to determine whether pharmaceutical prices have increased after correcting for therapeutic improvements. Then we describe the factors determining drug prices in the United States. Of particular importance are the roles of therapeutic advance and competition. Finally, we discuss a series of policy options for containing pharmaceutical expenditures. Some are directed at consumers, some at physicians, and still others at manufacturers. Current efforts to control pharmaceutical costs are a blend of all three approaches.

## The Problem of Drug Expenditures

The shares held by pharmaceuticals and other components of the U.S. health care system from 1960 through 2002 are shown in Figure 7.1.

Whereas the share of health care expenditures allocated to pharmaceuticals has risen in recent years, it is still far below the proportion spent on hospitals and physician services. This proportion declined from 1960 through the early 1980s but has increased more recently, particularly since 1994, and regained its earlier position of just over 10 percent of total health care expenditures.

Of these increased outlays on pharmaceuticals, only a portion is due to higher prices charged for existing drug products. Berndt estimates that only 22 percent of the growth in drug spending since 1997 has resulted from higher prices for existing drugs.[1] Still, price increases remain a relevant, if minor, factor for higher pharmaceutical expenditures.

To consider this matter, we review data from the Consumer Price Index (CPI) and its constituent parts, including pharmaceuticals and other health care services. Figure 7.2 shows time series data on the rate of increase in the overall CPI, the

## FIGURE 7.1. SHARE OF PERSONAL HEALTH EXPENDITURES, 1960–2002.

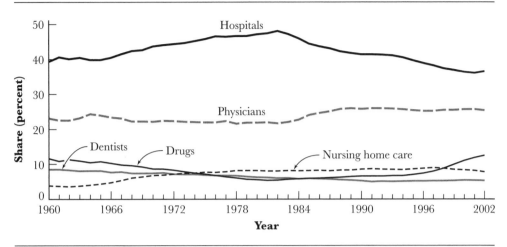

*Source:* Centers for Medicare and Medicaid Service, Office of the Actuary, National Health Statistics Group.

## FIGURE 7.2. RATE OF INCREASE FROM PREVIOUS YEAR (PERCENTAGE).

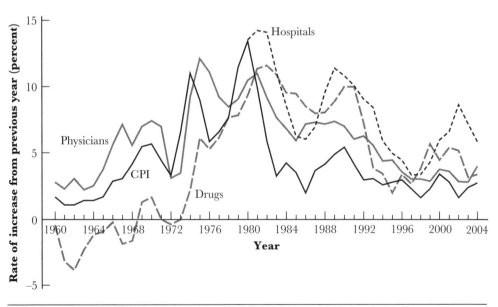

*Source:* Bureau of Labor Statistics, Consumer Price Index.

medical care component of the CPI, and also for its components (hospitals, physicians, dentists, and pharmaceuticals). The data shown are the annual rate of price change for the year prior to the indicated date.

These statistics show that the rate of price increase for health care exceeded that of the overall CPI for the entire period, but the rate of increase of pharmaceuticals is quite similar to that of the other health care components. Prior to 1980, the rate of increase of drug prices was below that of other health care components, but since then it has exceeded that of the other components, although it fell below the rate of change in hospital prices during the period for which data are available.[2]

If pharmaceuticals constitute only a small portion of overall health care expenditures, and if price increases have been similar to those of other components for many years, what explains continued public and congressional concern over drug prices and expenditures?

One answer to this query is that utilization has risen sharply, in part because of the country's aging population. Furthermore, drugs can do many more things today than in the past, so they are prescribed more frequently. Finally, direct-to-consumer (DTC) advertising may also lead to increased consumption. As a result of all of these factors, the number of prescriptions filled per year has risen dramatically, from 2 billion in 1993 to 3.4 billion in 2003.[3] Within some common therapeutic categories, the rise in quantity is even more dramatic. From 1993 to 1997, the number of antidepressant prescriptions filled increased by 111 percent, and that for cholesterol-lowering drugs rose by 162 percent. For oral antihistamines, this increase was fully 500 percent.[4]

The greater quantity of prescriptions filled is the primary factor behind recent increases in pharmaceutical spending. This includes both higher spending on new drugs, accounting for about 46 percent of the total increase since 1997, and higher quantities sold of existing drugs, which accounts for 32 percent of the total.[5] For the most part, therefore, higher spending is due to greater purchases of both new and existing drugs.

Another factor behind recent expressions of concern for these expenditures results from a fundamental difference between pharmaceuticals and other health service components: though most health care purchases are exclusively *services*, pharmaceuticals have both *service* and *manufactured* product components. The service role applies to knowledge of the therapeutic properties of the compound, gained from the research and development that lies behind all pharmaceutical products, and also to professional dispensing of the drug. However, the drug itself is a manufactured product, and most drugs are produced in volumes that take advantage of economies of scale in the manufacturing process. Production costs of drugs constitute less than half of total costs.[6] Because the prices charged for pharmaceuticals are much higher than production costs, it would theoretically be possible to reduce prices substantially and still cover manufacturing costs.[7]

To be sure, pharmaceutical margins must also cover the substantial research and marketing costs that accompany introduction of new drugs. At the same time, these are costs that generally have already been paid, and consumers may not see a link between them and what they are asked to pay. Further obscuring this linkage is the willingness of many pharmaceutical companies to sell the same or similar drugs at very different prices, through discounts to health insurers or health plans or to those in other countries.

Still another reason for public concern with pharmaceutical prices lies in the fact that most insurance plans cover well under 100 percent of the patient charges for drugs. Although more than four-fifths of total health care costs in the United States are paid by government or private insurers, third-party coverage for pharmaceuticals has historically been lower than that of hospital and physician services.[8] At the time of the Kefauver Committee hearings in the 1950s and 1960s, there was virtually no insurance coverage for drugs. In 1960, private insurance paid little of pharmaceutical expenses, and consumers paid directly out of pocket for 96 percent of their drug costs.[9] By 1999, the situation had changed and private health insurance covered an increasing proportion of total pharmaceutical expenditures. Out-of-pocket expenditures on pharmaceuticals fell to just 33 percent.[10] Still, the higher share of pharmaceutical expenditures paid directly means that consumers are less sheltered from drug costs than for other health care services, making them more visible to consumers.

For the elderly, the problem of high drug expenditures is more complicated. The universal health insurer for the elderly is the Medicare program, but Medicare's coverage of outpatient drugs did not begin until 2006. However, approximately 76 percent of seniors either qualify for Medicaid coverage (which covers outpatient drugs) or have private health insurance to supplement their Medicare coverage. Only 24 percent of the elderly have no extra drug coverage and have to pay out of pocket for their pharmaceuticals. For the rest, co-insurance or deductibles apply, where these payments are generally linked to the type of drug used to fill a prescription. For example, a prescription filled with a generic product may require only a $5 co-payment, while the co-payment for a branded product might be $20.

## Interpreting Pharmaceutical Price Data

Various reports, both public and private, disclose rapidly rising drug prices. A good example is a 1992 report by the U.S. Government Accountability Office (GAO), formerly the General Accounting Office. The GAO finds that "during the 1980s, prescription drug prices increased by almost three times the rate of general inflation and certain drugs increased in price by over 100 percent in five years."[11] This report reviews price data for a sample of widely used prescription drugs, and concludes: "Prices for nearly all 29 drug products increased more than the percentage changes for all three consumer price indexes for the six year period ending December 31, 1991. The maximum price increase for each product during this period generally exceeded 100 percent, with some prices increasing by 200 to 300 percent. . . . During this same period, the CPI for all items increased by 26.2 percent, the CPI for medical care by 56.3 percent, and the CPI for prescription drugs by 67 percent."[12]

These conclusions are incomplete. Since adoption of the 1984 law facilitating approval of generic drugs upon the originator's patent expiration, the importance of generics in pharmaceutical marketplaces has expanded rapidly. By 2000, fully 47 percent of pharmaceuticals dispensed, in terms of physical units, were for generic products, up from 40 percent as recently as 1993.[13] Today, about half of all drugs consumed in the United States are generics, and there has been little suggestion that high prices for these products are a problem.

An equally important factor is the role of large buyers who purchase pharmaceuticals to furnish them to their subscribers. These buyers include health insurance companies, HMOs, and some large employers who supply required drugs directly to their employees. As we describe later, these purchasers typically receive a substantial discount or rebate off the price established by the drug company. Since discounts or rebates are typically not disclosed, most discussions of pharmaceutical prices simply ignore them and thereby report higher prices than those that are actually paid.

## The Effect of Generic Products on Prices

Not only are generic products priced substantially below their branded counterparts; generic prices generally decline over time as the number of generic producers increases. For most products, the share of total sales for generics of a particular molecule expands greatly following patent expiration. Griliches and Cockburn observe that within two years of a branded drug's patent expiration, its market share of product revenues generally falls by 50 percent.[14] If this picture is broadly correct, then the increasing role of generic products in pharmaceutical markets has surely led to a declining average price for most products (including both the branded and the generic versions) following patent expiration and the entry of generic producers. A relevant question therefore is how the influence of generic entry, leading generally to lower prices, affects the claim by so many observers that pharmaceutical prices have sharply increased.

To answer this question, one first needs to decide whether the generic version of a drug is appropriately considered the same product as its branded counterpart. How one should appraise the statistical conclusions of many of these studies depends critically on this answer. In its computations, the Bureau of Labor Statistics (BLS) assumes that branded products are inherently different from their generic versions.[15] It notes that both patients and physicians frequently react differently to the two types of product despite their bioequivalence. On this basis, it treats these products as distinct entities and reports their price changes separately. Thus the BLS data does not incorporate the increasing use of lower-priced generic drugs in its published price series.[16]

In contrast, there is the implicit judgment of the Food and Drug Administration (FDA) that generic and branded versions of the same molecule are therapeutically identical. On this basis, one could prepare price series that include both incumbent and generic drugs that are linked according to their relative quantities. If this procedure is carried out for many individual products, average prices often decline.[17]

However, one cannot say that the FDA position is entirely correct and that the BLS position is entirely wrong, because a substantial number of buyers do in fact consider generic and branded products distinct. In their study of these issues, Griliches and Cockburn account for these views and construct adjusted price series. As might be expected, they report price series that lie between those based on the two extreme assumptions.[18] For the most part, their price series constructed for individual drugs show some price decline after introduction of generics, although less than price series based on the assumption that branded and generic versions are the same product.

## Launch Prices and Drug Price Changes

In addition to the issue of generic substitutability, the pricing strategies employed in the years following product introduction are also important. Two strategies are used: "skimming" and "penetration." The former involves setting a high introductory price but then reducing it over time, while the latter is the reverse, setting a low introductory price and increasing it over time. Clearly, prices of pharmaceutical products more frequently show a *declining* trend where a skimming strategy is common, but an *increasing* trend where penetration is employed.

Both pricing strategies are found in this industry. Skimming is more typically found with drugs representing a major therapeutic advance, while penetration is more commonly used for imitative products.[19] As a result, one is more likely to find rising drug prices when imitative products are introduced but declining prices when innovative products are seen. Therefore, rising prices may be a consequence of *low* (penetration) launch prices, while more moderate price trends may result from *high* (skimming) launch prices.

## Drug Prices and Quality Improvement

Branded pharmaceutical products compete not just with their generic substitutes but also among themselves. Even though a drug may be similar to others in its therapeutic category, it can differ in terms of side effects and adverse interaction profiles; higher introductory prices can frequently be explained by such improvements.[20] Indeed, a higher price for a new product generally reflects product improvement.

To investigate this issue, Berndt and his colleagues estimated a series of hedonic regression equations in which various attributes were used as proxies for the relative quality of a number of products. Through this technique, the authors were able to measure price trends while holding quality level constant. For the years between 1980 and 1996, and dealing only with antidepressant drugs, they report average price increases under three scenarios: the increase measured without accounting for generics or quality change, 7.11 percent; the increase including generics but without incorporating the improved quality of new products, 4.73 percent; and the increase incorporating both effects, 4.33 percent. Although the correction for generics was far more significant for the entire period they studied, they noted that there were particular years when the correction for quality change associated with new products was a more important factor than the increasing role of generics.[21]

Comanor, Schweitzer, and Carter also employed hedonic methods to study the separate effects of generic introduction and product attributes on drug prices. Their analysis was carried out for five pharmaceutical classes. They report that generics, as expected, lead to *lower* drug prices but that greater efficacy, reduced interaction leading to greater safety, and increased convenience in drug regimen tended to *increase* drug prices.[22]

## Measuring Prices When New Drugs Replace Old Ones

The BLS computes the overall CPI as well as its constituent parts as a Laspeyres index, which compares the cost of a given bundle of goods (often referred to as the "market basket") purchased at current prices to the cost of that same bundle purchased at base-year prices.[23] This market basket, however, must be adjusted periodically to reflect current expenditure patterns; otherwise the index would have ever less relationship with the actual goods purchased by consumers. In health care, new treatments for old problems, such as coronary artery disease or renal failure, have totally replaced techniques in use only a few years ago. In many cases, there are new therapies available for problems that were previously untreatable. If new and improved drugs replace older ones but at a higher price, the appropriate price index should account for quality improvement as well as price increase. If price indices fail to account adequately for quality improvement, measures of price changes are biased upward.

The method used by the BLS to measure price changes is designed to track prices for a fixed market basket, or one that changes slowly. When items in the market basket change through shifts in consumer demand, the BLS uses a "linking" technique through which the price index of a new market basket replaces the index for an older one. For example, if a new product, such as a more powerful antihypertensive drug, replaces an existing but less expensive one, price indices including the old and new products are each calculated, and the new index (with the higher-priced product) is scaled downward to equal the older one. The index including the new item then replaces the prior index in future calculations. No attempt is made to assess whether an improved drug is more or less expensive than would be justified by the quality change represented by its introduction. The price index merely tracks the prices of all items in the market basket and then recalculates the price index when a new product is included.

Failure to capture the effect of quality change is especially serious for pharmaceuticals, where turnover of products is rapid and new products frequently are an improved version of older ones, with greater efficacy, fewer side effects, or a more convenient regimen. The question of whether increases in drug prices exceed, fall behind, or accurately reflect quality changes is left unanswered.

## Prices and Margins: Differences Between Manufacturer and Retail Prices

There is also an important distinction between the prices set by pharmaceutical manufacturers and those ultimately paid by consumers. The difference between retail and manufacturer prices is the distribution margin, which includes the costs and profits of the dispensing pharmacy (as well as the wholesaler if one is involved in distributing the product). In many discussions of pharmaceutical costs, there is an implicit assumption that distribution margins are constant across products, such that whatever price is charged by the manufacturer is passed on to consumers, with merely a fixed amount added to cover distribution costs.

However, this picture is not generally accurate. Steiner in particular has disclosed "the inverse association between the margins of manufacturers and [those of] retailers."[24] His study offers empirical evidence on this relationship as well as the reasons for it. Salehi and Schweitzer[25] also report that the relationship applies to pharmaceuticals. Branded pharmaceuticals, which typically embody a high manufacturing margin, have lower distribution margins, while generic products with lower margins at the manufacturing stage generally have much higher distribution margins. As a result, price differences between branded and generic products are greater at the manufacturing stage of production than at retail.

## International Price Comparisons

International comparisons have also contributed to widespread concern that drug prices are excessive in the United States. For example, the GAO has published studies comparing U.S. drug prices with those in the United Kingdom and Canada.[26] These reports find that cash prices for the same branded products are generally higher in the United States than elsewhere. The GAO studies are subject to many of the same conceptual and methodological problems that were discussed earlier.

It is of particular signficance that the GAO studies fail to account for generic substitution in any comprehensive way. Even though their comparison of relative prices for a particular branded drug may be correct, they do not often reflect differences in the actual prices facing consumers since generics are typically more important in the United States than elsewhere. As we have noted, the share of the market accounted for by generic drugs in the United States has grown substantially and now comprises about half of all drug units (doses) sold.[27] Simply comparing the prices of specific branded products without including the prices of generic products therefore gives a misleading picture of the relative costs to consumers of filling a doctor's prescription.

For example, suppose that half of U.S. prescriptions for Cimetidine, a popular H2 blocker for gastric reflux and ulcers, are filled by the generic version, the price of which is $104 per hundred, while the price of the branded product, Tagamet, is $167. The average price is $135.50. Suppose further that the prices of both versions of the drug are lower in Canada, with Tagamet at $150 and the generic at $100. If the generic version's market share is only 20 percent in Canada, the average price there is $140, which is higher than the average U.S. price, even though the prices charged for both products are lower in Canada.

Another important problem with the GAO approach is that it relies on established nominal prices, which do not account for the many discounts and rebates present in the United States that are generally granted to large buyers. Even if these nominal prices accurately describe charges to pharmacies, which are then applied to cash customers, they do not reflect the transaction prices used for other classes of buyers, who in fact constitute the largest segment of demand. This factor is important because these discounts appear more widespread in the United States than in Britain or Canada.

Finally, the GAO reports fail to deal with drug consumption patterns varying among the three countries studied. Not only are drugs used differently in each country, but even the same drugs are taken in a variety of forms and dosages.[28] The GAO approach avoids the issue by asking a narrower question: Are wholesale prices higher in the United States than in Britain or Canada specifically for the highest-selling American drugs? This approach is likely to compare prices of highly popular U.S. products with those of less commonly used drugs in other countries, which is different from asking if drugs in general cost more in the United States than elsewhere.

In response to the GAO reports, Danzon and Chao carried out a more complete analysis of international drug price comparisons.[29] They included all drugs sold in nine countries, incorporating over-the-counter drugs that substitute for prescribed drugs; they also used data on average transaction prices at the manufacturer level. The authors found that price differences between countries depend greatly on how the comparison is framed—particularly which country's quantity weights are used to construct the price index. Comparison also depends on whether one examines price per gram of active ingredient or price per "standard unit" (per capsule, per milliliter of liquid, and so on). Although by most measures average U.S. drug prices exceed those in most other countries, this result does not always apply, and it does not include the more significant role played by generic products in the United States.

## Determining Drug Prices

We now turn to the causative factors that determine pharmaceutical prices. The R&D costs required to introduce a new drug are substantial, frequently in the hundreds of millions of dollars per drug. Researchers at the Tufts Center for Drug Development report that these costs reached $802 million per new drug introduced in 2002.[30]

Research costs include not only direct expenditures on research and testing but also the time costs incurred from the substantial differences between the dates that the outlays are made and the revenues received. Part of this lag represents the extended time that it takes for a drug to reach the stage of FDA application, and part is the time spent waiting for the FDA to evaluate a new product.

Furthermore, R&D outlays are typically made before a single prescription is filled. As a result, they are a classic example of sunk costs, which do not vary with output. R&D costs, like those on fixed plant and equipment, have already been incurred well before the product is sold, so they cannot influence actual market prices. Whether these costs are high or low, the optimal price charged by the pharmaceutical company is the same.

Similarly, most marketing costs are made in the early years of a product's life cycle and designed to introduce it to the medical community. As with research costs, they do not generally vary with output and are therefore sunk costs.

The variable costs in this industry lie at the manufacturing stage. For a large research-intensive company, however, production costs are generally less than half the value of the product.[31] Marginal costs for most drugs are relatively low and explain little about the prices that are charged.

Research and development, marketing, and manufacturing costs are all factors reflecting conditions on the supply side of the market. None of them has a major impact on pharmaceutical prices. Instead, prices depend predominantly on demand-side considerations. The prices charged for pharmaceuticals are determined largely by how valuable they are to consumers and what consumers are willing to pay for them. The critical factor is "willingness to pay," which in turn depends on various factors. At this point, we consider these factors and review some available evidence on their importance.

## Therapeutic Advance

The demand-side factor most important in determining the price of a pharmaceutical is its therapeutic advance compared to products already on the market. Doctors, patients, and HMOs are willing to pay a larger amount for an improved product compared to one without a substantial therapeutic advance. With increased willingness to pay, sellers can set higher prices without driving customers away.

The relative importance of *demand* in comparison to *supply* factors can be explored with the help of a simple example. Suppose drug A has been under development for many years. Costs have been high because its preclinical tests had to be redone, and clinical tests were also fraught with problems and took longer than expected. When its final (phase three) trials are completed, the manufacturer learns to its surprise that the new product is no more effective than competing drugs already on the market. In contrast, drug B follows another path. Its development and clinical trials go smoothly and quickly; best of all, the phase three trials show it to be more effective than existing therapies.

Which product, A or B, will be priced above drugs already on the market? Although Drug A has higher R&D costs, therapeutic equivalence to existing drugs leaves it unable to command a higher price. On the other hand, drug B yields improved therapy, which leads physicians and patients to be more willing to pay a higher price. Lower R&D costs have no affect on the price that the seller can set. What is significant, therefore, is relative effectiveness more than relative costs.

To explore empirically the importance of therapeutic advance, Lu and Comanor examined the price premium for new products compared to their existing rivals, evaluating the ratio of median price of new drugs to existing drugs. Among acute drugs that represent an important therapeutic advance, the price ratio for new drugs relative to existing drugs was 2.97, and 2.29 for chronic drugs. Among drugs representing a modest therapeutic advance, the ratios were 1.72 and 1.19, respectively. Finally, among drugs representing little or no therapeutic advance, the ratios were 1.22 and 0.94.[32]

These data show that the launch prices of drugs that embody an important therapeutic gain are two to three times greater than those of existing drugs for the same conditions. In contrast, drugs with moderate gains are priced at about one and one-half times greater, while products with little or no therapeutic advance are generally priced at or near the same level as existing products.

## Competitive Forces

For any new product introduced—whether it embodies a small or large therapeutic advance—there are typically existing products used for similar indications. These alternate products are those physicians would prescribe in the absence of the new product and are the rival products with which a new one must compete. This set of products, which defines a relevant economic market, rests on specific therapeutic indications and is much narrower than the conventional classification of a therapeutic category. Classifications such as antibiotics or hypertensives are so broad that they include pharmaceuticals with quite differing indications and hence products that do not actually compete with one another.

If there are alternative products available for similar indications, prescribing physicians must select among rival drugs. Physician and patient willingness to pay for specific drugs is influenced by any price differences that exist. In this case, sellers can hope to increase sales by cutting prices, and the more rival products that compete in the market, the more price cutting will occur.

The Lu and Comanor study found that launch prices are substantially lower when there are more branded rivals in direct competition, and subsequent price changes are lower as well. Despite frequent disdain for imitative products on the part of industry critics,[33] they play an essential role in promoting more competitive behavior and leading to lower final prices. New imitative products are an important competitive factor in the pharmaceutical marketplace.

Generic pharmaceuticals also have an important impact on market competition and price level. Generic producers typically start production after the relevant patent has expired. They do so by gaining FDA approval of an abbreviated new drug application (ANDA), which requires simple demonstration of bioequivalence to the original product. The prices set by generic producers are much lower than those charged by the original developer of the product because they compete largely by price. Moreover, the prices of generic products are also affected by the number of sellers. With more sellers, price competition becomes more vigorous, and prices decline below the level found when there was only a single generic entrant.

A study of anti-infectives found that the largest price effects occurred when the fourth and fifth generic firms entered. Average prices per prescription declined from nearly $30 with two or three sellers to less than $20 with the presence of a fourth rival, and eventually approached $4 for products with forty or more sellers.[34]

The reported decline in average price took place despite the fact that prices charged for the original branded products are typically *raised* rather than reduced once entry occurs.[35] The original manufacturers do not typically compete with generic entrants on the basis of price but often find it more profitable to concentrate on that segment of the market that includes brand-loyal customers. Such buyers are physicians and patients who know a particular brand and prefer it, so they continue to use it despite the presence of a lower-priced substitute. After generic manufacturers enter production, the price differential expands as the prices charged for the original branded products increase.

## Insured and Cash Buyers

As has been noted, a growing proportion of pharmaceutical purchases are made by insured patients such that a declining share is actually paid out of pocket. Currently, only about one-third of total drug expenditures are paid directly by consumers; the rest is paid through private or government insurance. There are thus two separate channels for drug expenditures with contrasting pricing practices in each.

The larger channel, representing about two-thirds of total expenditures, includes insured patients. Actual purchases are made by an intermediary, which can be a government agency, private insurance company, or HMO; this frequently involves the assistance of a pharmacy benefit manager (PBM) to help organize the complicated system of pricing and distribution. The transaction price is negotiated between the drug manufacturer and the intermediary or PBM. In most circumstances, moreover, manufacturers grant substantial (and secret) rebates and discounts to these buyers; their net prices are often much lower than those charged to cash buyers.[36] For this reason, the pricing studies that rely on reported prices can be misleading when applied to insured patients.

For these patients, the out-of-pocket price for a pharmaceutical product is set not by the drug manufacturer but rather by the insurance company, HMO, or government agency. Their co-pay is the relevant price, and it is this price that influences their purchasing decision.[37] Furthermore, in most cases this co-pay is not based on the amount actually paid by the intermediary for the specific product. For this reason, insured patients are largely insulated from whatever prices are charged by the manufacturers.

For many health plans, co-pays are tied to the formulary, which is a restrictive list of approved products. Many plans currently use three-tiered formularies, where the health plan sets a relatively low co-payment for generics, a moderate co-payment for the branded version of a drug whose manufacturer has agreed to a large discount in the wholesale price (this product is often called the "preferred brand"), and imposes the largest co-payment on all other branded products in the particular drug class. The expectation on the part of the health plan is that physicians will be pressured by their patients to select products with lower co-payment, thus allowing the health plan to reduce drug costs.

This effect has not been tested by researchers, but two studies have shown that patients are not very willing to switch drug products when their former product is placed in the more expensive co-payment category.[38] However, it is also possible that patients already familiar with a particular drug may be more insensitive to price changes for the drug while those who are newly introduced to a drug class are more eager to purchase the cheapest product available. This argument suggests that the physician-patient demand elasticity may depend on whether the patient has used the drug in the past. In this case, both physician and patient may recognize the possibility of costs and risks associated with switching away from a drug that "works" to a lower-priced alternative. In contrast, new patients to a drug class do not face the same switching costs.

Whereas the prices paid by intermediaries can affect health insurance premiums and thereby insured patients indirectly, the fact that pharmaceuticals account for only about 10 percent of health care expenditures means that these premiums are largely determined by other factors. For the larger channel of pharmaceutical distribution and expenditures, actual prices are generally lower than the prices widely reported. Furthermore, these prices are not paid directly by the patients.

In contrast, the smaller channel of distribution does involve cash prices, which are borne directly by patients. Of all prescriptions written, only 15–20 percent are paid out of pocket for branded products.[39] This is not an inconsequential proportion (and prices can be high for these buyers), but it does not represent a dominant share of pharmaceutical sales. Thus the problem of high drug prices, as they have an impact on consumers, largely applies to such purchases.

For uninsured patients who purchase pharmaceuticals much as they do other consumer goods, demand is often fairly price-elastic. Although the buyer is limited to a prescribed product, he or she can influence the physician's prescribing decision by calling attention to the prices of alternate products. Where a generic version of the drug is available, patients can also ask the pharmacist to substitute it for the branded product. The patient always has the option of not filling the prescription—which occurs in a large number of cases.[40]

In effect there are different price-setting mechanisms in place for the two distinct distribution channels. The channels need to be approached independently. Although some factors apply to both, there are many factors that affect only one or the other.

## The Role of the Pharmacy Benefit Manager

The PBM is relevant for the larger, insured distribution channel. For these sales, the PBM plays an important role and has a major effect on the prices paid to drug manufacturers by HMOs, health insurance companies, and many large employers. The beneficiaries of these buyers obtain their prescribed pharmaceuticals from local pharmacies, where their payment is the co-pay.

The affiliated PBM has contractual relations not only with the large buyer clients but also with drug manufacturers and pharmacies. For the pharmacies, these outlets are reimbursed for the drugs provided to their clients' beneficiaries. The reimbursement amount is determined by the amount paid by the pharmacy for the pharmaceutical, and also the co-payment received from the consumer. Reimbursement typically includes a dispensing fee in addition to a profit margin.

To cover this outflow, the PBM receives payments from two sources. The first and primary revenues are received from the affiliated contractor: the payer who provides for the particular patient. The payment made for the drug reimburses the PBM for payment to the pharmacy, minus a share of any rebates received by the PBM from the drug company. Absent any rebate, this payment merely equals the cash price. Without rebate, the payer would pay the same amount as any cash purchaser (albeit through a circuitous route).

What sets the stage for large payers to pay lower prices than cash customers are the rebate payments made by the drug manufacturers to PBMs. In most cases, drug companies rebate a portion of the payments received from pharmacies for their products to the PBMs who support these sales. These rebates are the subject of negotiation between the PBM and the manufacturer and can differ with the product and the buyer. In effect, the manufacturer receives a net price for the product, which equals the cash price minus the rebate. Finally, depending on the contractual arrangements between the PBM and the payers, a portion of the rebates received by the PBM are remitted to the supporting payer.

From the vantage point of the parties concerned, this complicated system has various advantages. For the drug manufacturer, the system permits it to separate product flows from payment flows in a way not commonly found in the American economy. Generally, products are shipped by a manufacturer to a wholesaler and then to a retailer; payment flows move in the reverse sequence. The presence of rebates permits manufacturers effectively to charge varying prices to buyers and thereby create a complicated system of differential pricing. The system is feasible because the ultimate consumer of these products does not typically bear the predominant share of their costs.

Similarly, the payers benefit by receiving a lower price for the drugs furnished to their beneficiaries compared to cash buyers. These buyers gain this advantage thanks to their greater bargaining power or more elastic demand.

Finally, insured or covered patients benefit from the availability of prescribed medicines at lower prices. Their effective price is merely the co-payment, although the same products are available through the same pharmacies to other buyers who must pay the higher cash price.

A major source of the rebates obtained by PBMs is their ability to switch consumers between alternate products. For pharmaceuticals as for most other products, a manufacturer is often willing to accept a lower price in return for increased sales. As a result, PBMs who promise to expand sales for one product at the expense of another are rewarded with lower prices, which in this system take the form of higher rebates. To receive a higher rebate, a PBM seeks to switch patients from one product to another. The switching process often involves contacting the prescribing physicians by telephone and requesting a change to another product for an individual patient.

The process of switching customers among competing products is the same one that generates a large share of the rebates received by PBMs. This switching process creates two sets of concerns. The first is division of rebates between the PBMs and the payers; the second is the effect of the switching process itself on the patient and the physician.

Since PBMs necessarily receive information on an individual physician's prescriptions for specific patients, they can use it to influence the prescribing decision. PBM representatives commonly seek to persuade physicians to shift their patients to drugs that offer a larger rebate. The physician, of course, has the final word, but these efforts are often quite effective and account for the large sums received by PBMs.

Although the contractual relationships between PBMs and drug manufacturers are complex, there are commonalities running through them. Rebates are typically larger as product sales increase, relative to either some benchmark or its share of product category sales. As an example, a rebate percentage may increase from 4 to 8 percent as the product's share of sales to particular customers increases from 30 to 45 percent.

A striking feature of the rebate process is that it is designed specifically to place one product at a more advantageous position than another. However, since one product's gain is achieved at the expense of another, producers of the latter have an incentive to respond. If there are sufficient PBMs to service competing manufacturers, then the rebate percentage should increase to a competitive level. Note that since higher rebates imply lower prices, this process can lead to competitive pricing. Alternatively, if there are only a few PBMs, then a manufacturer's affiliation with a PBM may have a substantial effect on market shares, with some drug companies offering larger rebates and gaining increased shares. In this case, there can be a wide disparity in rebates paid between products, PBMs, and payers.

## Differential Pricing

Where prices depend on demand conditions and where there are clear distinctions among types of buyer, we expect to find different prices charged to different buyers. The economist's model of price discrimination presents a clear description of this process and indicates that prices depend on the relevant price elasticity of demand. Where the elasticity differs with the class of consumer, final price differs as well. This pattern is pervasive throughout the pharmaceutical industry.

Even though pharmaceutical companies establish a list price for each drug, called the average wholesale price or AWP, many (or most) sales are made by discounting that price. These discounts can be substantial. A survey of drug prices in one area found that the average price charged for a selection of well-known products sold to hospitals was only 19 percent of that charged to a local pharmacy.[41] Since hospital demand for specific products is likely to be more elastic than for an individual pharmacy, which must stock a large number of products in order to fill individual prescriptions, hospital prices should be lower than those charged to pharmacies. Where prices are demand-driven, demand elasticities are reflected in price differences.

These discounts may also differ for individuals and chain store pharmacies, and between hospitals and HMOs. An important feature of the pharmaceutical industry is that there is no single price for an individual product even at a specific point in time; prices depend on the demand conditions presented by particular buyers.

Generic products entering the marketplace typically appeal more to some buyers than to others. For example, HMOs and hospital pharmacies are more likely to use generic drugs because they have the knowledge and expertise required to evaluate them, in contrast to individual physicians. One expects therefore that generic rivals will make greater sales to some buyers than to others. That being so, producers of branded products respond to generic competition more strongly in some market segments than in others. By setting much lower prices where generic competition exists, but keeping prices at their original level or even higher where generic competition is less important, the sellers of many branded products have been able to maintain a large proportion of their original sales.

The evidence that major pharmaceutical firms have followed this type of strategy is that they are sometimes able to maintain a substantial market share following patent expiration and generic entry. By the sixth year after patent expiration, average market shares for thirty-five products between 1984 and 1987 were fully 62 percent in physical units and 85 percent in dollar sales compared to the previous level.[42] The strategy of charging lower prices where firms face strenuous competition but higher prices where they do not is used by many drug companies to maintain sales and market share.

# Approaches for Containing Pharmaceutical Costs

Pharmaceutical companies have sought to maintain or expand revenues, but health care consumers, providers, and insurers have looked for methods to limit drug expenditures. Here as elsewhere, buyers and sellers face opposing incentives. Some buyers seek to reduce the quantity of drugs consumed, but most look for means to lower the price paid for a specific product or to redirect patients toward lower-priced alternatives. These methods can be divided into those focused on consumer behavior, physician prescribing patterns, and manufacturer actions. At this point, we review some of the measures that have been used.

### Patient-Focused Measures

Consumer behavior can be altered through economic incentives or education. Economic incentives typically mean cost sharing, through which patients bear more of the financial consequences of their actions by paying a larger share of drug costs. As the out-of-pocket cost of drugs increases, the quantity purchased declines, with patients either going without the prescribed drugs or shifting to less expensive alternatives such as generic products or over-the-counter options.

Cost sharing is sometimes criticized as being an overly blunt instrument, because it may discourage use of necessary as well as unnecessary therapies. The RAND Health Insurance Experiment studied the effect of cost sharing on consumption of prescribed drugs. Leibowitz and her colleagues reported that pharmaceutical expenditures by individuals without cost sharing were as much as 60 percent higher than for those with cost sharing.[43] These authors also found that consumers were generally more likely to reduce purchases of discretionary rather than essential drugs in response to increased cost sharing.

An alternative to economic incentives in dealing with consumer behavior is patient education. An example of this type of program is informing patients that generic drugs are equivalent to branded products. Another is explaining to patients that extensive use of certain drugs, such as antibiotics, is unnecessary and may even be harmful, thereby lowering the quantity purchased. Such programs can reduce consumer demand for specific products, but they are unlikely to limit very much the aggregate demand for pharmaceuticals. Many patients still expect a prescription at the conclusion of each physician visit, and physicians respond accordingly.

## Provider-Focused Measures

Despite the presence of consumer-oriented programs, most efforts at cost containment for pharmaceuticals are directed at those who make the decision on drug therapy: the physician, hospital, or managed care provider. Because physicians, particularly those in private practice, have few incentives to limit pharmaceutical costs, physician-directed policies are not much different from those aimed at consumers. When financial constraints are removed from patients, they are also generally removed from their physicians.

However, physicians are also the subject of education programs that seek to improve the quality of prescribing and reduce overall drug expenditures. These programs are present especially in HMOs and other managed care programs; they have great potential because the pace of new-drug introduction is rapid and physicians have difficulty keeping abreast of new therapeutic options. Without such programs, the primary means the physician has for learning about new products is pharmaceutical company marketing efforts, which are designed to increase rather than reduce spending on pharmaceuticals.

Physicians have few incentives to limit costs; this is not so for the organizations that actually pay for pharmaceuticals. Generic versions of drugs are generally favored, and newer, more expensive drugs often discouraged.[44] In addition, these payers promote the shift of certain products to over-the-counter status. These drugs can be obtained without a visit to the physician's office, and such products are typically not reimbursed.

Furthermore, hospitals, HMOs, and government reimbursement plans have adopted formularies designed explicitly to restrict the drug choices available to physicians in order to reduce costs. These lists of approved drugs depend in principle on the relative cost and effectiveness of alternative products. Though nearly every formulary program permits exceptions, the burden of obtaining an exemption is often great enough to discourage a physician from doing so unless he or she feels that a nonlisted drug is absolutely necessary.[45]

Formularies, however, have the potential for increasing rather than decreasing health care costs if they are so restrictive that patients are prescribed less-effective drugs. Even expensive drugs are generally less costly than a physician visit or hospital episode such that using suboptimal drugs may be penny wise but pound foolish. The question of whether or not a formulary lowers or raises drug or overall health care costs depends on the relative prices of the drugs included and excluded from the formulary, the number of patients who use the more expensive product when it is not necessary, and the treatment ramifications for patients who are switched to a less expensive drug when they need the more expensive one. Sloan and Gordon found that "limiting the number of drugs [through a formulary] appears to have been a very good idea for gastrointestinal disease patients and for those with asthma, but a bad one for coronary disease patients."[46] In the latter case, total medical costs actually increased with adoption of the formulary. Other studies have also shown that Medicaid formularies are not effective in lowering drug expenditures or reducing overall health care costs.[47]

## Manufacturer-Focused Measures

A more direct approach to cost containment is the exercise of a payer's monopsony power to limit the prices charged by pharmaceutical manufacturers. These actions are frequently adopted by governments offering coverage for pharmaceuticals in their national programs. Increasingly, foreign governments and insurance funds have sought to reduce drug prices as a means of cost control. In most countries, the question is not whether to fix prices but how to do so, and in particular how to set prices without removing the incentive to develop new and improved pharmaceuticals. A typical response is to permit use of a product and reimburse costs in accordance with its relative therapeutic benefits. Ideally, this objective leads to the same prices as those set in a competitive market. Regulatory objectives are thereby similar to those enforced by competitive markets.

Australia has progressed further than most other countries in attempting to calculate the cost-effectiveness of new drugs and setting reimbursement rates accordingly.[48] Canada uses this model at the national level as well. Britain, on the other hand, incorporates the profitability of the pharmaceutical company into its calculation of the National Health Service price for new products.

Advertising is often suggested as a cause of rising pharmaceutical expenditures. With the FDA's relaxation of prohibitions against direct-to-consumer advertising, this particular marketing approach is increasingly visible to the general public. The criticism of DTC advertising is that it influences prescribing and consumption decisions adversely—that is, against patient interests. Even though the FDA monitors advertising carefully to guard against unsubstantiated claims, it has followed the guidance of the Federal Trade Commission in recognizing that advertising is inherently biased in favor of the sponsor's product (for any product or service); one should not expect different behavior on the part of pharmaceutical advertisers.

Firms are permitted to present information regarding their products that is favorable, and leave it to other producers to do the same for their own products. If there is a need for unbiased information on competing products, it should be provided separately. In the case of pharmaceuticals, there are already a number of independent newsletters, some directed to physicians and others to patients, that compare alternative therapies. The potential of the Internet to expand this sort of information is considerable.

Prescribing quality would also be improved if the NIH sponsored more head-to-head clinical trials of competing drugs within a class so that competing claims could be evaluated. Drug firms, which sponsor most drug trials in connection with the drug approval process, have little incentive to conduct multiproduct trials, but such trials are precisely what physicians and health plans need.

# The Link Between Pharmaceutical Expenditures and Research

The most serious questions raised in discussion of pharmaceutical cost containment concern whether success can be achieved without sacrificing the large investment in R&D for new products made by major drug companies. If cost containment is pursued too severely, the fear is that these efforts will diminish the returns from innovation and that lower spending on R&D will result.

The answer to this question was sought in a recent paper by Scherer, who explored the link between pharmaceutical profitability and R&D expenditures.[49] Since these outlays are largely financed from internally generated funds, research levels are likely to depend on gross industry margin, which is the difference between firm receipts and direct costs. Finding substantial "cyclical co-movement in pharmaceutical industry gross margins and R&D outlays," Scherer concluded: "As profit opportunities expand, firms compete to exploit them by increasing R&D investments, and perhaps also promotional costs, until increases in costs dissipate most, if not all, supranormal profit returns. . . . This interpretation . . . has self-evident implications for policy interventions aimed at reducing industry prices and profits."[50]

# Conclusions and Directions for Future Research

Recent trends in pharmaceutical prices can be examined from various vantage points. That the prices of the most advanced drugs have increased over time is certainly correct, although this result turns largely on the increasing benefits of the new products. This result is especially strong when branded products are considered to be different from and perhaps superior to their generic counterparts. On the other hand, prices for the same-quality products have tended to decline over time. Since "inflation" traditionally describes price changes for the same or similar products, one cannot conclude from recent experience that there has been much pharmaceutical price inflation. What has occurred instead is that the prices of newer products (especially their branded versions) have increased substantially, even while prices of competing products and generic alternatives have declined.

Our picture of drug price control is a mixed one. The share of health expenditures devoted to pharmaceuticals is relatively low, and there is a history of moderate price increases, although with some acceleration, in recent years. Furthermore, in the last few years there have been rapid changes in the market for drugs, with increasing importance for provider-driven rather than patient-driven competition. These changes have had a growing impact on both average rates of price increase and patterns of price dispersion for pharmaceuticals. The increased segmentation of pharmaceutical markets on the basis of insurance coverage also means that the *average* price level conveys less information about what is actually taking place. Traditional measures of price changes are inadequate and tend to inflate the actual rate of increase; international comparisons also yield inconclusive results.

A critical policy issue for the cost of pharmaceuticals is whether uniform pharmaceutical prices should be mandated for various customer classes. If this type of proposal were enacted, whether through legislation or judicial decision, pricing practices would change sharply. Berndt has pointed out that under these conditions the vigor of competition in many pharmaceutical markets would diminish sharply, and we could expect to find higher overall prices.[51] This type of policy change would increase the cost of pharmaceuticals.

This overview of the major factors determining the cost of pharmaceuticals illustrates three important areas where additional information would assist policy analysts. The first is the need to understand better the relationship between drug price and quality level. Preliminary data show that prices are positively affected by a drug's therapeutic advance, but the extent of this relationship is not well explored. This question is especially important because of our present inability to account for quality improvement in measures of pharmaceutical price increase.

Second, we know little about how the quality level for a drug is determined. Until recently, the FDA assigned a three-level quality improvement score to each drug for which marketing approval was sought. This designation was crude at best, and sometimes contradicted by the marketplace. However, the FDA currently does not provide even these designations, and there is no agreed-on measure of the extent of therapeutic improvement represented by new drugs.

Third, we need a better understanding of the extent of competition in pharmaceutical markets. This factor is especially critical, because we are now observing another wave of consolidation in the pharmaceutical industry. Better understanding of the appropriate breadth of pharmaceutical markets is also needed. How much rivalry is there within or across therapeutic categories? Understanding of how pharmaceutical markets are structured and interact would assist in creating appropriate public policies for this industry.

# Notes

1. Berndt, E. R. "The U.S. Pharmaceutical Industry: Why Major Growth in Times of Cost Containment?" *Health Affairs,* Mar.–Apr. 2001, *20,* p. 107.
2. Department of Health and Human Services. *Health United States, 1999.* Hyattsville, Md.: National Center for Health Statistics, 1999.
3. Kaiser Family Foundation. "Prescription Drug Trends—Update." (Publication no. 3057-03.) Menlo Park, Calif.: Kaiser Family Foundation, Oct. 2004.
4. National Institute for Health Care Management. "Issue Brief: Factors Affecting Growth of Prescription Drugs Expenditures." Washington, D.C.: National Institute for Health Care Management, 1999.
5. National Institute for Health Career Management (1999). Berndt (2001) notes that "new drugs" in this data set includes new generic versions of existing products, so the importance of this factor is overstated somewhat.
6. Comanor, W. S., and Schweitzer, S. O. "Pharmaceuticals." In W. Adams and J. W Brock (eds.), *Structure of American Industry* (9th ed.). Upper Saddle River, N.J.: Prentice-Hall, 1995.
7. Comanor and Schweitzer (1995).
8. Health Insurance Institute of America. *Source Book of Health Insurance Data, 1993.* Prepared for the National Center for Health Statistics. *National Health Expenditure Survey, 1996.* Washington, D.C.: National Center for Health Statistics, 1996.
9. Danzon, P. M., and Pauly, M. V. "Health Insurance and the Growth in Pharmaceutical Expenditures." *Journal of Law and Economics,* Oct. 2002, *45*(2, Part 2), 587–614.
10. Danzon and Pauly (2002).
11. U. S. General Accounting Office. *Prescription Drugs Changes in Prices for Selected Drugs.* (GAO/HRD-92-128.) Washington, D.C.: GAO, 1992, p. 1.
12. U. S. General Accounting Office (1992), p. 2.
13. Pharmaceutical Research and Manufacturers Association. *Annual Report 2004–05.* Washington, D.C.: Pharmaceutical Research and Manufacturers Association, 2004; and National Institute for Health Care Management (1999).
14. Griliches, Z., and Cockburn, I. M. "Generics and New Goods in the Pharmaceutical Price Indexes." *American Economic Review,* Dec. 1994, p. 1218.
15. Griliches and Cockburn (1994).
16. In May 1996, the Bureau of Labor Statistics announced that it was changing its procedures for constructing the price index for pharmaceuticals and would henceforth use linking procedures that treated generics and their branded counterparts as perfect substitutes. However, these changes are sufficiently recent that we cannot determine their impact on reported price series at the current time.

17. Griliches and Cockburn (1994).
18. Griliches and Cockburn (1994).
19. Lu, Z. J., and Comanor, W. S. "Strategic Pricing of New Pharmaceuticals." *Review of Economics and Statistics,* Feb. 1998, p. 116.
20. Lu and Comanor (1998); and Comanor, W. S., Schweitzer, S. O., and Carter, T. "A Hedonic Model of Pricing Innovative Pharmaceuticals." In M. R. DiTommaso and S. O. Schweitzer (eds.), *Health Policy and High-Tech Industrial Development: Learning from Innovation in the Health Industry.* Cheltenham: Edward Elgar, 2005.
21. Berndt, E. R., Cockburn, I. M., and Griliches, Z., Keeler, T. E., and Baily, M. N. "Pharmaceutical Innovations and Market Dynamics: Tracking Effects on Price Indexes for Antidepressant Drugs." *Brookings Papers on Economic Activity: Microeconomics,* 1996, p. 174.
22. Comanor, Schweitzer, and Carter (2005).
23. Feldstein, P. J. *Health Care Economics* (4th ed.). Albany, N.Y.: Delmar, 1993.
24. Steiner, R. L. "The Inverse Association Between the Margins of Manufacturers and Retailers." *Review of Industrial Organization,* 1993, *8,* 717–740.
25. Salehi, H., and Schweitzer, S. "Economic Aspects of Drug Substitution." *Health Care Financing Review,* 1985, *6*(5), 59–68.
26. U.S. Congress, General Accounting Office. "Prescription Drugs: Companies Typically Charge More in the United States Than in Canada." (GAO/HRD-92-110.) Washington, D.C.: GAO, Sept. 30, 1992; and U.S. Congress, GAO. "Prescription Drugs: Companies Typically Charge More in the United States Than in the United Kingdom." (GAO/HEHS-94-29.) Washington, D.C.: GAO, Jan. 12, 1994.
27. Pharmaceutical Research and Manufacturers Association (2004).
28. Payer, L. *Medicine and Culture: Varieties of Treatment in the United States, England, West Germany, and France.* New York: Penguin, 1988.
29. Danzon, P., and Chao, L.-W. "Cross-National Price Differences for Pharmaceuticals: How Large, and Why?" *Journal of Health Economics,* 2000, *19,* 159–195.
30, DiMasi, J. A., Hansen, R. W., and Grabowski, H. G. "The Price of Innovation: New Estimates of Drug Development and Costs." *Journal of Health Economics,* 2003, *22*(2), 151-185.
31. Comanor and Schweitzer (1995).
32. Lu and Comanor (1998).
33. Kessler, D., Rose, J. L., Temple, R. J., Schapiro, R., and Griffin, J. P. "Therapeutic Class Wars: Drug Promotion in a Competitive Marketplace." *New England Journal of Medicine,* 1994, *331,* 1350–1353.
34. Wiggins, S. N., and Maness, R. "Price Competition in Pharmaceuticals: The Case of Anti-Infectives." *Economic Inquiry,* 2004, *42*(2), 247–263.
35. Frank, R., and Salkever, D. "Pricing Patent Loss and the Market for Pharmaceuticals." *Southern Economic Journal,* Oct. 1992, *50,* 165–179.
36. These lower prices are clearly indicated in Comanor, Schweitzer, and Carter (2005).
37. For evidence on this point, see Esposito, D. *You Get What You Co-Pay for: The Influence of Patent Co-Payments on the Demand for Drugs.* Doctoral dissertation, Department of Economics, University of California, Santa Barbara, June 2003.
38. Huskamp, H. A., and others. "The Effect of Incentive-Based Formularies on Prescription Drug Utilization and Spending." *New England Journal of Medicine,* 2003, *349,* 2224–2232; and Goldman, D. P., and others. "Pharmacy Benefits and the Use of Drugs by the Chronically Ill." *Journal of the American Medical Association,* 2004, *291,* 2344–2350.
39. One-half (the share of branded products) of one-third (the share of uninsured, cash customers) equals one-sixth, or nearly 17 percent of all prescriptions.

40. Cooper, J. K., Love, D. W., and Raffoul, P. R. "Intentional Prescription Nonadherence (Noncompliance) by the Elderly." *American Geriatrics Society*, 1982, *30*, 329; and Clark, L. T. "Improving Compliance and Increasing Control of Hypertension: Needs of Special Hypertensive Populations." *American Heart Journal*, 1991, *121*, 664.

41. Fritz, S. "Prescription Drug Pricing Hurting the Poor, Elderly Health." *Los Angeles Times*, Jan. 30, 1994.

42. U.S. Congress, Office of Technology Assessment. *Pharmaceutical R&D: Costs, Risks and Rewards.* (OTA-H-522.) Washington, D.C.: U.S. Government Printing Office, Feb. 1993.

43. Leibowitz, A., Manning, W. G., and Newhouse, J. P. "The Demand for Prescription Drugs as a Function of Cost-Sharing." *Social Science and Medicine*, 1985, *21*, 1063–1069.

44. Harris, B. L., Stergachis, A., and Ried, L. D. "The Effect of Drug Co-Payments on Utilization and Cost of Pharmaceuticals in a Health Maintenance Organization." *Medical Care*, 1990, *28*(10), 907–917.

45. Grabowski, H. G., Schweitzer, S. O., and Shiota, S. R. "The Medicaid Drug Lag: Adoption of New Drugs by State Medicaid Formularies." *Pharmacoeconomics*, 1992, *1*(supp.), 32–40.

46. Sloan, F. A., Gordon, G, and Cocks, D. L. "Do Hospital Drug Formularies Reduce Spending on Hospital Services?" *Medical Care*, 1993, *31*(10), 851–867.

47. See Schweitzer, S. O., and Shiota, S. R. "Access and Cost Implications of State Limitations on Medicaid Reimbursement for Pharmaceuticals," *Annual Review of Public Health*, 1992, *13*, 399–410; and Moore, W. J., and Newman, R. J. "Drug Formulary Restrictions as a Cost-Containment Policy in Medicaid Programs." *Journal of Law and Economics*, Apr. 1993, *36*, 71–97.

48. U.S. Congress, Office of Technology Assessment (1993).

49. Scherer, F. M. "The Link Between Gross Probability and Pharmaceutical R&D Spending." *Health Affairs*, Sept.–Oct. 2001, *20*, pp. 216–220.

50. Scherer (2001), p. 220.

51. Berndt, E. R. *Uniform Pharmaceutical Pricing: An Economic Analysis.* Washington, D.C.: American Enterprise Institute, 1994.

PART THREE

# QUALITY OF HEALTH CARE

CHAPTER EIGHT

# MEASURING OUTCOMES AND HEALTH-RELATED QUALITY OF LIFE

Patricia A. Ganz
Mark S. Litwin
Ron D. Hays
Robert M. Kaplan

In the first installment of a six-part series on the quality of health care that appeared in the *New England Journal of Medicine* in 1996, David Blumenthal culled several definitions to support his premise that medical outcomes are a critical component of quality.[1] One of the earliest attempts to define quality came from the American Medical Association, which in the mid-1980s stated that high-quality care was that "which consistently contributes to the improvement or maintenance of quality and/or duration of life."[2] Blumenthal went on to note that the Institute of Medicine held in the 1990s that quality consists of the "degree to which health services for individuals and populations increase the likelihood of desired health outcomes."[3] He contended that the most important new development in our current understanding of medical outcomes was the recognition that it is patients who define which outcomes are most important and whether or not they have been achieved. "Using psychometric techniques," he argued, "researchers have developed better measures of patients' evaluations of the results of care, thus allowing patients' views to be assessed with greater scientific accuracy."[4]

Blumenthal's emphasis on quality of life in the context of quality of care underscored a body of research that has grown rapidly over the last thirty years. Figure 8.1 summarizes the number of publications, under the topic of quality of life, identified in PubMed between 1972 and 2003. In 1972, PubMed did not identify any publications under the quality-of-life topic heading, over the next thirty years, the number of articles that use the quality-of-life key word grew dramatically. In

## FIGURE 8.1. QUALITY-OF-LIFE PUBLICATIONS BY YEAR.

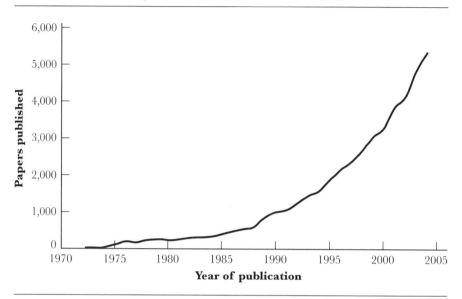

2004, it identified 5,399 articles. In these three decades, the tools for quality-of-life measurement became more refined, allowing sophisticated analysis of patients' perceived outcomes in a variety of illnesses. Today, health-related quality of life (HRQL) is studied in a variety of subjects throughout the stages of life[5] and as a measure of community health.[6]

This work has largely been built on a stage set by Paul Ellwood in his 1988 Shattuck lecture[7] in which he advocated using a technology of patient experience, drawing on a common patient-understood language of health outcomes. He proposed that "outcomes management would draw on four already rapidly maturing techniques. First, it would place greater reliance on standards and guidelines that physicians can use in selecting appropriate interventions. Second, it would routinely and systematically measure the functioning and well-being of patients, along with disease-targeted clinical outcomes, at appropriate time intervals. Third, it would pool clinical and outcome data on a massive scale. Fourth, it would analyze and disseminate results from the segment of the data base most appropriate to the concerns of each decision maker." Later, Ellwood went on to say that "the centerpiece and unifying ingredient of outcomes management is the tracking and measurement of function and well-being or quality of life. Although this sounds like a hopelessly optimistic undertaking, I believe that we already have the ability to obtain crucial, reliable data on quality of life at minimal cost and inconvenience."[8]

Ellwood's support for active inclusion of quality-of-life data as a key component of outcomes management lends important support to advancement of the field; however, more than a decade later this form of outcome assessment is still in its adolescence. Despite its appeal, quality-of-life data must be collected prospectively and cannot be retrieved from the administrative databases that are commonly used by health services researchers.

## Definition, Conceptualization, and Measurement of Quality of Life

Great energy has traditionally been expended by clinicians and other health care professionals attempting to lengthen the duration of survival in patients with various chronic diseases.[9] During the last few decades, dramatic advances in diagnosis, management, and overall understanding of the mechanisms of human disease have refined the treatment approaches to many medical conditions such that patients are now living longer with their disease. This is particularly true in oncology, where some patients live for years after their initial diagnosis.[10]

Historically, evaluation of the success of medical therapies has focused on specific clinical parameters and survival. However, the recent surge of interest in patient-centered endpoints has generated great support for the medical-outcomes movement. Not only clinicians but also payers and managers are interested in assessing outcomes to begin measuring quality of care. Indeed, some would argue that the thrust of the outcomes movement stems largely from outside the biomedical establishment, as clinicians are held ever more accountable to external authorities. To understand better how medical outcomes fit into the framework of health services research, it is necessary to focus on assessing quality of care.

In the well-known Donabedian model,[11] health care quality is examined in three parts: structure, process, and outcomes of care.

*Structure* of care refers to how medical and other services are organized in a particular institution or delivery system. It may include such diverse variables as specialty mix in a multiphysician medical group, access to timely radiological files in a hospital, availability of pharmacy services in a hospice program, or convenience of parking at an outpatient surgery center. It may also involve nonmedical support services such as coordination of care, social work, home care, daily assistance for the disabled, or clothing and housing for the socially disadvantaged.

*Process* of care refers to the content of the medical and psychological interactions between patient and provider. It may include variables such as whether or not a blood culture is ordered for a baby with a fever, the nature of the treatment prescribed for a patient with abdominal pain, how much compassion a doctor demonstrates when presenting a negative diagnosis with a patient, how many times a psychologist interrupts a client during a session, or whether a nurse regularly turns a bedridden patient to prevent bedsores.

*Outcomes* of care refer to specific indicators of what happens to the patient once care has been rendered. This may include clinical variables, such as blood sugar level in a diabetic, blood pressure in a hypertensive, abnormal chest X ray during treatment for pneumonia, or kidney function after transplantation. It may also include complications of treatment, such as bleeding after colonoscopic biopsy, allergic reaction to an antibiotic or injection of iodinated contrast material, graft occlusion after cardiac bypass surgery, infant mortality following emergency Cesarean delivery, or hospital death rate.

Outcomes of care may also include health-related quality of life (HRQL), another variable commonly studied in the field of medical outcomes research. The general concept of quality of life encompasses a range of human experience: access to the daily necessities of life such as food and shelter, intrapersonal and interpersonal response to life events, and activities associated with professional fulfillment and personal happiness.[12] A subcomponent of overall quality of life relates to health, so HRQL focuses on the patient's own perception of well-being, health, and the ability to function as a result of health status or disease experience. The World Health Organization defines health as a "state of complete physical, mental, and social well-being and not merely the absence of disease."[13] Because disease may affect both quantity and quality of life, the various components of well-being must be addressed in treating patients. In the Donabedian framework, HRQL is considered an important outcome variable. Figure 8.2 presents a framework described by Patrick and Bergner for the theoretical relationships among HRQL concepts, disease, the environment, and prognosis.[14]

Although quantity of life is relatively easy to assess (as survival or disease-free interval, in days, months, years), measuring quality of life presents more challenges primarily because it is less familiar to most clinicians and researchers. Proper measurement of such variables is often quite costly. To quantify what is essentially a subjective or qualitative phenomenon, the principles of psychometric test theory are applied.[15] Typically, HRQL data are collected with self-administered questionnaires, called instruments. These instruments contain questions, or items, that are organized into scales. Each scale measures an aspect, or domain, of HRQL. Some scales comprise dozens of items, while others may include only one or two items.

HRQL instruments may be general or disease-targeted. General HRQL domains address the essential or common components of overall well-being, while disease-targeted domains focus on the impact of particular organic dysfunctions that affect HRQL.[16] Generic HRQL instruments typically address general health perception; sense of overall well-being; and function in the physical, emotional,

## FIGURE 8.2. CONCEPTUALIZATION OF HRQL.

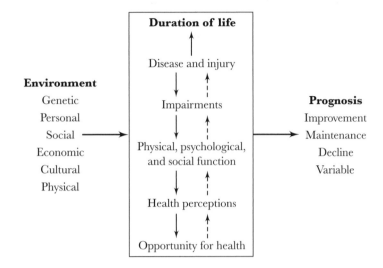

*Source:* Adapted from Patrick, D., and Bergner, M. "Measurement of Health Studies in the 1990s." *Annual Review of Public Health,* 1990, *11,* 174.

and social domains. Disease-targeted HRQL instruments focus on special or directly relevant domains, such as anxiety about cancer recurrence, dizziness from antihypertensive medication, or suicidal thoughts during depression therapy.

Many HRQL instruments are available. At least one journal, *Quality of Life Research,* is dedicated exclusively to presenting this research. Hence, an abundance of literature exists on general HRQL, and a significant body of work has been published on HRQL in patients with various conditions.[17]

## Psychometric Evaluation of HRQL Instruments

Developing and evaluating new instruments and scales is a long and arduous process; it should not be undertaken lightly. Simply drawing up a list of questions that seem appropriate is fraught with potential traps and pitfalls. Two important characteristics to assess in new instruments are reliability and validity. *Reliability* is the term used to indicate the amount of measurement error in a test instrument. If a measure were applied in exactly the same situation at two points in time, the same results would be expected. For example, if you use a ruler to measure the width of this book on several occasions, you would expect the same number of inches on each application. If you get a varying width, something about the measurement process is unreliable. Assuming no changes in health, the reliability of HRQL measures is assessed by their ability to produce the same scores on repeated administration. *Validity* indicates the extent to which the instrument measures what it is intended to measure. Validity of HRQL instruments is evaluated by examining the extent to which the associations (correlations) of the measures with other variables are consistent with prior hypotheses (construct validity). Reliability and validity should be established before using an instrument; therefore it is preferable to use established HRQL instruments if they are available and conceptually appropriate.

When scales and instruments are developed, they are first pilot-tested to ensure that the target population can understand and complete them with ease. Pilot testing reveals problems that might otherwise go unrecognized by researchers. For example, patients may not understand many terms that are commonly used by medical professionals. This may result in missing data if patients leave questions blank. Furthermore, since older patients may have poor eyesight, pilot testing in this group often identifies easily corrected visual barriers such as type size and page layout. In addition, self-administered instruments with complicated skip patterns ("If you answered yes to item 16b, continue with item 16c; if you answered no to item 16b, skip to item 19a") may be too confusing for even the most competent patients to follow. This too can result in missing data and introduce difficulties in the analysis. Pilot testing is a necessary and valuable part of instrument development; it serves as a reality check for scale developers.

## Caveats on Collecting HRQL Data

Once an instrument is thoroughly tested and has evidence supporting its reliability and validity, it must be administered in a manner that minimizes bias. Quality-of-life data cannot and should not be collected from patients directly by the treating health care provider; patients often favor socially desirable responses under such circumstances.[18] This introduces measurement error. No matter how objective the treating clinician may claim to be, it is impossible for him or her to collect objective and unbiased outcome data through direct questioning. Variations in phrasing, inflection, eye contact, rapport, mood, and other factors are difficult or impossible to eliminate. Third parties impartial to the results should collect the data using established psychometric scales and instruments.

## Future Directions in Applying HRQL Assessment

There is a need for basic descriptive information on the HRQL of differing patient groups, simply from an epidemiological perspective. Characterizing the fundamental elements of HRQL for these individuals requires studying their health perception and how daily activities are affected by general health and specific illness. Physical function and emotional well-being form the cornerstone of this approach, but research should also further explore issues such as eating and sleeping habits, anxiety and fatigue, depression, rapport with the clinician, presence of a spouse or partner, and social interaction. Characterization of these domains often addresses not only the actual functions but also the relative importance of these issues to patients.

Beyond the descriptive analysis, HRQL outcomes need to be compared in patients undergoing various types of therapy for the same condition. From the perspective of health policy, both general and disease-targeted HRQL should be measured to facilitate comparison among common diseases or conditions. HRQL outcomes may also be correlated with medical variables such as comorbidity; or sociodemographic variables such as age, race, gender, education, income, insurance status, geographic region, and access to health care. In this context, HRQL may be associated with many factors other than the traditional medical variables.

Research initiatives must rely on using established HRQL instruments with accepted psychometric characteristics and independent data collection procedures. The basic science of measurement of HRQL is well established[19] and is being widely adopted. However, integration of HRQL among other health services outcomes is still in its infancy. Indeed, the potential value of HRQL methods in health management organizations has yet to be fully realized. This affords a unique opportunity for simultaneous, coordinated introduction of such measurement techniques in both the clinical and the administrative spheres.

## Quality-Adjusted Life Years

Traditional measures of health outcome are very general. They include life expectancy, infant mortality, and disability days. The difficulty with these indicators is that they do not reflect most of the benefits of health care. For example, life expectancy and infant mortality are good measures because they allow comparison between programs with differing specific objectives. The difficulty is that neither is sensitive to minor variations in health status. Treatment of most common illnesses may have relatively little effect on life expectancy. Infant mortality, although sensitive to socioeconomic variations, does not register the effect of health services delivered to people who are older than one year.[20]

Survival analysis is an attractive generic measure of health status. It gives a unit of credit for each year of survival. Suppose, for example, that a person has a life expectancy of eighty years and dies prematurely at age fifty. In survival analysis, the person is scored as 1.0 for each of the first fifty years and zero each year thereafter. The problem is that years with disability are scored the same as years in perfect health. For example, a person with severe arthritis who is alive is scored exactly the same as someone in perfect health. Adjusted survival analysis has been proposed to address this problem. Using this method, we can summarize outcomes in terms of quality-adjusted life years (QALYs). In quality-adjusted survival analysis, years of wellness are scored on a continuum ranging from 0 for dead to 1.0 for optimum function.[21]

QALYs are a measure of life expectancy with adjustment for quality of life.[22] QALYs integrate mortality and morbidity to express health status in terms of equivalents of well-years of life. If a woman dies of breast cancer at age fifty and one would have expected her to live to age seventy-five, the disease was associated with twenty-five lost life years. If one hundred women died at age fifty (and also had life expectancy of seventy-five years), 2,500 (100 × 25 years) life years would be lost. For example, death is not the only outcome of concern in cancer patients. Many adults suffer from the disease leaving them somewhat disabled over a long period of time. Although they are still alive, the quality of their lives has diminished. QALYs take into consideration the quality-of-life consequences of these illnesses.

For example, a disease that reduces quality of life by one-half takes away 0.50 QALYs over the course of one year. If it affects two people, it takes away one year (2 × 0.50) over a one-year period. A pharmaceutical treatment that improves quality of life by 0.2 for each of five individuals results in the equivalent of one QALY if the benefit is maintained over a one-year period. The basic assumption is that two years scored as 0.5 add up to the equivalent of one year of complete wellness. Similarly, four years scored as 0.25 are equivalent to one completely well year of life. A treatment that boosts a patient's health from 0.5 to 0.75 produces the equivalent of 0.25 QALYs. If applied to four individuals, and the duration of the treatment effect is one year, the effect of the treatment would be equivalent to one completely well year of life. This system has the advantage of considering both benefits and side effects of programs in terms of the common QALY units. Although QALYs are typically assessed for patients, they can also be measured for others, including care givers who are placed at risk because they experience stressful life events. The Institute of Medicine recommended that population health metrics be used to evaluate public programs and to assist the decision-making process.[23]

## Cost-Effectiveness Decisions

In addition to health benefits, programs also have costs. Resources are limited and good policy decisions require allocations that maximize life expectancy and health-related quality of life. Methodologies for estimating costs have now become standardized.[24] From an administrative perspective, cost estimates include all costs of treatment and costs associated with caring for any side effects of treatment. From a social perspective, costs are broader and may include costs for family members who are not working in order to provide care. Comparing programs for a given population with a given medical condition, cost-effectiveness is measured as the change in costs of care for the program compared to the existing therapy or program, relative to the change in health measured in a standardized unit such as QALYs. The difference in costs over the difference in effectiveness is the *incremental cost-effectiveness,* usually expressed as the cost per QALY. Since the objective of all programs is to produce QALYs, the cost per QALY can be used to show the relative efficiency of various programs.[25]

Figure 8.3 compares programs that have been analyzed using cost per QALY. Some traditional interventions, such as mammography for women age forty to fifty, may cost as much as $240,000 to produce a QALY.[26] Screening programs, such as testing for high cholesterol, may also require many resources to produce a QALY.[27] On the other hand, public health programs such as tobacco control may produce a QALY at very low cost.[28] The figure shows a hypothetical "pay line." It might be argued that programs to the left of the pay line should be funded but those with a cost-per-QALY ratio to the right of the line be examined more carefully.

Contrary to the portrayal of cost-effectiveness analysis in the popular media, the purpose of the analysis is not to cut costs but rather attempt to identify which interventions produce the greatest amount of health using the resources that are available. Because of the confusion about cost-effectiveness analysis, the Office of Disease Prevention and Health Promotion in the Public Health Service appointed a panel to develop standards for such analysis. Their standards were published in 1996.[29]

The primary appeal of these approaches to summarizing the quality of various health states is their simplicity. By using QALYs, clinicians, managers, payers,

## FIGURE 8.3. COST-PER-QALY RATIOS.

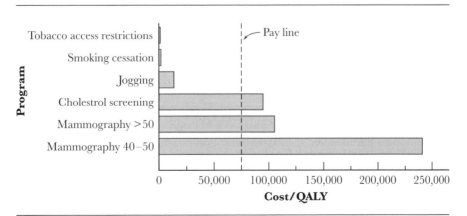

and investigators can compare outcomes and health service utilization among individuals or populations with a uniform unit of measurement that is easily quantified. However, these approaches raise important ethical concerns for the physician providing care to an individual patient.[30] Although a range of variables contribute to the physician's recommendations for treatment (or no treatment), there is nothing more relevant to decision making than the patient's own assessment of quality of life. Even if a treatment may be life-saving, ethical principles suggest that the patient's preference regarding treatment must be respected. If the patient feels that his or her quality of life is so poor that no treatment would make it better, then we should respect the patient's wishes.

## Feedback to Patients

To give better information to patients facing such decisions, it is important to have HRQL outcome data on individual treatments to facilitate clinical decision making. Specific examples of currently available information include the finding that HRQL is better when chemotherapy is given continuously rather than intermittently in women with advanced breast cancer,[31] or that the HRQL of women receiving breast conservation treatment is no different than it is for women undergoing mastectomy.[32] In addition, new information has recently become available to understand HRQL in men treated for localized prostate cancer.[33] However, there are limited data of this type. We need to expand our database on HRQL outcomes to improve information for managers, payers, health care executives, and policy makers involved in the process of distributing limited health care resources, as well as to physicians and patients involved in clinical decision making.

# Contributions from the Literature

In this section, we review seminal research in health services where HRQL methods were developed or incorporated as important outcomes. Although this section is not exhaustive, we present an historical framework for research in this area.

## Alameda County Human Population Laboratory Studies

Four decades ago, Lester Breslow and colleagues recruited a probability sample of adults from Alameda County, California, to examine the health status and well-being of a community. This research program conceptualized health in broader terms than the traditional categories of disability and disease. Their work drew heavily on the World Health Organization (WHO) definition of health to guide their assessment of the population, focusing on the physical, emotional, and social dimensions of well-being.[34] Although they examined some social indicators (such as employment, income, and marital status) in their study sample, the focus of their work was on the self-reported evaluation of the three dimensions of well-being (physical, mental, and social) identified in the WHO definition of health. The measurement methods available at the time were less developed psychometrically than now, but the investigators consistently demonstrated the reliability and validity of their self-report surveys[35] and were able to evaluate these three dimensions of health. They established the feasibility of asking people about their HRQL and demonstrated similar responses to personal interview, telephone, and mailed questionnaires as strategies for data collection. Further, they showed that data from the three administration strategies were nearly interchangeable.

In addition to the conceptually and methodologically pioneering work of this group, this research program made several critical observations:

- Those who were employed were healthier than those who were out of work or retired.[36]
- Separated persons were less physically healthy than those in other marital-status groups.[37]
- There is a positive association between physical health status and mental health status, independent of sex, age, or income adequacy.[38]
- There is a positive association between socioeconomic status and mental health.[39]
- Certain common health habits (hours of sleep, exercise, abstention from alcohol and tobacco) are positively related to physical health status,[40] and these personal health habits are inversely related to subsequent mortality[41] and disability.[42]

## The RAND Health Insurance Experiment

The RAND Health Insurance Experiment (HIE) was one of the first large health services research intervention trials. It was conceived in the early 1970s, at a time when there was considerable discussion about national health insurance reform and new approaches to limiting the rapidly expanding health care budget.[43] The HIE randomly assigned 2,005 families (3,958 individuals between fourteen and sixty-one years of age) to health insurance plans that provided free care, varying degrees of co-payment, or care through a health maintenance organization.[44] In addition to examining the cost of care and utilization of services, this comprehensively designed study looked at a number of important health outcomes, among them physiological measures (for example, blood pressure, far vision), health habits (smoking, weight, cholesterol level), and self-reported measures of health status (physical functioning, role functioning, mental health, social contacts, health perception). The high standards set for reliable and valid measures of health status in the RAND HIE led to extensive exploration of the conceptualization of health and the methodologies required for measuring HRQL.

Although it is not possible in this chapter to examine all of the advances in measurement of HRQL that were developed as part of the RAND HIE, a few key concepts and measures should be described. The methodological aspects of this work were spearheaded by John E. Ware, Jr., and are best captured in a paper published in 1984.[45] Ware noted that the "attention of society, government and health care providers has broadened beyond survival and biomedical status into the areas of behavioral and psychosocial outcomes. There also seems to be a shift in the objectives of health care toward more socially relevant health and quality-of-life outcomes and increased awareness of the interest in the psychological and economic costs of disease and disability."[46]

Ware also noted the methodological advances that made it possible to have patients evaluate these matters through self-report measures.

Ware carefully clarifies that "quality of life encompasses personal health status and other factors such as family life, finances, housing and jobs," such aspects being the content of much of the social indicators research movement; however, not all of these factors are expected to be influenced by the health care system.[47] Therefore, he suggests, it is more important to consider the concept of health status as separate from the larger arena of quality of life, with health representing proper functioning and well-being (hearkening back to the WHO definition of health).[48] In this explication of a framework for measurement of health-related quality of life, Ware identifies the dimensions seen in Figure 8.4: the disease, personal functioning, psychological distress and well-being, general health perceptions, and social and role functioning.[49]

Using this framework, the RAND investigators developed a number of large questionnaire batteries to examine each dimension of HRQL. These questionnaires were developed and evaluated specifically for the HIE and were then used as critical outcome measures. Detailed descriptions of these measures are available as separate reports prepared through the RAND Corporation, and also through many publications.

One of the most widely used measures is the Mental Health Inventory (MHI), described by Veit and Ware in 1983.[50] In contrast to existing psychological measures designed to diagnose mental illness, the MHI was developed to look at psychological distress and well-being in the general population. Ware and associates drew heavily on existing measures of well-being in developing the MHI. However, they performed much additional work to conceptualize the issues of importance to this domain of HRQL and were careful to separate mental health from physical health. What resulted was a thirty-eight-item index of mental health that

## FIGURE 8.4. FRAMEWORK FOR MEASURING HEALTH STATUS.

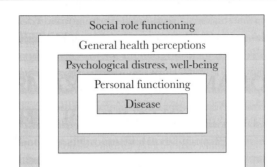

*Source:* Adapted from Ware, J. E., Jr. "Methodology in Behavioral and Psychosocial Cancer Research: Conceptualizing Disease Impact and Treatment Outcomes." *Cancer,* 1984, *53*(10 Suppl.), 2316–2326.

could be separated into two main constructs: (1) psychological distress (anxiety, depression, loss of behavioral or emotional control) and (2) psychological well-being (general positive affect, emotional ties). Elegant psychometric evaluation of this measure was completed as part of the HIE.[51]

There are many important legacies from the RAND Health Insurance Experiment. From the point of view of quality-of-life research, conceptualizing HRQL as a key outcome of health care is critical. In addition, the HIE developed reliable and valid tools for measuring the dimensions of HRQL. However, in addition to the tools themselves, data from this study also constitute important reference points for the relative value of specific changes in scores. That is to say, what does a change in quality-of-life score mean? Data on life events captured in the RAND HIE in relation to change scores for the measures of health-related quality of life provide intervention-based validity for the quality-of-life scores. The reader is referred to a review by Testa and Nackley[52] for an excellent discussion of this issue. Efforts to understand the meaning of differences in HRQL scores continue today, focusing on estimation of clinically important or minimally important differences.[53]

### The Medical Outcomes Study

The Medical Outcomes Study (MOS) is another example of a major health services research study that in its design and conceptualization included health-related quality of life as a key outcome of care[54] (see Table 8.1). Many of the key investigators for this study had been involved in the RAND HIE. Again, Ware and colleagues at RAND were central figures in developing the health outcome measures for the MOS. Thus it is not surprising that the measures of functional status, health, and well-being draw heavily on the prior measures developed for the Health Insurance Experiment.[55]

## TABLE 8.1. CONCEPTUAL FRAMEWORK FOR THE MEDICAL OUTCOMES STUDY.

| Structure of Care | Process of Care | Outcomes |
|---|---|---|
| *System Characteristics* | *Technical Style* | *Clinical End Points* |
| Organization | Visits | Symptoms and signs |
| Specialty mix | Medications | Laboratory values |
| Financial incentives | Referrals | Death |
| Workload | Test ordering | |
| Access and convenience | Hospitalizations | *Functional Status* |
| | Expenditures | Physical |
| *Provider Characteristics* | Continuity of care | Mental |
| Age | Coordination | Social |
| Gender | | Role |
| Specialty training | *Interpersonal Style* | |
| Economic incentives | Interpersonal manner | *General well-being* |
| Beliefs and attitudes | Patient participation | Health perceptions |
| Preferences | Counseling | Energy and fatigue |
| Job satisfaction | Communication level | Pain |
| | | Life satisfaction |
| *Patient Characteristics* | | |
| Age | | *Satisfaction with Care* |
| Gender | | Access |
| Diagnosis or condition | | Convenience |
| Severity | | Financial coverage |
| Comorbid conditions | | Quality |
| Health habits | | General |
| Beliefs and attitudes | | |
| Preferences | | |

*Source:* Adapted from Tarlov, A. R., and others. "The Medical Outcomes Study: An Application of Methods for Monitoring the Results of Medical Care." *JAMA,* 1989, *262*(7), 925–930.

The self-report measures of HRQL used in the MOS were quite lengthy.[56] However, one of the major methodological advances from this project was the realization that shorter measures might be as effective as the lengthier measures traditionally used in this type of research. Longer measures lead to added precision, but they also increase the burden on the respondent and the likelihood of missing data. Furthermore, they are too cumbersome for most clinical settings. An additional conceptual breakthrough was developing a generic HRQL tool that could facilitate comparing common diseases across specific dimensions of HRQL. Noteworthy results from this research include development of the MOS short form, first published as a twenty-item questionnaire[57] and later an expanded version known as the MOS Short Form 36 or RAND 36-Item Health Survey 1.0.[58] The short forms of the MOS instruments are widely used in a variety of research and clinical settings to examine health outcomes of care.[59] These measures have been translated for use in multinational studies as well as national studies that include diverse populations.[60]

In recent years, the goal of parsimony in instrument selection has generated interest in an even shorter form of the MOS instrument, known as the SF-12.[61] This twelve-item questionnaire summarizes HRQL in two domains: the mental component summary and the physical component summary. Although there is some sacrifice in richness of the data, the SF-12 summary scales are equivalent to the SF-36 counterparts.

Because of the desirability of preference-based scores for cost utility analyses and other applications, attempts have recently been made to estimate preference scores from the SF-36. Fryback[62] derived regression equations to predict the Quality of Well-Being Scale (QWB) from the SF-36. A six-variable regression model accounted for 57 percent of the variance in QWB scores. Nichol and colleagues[63] used a similar method to predict HUI-2 preference scores from the SF-36 in a sample of 6,921 patients with Kaiser health insurance. Fifty percent of the variance (adjusted R-squared) in the HUI-2 was accounted for, and each of the SF-36 scales had a significant and unique positive association with the HUI-2 in the regression model.

In selecting HRQL instruments, investigators are well-advised to consult www.proqolid.org, an outstanding source of information on new and existing HRQL measurement tools for a variety of clinical conditions. In addition, investigators are directed to the work of M. Staquet and colleagues, who proposed uniform guidelines for reporting HRQL data from clinical trials.[64]

Another approach to deriving a preference-based score is a six-dimensional health classification scheme using a subset of items from the SF-36.[65] Multiattribute utility theory was used to derive preference weights for nine thousand health states based on ratings by a sample of 166 health professionals, health service managers and administrators, staff at the University of Sheffield medical school, under-graduates, and patients at hospital outpatient clinics. Visual analog and standard gamble estimating equations were developed to predict the preference scores. A larger study of 611 people from the UK general population was subsequently used to derive more definitive weights.[66]

## Efficacy Studies

Quality of life has long been an implied outcome of treatment for a variety of common, chronic medical conditions. For a disease such as rheumatoid arthritis, subjective assessment of response to anti-inflammatory agents (pain relief, in-creased mobility) has been critical in evaluating new treatments.[67] In the case of antihypertensive treatments, side effects from medication may interfere with com-pliance and affect successful control of this clinically silent condition.[68] Cancer treatments are another area where quality-of-life outcomes are salient.[69] Ran-domized clinical trials of treatment efficacy are the most compelling studies in which quality-of-life measures have been used.

Several authors have used quality of life measures to estimate the effectiveness of clinical interventions. However, most of these analyses use subjective estimates of clinical outcomes because the studies did not incorporate quality-of-life mea-sures. Recently, two excellent examples of policy analysis associated with prospec-tive randomized clinical trials were published. In each case, the quality-of-life measurement was incorporated into the study protocol and the cost-effectiveness analysis was part of the study planning. These studies were the Diabetes Preven-tion Program (DPP) and the National Emphysema Treatment Trial (NETT).

## Diabetes Clinical Trial

In the DPP, patients at risk for type II diabetes were randomly assigned to one of three conditions: intensive lifestyle modification, metformin, or placebo.[70] The DPP included 3,234 adults with impaired glucose tolerance. The intensive lifestyle in-tervention was designed to reduce the initial body weight by 7 percent through reg-ular physical activity and diet. The metformin group took one 850 mg tablet each day. The placebo group also took one tablet per day. The patients were evaluated prior to randomization and at annual intervals over the course of three years.

Quality of life was measured using the QWB. The measure was chosen because it can be used to estimate QALYs. Over the course of three years, those randomly assigned to the lifestyle intervention accrued 0.050 more QALYs than those assigned a regular dose of metformin. Among the three interventions, the lifestyle approach was the most expensive (total cost US$27,065 in year 2000 dollars). Metformin was less expensive ($25,937), while the placebo was the least expensive option ($23,525).

Figure 8.5 summarizes the cost per QALY for the lifestyle and metformin conditions from a health care system perspective. The figure shows the cost per QALY attributable to the interventions in comparison to placebo and to doing nothing. Although both interventions offer significant benefits over placebo or doing nothing, the cost per QALY for the lifestyle invention was significantly lower than that for metformin. In other words, even though the lifestyle intervention was more expensive, it offers significantly better value for money.

The second example is an evaluation of surgery for emphysema. Emphysema is the dominant cause of chronic obstructive pulmonary disease (COPD), which is the fourth leading cause of death and a major cause of disability in the United States.[71] COPD is caused by loss of elastic recoil of lung tissue in addition to chronic inflammation in airways. Lungs often become hyperinflated and there is an increase in the functional residual capacity. Hyperinflation may place greater strain on the muscles of respiration, increasing the effort required to breathe and reducing capacity for exercise. COPD is associated with activity limitations, premature death, and reduced quality of life.[72] Despite major advances in diagnosis and medical therapeutics, standard medical therapy often has little effect on life quality.[73] Thus many patients seek surgical treatments that may produce more dramatic improvements.

Lung volume reduction surgery (LVRS) is an intervention designed to reduce the volume of the hyperinflated lung. The procedure was introduced in the 1950s,

## FIGURE 8.5. COST PER QALY IN DPP.

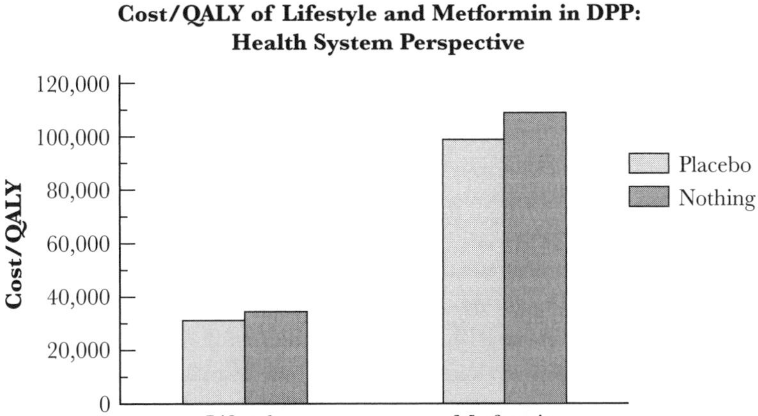

Source: Data from DPP Group 2003, *Diabetes Care, 26,* 2518.

but one in six patients died from the surgery. As a result, the procedure was abandoned by the late 1950s.[74] An improved procedure was reintroduced in the 1990s, and the initial results were encouraging. Shortly thereafter, patient testimonials and marketing efforts resulted in popular enthusiasm for the procedure and pressure for Medicare to pay for it.[75] A report commissioned by the Center for Medicare and Medicaid Services (CMS) cited a paper noting that more than twelve hundred LVRS procedures had been performed on Medicare beneficiaries.[76] Further, the rate of growth was exponential.[77] On the other hand, the technology assessment raised significant questions about the benefits of the procedure. For example, it was noted that about one-quarter of the Medicare beneficiaries who received LVRS died within one year.[78] In response to these concerns, Medicare decided to halt payment for the procedure until it could be studied.

The National Emphysema Treatment Trial is a multicenter randomized clinical trial designed to evaluate LVRS.[79] Subjects with moderate to severe emphysema were randomly assigned to usual medical therapy alone or to usual medical therapy plus LVRS. All patients in the trial participated in pulmonary rehabilitation prior to randomization.

Quality of life was one of the primary outcome measures because surgery was not expected to improve life expectancy. HRQL was measured using four methods, two generic and two disease-specific. One measure was chosen because it could be used to estimate QALYs in cost-effectiveness analysis. The study was unusual because it included a prospective plan for policy analysis.

The NETT trial randomized 1,218 patients to either maximum medical therapy or to the combination of maximal medical therapy plus LVRS.[80] Over the first twelve months of the study, LVRS patients had significantly more hospital days, ambulatory care days, and nursing home admissions. However, utilization began to change by the thirteen-to-twenty-four-month interval. During the second year, those in the maximal medical arm used more hospital days and had more emergency room visits. In the third year, utilization was equivalent between the two groups. Figure 8.6 summarizes the cumulative QALYs per person over the first three years of the project. After one year, the groups differed but the effect was nonsignificant. However, by year two the groups began separating, and this difference grew by year three.

Cost per QALY was evaluated three years following randomization.[81] Using best estimates for cost, mortality, and quality of life, it was concluded that LVRS was more expensive than maximal medical therapy ($98,952 vs. $62,560). However, QALYs were also greater in the LVRS arm (1.463 vs. 1.271). Thus the incremental cost per QALY was approximately $190,000.

To capture potential long-term gains, the analysis also estimated projected benefits over an extended period of time. The analyses suggested that at five years

## FIGURE 8.6. MEAN CUMULATIVE QALYS, YEARS 1–3.

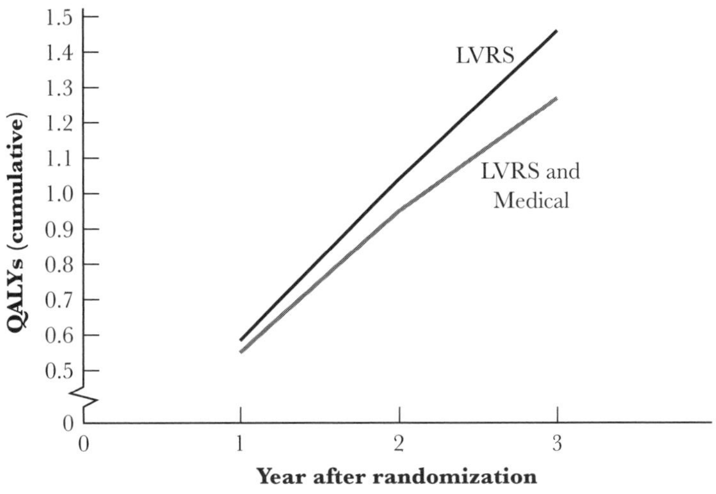

the incremental cost per QALY was $88,000 for nonhigh-risk patients; at ten years it was $53,000.[82]

The NETT trial demonstrated that the cost-effectiveness of LVRS is comparable to several other surgical procedures. The relative cost-effectiveness of LVRS is particularly impressive if benefits of the procedure are projected into the future. The NETT was a milestone study because the cost-effectiveness analysis was planned and executed as a companion to the RCT. Further, the NETT trial allowed rapid diffusion of the findings.[83] The trial and cost-effectiveness analysis were used as the basis of Medicare policy funding LVRS surgery. By early 2004, Medicare coverage for LVRS was approved. The trial offers an excellent example of rapid translation from research to policy.

These two examples demonstrate the importance of evaluating quality-of-life endpoints in efficacy studies because they provide an additional outcome that includes the patient perspective. This is most important in therapeutic situations where the toxicity of treatment is high and the benefits may be few.

Quality-of-life assessment has been widely adopted by the pharmaceutical industry as a component of the drug approval process.[84] These assessments are also an expanding part of large clinical treatment trials for patients with cancer and AIDS. We are still in the early phases of experience with HRQL as an outcome in such large-scale and long-term trials. Recently, there has been a move toward more abbreviated quality-of-life outcome measures for integration into large multicenter trials.[85] In these situations, the burden on respondents and staff is an important consideration. It is hoped that these shorter forms will be equally sensitive to measuring difference in quality-of-life outcomes. Many studies are under way currently, and results should be forthcoming in the next few years.

## Effectiveness Research

The newest aspect of health services research is in the area of effectiveness. Certain clinical topics do not lend themselves to randomized clinical trials because of ethical concerns, inability to control adequately for contravening factors, and various other reasons. In these clinical areas, consensus has arisen that descriptive studies are most appropriate to improve our understanding. These studies primarily address effectiveness. In contrast to controlled clinical trials that examine efficacy, effectiveness research studies the outcomes of treatment as they are actually practiced in clinical settings. To this end, in the 1990s the Agency for Health Care Policy and Research (now known as the Agency for Healthcare Research and Quality, or AHRQ) funded a number of patient outcome research teams (PORT) to investigate common medical treatments and procedures.[86] Although this research effort emphasized literature review of efficacy studies as well as examination of practice variations using administrative databases, it has also been an opportunity to collect quality-of-life outcome data from patients undergoing various procedures. The PORTs have not conducted clinical trials; hence their primary contribution has been in shaping the clinical effectiveness and outcomes literature.[87]

In summarizing the initial work in this area, the agency concluded that although the effectiveness initiative was relatively inexpensive to conduct, it provided primarily observational data for development of hypotheses for future research. Specifically, "It is increasingly clear that limitations of observational designs prevent these studies from providing definitive answers to many questions of comparative clinical effectiveness. More experience has also confirmed that changing practice and realizing savings in health care are not easily achieved. Research and experience have demonstrated that development and dissemination of even high quality, highly credible information is often insufficient to alter practices. Enhanced knowledge must be linked with supportive practice environments and incentives for change."[88] Thus the second generation of PORT studies (PORT II) often evaluated randomized designs within real-world clinical situations.

For example, Schoenbaum[89] studied 375 male and 981 female patients with current depression treated in forty-six clinics at six nonacademic managed care organizations, who were randomized to usual care or one of two interventions designed to increase the rate of effective depression treatment (medication management or psychotherapy). The average health care costs increased $429 ($424) for the medication intervention group and $983 ($275) for the psychotherapy group among men and women, respectively. The estimated cost per QALY for men ranged between $16,600 and $42,600 for the interventions, while for women costs per QALY were $23,600 or below for the medication intervention and $12,500 or below for psychotherapy.

# Future Research and Policy Issues

A great deal of work remains in order to operationalize research in outcomes and HRQL to inform health policy in the United States.

## Incorporating HRQL Endpoints

How can HRQL endpoints be effectively incorporated in research, clinical care, and policy decisions?

Several workshops among health services researchers[90] sponsored through the National Institutes of Health (NIH) and the National Cancer Institute (NCI)[91] have emphasized the need for incorporating HRQL endpoints into research and clinical care settings. The technologies, though not yet perfect, are much more accessible and feasible than just a short time ago. Scannable, user-friendly instruments are available, and normative databases are being developed rapidly. Health care consumers and providers would like access to HRQL outcomes information.

As has been emphasized by several prominent health services researchers,[92] it is the patient outcome that must drive our policy decisions. Prolonged survival with poor quality of life may not be desirable to patients. Consumers are anxious to have information about the HRQL impact of new treatments. If there is uncertainty about the efficacy or effectiveness of a treatment or choices among treatments, then HRQL endpoints will take on paramount importance.

Only through a concerted effort to collect primary HRQL data can this outcome be considered as a primary endpoint. All studies of efficacy and effectiveness must include patient-rated measures of HRQL whenever there is a potential quality-of-life question. Common core measures should be shared across studies so that relevant comparisons can be made. An example of how this might be done is the new NIH-sponsored Roadmap Initiative project on Dynamic Assessment of Patient-Reported Chronic Disease Outcomes.[93] The primary objective of this five-year, $25 million effort is creation of a Patient-Reported Outcomes Measurement Information System (PROMIS) to facilitate computer-based assessment of self-reported symptoms and other domains of health-related quality of life across a range of chronic diseases.[94]

However, we must not fail to ask critical questions related to new therapies, to better understand their relevance to patients. For enough data to materialize, these measures of HRQL must be considered routine and not exceptional. The additional costs of data collection should be borne by funding agencies, insurers, and providers so that the value of new tests or procedures can be fully evaluated.

## HRQL Endpoints and Changing Health Policy

Are HRQL endpoints sufficient to force a change in health policy?

In asking this about HRQL outcomes, we must ask whether statistically significant changes in evaluating HRQL are *clinically* significant. To obtain more precise evaluation of the quality of our tools, it is necessary to reference or calibrate our HRQL instruments against known outcomes of clinical importance to patients, purchasers of health care, and health care providers. For this work to proceed, we must invest in collecting important clinical information along with our HRQL data. Research in HRQL needs to be supported to extrapolate effectively from the HRQL endpoint to decisions on public health policy. Short-term management applications include using HRQL endpoints and other outcomes and effectiveness research as critical measures in the quality assurance (QA) arena.

## Advancing the HRQL Research Agenda

As Andersen, Davidson, and Ganz[95] have described, "There are symbiotic relationships between Health Services Research (HSR) and Quality of Life (QOL) studies." First, the HSR paradigm gives guidance for including structure and process in designing QOL studies. HSR suggests what leads to QOL improvement. It supplies ways to conceptualize, and relates the many important forces that contribute to, QOL in addition to specific clinical interventions. Second, QOL is an important outcome in the HSR paradigm. Early studies in HSR did not focus primarily on QOL as an outcome indicator. Health service utilization was investigated as a means to improve access to care and change the organization and delivery of care, rather than as a direct vehicle to enhance health status and QOL. Quality of life, however, is a key outcome in the emerging model of HSR.[96]

Until recently, and with the exception of a few studies already cited, HRQL was included infrequently in traditional health services research. The expansion and development of HRQL measurement has emerged primarily from clinical research. What is needed urgently is careful and appropriate inclusion of HRQL outcomes in traditional health services research. Similarly, researchers in clinical settings who are measuring HRQL should account for the structure and process of care in designing their research and data collection. As suggested by Andersen and colleagues, "This era of health care reform calls for a paradigm shift, away from the heroic and costly therapeutic measures that extend the quantity of life, to a patient or consumer-focused approach aimed at health promotion and disease prevention, using QOL measures as the ultimate criteria for success."[97] As indicated throughout this chapter, the potential for accomplishing this goal is on the horizon.

# Notes

1. Blumenthal, D. "Part 1, Quality of Care—What Is It?" *New England Journal of Medicine,* 1996, *335*(12), 891–894.

2. Council on Medical Service, American Medical Association. "Quality of Care." *Journal of the American Medical Association,* 1986, *256*(8), 1032–1034.

3. Lohr, K. N., Donaldson, M. S., and Harris-Wehling, J. "Medicare: A Strategy for Quality Assurance, Part V: Quality of Care in a Changing Health Care Environment." *Quality Review Bulletin,* 1992, *18*(4), 120–126.

4. Blumenthal (1996).

5. Liao, Y., McGee, D. L., Cao, G., and Cooper, R. S. "Quality of the Last Year of Life of Older Adults, 1986 vs. 1993." *Journal of the American Medical Association,* 2000, *283*(4), 512–518; Wolfe, J., and others. "Symptoms and Suffering at the End of Life in Children with Cancer." *New England Journal of Medicine,* 2000, *342*(5), 326–333.

6. Centers for Disease Control and Prevention. "Community Indicators of Health-Related Quality of Life—United States, 1993–1997." *Journal of the American Medical Association,* 2000, *283*(16), 2097–2098.

7. Ellwood, P. M. "Shattuck Lecture—Outcomes Management: A Technology of Patient Experience." *New England Journal of Medicine,* 1988, *318*(23), 1549–1556.

8. Ellwood (1988).

9. Tarlov, A. R. "The Coming Influence of a Social Sciences Perspective on Medical Education." *Academic Medicine,* 1992, *67*(11), 724–731.

10. Ganz, P. A. "Quality of Life and the Patient with Cancer: Individual and Policy Implications." *Cancer,* 1994, *74*(4 Suppl.), 1445–1452.

11. Donabedian, A. *The Definition of Quality and Approaches to Its Assessment.* Ann Arbor, Mich.: Health Administration Press, 1980.

12. Patrick, D. L., and Erickson, P. "Assessing Health-Related Quality of Life for Clinical Decision-Making." In S. R. Walker and R. M. Rosser (eds.), *Quality of Life Assessment: Key Issues in the 1990s.* Dordrecht, Kluwer Academic, 1993.

13. WHO. *Constitution of the World Health Organization: Basic Documents.* Geneva: WHO, 1948.

14. Patrick, D. L., and Bergner, M. "Measurement of Health Status in the 1990s." *Annual Review of Public Health,* 1990, *11*, 165–183.

15. Tulsky, D. S. "An Introduction to Test Theory." *Oncology,* 1990, *4*(5), 43–48.

16. Patrick, D. L., and Deyo, R. A. "Generic and Disease-Specific Measures in Assessing Health Status and Quality of Life." *Medical Care,* 1989, *27*(3 Suppl.), S217–S232.

17. McDowell, I., and Newell, C. *Measuring Health: A Guide to Rating Scales and Questionnaires.* New York: Oxford University Press, 1996; Patrick, D. L., and Erickson, P. *Health Status and Health*

*Policy: Allocating Resources to Health Care.* New York: Oxford University Press, 1993; Spilker, B. *Quality of Life Assessments in Clinical Trials.* New York: Raven Press, 1990.

18. Tannock, I. F. "Management of Breast and Prostate Cancer: How Does Quality of Life Enter the Equation?" *Oncology,* 1990, *4*(5), 149–156.

19. Guyatt, G. H., Feeny, D. H., and Patrick, D. L. "Measuring Health-Related Quality of Life." *Annals of Internal Medicine,* 1993, *118*(8), 622–629.

20. Stein, R. E., Stanton, B., and Starfield, B. "How Healthy Are U.S. Children?" *Journal of the American Medical Association,* 2005, *293*(14), 1781–1783.

21. Kaplan, R. M., Ake, C. F., Emery, S. L., and Navarro, A. M. "Simulated Effect of Tobacco Tax Variation on Population Health in California." *American Journal of Public Health,* 2001, *91*(2), 239–244.

22. Kaplan, R. M. "Quality of Life Assessment for Cost/Utility Studies in Cancer." *Cancer Treatment Reviews,* 1993, *19* (Suppl. A, 1), 85–96; Russell, L. B. "Modeling for Cost-Effectiveness Analysis." *Statistics in Medicine,* 1999, *18*(23), 3235–3244; Weinstein, M. C., and others. (1996). "Recommendations of the Panel on Cost-Effectiveness in Health and Medicine." *Journal of the American Medical Association,* 1996, *276*(15), 1253–1258.

23. Field, M. J., and Gold, M. R. *Summarizing Population Health.* Washington, D.C.: Institute of Medicine, National Academy Press, 1998.

24. Gold, M. R. *Cost-Effectiveness in Health and Medicine.* New York: Oxford University Press, 1996.

25. Gold (1996).

26. Eddy, D. M. "Screening for Breast Cancer." Annals of Internal Medicine, 1989, *111*(5), 389–399.

27. Taylor, W. C., Pass, T. M., Shepard, D. S., and Komaroff, A. L. "Cholesterol Reduction and Life Expectancy: A Model Incorporating Multiple Risk Factors." *Annals of Internal Medicine,* 1987, *106*(4), 605–614. [Published erratum in *Annals of Internal Medicine,* Feb. 1988, *108*(2), 314].

28. Kaplan, Ake, Emery, and Navarro (2001).

29. Gold (1996).

30. Dean, H. E. "Political and Ethical Implications of Using Quality of Life as an Outcome Measure." *Seminars in Oncology Nursing,* 1990, *6*(4), 303–308.

31. Coates, A., and others. "Improving the Quality of Life During Chemotherapy for Advanced Breast Cancer: A Comparison of Intermittent and Continuous Treatment Strategies." *New England Journal of Medicine,* 1987, *317*(24), 1490–1495.

32. Ganz, P. A., and others. "Breast Conservation Versus Mastectomy: Is There a Difference in Psychological Adjustment or Quality of Life in the Year After Surgery?" *Cancer,* 1992, *69*(7), 1729–1738.

33. Litwin, M. S., and others. "Quality-of-Life Outcomes in Men Treated for Localized Prostate Cancer." *Journal of the American Medical Association,* 1995, *273*(2), 129–135.

34. WHO (1948); Breslow, L. "A Quantitative Approach to the World Health Organization Definition of Health, Physical, Mental and Social Well-Being." *International Journal of Epidemiology,* 1972, *1*(4), 347–355.

35. Breslow (1972).

36. Belloc, N. B., Breslow, L., and Hochstim, J. R. "Measurement of Physical Health in a General Population Survey." *American Journal of Epidemiology,* 1971, *93*(5), 328–336.

37. Belloc, Breslow, and Hochstim (1971).

38. Berkman, P. L. "Measurement of Mental Health in a General Population Survey." *American Journal of Epidemiology,* 1971, *94*(2), 105–111.

39. Berkman (1971).

40. Belloc, N. B., and Breslow, L. "Relationship of Physical Health Status and Health Practices." *Preventive Medicine*, 1972, *1*(3), 409–421.

41. Belloc and Breslow (1972).

42. Breslow, L., and Breslow, N. "Health Practices and Disability: Some Evidence from Alameda County." Preventive Medicine, 1993, *22*(1), 86–95.

43. Starr, P. *The Social Transformation of American Medicine*. New York: Basic Books, 1982.

44. Brook, R. H., and others. "Does Free Care Improve Adults' Health? Results from a Randomized Controlled Trial." *New England Journal of Medicine*, 1983, *309*(23), 1426–1434; Newhouse, J. P., and others. "Some Interim Results from a Controlled Trial of Cost Sharing in Health Insurance." *New England Journal of Medicine*, 1981, *305*(25), 1501–1507; Manning, W. G., and others. "A Controlled Trial of the Effect of a Prepaid Group Practice on Use of Services." *New England Journal of Medicine*, 1984, *310*(23), 1505–1510.

45. Ware, J. E., Jr. "Methodology in Behavioral and Psychosocial Cancer Research: Conceptualizing Disease Impact and Treatment Outcomes." *Cancer*, 1984, *53*(10 Suppl.), 2316–2326.

46. Ware (1984).

47. Ware (1984).

48. WHO (1948).

49. Ware (1984).

50. Veit, C. T., and Ware, J. E., Jr. „The Structure of Psychological Distress and Well-Being in General Populations." *Journal of Consulting and Clinical Psychology*, 1983, *51*(5), 730–742.

51. Veit and Ware (1983).

52. Testa, M. A., and Nackley, J. F. "Methods for Quality-of-Life Studies." *Annual Review of Public Health*, 1994, *15*, 535–559.

53. Wyrwich, K. W., and others. "Estimating Clinically Significant Differences in Quality of Life Outcomes." *Quality of Life Research*, 2005, *14*(2), 285–295.

54. Tarlov, A. R., and others. "The Medical Outcomes Study: An Application of Methods for Monitoring the Results of Medical Care." *Journal of the American Medical Association*, 1989, *262*(7), 925–930.

55. Stewart, A. L., and Ware, J. E. (eds.). *Measuring Functioning and Well-Being: The Medical Outcomes Study Approach*. Durham, N.C.: Duke University Press, 1992.

56. Stewart and Ware (1992).

57. Stewart, A. L., Hays, R. D., and Ware, J. E., Jr. "The MOS Short-Form General Health Survey: Reliability and Validity in a Patient Population." *Medical Care*, 1988, *26*(7), 724–735; Stewart, A. L., and others. "Functional Status and Well-Being of Patients with Chronic Conditions: Results from the Medical Outcomes Study." *Journal of the American Medical Association, 1989, 262*(7), 907–913.

58. Ware, J. E., Jr., and Sherbourne, C. D. "The MOS 36-Item Short-Form Health Survey (SF-36). Part I: Conceptual Framework and Item Selection." *Medical Care*, 1992, *30*(6), 473–483; Hays, R. D., Sherbourne, C. D., and Mazel, R. M. "The RAND 36-Item Health Survey 1.0." *Health Economics*, 1993, *2*(3), 217–227.

59. Meyer, K. B., and others. "Monitoring Dialysis Patients' Health Status." *American Journal of Kidney Disease*, 1994, *24*(2), 267–279; Jacobson, A. M., De Groot, M., and Samson, J. A. "The Evaluation of Two Measures of Quality of Life in Patients with Type I and Type II Diabetes." *Diabetes Care*, 1994, *17*(4), 267–274; Jette, D. U., and Downing, J. "Health Status of Individuals Entering a Cardiac Rehabilitation Program as Measured by the Medical Outcomes Study 36-Item Short-Form Survey (SF-36)." *Physical Therapy*, 1994, *74*(6), 521–527.

60. Aaronson, N. K., and others. "International Quality of Life Assessment (IQOLA) Project." *Quality of Life Research*, 1992, *1*(5), 349–351.

61. Ware, J. E., Kosinski, M., and Keller, S. D. *SF-12: How to Score the SF-12 Physical and Mental Health Summary Scales* (1st ed.). Boston: Health Institute, New England Medical Center, 1995.

62. Fryback, D. G., and others. "Predicting Quality of Well-Being Scores from the SF-36: Results from the Beaver Dam Health Outcomes Study." *Medical Decision Making*, 1997, *17*, 1–19.

63. Nichol, M. B., Sengupta, N., and Globe, D. R. "Evaluating Quality-Adjusted Life Years: Estimation of the Health Utility Index (HUI2) from the SF-36." *Medical Decision Making*, 2001, *21*(2), 105–112.

64. Staquet, M., Berzon, R., Osoba, D., and Machin, D. "Guidelines for Reporting Results of Quality of Life Assessments in Clinical Trials." *Quality of Life Research*, 1996, *5*(5), 496–502.

65. Brazier, J., Usherwood, T., Harper, R., and Thomas, K. "Deriving a Preference-Based Single Index from the UK SF-36 Health Survey." *Journal of Clinical Epidemiology*, 1998, *51*(11), 1115–1128.

66. Brazier, J., Roberts, J., and Deverill, M. "The Estimation of a Preference-Based Measure of Health from the SF-36." *Journal of Health Economics*, 2002, *21*(2), 271–292.

67. Potts, M. K., Mazzuca, S. A., and Brandt, K. D. "Views of Patients and Physicians Regarding the Importance of Various Aspects of Arthritis Treatment, Correlations with Health Status and Patient Satisfaction." *Patient Education and Counseling*, 1986, *8*, 125–134.

68. Croog, S. H., and others. "The Effects of Antihypertensive Therapy on the Quality of Life." *New England Journal of Medicine*, 1986, *314*(26), 1657–1664; Testa, M. A., and others. "Quality of Life and Antihypertensive Therapy in Men: A Comparison of Captopril with Enalapril. The Quality-of-Life Hypertension Study Group." *New England Journal of Medicine*, 1993, *328*(13), 907–913.

69. Coates (1987); Ganz (1992); Litwin and others (1995).

70. Diabetes Primary Prevention Group. "Within-Trial Cost-Effectiveness of Lifestyle Intervention or Metformin for the Primary Prevention of Type 2 Diabetes." *Diabetes Care*, 2003, *26*(9), 2518–2523.

71. "National Vital Statistics Report." 2004. [www.cdc.gov/nchs/fastats/copd.htm] (accessed Oct. 15, 2004).

72. Pauwels, R. A., and Rabe, K. F. "Burden and Clinical Features of Chronic Obstructive Pulmonary Disease (COPD)." *Lancet*, 2004, *364*(9434), 613–620.

73. Sutherland, E. R., and Cherniack, R. M. "Management of Chronic Obstructive Pulmonary Disease." *New England Journal of Medicine*, 2004, *350*(26), 2689–2697.

74. Brantigan, O. C., and Mueller, E. "Surgical Treatment of Pulmonary Emphysema." *American Surgeon*, 1957, *23*(9), 789–804; Lefrak, S. S., and others. "Recent Advances in Surgery for Emphysema." *Annual Review of Medicine*, 1997, *48*, 387–398.

75. Cooper, J. D., and others. "Results of 150 Consecutive Bilateral Lung Volume Reduction Procedures in Patients with Severe Emphysema." *Journal of Thoracic and Cardiovascular Surgery*, 1996, *112*(5), 1319–1329; discussion 1329–1330.

76. Huizenga, H. F., Ramsey, S. D., and Albert, R. K. "Estimated Growth of Lung Volume Reduction Surgery Among Medicare Enrollees, 1994 to 1996." Chest, 1998, *114*(6), 1583–1587.

77. Huizenga, Ramsey, and Albert (1998).

78. Huizenga, Ramsey, and Albert (1998).

79. Fishman, A., and others. "A Randomized Trial Comparing Lung Volume Reduction Surgery with Medical Therapy for Severe Emphysema." *New England Journal of Medicine*, 2003, *348*(21), 2059–2073.

80. Fishman and others (2003).

81. Ramsey, S. D., and others. "Cost Effectiveness of Lung Volume Reduction Surgery for Patients with Severe Emphysema." *New England Journal of Medicine*, 2003, *348*(21), 2092–2102.

82. Ramsey and others (2003).

83. Ramsey and others (2003).

84. Testa, M. A. "Parallel Perspectives on Quality of Life During Antihypertensive Therapy, Impact of Responder, Survey Environment, and Questionnaire Structure." *Journal of Cardiovascular Pharmacology*, 1993, *21*(Suppl. 2), S18–S25; Bombardier. C., and others. "Auranofin Therapy and Quality of Life in Patients with Rheumatoid Arthritis: Results of a Multicenter Trial." *American Journal of Medicine*, 1986, *81*(4), 565–578; Johnson, J. R., and Temple, R. "Food and Drug Administration Requirements for Approval of New Anticancer Drugs." *Cancer Treatment Reports*, 1985, *69*(10), 1155–1159.

85. Moinpour, C. M., and others. "Quality of Life Assessment in Southwest Oncology Group Trials." *Oncology*, 1990, *4*(5), 79–89; Wu, A. W., and others. "Applications of the Medical Outcomes Study Health-Related Quality of Life Measures in HIV/AIDS." *Quality of Life Research*, 1997, *6*(6), 531–554.

86. Heithoff, K. A., and Lohr, K. N. "Effectiveness and Outcomes in Health Care." In *Proceedings of an Invitational Conference by the Institute of Medicine*. Washington, D.C.: National Academy Press, 1990.

87. Goldberg, H. I., and others. "Deliberations on the Dissemination of PORT Products: Translating Research Findings into Improved Patient Outcomes." *Medical Care*, 1994, *32*(7 Suppl.), JS90–JS110.

88. "The Outcome of Outcomes Research at AHCPR: Final Report." (Summary.) Agency for Health Care Policy and Research, Rockville, Md, 1999. [http//www.ahrq.gov/clinic/out cosum.htm] (accessed September 6, 2006).

89. Schoenbaum, M., Sherbourne, C., and Wells, K. "Gender Patterns in Cost Effectiveness of Quality Improvement for Depression: Results of a Randomized, Controlled Trial." *Journal of Affective Disorders*, 2005, *87*(2–3), 319–325.

90. Lohr, K. N. "Advances in Health Status Assessment: Overview of the Conference." *Medical Care,* 1989, *27*(3 Suppl.), S1–S11; Lohr, K. N. "Applications of Health Status Assessment Measures in Clinical Practice: Overview of the Third Conference on Advances in Health Status Assessment." *Medical Care*, 1992, *30*(5 Suppl.), MS1–MS14.

91. Nayfield, S. G., and Hailey, B. J. (eds) "Quality of Life Assessment in Cancer Clinical Trials." Bethesda, Md.: Department of Health and Human Services, 1990; Furberg, C. D., and Schuttinga, J. A. (eds) "Quality of Life Assessment, Practice, Problems, Promise." Bethesda, Md.: Department of Health and Human Services, 1990.

92. Ellwood (1988).

93. "Dynamic Assessment of Patient-Reported Chronic Disease Outcomes." National Institutes of Health, 2004. [http://grants.nih.gov/grants/guide/rfa-files/rfa-rm-04–011.html] (accessed July 24, 2005).

94. "Dynamic Assessment of Patient-Reported Chronic Disease Outcomes" (2004).

95. Andersen, R. M., Davidson, P. L., and Ganz, P. A. "Symbiotic Relationships of Quality of Life, Health Services Research and Other Health Research." *Quality of Life Research*, 1994, *3*(5), 365–371.

96. Andersen, Davidson, and Ganz (1994).

97. Andersen, Davidson, and Ganz (1994).

CHAPTER NINE

# EVALUATING THE QUALITY OF CARE

Elizabeth A. McGlynn

In its seminal report, *Crossing the Quality Chasm,*[1] the Institute of Medicine (IOM) adopted this statement, originally developed by the Advisory Commission on Consumer Protection and Quality in the Health Care Industry[2]: the purpose of the health care system is "to continually reduce the burden of illness, injury, and disability, and to improve the health and functioning of the people of the United States."

Evaluations of health care quality provide a concrete assessment of the degree to which the U.S. health care system is successfully achieving this purpose and can be used to track whether quality improvement interventions are effective.

The main purpose of this chapter is to review a variety of methods for assessing quality of care and summarize some of what is known about the current level of quality in the United States. We begin by describing the multiple dimensions on which quality may be evaluated and criteria for selecting assessment topics. Next, we present a conceptual framework for organizing evaluations of quality. Finally, we offer definitions, methods, and key results within this framework.

We have made significant advances in the last decade in recognizing the importance of routinely measuring quality and developing the tools necessary to evaluate performance at all levels of the health care system. In the future, we must find ways to integrate quality measurement at the point of care delivery so that we can make substantial progress in closing the quality chasm that currently exists.

## The Multiple Dimensions of Quality

Quality is a multidimensional concept reflecting the variety of perspectives held by the multiple participants in the health care system. The IOM has defined six domains of performance that capture these dimensions[3]:

1. Safe: service delivery that is free of accidental injury
2. Effective: providing services based on scientific knowledge to all who could benefit, and refraining from offering services to those not likely to benefit
3. Patient-centered: delivery of services in a manner that demonstrates respect for and honors patients' individual preferences and values
4. Timely: services that are free from undesirable and unnecessary delays
5. Efficient: services that are delivered without waste of resource inputs
6. Equitable: a pattern of care delivery that does not vary by factors unrelated to individual health needs (such as age, gender, race, income, education, location)

The IOM's six aims for improvement in the functioning of the health care system are currently used by most groups to define the scope of their quality measurement activities. These aims should not be viewed as mutually exclusive; measures of performance in many cases will cut across these domains.

## Criteria for Evaluating Quality Measures

It is neither feasible nor desirable to measure everything that occurs in the health care system. Quality assessment or monitoring is conducted by selectively examining specific aspects of performance across each of the six dimensions of the health delivery system. Criteria for selecting a set of performance measures are used by most groups undertaking this exercise. Although the criteria may differ somewhat, most can be categorized as addressing (1) importance, (2) scientific support, (3) usability, or (4) feasibility.[4] Each of these is briefly described.

A topic or measure of quality is deemed important if at least one user group could make use of the results. The potential uses of measures include making policy decisions (on the part of private or public groups), shaping clinical decisions (the focus for quality improvement programs), choosing where to go for health care services, or determining the structure of payment for particular providers. Importance may be defined in a variety of ways, among them how common a particular problem is (disease prevalence, utilization rate), the impact the problem has on the health system (cost of care, major determinant of death or disability), the likelihood that improvement could affect the health and well-being of the population, whether the area is likely to affect choices made by patients, the amount of variation in the attribute across the system, and the degree to which performance is substandard. How importance is evaluated reflects the likely use of the measure as well as the group responsible for obtaining the necessary information. For example, the IOM, under contract from the Department of Health and Human Services, developed a list of priority areas for quality improvement. Here is a list of areas identified by the group; this illustrates the results of one approach to selecting important topics for quality measurement.[5]

Asthma

Care coordination

Children with special health care needs

Diabetes

End of life with advanced organ system failure

Evidence-based cancer screening

Frailty associated with old age

Hypertension

Immunizations

Ischemic heart disease

Major depression

Medication management

Nosocomial infections

Obesity

Pain control in advanced cancer

Pregnancy and childbirth

Self management and health literacy

Severe and persistent mental illness

Stroke

Tobacco-dependence treatment in adults

Scientific support is used, sometimes indiscriminately, to refer to either the evidence that underlies a particular element of care delivery or the performance characteristics of the measure itself. For example, a group could decide to focus on heart disease because it is a leading reason for death across most age and gender groups in the population and because there are effective ways to prevent and treat the condition; these criteria are used to establish that heart disease is "important." In selecting measures related to effectiveness (one of the six IOM aims), the group will likely evaluate the areas in which scientifically rigorous studies have established that a particular care process (such as giving beta blockers to people who have had heart attacks) is likely to significantly improve outcomes (here, the likelihood that a patient will not have a subsequent cardiac event resulting in death or disability). Because this care process has been evaluated in randomized controlled clinical trials, the scientific support is considered to be at the highest level. However, there is an additional aspect of scientific support related to the measure itself. The question is whether it is possible to evaluate this care process in a way that is valid (measures the actual process of interest) and reliable (repeated measures would arrive at the same conclusion). Further, if the measure was intended to be used to compare performance at one facility to that at another, additional considerations would apply, such as whether the patient populations are similar enough to permit fair comparisons or whether adequate statistical adjustments have been made to account for differences (that is, adequate methods of risk or case-mix adjustment).

Usability refers to whether the information produced by a measure can be understood and acted on by the intended audience. For a measure to be useful, it has to be a key element in decision making, subjected to analysis that determines whether the results should be used in making a decision, and presented in a way that is understandable to the user and available when a decision has to be made. Relatively little attention has been paid to the influence of data presentation on the usability of the data (and the choices made). The methods by which performance information is presented (visual cues, ordering data, trending cues, and summarizing measures) can significantly affect the choices made by consumers; the addition of cues to help consumers evaluate health plan choices results in optimal decisions being made more frequently.[6] Greater attention to the usability dimension will be necessary in the future for all audiences.

Feasibility refers to the ease with which a measure can be implemented for routine use (as opposed to its use in a research study). Feasibility is largely determined by the availability of necessary data elements for constructing quality measures. In general, measures that can be constructed using administrative claims data are most easily implemented. Measures that require surveys, clinical information from medical records, or onsite observation are more costly and difficult to implement. Significant attention must be directed to improving the information infrastructure available for managing care and evaluating quality if we hope to monitor the performance of the U.S. health care system across all six of the IOM aims.

These criteria can be used hierarchically to evaluate potential quality measures. If a measure is not important, it makes no sense to evaluate the measure on the other criteria. If a measure is not scientifically sound, then it likely is not usable. If a measure is not usable, then it does not matter if it is feasible. Criteria such as these are frequently used to winnow a large number of competing measures down to a manageable set.

## A Conceptual Framework for Quality Assessment

A conceptual framework is a useful mechanism for defining the aspects of care that are evaluated in a quality assessment. The most commonly used conceptual framework in quality assessment is the one proposed by Avedis Donabedian.[7] He identified three dimensions of quality: structure, process, and outcomes (Figure 9.1). We have modified this framework to reflect how the IOM aims fit into this evaluation approach. We organize our review of quality assessment around these three dimensions. In each section, we present a definition of the quality dimension, discuss methods available for assessing that dimension, and summarize what is known about that aspect of quality of care in the U.S. health care system today.

### FIGURE 9.1. CONCEPTUAL FRAMEWORK FOR QUALITY ASSESSMENT.

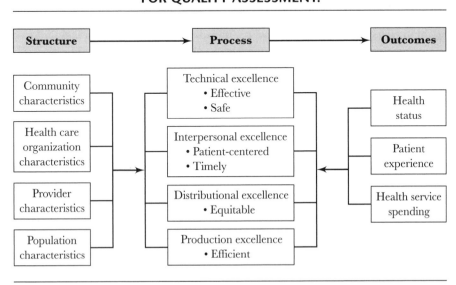

# Structure

Information about the structure of the health care delivery system is used most often to describe the context in which care is delivered and to explore potential explanations for variation in the pattern of care delivery. Structural measures are most often used as proxies for other, more-difficult-to-measure constructs such as safety and equity.

## Definition of Structural Quality

Structural quality refers to those stable elements of the health care delivery system in a community that facilitate or inhibit access to and provision of services. The elements include community characteristics (say, prevalence of disease), health care organization characteristics (such as number of hospital beds per capita, managed care penetration), provider characteristics (specialty mix, board certification status), and population characteristics (demographics, insurance coverage). Structural characteristics can be used to describe both the need for health care (prevalence or incidence of disease) and the capacity of the community or health care delivery system to meet those needs (availability of properly trained personnel).

## Methods of Structural Quality Assessment

For purposes of quality assessment, we are particularly interested in those elements of structure that (1) predict variations in the processes or outcomes of care and (2) are subject to change. For example, the characteristics of the population residing in a community may predict differences in processes of care or outcomes. Persons without health insurance or who are otherwise economically disadvantaged may experience barriers to accessing the health service system; such barriers might be suggested by a comparatively lower rate of using necessary services among certain populations. In turn, such reduction in utilization might be associated with less favorable outcomes. However, policy makers are unlikely to be able to change the characteristics of the population. The more appropriate focus for quality improvement is on reducing barriers to access, through changes in either the availability of insurance or characteristics of the health services delivery system (for example, number of public health clinics, hours of operation for other health providers). Because the relationship between the structure of the health services delivery system and the processes or outcomes of care is indirect, policy makers may find direct action on such measures more difficult than for results from measures of process quality or outcomes.

Community characteristics represent the context in which the health services delivery system operates; they offer one perspective for evaluating the adequacy of the service system to respond to community needs. The prevalence of disorders in the community, for instance, may be useful in estimating specific community needs. Information about the availability of health resources may be an indicator of the potential for meeting those needs. One common measure of resource availability is the physician-to-population ratio; the general tendency is to interpret a higher ratio as representing better quality (though this is not always the case).[8] The location of the community relative to health resources is another key indicator of the ease with which residents may obtain certain services; inner-city and rural residents may have to travel further than others to obtain services. Although an evaluation of community characteristics is not generally included in quality assessment, it may be an important precursor to understanding the particular quality challenges likely to be faced in a community.

Health care organization characteristics have been evaluated in terms of the capacity of the organization to provide high-quality services. Various factors—notably the quality of the physical plant and equipment, ownership, accreditation, staffing patterns, organizational culture, distribution of reimbursement by source of payment, organizational structure, and governance mechanisms—have been considered markers of the likelihood that an organization provides good quality of care. Most of these factors at best can be viewed as facilitating or inhibiting the likelihood of delivering good care; because these factors always appear in combination, it is difficult to evaluate the incremental effect each has on quality. The most commonly used organizational characteristic for evaluating quality is the volume of procedures performed; volume is used as a proxy for outcomes because it is much easier to measure and because evidence has previously established a relationship between these factors.

Provider characteristics have been included as explanatory factors in quality assessments, among them age (or years in practice), gender, race or ethnicity, medical school attended, location of residency training program, specialty, board certification status, job satisfaction, and method of compensation. Board certification is the professional indicator of quality; additional years of training and an examination are required to become board-certified. Various specialty boards are responsible for granting board certification. Overall, about 85 percent of licensed physicians receive initial board certification.[9] The American Board of Medical Specialties (ABMS), representing twenty-four specialty boards, is developing mechanisms to evaluate professional competence throughout a physician's career. The ABMS maintenance of certification initiative includes four elements: (1) professional standing, (2) lifelong learning and periodic self-assessment, (3) cognitive expertise; (4) performance in practice.[10] For physicians who were initially board-certified in 1990 or later (1987 for critical care medicine and 1988 for geriatric medicine), participation in the maintenance of certification program is required to continue to be board-certified. Renewal of certification occurs every ten years.

Population characteristics may be useful in predicting the likelihood that an individual receives high-quality care. Information may be used to identify individuals who are at risk for receiving lower-quality care; in particular, organizations that provide services to individuals at high risk should be aware of the special needs of these populations. Various population characteristics have been examined: sociodemographics, insurance coverage and type, presence of comorbid conditions, functional status, and so on.

Organizational accreditation is a common method of assessing structural quality. Several organizations conduct accreditation programs. Generally accreditation requires that an onsite survey team inspect the facility and verify that the organization meets standards. The Joint Commission on the Accreditation of Healthcare Organizations (JCAHO) accredits hospitals, health care networks, clinical laboratories, and organizations that offer home care, long-term care, behavioral health care, and ambulatory care. The National Committee for Quality Assurance (NCQA) accredits managed care organizations, managed behavioral health care organizations, credentials verification organizations, physician organization certification, and preferred provider organizations. The American Accreditation Healthcare Commission accredits utilization review programs, preferred provider organizations, and managed care organizations.

## What Do We Know About Structural Quality?

In this section we offer some highlights from research on structural quality to illustrate the use of common approaches to measurement of this construct.

***Community Characteristics.*** Although the characteristics of communities in the United States vary widely, there is little evidence of a systematic relationship between those characteristics and the processes or outcomes of care. A study of the Medicare population in the United States found substantial variation in the amount spent on health care in the last six months of life; however, higher spending was not generally associated with better quality of preventive services or care for heart attacks.[11] In fact, areas in the lowest quintile of spending performed best on eight of the ten measures of quality. The study also found that as spending at the end of life increased, the relative risk of death also increased; there was no relationship between the level of spending and decline in functional status or satisfaction.[12] Similarly, a comprehensive study of the quality of care delivered in twelve diverse metropolitan areas in the United States (Boston; Cleveland; Greenville, South Carolina; Indianapolis; Lansing, Michigan; Little Rock, Arkansas; Miami; Newark, New Jersey; Orange County, California; Phoenix, Arizona; Seattle; and Syracuse, New York) found remarkably little variation. The health care markets in these metropolitan areas vary by median income ($19,672–$32,890), the proportion of the population living below the poverty line (10–25 percent), the proportion of the nonelderly who do not have health insurance (8.1–23.0 percent), the number of hospital beds per thousand population (1.6–5.0), the number of physicians per thousand population (1.7–3.3), and the penetration of managed care (13–52 percent). Despite these differences in the economic and resource profile of the communities, the proportion of recommended care received overall ranged from 51 percent in Little Rock and Orange County to 59 percent in Seattle.[13] The absence of a relationship between the amount of money spent on health care and the quality of care received has fueled efforts to identify sources of waste or inefficiency in delivery of health services. If substantial amounts of waste were eliminated, the United States could use the savings to either reduce health care expenditures or increase access to care for underserved populations.

***Health Care Organization Characteristics.*** The relationship between the volume of procedures performed in an institution or by a provider and the outcomes of those procedures has been studied extensively, with mixed results. One review of 135 studies published between 1980 and 2000 reported statistically significant relationships between outcomes and hospital volume (71 percent of studies) and physician volume (69 percent of studies).[14] The magnitude of the relationship varied with the type of service or procedure; AIDS treatment and surgery for pancreatic cancer, esophageal cancer, abdominal aortic aneurysm, and pediatric cardiac problems demonstrated the largest difference in outcomes related to volume. In examining some of the methodological issues, the authors noted that studies using risk adjustment models based on clinical data were less likely to find significant differences than those using risk adjustment models based on administrative data. Another review of seventy-six studies published between 1990 and 2000 selected the study most likely to produce an unbiased estimate of the relationship between volume and mortality for each of the thirty-four diagnoses or interventions investigated.[15] The review found a significant relationship between hospital volume and mortality in about two-thirds of the studies (twenty-two of thirty-three) and in about half of the studies (six of fifteen) of physician volume and mortality. Consistent with the other review, the volume-outcome relationship was particularly strong for pancreatic cancer. These results have encouraged private purchasers, led by the

Leapfrog Group, to advocate selective referral on the basis of volume. Two recent studies examining such policies, however, suggest caution. A study of the volume-outcome relationship for coronary artery bypass graft (CABG) surgery found that low-volume hospitals were more likely to operate on higher-risk patients and in urgent circumstances.[16] Further, no relationship between volume and outcome was found for patients under age sixty-five and those at low operative risk. The authors estimated that fewer than forty-five deaths (less than 1 percent) could be averted through eliminating CABG procedures done at the one hundred hospitals with the lowest volumes. A study of the relationship between the volume of very low birth weight (VLBW) babies admitted to a hospital and mortality found that only 9 percent of the variation in mortality was explained by volume.[17] Rankings based on risk-adjusted mortality were more reliable, predicting 34 percent of the variation in outcomes. The Leapfrog Group, a consortium of large purchasers of health care services (employers and government), has established standards for selective referral to high-volume facilities as a means of improving the quality and safety of care for its members.[18] In the absence of acceptable risk-adjusted outcome measures, Leapfrog recommends using volume as a proxy for safety.

The presence of computerized physician order entry (CPOE) systems in hospitals is another structural measure recommended by the Leapfrog Group to evaluate safety. A systematic review of the literature found five randomized trials that evaluated the effect of CPOE on medication safety; two reported a significant reduction in the rate of serious medication errors.[19] The authors concluded that most studies did not have sufficient power to detect differences in adverse drug events and had evaluated homegrown systems rather than commercial products. Nonetheless, there is considerable encouragement by large employers for hospitals to implement such systems. A recent study conducted at the University of Pennsylvania found that many errors persisted even after implementation of CPOE, and other problems were introduced as a result of the system.[20] Examples of problems with the system that may contribute to increased medication errors are fragmented displays, pharmacy inventory displays mistaken for dosage guidelines, orders placed in paper charts rather than in the CPOE system, separation of functions that can result in double dosing and incompatible orders, and inflexible ordering formats.

Another measure of safety is the patient safety culture in an organization. Under a contract from the Agency for Healthcare Research and Quality, Westat has developed a standardized survey, the Hospital Survey on Patient Safety Culture, which is administered to hospital staff.[21] Preliminary benchmarks on twelve composite scores from twenty hospitals are available on the AHRQ Website. For example, the benchmark composite score for overall perceptions of safety is 56 percent (the average proportion of staff responding with "strongly agree" or "agree" to four questions). The benchmark scores for other composite scales range from 43 percent (nonpunitive response to error) to 71 percent (supervisor manager expectations and actions promoting patient safety and organization learning—continuous improvement).

Few studies have examined the relationship between accreditation status and process quality or outcomes. One study of JCAHO accreditation found that although hospitals not participating in accreditation surveys had lower-quality care, the level of accreditation (such as commendation) was not associated with the rate of effective care for heart attacks (for instance, use of aspirin and beta blockers) or better mortality outcomes.[22] The authors of the study made several recommendations for improving the utility of accreditation as a marker of quality, including incorporating quality measures into the accreditation decision. NCQA does incorporate quality measures into its accreditation decisions for health plans and reports higher performance on almost all process quality measures in accredited plans compared to nonaccredited plans.[23] As part of the accreditation requirements, health plans seeking NCQA accreditation must publicly report the results of their quality measures.

*Provider Characteristics.* As discussed earlier, board certification is commonly used as a structural measure of physician quality. A review of studies published between 1966 and 1999 found relatively few evaluated the relationship between board certification status and outcomes. The thirteen studies that met criteria for inclusion in the review reported thirty-three separate findings; sixteen findings demonstrated better outcomes among board-certified physicians, three reported that board-certified physicians had worse outcomes, and fourteen showed no association.[24] Board certification is frequently reported by organizations furnishing evaluation of physician quality.

*Population Characteristics.* Equity is most often evaluated by comparing the experience of patients in population subgroups (race, income, insurance, education, gender). A review of the literature on disparities in provision of health services found lower quality and intensity of services delivered to racial and ethnic minorities across a range of conditions and interventions.[25] Studies that controlled for sociodemographics, insurance status, and health status found that these disparities were smaller though rarely eliminated. The review notes that insurance status is a particularly important predictor; people with private insurance generally receive higher-quality care than those with either public insurance or none. To some degree, the observed disparities are a function of the settings in which individuals in ethnic and racial minority groups receive care (such as nonteaching hospitals, or public hospitals and clinics). Patients receiving care in military facilities and, less consistently, in the Veterans Administration health care system, were less likely to experience inequity in delivery of care. Considerable policy attention is currently being devoted to interventions that reduce or eliminate disparities in health care delivery.

# Process

Comparison of organizations for consumer choice or accountability is dominated by process quality measures because they occur more frequently than negative outcomes and are consistent with the structure of clinical practice guidelines.

## Definition of Process Quality

Process quality refers to what occurs in the interaction between a patient and a provider. Donabedian identified two dimensions of process quality: technical excellence and interpersonal excellence.[26] The former means that the intervention was effective (that is, only those services were provided that, according to scientific evidence, are likely to benefit patients) and that it was provided safely. The latter means the intervention was patient-centered and delivered in a timely manner. We offer two amendments to Donabedian's definition of technical quality to align more clearly with the IOM aims: distributional excellence and production excellence. Distributional excellence means that care processes are delivered equitably; that is, they do not vary by population characteristics that are unrelated to health needs. Production excellence means that services are provided in an efficient manner that is not characterized by substantial waste of resources.

For purposes of technical quality assessment, we are primarily interested in those processes of care that are likely to produce optimal outcomes: either improvement in health or reduction in the rate of decline in functioning. The best evidence of the relationship between processes and outcomes is from randomized controlled trials because they can prove conclusively the efficacy of an intervention (the potential to produce desired outcomes under ideal circumstances). Evidence from other scientific methods, though not as conclusive, is often used to demonstrate the importance of a variety of interventions in medical care. In assessing interpersonal and distributional quality, we are interested in those processes that are more likely to improve outcomes, particularly health and patient experience outcomes. Production excellence measures should predict better economic outcomes.

## Methods of Process Quality Assessment

We discuss four methods used to evaluate the quality of medical care processes: (1) appropriateness of an intervention, (2) adherence to practice guidelines or standards of care, (3) practice profiling, and (4) consumer reports or ratings. These four methods share some features, but we discuss them separately to emphasize a number of methodological considerations.

***Appropriateness.*** Appropriateness of an intervention means that, for individuals with particular clinical and personal characteristics, the expected health benefit from doing an intervention (diagnostic or therapeutic procedure) exceeds the expected health risk by a sufficient margin so that the intervention is worth doing. RAND and UCLA have pioneered a method of assessing the appropriateness with which a variety of interventions are evaluated.[27] The basic method involves five steps:

1. *Review the literature.* A detailed literature review is conducted to summarize what is known about the efficacy, utilization, complications, cost, and indications for the subject intervention. Where possible, outcome evidence tables are constructed for clinically homogeneous groups.

2. *List indications.* A preliminary list of indications is developed for the intervention that categorizes patients in terms of their symptoms, past medical history, results of previous diagnostic tests, and clinically relevant personal characteristics (such as age). The indications list is designed to be detailed enough that patients within an indication are homogeneous with respect to the clinical appropriateness of performing a procedure; the indications are comprehensive enough that all persons presenting for the procedure can be categorized.

3. *Convene a panel to select indications.* A nine-person multispecialty panel is assembled to assume responsibility for developing and rating the final set of indications. The panel is chosen to be diverse with respect to geographic location, practice style, and other characteristics. Both "doers" and "nondoers" of a procedure are included on the panel.

4. *Rate the indications.* The indications are rated using a modified Delphi process. In the first round, panelists individually rate the indications (the literature review prepared in step one is made available); the panelists may also recommend changes to the structure of the indications. In the second round, the panel meets face-to-face for a discussion of the results from the first round and makes final ratings. The indications are rated from 1 to 9, where 1 means that the procedure is very inappropriate for persons within an indication and 9 means that the procedure is very appropriate for persons within an indication. The median

panel rating is used to determine the appropriateness rating for each indication; a median rating of 1–3 is considered inappropriate, 4–6 is equivocal or of uncertain value, and 7–9 is appropriate. There is also a requirement that the panel have a reasonable and statistically determined level of agreement among themselves.

5. *Evaluate appropriateness of interventions.* The appropriateness with which interventions are used can then be evaluated. Generally, information is abstracted from the medical record (inpatient or outpatient) because of the level of clinical detail required to assign patients to indications. An alternative approach that has been applied when appropriateness is assessed prospectively is to interview both the patient and the physician.

The appropriateness method is used to develop valid quality indicators for evaluating adherence to evidence-based medicine. The reliability and validity of the appropriateness method has been extensively evaluated. The test-retest reliability of individual panel members' ratings and the reproducibility of overall panel ratings have been found comparable to the levels of common diagnostic tests.[28] The content and construct validity of ratings of appropriateness is supported by the studies done.[29] For example, regression analysis performed on indications for patients with chronic stable angina undergoing coronary angiography demonstrated that the procedure was more likely to be considered appropriate (1) as severity increased, (2) among patients who had failed medical therapy, and (3) among patients who had positive findings on noninvasive tests.[30]

The ratings of each indication are the explicit standards by which care is evaluated. The indications can be linked to the quality of scientific evidence, and ratings can be updated as knowledge changes. Sensitivity analyses can be used to evaluate the importance of certain factors in the indication structure in determining appropriateness. For example, in our study of appropriateness of hysterectomy, we found that among women who wanted to maintain fertility, the expert panel required considerable evidence of efforts to find an alternative solution to the presenting problem before the hysterectomy was considered appropriate.[31] Because there are no national averages established for the expected appropriateness of care, most of the comparisons have been made among groups (hospitals, managed care organizations) participating in a study.[32]

Most studies of appropriateness were conducted in the 1980s and early 1990s, when overuse was the major quality issue. Although the appropriateness method can be used to evaluate both underuse and overuse, its application to the problem of overuse is more common. As initiatives to control rising health care costs were implemented (such as managed care), concern shifted to underuse of services. The pendulum is once again swinging back toward concern about overuse, which may give rise to a new generation of appropriateness studies. The appropriateness method represents one method for evaluating the IOM domains of effectiveness and safety.

*Adherence to Guidelines.*  Adherence to practice guidelines or professional standards is a method of process quality assessment that evaluates the extent to which care is consistent with professional knowledge, either by examining adherence to specific practice guidelines or by evaluating whether care meets certain professional standards. The AHRQ defines clinical practice guidelines as "systematically developed statements to assist practitioner and patient decisions about appropriate health care for specific clinical conditions."[33] Practice guidelines are often formulated graphically as decision algorithms to reflect the complexity of clinical decision making. Adherence to guidelines is the method used to evaluate the IOM domains of effectiveness and safety.

From 1992 to 1996, AHRQ funded development of practice guidelines[34] and published a monograph on various methodological approaches to development of clinical practice guidelines.[35] More recently, AHRQ funded several evidence-based practice centers to conduct systematic review of the literature that can be used by others to develop practice guidelines.[36] Today, most specialty societies develop practice guidelines in their area of clinical expertise. The federal government maintains a Web-based clearinghouse of guidelines from a variety of sources.[37] The U.S. Preventive Services Task Force is one of the leading organizations developing guidelines for use of preventive care services (immunizations, Pap smears, mammograms). The most recent reports from this group can be found on the Web.[38] Because of the relative ease of evaluating adherence to preventive service standards, they represent a common basis for quality assessment. One argument that is frequently raised in objection to using the rate of adherence to preventive service recommendations as a marker of quality is the role of patient compliance in seeking such services. Despite this concern, preventive service use remains one of the leading quality indicators currently in use.

For purposes of quality assessment, it is almost always necessary to translate guidelines into review criteria by establishing operational definitions of adherence and nonadherence to the guidelines, as well as definitions for key clinical concepts employed in the guidelines. Many practice guidelines, for example, contain vague clinical terms ("mild," "moderate," "severe") that must be explicitly defined in order to evaluate whether a particular patient qualifies for an element of the guidelines and then to assess adherence to the guideline. The performance expectation is generally 100 percent adherence to the guideline, and comparisons are made either among similar groups or compared to a benchmark.

Three data sources are used to determine the degree of adherence to practice guidelines: administrative data, medical records, and patient surveys. Administrative data are generated to pay claims for reimbursement under health insurance plans. Because claims are filed only for those services included in a benefit package, administrative data can be used to evaluate quality only where the service is covered and when the conditions for appropriate use can be ascertained from such data sources; preventive services are often evaluated using claims data. Medical record data are used when greater clinical detail is required to determine the population that should be receiving an intervention or to evaluate some types of intervention; medical records are used for assessing elements of chronic disease care, particularly if severity of disease is necessary for determining the needed interventions. Surveys are used to obtain patient reports on interventions such as immunization, mammography, and cholesterol testing that are indicators for technical process quality. The National Immunization Survey, for example, tracks the rate of immunizations for children in the first two years of life. Such reporting is particularly useful if the intervention is likely to be remembered accurately by consumers and if the intervention is difficult to identify in other data sources.

***Practice Profiling.*** Practice profiling is a method for comparing the patterns of cost, utilization, and quality of processes among providers. The method usually compares practice patterns to an empirical norm (say, the average of other physicians in the organization). Profiles are generally constructed as a rate of occurrence of some process (such as office visit, service, surgical procedure, laboratory test) over a specified period of time for a defined population.[39] What distinguishes profiling from most appropriateness or guideline adherence approaches is that a clear standard does not exist or the review is not condition-specific; rather, it may cover a broader range of practice patterns (such as hospital admission rate). Profiles can be constructed at any level in the health delivery system: nationally; regionally; or by health plan, specialty, medical group, or individual physician. Profiling is most often used to examine utilization of a variety of services: hospital admission, ambulatory visit, laboratory test use, referral pattern, diagnostic test use, medication prescription. Profiling methods are used to assess the IOM domain of efficiency, and in some cases equity.

In the past, profiling was used for internal quality improvement and cost containment more often than for external reporting of performance. One consequence of this is that there are fewer reports in the literature about the results of profiling analyses. There are, however, a few articles emphasizing some of the critical issues that must be addressed if profiling is to be used routinely for quality assessment.[40] Perhaps the most important issue that arises is the need for case-mix or severity adjustment (differences in severity, prevalence of diseases, and other characteristics of the populations being compared). The methods for case-mix adjustment, particularly in an ambulatory setting, are in a developmental stage.

In addition, much of the clinical information that is typically required for case-mix adjustment cannot be found among claims data; this implies that supplemental data are required in order to make adequate adjustments. One study of referral patterns found that adjusting for the age and sex distribution of patients in a physician's panel reduced the coefficient of variation in referrals by more than 50 percent.[41] When a case-mix adjustment was applied, 75 percent of physicians identified as outliers under the age and sex adjustment method were no longer classified as outliers.

This problem is particularly important to solve for the purpose of external comparison, but even internal uses of profiling would benefit substantially from improved adjustment methods (as when physicians in a health plan are profiled). For example, the Medical Outcomes Study found that patients of cardiologists were older, had lower functional status and well-being scores, and had more chronic diagnoses than patients of general internists; patients of family practitioners were younger and had better functional status and fewer chronic conditions than patients of general internists.[42] These case-mix characteristics were associated with differences in rate of hospitalization, physician visit, and prescription drug use. Internal plan comparisons should account for these variations.

The other challenge for profiling is the problem of sample size. There is considerable interest in using profiling techniques to examine the practice patterns of individual physicians. However, one must have an adequate number of observations on each physician to determine whether the differences observed are statistically significant. Among other things, this implies that common processes (such as use of screening mammography) are more suitable for profiling than rarer processes (using adjuvant chemotherapy for breast cancer treatment). Among processes, greater aggregation is more suitable than less (using all laboratory tests versus using a single test).

Today, large employers and health plans are using profiling methods to construct tiered networks of providers on the basis of relative resource use (such as establishing lower co-payment amounts for patients using providers whose practice is deemed more "efficient") and to reward providers whose profiles suggest they use resources less intensively. Most of the profiling tools in use today are proprietary and rely on claims data.

**Consumer Ratings.**  Consumer ratings are the most appropriate method for evaluating the interpersonal quality of care (that is, the IOM domains of patient-centeredness and timeliness). Surveys of individuals are the most common method for eliciting information from individuals about their health care. Two types of information are generally sought: (1) reporting of events and (2) ratings of care. We discuss reporting of events (patient experience) here and ratings of care (patient satisfaction) under the outcomes section.

Consumer reports are used to evaluate a variety of access issues, among them waiting time for an appointment or to see the doctor, distance to the nearest health facility, hours of operation, ability to see the provider one wants to see, and other similar questions regarding the consumer's experience in trying to obtain services. Consumers may also report on what the physician did during an encounter (explain options, furnish requested information, counsel about health habits). Patients' ability to report on events varies with the time frame (a shorter time span produces more reliable information) and the type of event (invasive events such as surgery may be more memorable than health promotion counseling).

In an effort to standardize the survey methods used to elicit information from consumers, in 1995 AHRQ awarded cooperative agreements to RAND, Harvard, and Research Triangle Institute to develop the Consumer Assessment of Health Plans Survey (CAHPS).[43] There are now five separate CAHPS instruments available for health plans, ambulatory care, hospitals, nursing homes, and dialysis facilities.

## What Do We Know About Process Quality?

It is beyond the scope of this chapter to summarize all of the literature regarding process quality. However, we include some key results that have been published in each of the IOM domains. Together they illustrate application of the methods described here for measuring process quality.

*Technical Excellence: Effectiveness.* The most comprehensive assessment of health care quality ever undertaken reported that American adults receive just 55 percent of recommended care for the leading causes of death and disability and for the main reasons they seek health care services.[44] The study analyzed performance on 439 indicators of effectiveness across thirty chronic and acute health problems as well as preventive care. Few differences were found in the likelihood that people received needed preventive care or care for common chronic and acute health problems. Deficits were reported across the continuum of care from screening (52 percent) to diagnosis (56 percent), treatment (58 percent), and follow-up (59 percent). The quality of care did vary substantially by health condition. For example, 68 percent of recommended care was delivered for patients with coronary artery disease, compared to 25 percent for atrial fibrillation. Among patients with a diagnosis of depression noted in the medical record, just 58 percent of recommended care was delivered. People with diabetes received 45 percent of recommended care, which is of particular concern given the increased prevalence of diabetes related to the epidemic of obesity in America. A higher rate of failure to deliver needed care (underuse) was reported compared to delivering care that was of no benefit or potentially harmful to the patient (overuse).

Beginning in December 2003, Congress required the AHRQ to produce an annual report on health care quality in the United States.[45] The section on effectiveness addresses care related to cancer, diabetes, end stage renal disease, heart disease, HIV/AIDS, maternal and child health, mental health, respiratory diseases, and nursing home and home health care; both process and outcome measures are reported. A few results are highlighted here.

The rates of screening for cancer vary from 33.3 percent for one colorectal cancer screening method (fecal occult blood testing) to 70.3 percent for breast cancer screening (mammography) and 81.4 percent for cervical cancer screening (Pap smears). For diabetes, the report indicates that only one-third of adults received all five recommended care processes (blood sugar test, lipid profile, retinal examination, foot examination, and influenza vaccine). Although in 1999–2000 more adults reported they had received cholesterol screening than in 1988–1994, just one-quarter of those with a high cholesterol level are taking medication for the problem. Counseling about healthy eating and the importance of physical activity are important interventions for preventing children from becoming overweight. In 2001, 36 percent of children had been counseled about healthy eating and 22.8 percent about exercise in the prior year; 70.7 percent had their height and weight measured. Effective management of asthma in children can prevent hospitalization; profiling the rate of hospitalization for children with asthma yields an indication of how well it is managed. In 2001, the rate of hospitalization for asthma varied from 98 per 100,000 population in the best-performing states to 261.5 per 100,000 population in the worst-performing states.

NCQA produces an annual report on the effectiveness of care delivered to people enrolled in health plans.[46] In 2004, NCQA collected standardized information from 563 health plans on about twenty-six effectiveness-of-care measures across preventive, chronic disease, and acute condition care. A few results are highlighted here.

Between 2000 and 2004, the proportion of adolescents in these plans who are receiving recommended immunizations has increased from 36.8 percent to 58.7 percent. The proportion of smokers reporting they were advised by their provider to quit has remained about the same (approximately two-thirds). The proportion of persons with diabetes receiving blood sugar monitoring averaged 74.8 percent in Medicaid plans, 84.6 percent in commercial plans, and 87.9 percent in Medicare plans. Beta blockers were received by a high proportion of patients who had heart attacks (94.3 percent). Among children making a visit for a sore throat, 70.7 percent in commercial plans were tested for the presence of a bacterial infection prior to receiving antibiotics, compared to 53.8 percent in Medicaid plans. About 20 percent of children who had a visit for a cold inappropriately received antibiotics.

Results of quality measures in hospitals became publicly available for the first time through the Centers for Medicare and Medicaid Services (CMS) in late 2003 and JCAHO in July 2004. Effectiveness measures are reported for three clinical areas: heart attack, heart failure, and pneumonia. Performance for heart attack care is high on average, ranging from 80 percent of patients with left ventricular systolic dysfunction receiving ACE inhibitors to 95 percent of patients receiving aspirin at both admission and discharge.[47] Heart failure care ranged from 55 percent of patients receiving appropriate discharge instructions to 88 percent of patients receiving an assessment of left ventricular function. For pneumonia, 50 percent of patients who had not previously received a pneumococcal vaccine received one; 99 percent of patients had their oxygen status assessed. Significant improvement was reported for most measures between the first quarter of 2002 and the last quarter of 2004.

*Technical Excellence: Safety.*  Safety is most often assessed using structure or outcome measures; however, appropriate use of medications is a common process measure of safety. In 2000, 13.5 percent of elderly Americans received at least one of thirty-three medications known to be potentially harmful for them.[48] Research has identified eleven medications that should never be prescribed to elderly persons; in 2000, 2.4 percent of the elderly received at least one of these medications. The elderly are at increased risk of experiencing drug-drug interactions because they typically receive medications from multiple physicians. In 2001, 25.5 percent of the elderly reported in a national survey that the doctor they usually saw for care did not ask them about medications prescribed by other doctors they had seen.

*Interpersonal Excellence: Patient-Centeredness.*  Consumer ratings and reports are the principal means by which patient-centeredness is evaluated. The National CAHPS Benchmarking Database (NCBD) reports results from a number of standardized measures of patient-centered care. In 2004, 223 commercial plans, 149 Medicaid plans, and 288 Medicare plans supplied their results to the NCBD.[49] The report presents results on four composite measures of patient-centeredness. In 2004, 75 percent of commercial enrollees, 64 percent of Medicaid enrollees, and 81 percent of Medicare enrollees reported they did not have a problem getting needed care. Medicaid enrollees were most likely to report experiencing a big problem getting needed care (15 percent). Enrollees in all plan types were less likely to report that their doctors always communicated well (59 percent for commercial, 58 percent for Medicaid, and 68 percent for Medicare enrollees). The proportion reporting that office staff were always courteous and helpful ranged from 63 percent for Medicaid enrollees to 78 percent for Medicare enrollees. The majority of enrollees reported they did not have a problem getting needed information and help from their health plan (64 percent for commercial, 68 percent for Medicaid, and 73 percent for Medicare enrollees).

*Interpersonal Excellence: Timeliness.* The NCBD reports one composite measure related to timeliness; it summarizes four separate questions about how often consumers received different types of health care in a timely manner.[50] Overall, 46 percent of commercial enrollees, 42 percent of Medicaid enrollees, and 57 percent of Medicare enrollees reported that they always received timely care. Medicaid enrollees were more likely to report having problems getting needed help or advice during office hours; 21 percent said they never or sometimes got help when they called, compared to 12 percent for commercial and 9 percent for Medicare enrollees. Similar findings were reported for whether care was obtained as soon as desired for an illness, injury, or other health problem; 21 percent of Medicaid enrollees (compared to 12 percent of commercial and 10 percent of Medicare enrollees) reported they never or sometimes got this type of care as soon as they wanted. For other appointments, such as for preventive care, 23 percent of Medicaid enrollees, 17 percent of commercial enrollees, and 9 percent of Medicare enrollees reported they never or sometimes got an appointment as soon as they wanted. Only 20 percent of commercial, 18 percent of Medicaid, and 25 percent of Medicare enrollees reported they were always taken to the examination room within fifteen minutes of their scheduled appointment time.

Timeliness can also be a factor in delivery of clinical care processes. Three of the publicly reported hospital measures evaluate the number of minutes it takes from the time a patient arrives at the hospital to the time a needed care process is delivered; timeliness is critical to good outcomes in these areas. For patients admitted with a heart attack, hospitals in the bottom quartile of performance averaged 138 minutes to deliver thrombolytic therapy in the third quarter of 2002 and 63 minutes by the second quarter of 2004; by comparison, hospitals in the top quartile declined from 49 minutes on average to 24 minutes.[51] Time to percutaneous coronary intervention for heart attack patients improved from 881 minutes in the bottom quartile of hospitals in the third quarter of 2002 to 340 minutes in the second quarter of 2004. Time to initiation of antibiotics among patients admitted with pneumonia improved from 380 minutes in the bottom-quartile hospitals in quarter three of 2002 to 254 minutes in quarter two of 2004.

*Distributional Excellence: Equity.* The National Healthcare Disparities Report (NHDR) is produced annually by AHRQ to summarize current disparities in delivery of health services on the basis of race, ethnicity, and socioeconomic status, and among priority populations (such as persons with special health care needs, the elderly, residents of rural areas, children, and women).[52] Results are reported for the IOM categories of effectiveness, safety, patient-centeredness, and timeliness.

The 2004 report emphasized three themes: (1) disparities are pervasive across all of the groups identified by the report; (2) improvement is possible, judging by the success of programs that have made closing the disparity gap a priority; and (3) considerable gaps exist in the information base necessary to track the presence of disparities and the relative success of programs in eliminating these disparities. A few highlights from the report related to process quality are presented here.

In 2001, blacks were 38 percent less likely to receive all five recommended care processes for diabetes, controlling for age, gender, income, education, insurance, and residence; Hispanics were 33 percent less likely to receive these services. Differences among income groups were not statistically significant.

Disparities in the rate of immunization are found across all age groups. White children were more likely to receive all recommended vaccines (76.6 percent) compared to black children (68.8 percent); Asian children were vaccinated at about the same rate as whites (79.2 percent). Children living in families with income less than 100 percent of the poverty line were significantly less likely to receive all childhood vaccinations compared to those living in families with income above 400 percent of the poverty line (69.3 percent vs. 81.6 percent). Vaccination rate does not appear to vary by race among adolescents, except for a lower rate of measles-mumps-rubella vaccine among black adolescents. Immunization patterns among adults were comparable; black high-risk nonelderly adults and the elderly were less likely to receive influenza vaccine compared to whites (25.2 percent versus 21.4 percent), although considerable room for improvement is evident among all groups. Elderly persons who are black or Asian are less likely to receive pneumococcal vaccine than whites (56.6 percent for whites, 33.6 percent for blacks, 28.2 percent for Asians).

Profiling methods are frequently used to evaluate disparities in provision of needed services (overuse) or to identify potential underuse of needed services. Inappropriate prescribing of antibiotics was more common among whites than blacks, occurring in 195.4 visits per 10,000 population versus 153.2 visits per 10,000 population. Some patterns of hospitalization suggest underuse of needed services in the outpatient setting. Blacks are significantly more likely to be hospitalized for asthma than whites. The asthma hospitalization rate for black children is 55.9 per 10,000 population versus 16.2 for white children. The same disparities exist among adults, although the hospitalization rate is considerably lower than what is found in children; black adults had 21.4 hospitalizations per 10,000 population compared to 8 per 10,000 for white adults. Hospitalization for congestive heart failure occurs almost twice as frequently for blacks as for whites (5.0 per 1,000 population versus 2.6 per 1,000). The differences are greatest in the forty-five-to-sixty-four-year-old population (7.6 per 1,000 among blacks versus 1.9 per 1,000 for whites).

***Production Excellence: Efficiency.*** Efficiency is a relatively new addition to the definition of quality, and there are few systematic studies available that rigorously document the relative use of resources to produce a specific health care service. Recent studies by Fisher and colleagues using Medicare data demonstrate substantial differences in spending on hospital and physician services among similar patient cohorts.[53] For example, use of services for patients following a heart attack was 77 percent higher in the highest quintile region compared to the lowest; similar ratios were reported for patients following an initial episode of colorectal cancer (59 percent higher in the top versus the bottom quintile) and hip fracture (69 percent higher in the top). In each cohort, about half of the spending was on hospital services and half on physician services. These differences in spending did not produce a higher rate of effective care.

# Outcomes

Many people argue that outcomes are the only legitimate way to evaluate quality. This section highlights some of the benefits and challenges inherent in using outcomes to assess quality.

## Definition of Outcomes

Outcomes can be defined as the result of efforts to prevent, diagnose, and treat various health problems encountered by the population. Outcomes are seen by many as the bottom-line measure of the degree to which the health care delivery system is achieving its purpose. A range of potential dimensions can be included in the broad category of outcomes. In Figure 9.1, for example, we list health status (clinical and functional), patient experience, economic, and provider experience as examples of types of outcome used to assess the performance of the health system.

Clinical status refers to biological, physiological, and symptom-based aspects of health; examples are blood pressure, blood sugar level, cholesterol level, lung function, and mortality. These are the outcomes that are generally of interest to physicians because they are most directly amenable to treatment. Functional status captures multiple dimensions, among them physical, mental, role, and social functioning. Assessments of functional status typically ask respondents to indicate the frequency or extent to which physical or mental disorders interfere with their ability to perform their usual activities. Functional status is of greatest interest to consumers because it represents how changes in clinical status affect their everyday life. Consumer satisfaction assesses the extent to which experiences in the health service system were consistent with expectations and were acceptable to those receiving care.

There are two key challenges in using outcome assessments for evaluating the quality of care. Both challenges reflect the fact that the outcomes we observe are produced through the interaction of a variety of factors in and outside of the health service delivery system. First, to use outcomes to make externally valid comparisons among health plans or providers, adequate methods must be employed to control for differences in the severity of illness or the health profile of the populations being compared. A familiar example of an initial failure to do this was the release by the Health Care Financing Administration (HCFA) of hospital mortality data. Initially, the data were not adjusted for differences in the severity of illness for patients, and not surprisingly some of the hospitals that had the worst performance records were those serving the sickest patients (for example, hospices for the terminally ill).[54] In response to complaints from hospitals and physicians about deficiency in the measures and lack of uptake from consumers, HCFA ceased publication of hospital mortality data in 1993.[55] There is still considerable controversy as to whether the severity adjustments introduced by HCFA subsequent to the initial release were adequate, but the addition of severity adjustments substantially improved the discriminant validity of the model.[56]

The second key challenge for the use of outcomes data is the issue of attribution—that is, determining the extent to which the health plan or physician that is currently being evaluated is responsible for the observed outcomes. Health outcomes are affected by a variety of factors, not all of which can be modified by the health delivery system. One study estimated that 40 percent of mortality can be attributed to behavioral factors, 20 percent to social circumstances and environmental exposures, 30 percent to genetics, and 10 percent to inadequacies in medical care.[57] Because these factors may be distributed differently among populations enrolled in health plans and those seeking care from primary care physicians, these external effects must be controlled for in statistical analyses in order to understand the extent to which variations in the quality of care contribute to the observed variations in outcomes. For interventions that take place over a long period of time (chronic disease care), outcomes observed in the current time period may be the result of action taken (or not taken) much earlier in the course of illness, and the actions might not have been undertaken by the physicians or health plan currently responsible for treating the patient. To the extent that individuals change providers frequently, discontinuity in service may further contribute to a less-than-optimal course of treatment. Who bears the responsibility for these complex series of events remains a question open to debate.

## Methods of Outcome Assessment

We consider three approaches to outcome assessment used to evaluate the quality of care delivered: (1) condition-specific; (2) generic; and (3) sentinel events, or adverse outcomes.

***Condition-Specific Approach.*** The condition-specific approach, sometimes referred to as a "tracer" condition approach, examines the outcomes for individuals who have a particular diagnosis (say, hypertension). The condition-specific approach is used to evaluate the IOM domains of effectiveness and equity. The outcomes for condition-specific approaches may emphasize clinical status (blood pressure control for hypertension), although disease-specific measures of functional status should also be assessed (for prostate cancer, treatment assessments should include incontinence, impotence, and bowel function). The advantage of condition-specific outcome assessment from a quality perspective is that it may most closely reflect a link to the processes of care delivered. For example, if one health plan has a higher proportion of individuals with hypertension whose blood pressure is outside the "controlled" range, one might reasonably conclude that the plan has problems in managing the disease (medication, diet, monitoring for complications). The difficulty with condition-specific approaches to quality assessment is that they require substantial investment in developing methods across a sufficient range of diseases to produce a picture of the overall quality of care delivered in a health plan or hospital.

Research suggests that quality is not consistent from condition to condition.[58] This implies that we are likely to observe variability in outcomes by condition; some organizations may have good outcomes for adult chronic diseases and be less successful in achieving good outcomes for chronic disease in childhood. One study of quality at the hospital level found that the relative rates of complications were similar within institutions, but there was less correlation between medical and surgical cases.[59] The other difficulty in the context of today's information systems is that one may not be able to easily identify individuals who have particular health problems so that population-based outcome assessments can be conducted.

***Generic Approach.*** The generic approach examines outcomes that can be assessed for all individuals, regardless of their health problems. The generic approach is used to evaluate the IOM domains of safety, patient-centeredness, and efficiency. Outcomes regarding mortality, general functional status, level of health care spending, and patient satisfaction are most commonly assessed in generic approaches.

The advantage to the generic approach is that it can be applied across the entire population enrolled in a health plan, receiving care from a hospital, or seeing a particular physician. The difficulty with this approach is that research has yielded considerably less understanding of the link between what is done in the medical care system and the resulting generic outcomes for the population. There is reason to believe that other factors (education, socioeconomic status) enter into determining these outcomes. Further, the need to control for variation in severity and case mix of a population in making comparisons of generic outcomes is extremely important, and few reliable methods for doing so currently exist.

Patient experience may be the most commonly evaluated generic outcome at the level of the health plan or hospital. Patient experience measures consumer ratings as to the quality and acceptability of care. CAHPS is the standardized set of instruments most commonly used to evaluate patient experience today.

*Sentinel Event Approach.* The sentinel event approach identifies some occurrence, usually an adverse outcome, that is likely to be associated with poor quality of care and tracks the frequency with which the event occurs. Sentinel events are used to evaluate the IOM domains of effectiveness, equity, and safety. Examples of adverse outcomes are mortality, early readmission to a hospital, complications of a surgical procedure (transfusion, reoperation), nosocomial infection in the hospital, suicide, adverse drug reaction (especially as a result of interactions among one or more drugs), and very low birthweight. Sentinel events can be useful for identifying potential problems, but it is almost always necessary to conduct further assessments to conclude whether an adverse event was "preventable" or not. The frequency with which adverse events occur affects their practicality for quality assessment. Events that occur rarely are less useful for quality monitoring because it is more difficult to determine whether differences are statistically significant.

## What Do We Know About Outcomes?

As with the literature on process quality, it is beyond the scope of this chapter to summarize everything that is known about the outcomes of care. Rather, we offer examples of some of the important findings from the published literature. This section is also organized to highlight application of outcomes methods to evaluating quality in the applicable IOM domains.

*Outcomes: Effectiveness.* Condition-specific outcomes are used to evaluate the effectiveness of care. For example, NCQA reports on the proportion of enrollees in health plans with hypertension who have their blood pressure controlled. In

2003, 62.2 percent of commercial enrollees, 61.4 percent of Medicare enrollees, and 58.6 percent of Medicaid enrollees with hypertension had their blood pressure controlled.[60] Substantial improvement in control has been demonstrated across all plan types since the measure was first reported in 2000. NCQA uses two outcome measures to assess effectiveness of care for diabetes: poor control of blood sugar (glycosylated hemoglobin) and control of cholesterol (lipids). In 2003, 32 percent of commercial, 48.6 percent of Medicaid, and 23.4 percent of Medicare enrollees with diabetes had a blood sugar level that was clearly too high. Lipid control was somewhat better; 60.4 percent of commercial, 47.8 percent of Medicaid, and 67.7 percent of Medicare enrollees with diabetes had their lipid level under 130 mg/dL. More recently, guidelines have emphasized a lower threshold definition of control—under 100 mg/dL. Using this definition, 34.7 percent of commercial, 27.8 percent of Medicaid, and 41.9 percent of Medicare enrollees had their lipids controlled. Outcome measure thresholds can change over time as new scientific evidence is acquired or more effective therapies become available.

Pain is a generic outcome measure being used by CMS to evaluate the effectiveness of care for postacute and chronic care residents of nursing homes.[61] In 2003, 22 percent of postacute care and 6.7 percent of chronic care nursing home residents reported they had moderate-to-severe pain in the past week. State variation in this rate among chronic care residents narrowed considerably from 22 percentage points (7 percent to 29 percent) in 2002 to 10 percentage points (3 percent to 12 percent) in 2003.

***Outcomes: Safety.*** Adverse events are a common method for measuring outcomes related to safety. Infections that are acquired while a patient is receiving care (generally in a hospital) are called nosocomial and represent a serious threat to patients who are already vulnerable because of the reason they were hospitalized. *Healthy People 2010* sets performance targets for five types of nosocomial infection; they are tracked through the National Nosocomial Infection Surveillance System. By 2002, targets in four of the five areas had been met.[62]

Another type of adverse event used to monitor safety is mortality, or complications following a surgical procedure. Both procedure-specific and generic adverse events are assessed. For example, 3.1 percent of surgical patients experience a urinary tract infection following surgery, 2.2 percent develop pneumonia, and 1 percent develop a venous thromboembolism (blood clot).[63] Complications following joint replacement surgery occur at much higher rates; average complication rates for Medicare patients are 9.4 percent for knee replacement, 9.5 percent for hip replacement for degenerative disorders, and 22.6 percent for hip replacement following hip fracture.

*Outcomes: Patient-Centeredness.* The NCBD makes available results for four overall ratings of patient experience with care: personal doctor, specialists, health care, and health plan. Respondents are asked to rate each category on a scale from 0 to 10, with 0 representing the worst possible and 10 the best possible in that category. In 2004, 53 percent of commercial, 58 percent of Medicaid, and 66 percent of Medicare enrollees rated their personal doctor a 9 or 10.[64] For specialists, 57 percent of commercial, 59 percent of Medicaid, and 67 percent of Medicare enrollees rated the physician a 9 or 10. Ratings of health care were similar to those for personal doctor (53 percent for commercial, 51 percent for Medicaid, and 67 percent for Medicare rating a 9 or 10). Health plan ratings were the lowest, with 41 percent of commercial, 50 percent of Medicaid, and 52 percent of Medicare enrollees rating their plan a 9 or 10.

*Outcomes: Efficiency.* Fisher and colleagues reported on the relationship between health care spending and risk of death following a hip fracture, treatment for colon cancer, and heart attack as well as over time for a general cohort of Medicare patients.[65] For each cohort, every 10 percent increase in the expenditure index was associated with an increase in the risk of death. The study found no relationship between increased spending and changes in functional status over time. Similarly, no statistically significant relationship was found between level of health care spending and patient satisfaction with care. A test for trend suggested there was less overall satisfaction with care and greater satisfaction with interpersonal care in higher-spending regions.

## Conclusion

Tremendous progress has been made over the past decade in developing methods for measuring quality, applying those methods in a variety of settings, and public reporting about the results. In areas where quality measurement is routinely applied and reported, progress is being made. However, significant deficits exist in the structural elements of care, processes of care, and outcomes. The consequences of failure to deliver effective health services are significant in terms of preventable disability and death as well as avoidable expenditures. Significant improvement in the quality of care delivered in the United States will require a substantial investment in the information infrastructure for the health care system. Where such investments have been made, greater progress is evident; nevertheless, few organizations today have adequate information infrastructures in place. The infrastructure investment must include mechanisms for regularly obtaining reports and ratings from patients.

The information infrastructure is necessary but not sufficient to improve quality. Performance must be evaluated across the multiple dimensions outlined by the IOM at all levels in the health care system, from individual providers up to the nation. Performance assessment systems must include a broad set of measures, or else the incentive for the health care industry will be to improve only the handful of areas measured. Further, information about performance should be made available regularly to all players in the health care system. For providers, having information available at the point of care increases the likelihood of needed services being delivered as the opportunities arise; this is likely to be both more effective and more efficient than the current system.

Increasing the information about performance that is routinely available also expands opportunities to pay high performers differentially. Currently, the payment system does not pay providers who deliver higher-quality care more than those who deliver lower quality. Offering such incentives is another way we might accelerate progress on delivery of high-quality care.

Each of these policy changes will facilitate redesign of the health care delivery system from one that is reactive and inefficient to one able to proactively and efficiently manage the health service needs of the population in achieving the highest levels of health and functioning possible.

# Notes

1. Committee on Quality Health Care in America, Institute of Medicine. *Crossing the Quality Chasm: A New Health System for the 21st Century.* Washington, D.C.: National Academy Press, 2001.

2. Advisory Commission on Consumer Protection and Quality in the Health Care Industry. "Quality First: Better Health Care for All Americans," 1998. [http://www.hcquality commission.gov/final] (accessed July 26, 2005).

3. Committee on Quality Health Care in America (2001).

4. McGlynn, E. A. "Selecting Common Measures of Quality and System Performance." *Medical Care*, 2003, *41* (Suppl.), I39–I47.

5. Institute of Medicine. *Priority Areas for National Action: Transforming Health Care Quality.* Washington, D.C.: National Academy Press, 2003.

6. Hibbard, J. H., Slovic, P., Peters, E., and Finucane, M. L. "Strategies for Reporting Health Plan Performance Information to Consumers: Evidence from Controlled Studies." *Health Services Research*, 2002, *37*, 291–313.

7. Donabedian, A. *Explorations in Quality Assessment and Monitoring. Vol. I: The Definition of Quality and Approaches to its Assessment.* Ann Arbor, Mich.: Health Administration Press, 1980.

8. Fisher, E. S., and others. "Associations Among Hospital Capacity, Utilization, and Mortality of U.S. Medicare Beneficiaries, Controlling for Sociodemographic Factors." *Health Services Research*, 2000, *34*, 1351–1362.

9. Horowitz, S. D., Miller, S. H., and Miles, P. V. "Board Certification and Physician Quality." *Medical Education*, 2004, *38*, 10–11.

10. Brennan, T. A., and others. "The Role of Physician Specialty Board Certification Status in the Quality Movement." *Journal of the American Medical Association*, 2004, *292*, 1038–1043.

11. Fisher, E. S., and others. "The Implications of Regional Variations in Medicare Spending. Part 1: The Content, Quality, and Accessibility of Care." *Annals of Internal Medicine*, 2003, *138*, 273–287.

12. Fisher, E. S., and others. "The Implications of Regional Variations in Medicare Spending. Part 2: Health Outcomes and Satisfaction with Care." *Annals of Internal Medicine*, 2003, *138*, 288–298.

13. Kerr, E. A., and others. "Profiling the Quality of Care in 12 Communities: Results from the CQI Study." *Health Affairs*, 2004, *23*, 247–256.

14. Halm, E. A., Lee, C., and Chassin, M. R. "Is Volume Related to Outcome in Health Care? A Systematic Review and Methodologic Critique of the Literature." *Annals of Internal Medicine*, 2002, *137*, 511–520.

15. Gandjour, A., Bannenberg, A., and Lauterbach, K. W. "Threshold Volumes Associated with Higher Survival in Health Care: A Systematic Review." *Medical Care*, 2003, *41*, 1129–1141.

16. Peterson, E. D., and others. "Procedural Volume as a Marker of Quality for CABG Surgery." *Journal of the American Medical Association*, 2004, *291*, 195–201.

17. Rogowski, J. A., and others. "Indirect vs. Direct Hospital Quality Indicators for Very Low-Birth-Weight Infants." *Journal of the American Medical Association*, 2004, *291*, 202–209.

18. Leapfrog Group for Patient Safety. "Evidence-Based Hospital Referral." [http://www.leapfroggroup.org/media/file/Leapfrog-Evidence-based_Hospital_Referral_Fact_Sheet.pdf] (accessed July 27, 2005).

19. Kaushal, R., Shojania, K. G., and Bates, D. W. "Effects of Computerized Physician Order Entry and Clinical Decision Support Systems on Medication Safety: A Systematic Review." *Archives of Internal Medicine*, 2003, *163*, 1409–1416.

20. Koppel, R., and others. "Role of Computerized Physician Order Entry Systems in Facilitating Medication Errors." *Journal of the American Medical Association*, 2005, *293*, 1197–1203.

21. Westat. "Comparing Your Results: Preliminary Benchmarks on the Hospital Survey on Patient Safety Culture (HSOPSC)." [http://www.ahrq.gov] (accessed July 28, 2005).

22. Chen, J., Rathore, S. F., Radford, M. J., and Krumholz, H. M. "JCAHO Accreditation and Quality of Care for Acute Myocardial Infarction." *Health Affairs*, 2003, *22*, 243–254.

23. National Committee for Quality Assurance (NCQA). "The State of Health Care Quality, 2004." [http://www.ncqa.org/communications/SOMC/SOHC2004.pdf] (accessed July 28, 2005).

24. Sharp, L. K., and others. "Specialty Board Certification and Clinical Outcomes: The Missing Link." *Academic Medicine*, 2002, *77*, 534–542.

25. Smedley, B. D., Stith, A. Y., and Nelson, A. R. (eds.). *Unequal Treatment: Confront Racial and Ethnic Disparities in Health*. Washington, D.C.: National Academy Press, 2003.

26. Donabedian (1980).

27. Brook, R. H. "The RAND/UCLA Appropriateness Method." In K. A. McCormick, S. R. Moore, and R. A. Siegel (eds.), *Clinical Practice Guideline Development: Methodology Perspectives*. (AHCPR publication no. 95-0009.) Rockville, Md.: Agency for Health Care Policy and Research, Public Health Service, U.S. Department of Health and Human Services, Nov. 1994; Brook, R. H., and others. "A Method for the Detailed Assessment of the Appropriateness of Medical Technologies." *International Journal of Technology Assessment*, 1986, *2*, 53–63.

28. Shekelle, P. G., and others. "The Reproducibility of a Method to Identify the Overuse and Underuse of Medical Procedures." *New England Journal of Medicine*, 1998, *338*, 1888–1895.

29. Shekelle, P. G., Chassin, M. R., and Park, R. E. "Assessing the Predictive Validity of the RAND/UCLA Appropriateness Method Criteria for Performing Carotid Endarterectomy." *International Journal of Technology Assessment in Health Care,* 1998, *14,* 707–727.

30. Kravitz, R. L., and others. "Validity of Criteria Used for Detecting Underuse of Coronary Revascularization." *Journal of the American Medical Association,* 1995, *274,* 632–638.

31. Bernstein, S. J., and others. *Hysterectomy: A Literature Review and Ratings of Appropriateness.* Santa Monica, Calif.: The RAND Corporation, 1992.

32. Leape, L. L., and others. "The Appropriateness of Use of Coronary Artery Bypass Graft Surgery in New York State." *Journal of the American Medical Association,* 1993, *269,* 753–760; Bernstein, S. J., and others. "The Appropriateness of Hysterectomy: A Comparison of Care in Seven Health Plans." *Journal of the American Medical Association,* 1993, *269,* 2398–2402.

33. The definition appears in the Foreword to each of the practice guidelines. See, for example, Urinary Incontinence Guideline Panel. *Urinary Incontinence in Adults: Clinical Practice Guideline.* (AHCPR publication no. 92-0038.) Rockville, Md.: Agency for Health Care Policy and Research, Public Health Service, U.S. Department of Health and Human Services, Mar. 1992, p. iii.

34. Guidelines were developed for a number of conditions, including acute pain management for operative or medical procedures and trauma; urinary incontinence in adults; prediction, prevention, and treatment of pressure ulcers in adults; management of functional impairment caused by cataracts in adults; detection, diagnosis, and treatment of major depression in primary care; screening, diagnosis, management, and counseling regarding sickle cell disease in newborns and infants; evaluation and management of early HIV infection; diagnosis and treatment of benign prostatic hyperplasia; management of cancer pain; diagnosis and management of unstable angina; evaluation and care of patients with left-ventricular systolic dysfunction; otitis media with effusion in young children; and acute low back problems in adults.

35. McCormick, K. A., Moore, S. R., and Siegel, R. A. (eds.). *Clinical Practice Guideline Development: Methodology Perspectives.* (AHCPR publication no. 95-0009.) Rockville, Md.: Agency for Health Care Policy and Research, Public Health Service, U.S. Department of Health and Human Services, Nov. 1994.

36. Reports from the evidence-based practice centers can be found at http://www.ahrq.gov/clinic/epcix.htm (accessed July 28, 2005).

37. National Guideline Clearinghouse. [http://www.guideline.gov] (accessed July 28, 2005).

38. Latest versions of the literature reviews and recommendations from the U.S. Preventive Services Task Force can be found at [http://www.ahrq.gov/clinic/prevenix.htm] (accessed July 28, 2005).

39. Lasker, R. D., Shapiro, D. W., and Tucker, A. M. "Realizing the Potential of Practice Pattern Profiling." *Inquiry,* 1992, *29,* 287–297.

40. Welch, H. G., Miller, M. E., and Welch, W. P. "Physician Profiling: An Analysis of Inpatient Practice Patterns in Florida and Oregon." *New England Journal of Medicine,* 1994, *330,* 607–612; Salem-Schatz, S., Moore, G., Rucker, M., and Pearson, S. D. "The Case for Case-Mix Adjustment in Practice Profiling: When Good Apples Look Bad." *Journal of the American Medical Association,* 1994, *272,* 871–874; McNeil, B. J., Pedersen, S. H., and Gatsonis, C. "Current Issues in Profiling Quality of Care." *Inquiry,* 1992, *29,* 298–307; Lasker, Shapiro, and Tucker (1992).

41. Salem-Schatz, Moore, Rucker, and Pearson (1994).

42. Kravitz, R. L., and others. "Differences in the Mix of Patients Among Medical Specialties and Systems of Care: Results from the Medical Outcomes Study." *Journal of the American Medical Association,* 1992, *267,* 1617–1623.

43. The history of this initiative can be found at [http://www.ahrq.gov/research/cahptrip.htm] (accessed July 28, 2005).

44. McGlynn, E. A., and others. "The Quality of Health Care Delivered to Adults in the United States." *New England Journal of Medicine*, 2003, *348*, 2635–2645.

45. Agency for Healthcare Research and Quality (AHRQ). "2004 National Healthcare Quality Report." 2004. [http://www.qualitytools.ahrq.gov] (accessed July 28, 2005).

46. NCQA (2004).

47. Williams, S. C., and others. "Quality of Care in U.S. Hospitals as Reflected by Standardized Measures, 2002-2004." *New England Journal of Medicine*, 2005, *353*, 255–264.

48. AHRQ (2004).

49. National CAHPS Benchmarking Database. *NCBD 2004 Chartbook*. Nov. 2004. [http://www.ahrq.gov] (accessed July 28, 2005).

50. National CAHPS Benchmarking Database (2004).

51. Williams and others (2005).

52. Agency for Healthcare Research and Quality. "National Healthcare Disparities Report 2004." [http://www.qualitytools.ahrq.gov] (accessed Aug. 1, 2005).

53. Fisher and others, Part 2 (2003).

54. Berwick, D. M., and Wald, D. L. "Hospital Leaders' Opinions of the HCFA Mortality Data." *Journal of the American Medical Association*, 1990, *263*, 247–249.

55. Galvin, R. S., and McGlynn, E. A. "Using Performance Measurement to Drive Improvement: A Road Map for Change." *Medical Care*, 2003, *41*(1, Suppl.), I48–I60.

56. Fleming, S. T., Hicks, L. L., and Bailey, R. C. "Interpreting the Health Care Financing Administration's Mortality Statistics." *Medical Care*, 1995, *33*, 186–201.

57. McGinnis, J. M., Williams-Russo, P., and Knickman, J. R. "The Case for More Active Policy Attention to Health Promotion." *Health Affairs*, 2002, *21*, 78–93.

58. McGlynn and others (2003).

59. Iezzoni, L. I., and others. "Using Administrative Data to Screen Hospitals for High Complication Rates." *Inquiry*, 1994, *31*, 40–55.

60. NCQA (2004).

61. AHRQ, National Healthcare Quality Report (2004).

62. AHRQ (2004).

63. AHRQ (2004).

64. National CAHPS Benchmarking Database (2004).

65. Fisher and others, Part 2 (2003).

CHAPTER TEN

# PUBLIC RELEASE OF INFORMATION ON QUALITY

Elizabeth A. McGlynn
John L. Adams

Information about the quality of care delivered by entities in the health care system—health plans, hospitals, medical groups—is becoming more routinely available. Although it remains easier to find out how well a variety of consumer products are likely to perform than it is to determine the reliability with which a specific physician or hospital will deliver evidence-based medicine, significant progress is being made. Publicly available information on quality (or, more broadly, performance) may be used by consumers and payers to choose among health plans, hospitals, and physicians, and by providers to improve their performance.[1] The motivation for improvement may be professional (providers want to perform at the top of the class), financial (incentives or disincentives tied to level of performance), or regulatory (reaching a baseline level of performance required to stay in business).

Changes in the organization and financing of care have also increased concern about variation in quality. In the unrestricted-choice model characterized by fee-for-service, individual providers were accountable for ensuring the delivery of high-quality health care. Physicians were trusted to be effective advocates for their patients' needs. However, as third-party purchasers and their agents began to use financial incentives to control costs and restrict choices, the perception (if not the reality) was that physicians could no longer act solely in the patient's interest. Recent introduction of high-deductible plans with catastrophic insurance (also known as consumer-directed health plans) is intended to make consumers more aware of differences among providers in the cost and quality of care.

Rising health care costs that appear to threaten the viability of some major American industries (such as automobile manufacturing) have caused purchasers to ask for evidence that they are getting good value for their money. These questions have been stimulated in part by evidence that serious deficits in quality exist. For example, the Institute of Medicine highlighted the problem of medical errors in hospitals and estimated that as many as ninety-eight thousand people die each year as a result of such errors.[2] A national study of the quality of medical care delivered found that American adults receive only 55 percent of recommended care for the leading causes of death, disability, and utilization.[3]

Taken together, these concerns and challenges lead to calls for more transparency about the performance of the health care system. The purpose of this chapter is to (1) describe the type of information that is currently being publicly released, (2) discuss some of the methodological issues that arise in producing information for public release, and (3) summarize what is known about the use of information on quality for consumer choice and quality improvement.

## Public Information on Quality

The breadth and depth of information about quality that is publicly available varies by type of entity. The most comprehensive information available nationally is about health plans, thanks to the efforts of the National Committee for Quality Assurance (NCQA) since the early 1990s. Information about hospitals only recently became more consistently available nationally. Information about medical groups and individual physicians lags behind. Table 10.1 lists the types of information available at each level in the health system and gives some examples of organizations that currently release data. This is not an exhaustive list, but one intended to demonstrate the leading approaches to making information about quality available to decision makers.

### Health Plans

NCQA is responsible for the widespread availability of information on the performance of managed care plans. NCQA annually collects and reports information on selected processes and outcomes of care, patient experiences with care, and accreditation. Most report cards on managed care plan performance are based primarily, or solely, on the information made public by NCQA; health plans voluntarily submit the data on which these reports are based.

Information on selected processes and outcomes of care is reported by plans using standardized specifications contained in a reporting system known as the

## TABLE 10.1. ILLUSTRATION OF
## PUBLIC INFORMATION RELEASED, BY ENTITY.

| Organizational Entity | Type of Information | Examples |
|---|---|---|
| Health plan | Process, outcomes of care | National Committee for Quality Assurance (NCQA), Centers for Medicare and Medicaid Services (CMS) [HEDIS] |
| | Patient experience with care | NCQA, CMS (CAHPS) |
| | | *Consumer Reports* |
| | Accreditation | NCQA |
| Hospital | Process of care | Hospital Quality Alliance, CMS, Joint Commission on Accreditation of Healthcare Organizations (JCAHO) |
| | Patient safety | JCAHO, Leapfrog |
| | Rankings by disease | *U.S. News & World Report* |
| | Mortality by procedure | New York, Pennsylvania, California |
| | Patient experience | California HealthCare Foundation |
| Medical group | Process, outcomes of care | Pacific Business Group on Health (PBGH), Minnesota Community Measurement |
| | Patient experience with care | PBGH |
| Physician | Mortality rate for coronary artery bypass graft surgery (CABG) | New York, Pennsylvania |
| | Process of care | Bridges to Excellence, NCQA Physician Recognition Program |

Health Plan Employer Data and Information Set (HEDIS). For HEDIS 2006, plans will be asked to report on their performance in calendar year 2005 on forty-nine measures of the effectiveness of care. They are shown in Table 10.2. In 2005 (the most recent year for which data are available), 491 health plans reported data for public release.[4]

## TABLE 10.2. LISTING OF THE HEDIS
## 2006 EFFECTIVENESS OF CARE MEASURES.

| Area | Measure Title | Measure Content |
|------|---------------|-----------------|
| Preventive care | Childhood Immunization Status | Proportion of 2-year-olds who are up to date on vaccines to prevent diphtheria, tetanus, polio, measles, mumps, rubella, haemophilus influenzae type b, hepatitis B, chickenpox, pneumonia |
| | Adolescent Immunization Status | Proportion of 13-year-olds who were up to date on vaccines to prevent measles, mumps, rubella, hepatitis B, chickenpox |
| | Colorectal Cancer Screening | Proportion of adults age 50 to 80 who have been screened for colorectal cancer using at least one of four methods |
| | Breast Cancer Screening | Proportion of women age 52 to 69 who have had a mammogram in the past two years |
| | Cervical Cancer Screening | Proportion of women 21 to 64 who have had a Pap smear in the past three years |
| | Chlamydia Screening in Women | Proportion of sexually active women 16 to 25 who have been screened for chlamydia |
| | Glaucoma Screening in Older Adults | Proportion of adults age 65 and older who have had a comprehensive eye examination |
| | Flu Shots for Adults | Proportion of adults 50 to 64 who received an influenza vaccination |
| | Flu Shots for Older Adults | Proportion of Medicare members 65 and older who received an influenza vaccination |
| | Pneumonia Vaccination Status for Older Adults | Proportion of Medicare members 65 and older who report having received a pneumococcal vaccine |
| | Physical Activity in Older Adults | Proportion of Medicare members who have talked with their doctor about physical activity and who have received counseling about engaging in physical activity |
| Comprehensive diabetes care | Measurement of Blood Sugar | Proportion of adults (18 to 75) with diabetes who have had at least one hemoglobin A1c (HbA1c) test in a year |
| | Poor Control of Blood Sugar | Proportion of adults with diabetes whose HbA1c is greater than 9% |
| | Lipid Screening | Proportion of adults with diabetes who have had their lipid level tested |

## TABLE 10.2.  LISTING OF THE HEDIS
## 2006 EFFECTIVENESS OF CARE MEASURES, Cont'd.

| Area | Measure Title | Measure Content |
|---|---|---|
| | Lipid Control (I) | Proportion of adults with diabetes whose lipid level (LDL-C) is < 130 mg/dL |
| | Lipid Control (II) | Proportion of adults with diabetes whose lipid level (LDL-C) is < 100 mg/dL |
| | Screening for Retinopathy | Proportion of adults with diabetes who have had a retinal eye examination |
| | Monitoring for Diabetic Nephropathy | Proportion of adults with diabetes who have been screened for or received medical attention for kidney disease |
| Heart disease care | Controlling High Blood Pressure | Proportion of adults age 46 to 85 with hypertension whose blood pressure is ≤ 140/90 mm Hg |
| | Beta Blocker After Heart Attack | Proportion of adults age 35 and older who receive a beta blocker following discharge from a hospital for a heart attack |
| | Persistence of Beta Blocker Treatment After a Heart Attack | Proportion of adults age 35 and older who continued to receive beta blockers at least six months following discharge from a hospital for a heart attack |
| | Cholesterol Management for Patients with Cardiovascular Conditions | Proportion of adults age 18 to 75 who had a heart attack, percutaneous transluminal coronary angioplasty, or CABG surgery who were screened for lipid levels and whose lipid levels (LDL-C) were < 130 mg/dL and < 100 mg/dL |
| Pulmonary care | Use of Appropriate Medications for People with Asthma | Proportion of members age 5 to 56 with persistent asthma who received a medication for long-term control of asthma |
| | Use of Spirometry in Assessment and Diagnosis of COPD[a] | Proportion of adults age 40 and older with new diagnosis of chronic obstructive pulmonary disease (COPD) whose lung function was evaluated using spirometry to confirm the diagnosis |
| Mental health care | Follow-up After Hospitalization for Mental Illness | Proportion of members age 6 and older who were seen in an outpatient setting within 7 and 30 days after being discharged from a hospital with a mental health disorder |
| | Antidepressant Medication Management | The proportion of adults age 18 and older who were seen at least three times in the 12 weeks following a new prescription for an antidepressant; the proportion who were still receiving an antidepressant 12 weeks and 6 months after being started on one |

## TABLE 10.2. LISTING OF THE HEDIS
## 2006 EFFECTIVENESS OF CARE MEASURES, Cont'd.

| Area | Measure Title | Measure Content |
|------|---------------|-----------------|
| | Follow-up Care for Children Prescribed Medication for Attention-Deficit/ Hyperactivity Disorder (ADHD) | Proportion of children age 6 to 12 years who had one follow-up visit within 30 days after being newly prescribed medication for ADHD; among those who continue to receive ADHD medication, the proportion who had two additional follow-up visits over the next 9 months |
| Other chronic disease care | Osteoporosis Management in Women Who Had a Fracture | Proportion of women age 67 and older who had a fracture, who had a bone mineral density test or prescription for a medication to treat osteoporosis in the 6 months following the fracture |
| | Disease Modifying Antirheumatic Drug (DMARD) Therapy in Rheumatoid Arthritis | Proportion of adults age 18 and older with rheumatoid arthritis who received a DMARD prescription |
| | Medical Assistance with Smoking Cessation | The proportion of adults age 18 and older who smoke and who received advice to quit from their clinician, who had a discussion about smoking cessation medications, and who discussed smoking cessation strategies |
| | Management of Urinary Incontinence in Older Adults | Proportion of Medicare members age 65 and older who have urinary incontinence and who have discussed the problem with their clinician and received treatment for the problem |
| Medication safety | Annual Monitoring for Patients on Persistent Medications[a] | Proportion of adults age 18 and older who are taking selected medications and who receive appropriate screening annually to monitor for side effects or to determine whether the dosage is clinically effective |
| | Drugs to Be Avoided in the Elderly[a] | Proportion of Medicare members age 65 and older who received at least one medication that should not be prescribed to older persons; proportion receiving two or more such medications |
| Functional status | Medicare Health Outcomes Survey | Proportion of Medicare members age 65 and older whose functional status declined over a two-year period, better, the same, or worse than expected |

[a]First-year measure

NCQA also collects and reports information on patients' experiences with care using a standardized survey known as the Consumer Assessment of Health Plans Survey (CAHPS).[5] The survey, developed by RAND, Harvard, and RTI under a cooperative agreement with the Agency for Healthcare Research and Quality (AHRQ), is fielded by independent vendors on behalf of participating health plans. Surveys are returned directly to the vendor, which prepares the results and sends the data to NCQA. The results can be reported as either single-item ratings (health plan, personal doctor or nurse, all health care) or multiple-item composites (getting needed care, getting care quickly, courteous and helpful office staff, customer service, claims processing). There are versions of health plan CAHPS for enrollees in commercial, Medicare, and Medicaid plans.

NCQA also accredits managed care plans using a set of standards that cover structural dimensions of the organization as well as indicators of performance based on a subset of HEDIS and CAHPS results. NCQA reports the overall accreditation outcome as excellent, commendable, accredited, provisional, or denied. Accreditation is also reported in consumer-oriented categories (access and service, qualified providers, staying healthy, getting better, and living with illness), using one to four stars. Both types of accreditation results are available on the NCQA Website (www.ncqa.org). Users can construct their own report card for a specific geographic area using the aggregate categories. Some detail about performance on select chronic disease indicators in the living-with-illness category is also available on the Website. Additional detail on other measures is available in NCQA's commercial product, Quality Compass.

In 2005, NCQA and *U.S. News & World Report* collaborated on producing "America's Best Health Plans," parallel to the annual report on hospitals.[6] The top fifty commercial, twenty-five Medicare, and twenty-five Medicaid plans were listed in the magazine. To arrive at the rankings, information was combined on multiple measures in four categories: access to care, member satisfaction, prevention, and treatment. Complete rankings on all health plans were reported on the Website (www.usnews.com/healthplans) along with a listing of health plans that did not participate in HEDIS or NCQA accreditation.

## Hospitals

Beginning late in 2003, information on how hospitals performed on a set of clinical quality measures was released publicly by the Centers for Medicare and Medicaid Services (www.cms.hhs.gov). The Joint Commission on Accreditation of Healthcare Organizations (JCAHO) released its first public report in July 2004 (www.qualitycheck.org). National data on ten measures of clinical quality were released by CMS in November 2004 through the efforts of a consortium called the Hospital Quality Alliance (HQA). Although public reporting among hospitals began as a voluntary effort, the Medicare Prescription Drug, Improvement, and Modernization Act of 2003 (which introduced prescription drug coverage for Medicare enrollees for the first time) added a financial incentive for hospitals to participate. Hospitals that reported the ten measures publicly in FY 2005 were eligible to receive a 0.4 percent annual reimbursement update. In FY 2006, hospitals that did not report and meet a set of data exchange and validation requirements would receive a reduction of 0.4 percent in their annual payment update. Virtually all eligible hospitals were participating by FY 2005. The measures being reported on hospitals in FY 2005 are shown in Table 10.3.

In addition to information available to consumers on the CMS and JCAHO Websites, insurers and large employers purchase reports on hospital quality performance from a number of private vendors. The results are generally made available through an insurance company portal or employer portal and may be the information most routinely seen by employed and insured populations. Most of these report cards depend on publicly available measures and data as their source, most notably the quality indicators (QIs) from AHRQ.[7] The QIs cover prevention (as an example, evidence of hospital admissions that could have been avoided through better outpatient management), quality of inpatient care (mortality rate by condition and procedure), and patient safety (avoidable complications, iatrogenic events).

At the state level, hospital mortality rates have been released for coronary artery bypass graft (CABG) surgery. Perhaps the leading example of this is New York State's Cardiac Reporting System, which releases risk-adjusted, in-hospital mortality rates for CABG surgery for all hospitals in New York. The Pennsylvania Health Care Cost Containment Council has also released public information on risk-adjusted, in-hospital mortality rates for the same surgery. The Pacific Business Group on Health (PBGH) led development of the California Coronary Artery Bypass Graft (CABG) Surgery Mortality Reporting Program, which released its first report in 2001 on 79 of the 118 hospitals that perform the surgery; hospitals voluntarily participated in the program (the New York and Pennsylvania efforts were mandatory). In 2001, the California state legislature mandated all hospitals to report their mortality rate following CABG surgery annually to the state Office of Statewide Health Planning and Development; the first report from the mandatory effort is due in December 2005. PBGH has also released data on risk-adjusted mortality rates following various transplant procedures for hospitals in California.

Accreditation status represents another type of information publicly available on hospital quality. JCAHO is responsible for conducting hospital accreditation in the United States. Hospitals that wish to serve Medicare beneficiaries must obtain accreditation, which means most hospitals in the United States seek it. The methods used by JCAHO to make accreditation decisions changed in 2004 with the adoption of the Shared Visions-New Pathways initiative. One innovative

## TABLE 10.3. SELECT QUALITY MEASURES
## PUBLICLY REPORTED ON HOSPITALS.

| Clinical Area | Description of Measure | Reporting Entity |
|---|---|---|
| Heart attack (acute myocardial infarction) (HQA) | Proportion of patients age 18 and older who receive aspirin within 24 hours of admission for a heart attack | Joint Commission on Accreditation of Health-careOrganizations (JCAHO), Hospital Quality Alliance |
| | Proportion of patients 18 and older discharged from a hospital with an aspirin prescription | JCAHO, HQA |
| | Proportion of patients discharged from a hospital following a heart attack who have left ventricular systolic dysfunction, who are prescribed an ACE inhibitor at discharge | JCAHO, HQA |
| | Proportion of patients receiving smoking cessation counseling or advice | JCAHO |
| | Proportion of patients receiving a beta blocker within 24 hours of admission for a heart attack | JCAHO, HQA |
| | Proportion of patients receiving a beta blocker on discharge following a heart attack | JCAHO, HQA |
| | Mean time from arrival at the hospital until initiation of thrombolytic therapy | JCAHO |
| | Mean time from arrival at the hospital until initiation of a percutaneous coronary intervention | JCAHO |
| | Adjusted mortality rate | JCAHO |
| Heart failure | Proportion of patients receiving comprehensive instructions at discharge for heart failure | JCAHO |
| | Assessment of left ventricular function | JCAHO, HQA |
| | Prescription of an ACE inhibitor at discharge among persons with left ventricular systolic dysfunction | JCAHO, HQA |
| | Smoking cessation or advice | JCAHO |
| Pneumonia | Oxygenation assessed within 24 hours of admission for pneumonia | JCAHO, HQA |
| | Pneumonia vaccine completed by discharge | JCAHO, HQA |
| | Blood cultures collected prior to initiation of antibiotics | JCAHO |
| | Smoking cessation counseling prior to discharge among those who smoke | JCAHO |
| | Mean time from arrival at hospital to initiation of antibiotics | JCAHO, HQA |

aspect of this new approach is the tracer methodology. Onsite surveyors select a patient from the list of those currently in the hospital and follow the person's experience through the entire stay, from admission through current status. On average, about eleven patient tracers are selected during the weeklong visit. Following the patient through the hospital process gives surveyors a different view of how well the various systems and procedures are operating within a hospital. As of December 2004, about forty-five hundred hospitals had been through the JCAHO accreditation process. Of these, 9 percent were accredited, 87 percent received provision accreditation, 1 percent received condition accreditation, and fewer than 1 percent received a preliminary denial of accreditation.

In the popular press, perhaps the most familiar report card on hospitals is *U.S. News & World Report*'s annual issue on "America's Best Hospitals." The magazine examines three major aspects of performance in developing its rankings: reputation, mortality rate, and annual surveys by the American Hospital Association. Rankings are calculated for all hospitals in each of seventeen specialty areas (cancer; digestive disorders; ear, nose, and throat; geriatrics; gynecology; heart and heart surgery; hormonal disorders; kidney diseases; neurology and neurosurgery; ophthalmology; orthopedics; pediatrics; psychiatry; rehabilitation; respiratory disorders; rheumatology; and urology). An Index of Hospital Quality (IHQ) is calculated for each hospital in twelve of the specialty areas. Reputation scores are based on a survey of thirty-four hundred board-certified physicians who are asked to rank the top five hospitals in the nation in their specialty (results are averaged for the most recent three years). Mortality scores are based on the ratio of observed to expected risk-adjusted mortality rates from Medicare data. The final category is composed of a variety of structural elements: whether the hospital is a member of the Council of Teaching Hospitals, availability of high-technology services, medical and surgical volume, nurse-to-patient ratio, availability of a state-certified trauma center and the level of that center, patient-community services index, availability of geriatric services, availability of obstetric care and birthing rooms, medical and surgical intensive-care beds, hospice and palliative care, National Cancer Institute designated cancer center, nurse magnet facility, and epilepsy center certification. The weights for combining these structural elements into a score for each specialty are based on factor analysis. Each of the three major components has an equal weight in determining the final overall ranking for each specialty.

## Medical Groups

As information on quality becomes available more systematically on managed care plans, interest in having such information at the medical group level has increased. Many consumers do not understand the role health plans play in ensuring provision of high-quality care and would prefer information closer to the point of service delivery. This is particularly true in areas, such as California, where medical groups are a dominant form of physician organization and many medical groups contract with multiple health plans.

PBGH, a coalition of large and small employers, has produced a series of report cards on 139 medical groups and independent practice associations in California. The report cards cover five major areas: patient rating of care, communicating with patients, getting treatment and specialty care, timely care and service, and coordinating patient care. The 2004 reports were based on responses from more than fifty thousand adults who were commercially enrolled members of HMOs and who responded to the California Consumer Assessment Survey. The results are presented in categories (excellent, good, fair, poor). Numeric results are also available (using bar graphs) for the individual items that make up the categorical results. Reports are available on a Website (www.healthscope.org) that also includes reports on health plans and hospitals in California.

Minnesota has initiated a statewide reporting system on medical groups. In 2004, MN Community Measurement reported results on more than fifty measures for fifty-two groups across six areas: asthma, children's health, depression, diabetes, hypertension, and women's health. The measures are technical process and outcomes measures based on guidelines from the Institute for Clinical Systems Improvement. The results are presented graphically with the point estimate and 95 percent confidence interval; comparisons to performance across all medical groups are also provided. The Website includes information for consumers about what they can do to improve their health in the target area as well as the role their provider plays (www.mnhealthcare.org).

## Physicians

Consumers are probably most interested in the quality of individual physicians, but little information is publicly available at this level yet. Most of the reports at the level of the individual physician have been developed for internal use by health plans or medical groups as part of determining compensation. Risk-adjusted mortality rate following CABG surgery is available at the individual physician level in New York and Pennsylvania and is expected in California by the summer of 2006.

NCQA has developed voluntary programs for recognizing provider performance in three areas: diabetes, heart and stroke, and physician office practice. The Diabetes Physician Recognition Program is cosponsored by the American Diabetes Association. Physicians can apply for recognition if they submit data on at least thirty-five patients with diabetes (if seeking individual recognition) or twenty-five patients per physician for groups seeking recognition. Physicians seeking recognition must complete an application and abstract data from medical records or administrative databases on eleven diabetes process and outcome measures; an optional patient survey is also part of the program. The Heart/Stroke Recognition Program is cosponsored by the American Heart Association and American Stroke Association and contains five clinical measures; a patient survey tool is not part of this program. The Physician Practice Connections Program recognizes physicians who have systems in place to offer evidence-based medicine, provide patient education and support, and manage the care of complex patients. There are nine modules in which assessments are conducted; recognition is furnished for participating in any module. For all of the recognition programs, physicians who have successfully met the thresholds established by NCQA are recognized on the NCQA Website with a seal.

## Report Cards on Other Entities

Report cards have been developed for other entities as well, notably nursing homes and dialysis centers.

The Centers for Medicare and Medicaid Services makes a report card available called Nursing Home Compare (www.medicare.gov/NHCompare). The results are based on data collected on all nursing home residents at specific intervals during their stay. The Website has a search tool that enables the user to identify nursing homes by state, county, city, zip code, or name. The first level of the report card gives general information about the nursing home, such as whether it participates in Medicare, how many beds are certified, whether the ownership is by a nonprofit or for-profit corporation, whether it is located in a hospital or part of a chain, and whether there are resident and family councils. The next level down has information about the number of quality measures for which data are available, the total number of deficiencies in health care that were identified, the nursing staff hours per resident per day, and the number of certified nursing assistant hours per resident per day. Performance on up to fifteen quality measures is covered, along with average performance in the state and the nation. There is additional detail on deficiencies, including the date the deficiency was corrected, the level of harm (on a 4-point scale), and the number of residents affected (few, some, many).

CMS also makes Dialysis Facility Compare available on its Website (on the site www.medicare.gov, go to Search Tools). Three quality measures are available: control of anemia, adequacy of hemodialysis, and patient survival (actual versus expected). In addition, there is information about the facility (address, date of initial Medicare certification, whether evening appointments are available, number of treatment stations, types of dialysis offered, facility ownership type) along with links to other Websites offering resources for patients with end stage renal disease and their families. The quality results are displayed on a bar graph and compare facility performance to that in the state overall and the nation. The data in the report are about two years old.

# Some Methodological Issues in Performance Reporting

Current report cards vary along a number of dimensions reflecting lack of agreement on (or lack of attention to) how best to communicate information to various audiences. The proliferation of such report cards in different formats, along with evidence that the methodological choices made are likely to influence how the information is received and used, underscore the need to promote greater rigor in developing these tools. We discuss here a number of methodological issues that are likely to be encountered (explicitly or implicitly) by report card developers and what is known about the importance of some of these issues.

## Number of Measures

As the amount of information collected on quality performance expands, attention shifts to how this information can be meaningfully transmitted to consumers. Both methodological and communications issues arise and interact. Cognitive psychology affords some insight into the amount of information humans can use in making a decision. Typically, five to seven "bits" of information are the maximum that can be held in short-term memory and incorporated into a single decision. Thus minimizing the amount of information on a report card facilitates use by the intended audience. However, a single number about performance (for example, overall hospital mortality or mortality following CABG surgery) may not be adequate to characterize all the important decision dimensions for consumers. Further, most studies of quality that examine multiple dimensions of performance find considerable heterogeneity in the results, suggesting that the user needs to be cautious in drawing inferences about the relationship between performance in the area reported and performance in an unreported area.[8] This balancing act between offering enough information but not too much continues to be debated among those producing report cards. Making information available on the Internet may be the best opportunity to tailor results for individuals. High-level aggregate results could be displayed on the first page of a Website, and then users could seek additional detail relevant to their own circumstances on subsequent pages.

## Display of Results

Report cards present results in a variety of formats, including giving results on individual performance measures versus summary scores for multiple measures. Some present both summary scores and individual results (for example, the PBGH medical group report card). A review of the literature on decision making suggests strongly that the scale approach is preferable because it serves the purpose of reducing the amount of information that consumers must consider in making a decision.[9] The authors note that there is an apparent contradiction between the amount of information people can typically use in making a decision and the desire frequently expressed by consumers for more information.

A study by one of those authors yielded an interesting insight into this conflict.[10] Handicappers for horse races were given the option of selecting five to forty variables from among eighty-eight possible, to predict the winners of horse races. Their confidence in prediction increased with the number of variables, but their accuracy did not improve. The handicappers were as accurate in predicting results with five variables as they were with forty; as the number of variables increased, the level of consistency decreased. The authors of the review article conclude that "the approach of giving consumers the maximum amount of information is not the most effective path to informed consumer choice."[11] Further, they report that in focus groups consumers "commonly respond that they find the information overwhelming and confusing and that they do not know how to bring all the pieces of information together into a decision."[12] In these focus groups, consumers were looking at report cards with about twenty measures or pieces of information (plan characteristics) on them; in some cases as many as thirty-eight plans were included.

Research on approaches to displaying information reveals that the type of presentation can affect both the interpretation of results and the relative weight placed on multiple dimensions.[13] The authors found that adding visual cues about performance (stars, stacked bar with stars, and so on) increased the weight placed on quality results compared to report cards without evaluation signals. Similarly, ordering plans according to quality performance increased the weight consumers place on this dimension in choosing among health plans. They also found that, if people were given information on time trends in performance, they weighted positive trends (improvement) more highly than absolute level of current performance. Finally, in this experiment, the authors found that participants had difficulty consistently weighting multiple performance measures in their choices and were unaware of the influence that data display had on their decision.

## Credibility of Data Source

One of the challenges for public reporting is the credibility of the data source. Users may be suspicious of information that is produced by the entity being evaluated. For example, a study of employer responses to a report card produced by a medical center found that 45 percent thought the report was hospital advertising.[14] Among consumers seeing the report, 30 percent thought it was hospital advertising or public relations.[15] Consumers, however, were more likely than employers to report that the information was useful in decision making.

Two approaches are commonly used to enhance the credibility of the information. In some cases, a third party collects and analyzes the data. This is true for JCAHO and NCQA accreditation and for the consumer surveys used by NCQA (CAHPS). The other approach is to audit the performance data. NCQA requires that HEDIS results, based on plans' analyses of their own administrative and medical record data, be audited by an outside group certified to perform this function. Auditors essentially look at both the integrity of the process used to produce the result and the reproducibility of the results in determining whether the information is accurate.

## Risk Adjustment

For comparison between entities to be fair, the data must be adequately adjusted for differences in the populations receiving services; this is known as risk or case-mix adjustment. A number of issues related to risk adjustment should arise when results are used to make comparison among entities. First, there is often lack of clarity around the factors that should be adjusted for in this application. For quality measurement, the key question is whether the factor inherently causes quality differences (for instance, people who have comorbid heart failure are more likely to die from a heart attack) or whether that factor is associated with quality differences but neither clinically or biologically causes the difference (as with race). Adjusting for the second type of factor can mask important differences in quality for subpopulations. Second, one must consider the adequacy of the data source for representing the factors of interest. For example, in New York State, comparison using administrative versus clinical data concluded that clinical data were superior, largely due to the importance of three clinical factors in predicting cardiac surgical outcomes (ejection fraction, reoperation, and 90 percent occlusion of the left main trunk) that were available only in the clinical dataset.[16] The adequacy of data sources varies considerably by the type of measure, with no single source being adequate for all dimensions of performance. Third, one must consider whether application of risk-adjustment methods significantly changes the conclusion one is likely to draw. The methods themselves are complex and create additional challenges for communicating results; if no significant differences are found, the complexity may not be justifiable.

Outcome data are more likely to require risk adjustment than process measures because a larger number of factors outside the control of the organization being evaluated contribute to observed performance.[17] The reports on hospital mortality have paid the greatest attention to risk-adjustment issues. Process measures may require less adjustment because the criteria used to define eligibility for an indicator generally exclude individuals for whom the process is not indicated. However, clinical data sources are better than others at excluding inappropriate candidates on the basis of comorbid conditions or other clinical considerations. Patient-reported information may be necessary to capture preferences, including refusals. Recent attention has been given to the role of case-mix adjustment with patient experience measures.[18]

## Missing Data

In our previous work on developing reporting strategies, we considered a number of potential solutions to handling missing data.[19] These issues are particularly important if one is developing scales (groups of measures), but some of the same issues may arise if one is reporting performance on single items. Reports based on surveys routinely face this issue because respondents may not answer all questions. One always has the option of noting nonresponse (NR) for entities that do not report on one or more measures, but it may be difficult for consumers to compare *NR* with an actual performance result. For this reason, we prefer some type of imputation strategy. Three are summarized here.

Mean imputation takes the average value of all entities that have reported on a measure and assigns this average to entities whose results were missing for the measure. Imputing the mean value maintains the mean of the observed values and is a conservative approach suggesting that in the absence of other information we assume an entity's performance is average.

Regression imputation is a more sophisticated approach to imputing the means because it uses more information to estimate what the entity's performance might have been, given other characteristics (for example, number of enrollees or profit status) or performance on other measures. This method is likely to estimate a missing value closer to the true performance than simple mean imputation. There are also more modern methods of imputation (for instance, multiple imputation) used in statistical analysis. Their failure to be adopted for performance reporting may be a consequence of the difficulty in explaining these complex methods to lay audiences.

We can also impute zero, or the lowest observed value, for plans not reporting results. Both represent a more punitive approach to dealing with missing data. In previous work, we used the lowest observed value because it represented real performance (compared with zero, which is unlikely) and because most entities that report results could likely outperform the worst entity. This approach, which may be most useful in voluntary reporting programs, is designed to encourage complete reporting by penalizing entities that fail to report.

Report cards that present summary scales must choose an imputation method. Because the method used is likely to affect the results, it would be preferable for report card developers to indicate the method they used to deal with missing data.

Most report cards are not explicit about the methods used to address problems with missing data.

## Aggregation Issues

If a report card developer chooses to present scales, a number of other analytic issues arise in constructing the aggregate or composite scales. Conclusions can vary with the choices in these areas.

***Choosing an Organizing Framework.*** There are two strategies for creating a framework. The first approach, which might be called "bottom-up," starts with the individual measures that are available and creates summary categories that maximize the number of measures used. This can be done quantitatively, using factor analysis or other methods designed to identify patterns in data, or it can be done qualitatively by obtaining expert opinion.

The second approach, which might be called "top-down," starts with the information that potential users would like to have to make decisions and identifies measures that communicate the desired information. The Foundation for Accountability did considerable work in this area, which contributed to the frameworks used by NCQA and others. The methods for identifying what information the target audience wants may include surveys, focus groups, or semistructured interviews.

The bottom-up approach is more frequently associated with research or decision analysis. This approach has the advantage of trying to use all available information. Since the approach is empirically driven, another advantage is the opportunity to identify patterns in data that might otherwise escape notice. The disadvantage of this approach, particularly if done quantitatively (say, using factor analysis), is that it may produce results that are difficult to interpret and not valued by the intended audience. In analyzing Medicare plan performance data using factor analysis, we found some of the resulting groups impossible to interpret.[20]

The top-down approach is more audience-sensitive because it identifies attributes that are important to those making the decision. Because decision makers generally come to a task with some questions already in mind, an optimal top-down approach organizes information into categories that respond to the questions on the mind of the potential user. The disadvantage of this approach is that there may be categories of interest to decision makers for which few measures currently exist, if any.

***Scaling.*** Individual measures that are combined to create summary categories may have differing means and variances. This potentially presents a problem for scaling in that it can permit some measures to have a greater (or lesser) effect on the results because of their distributional properties.

Standardization is a simple calculation, but it is frequently misunderstood owing to its similarity to related statistical calculations. The idea is to transform item scores so that entities are ranked on a comparable scale across items. This prevents an item with a large range (say 0–100) from completely dominating an item with a small range (say, 0–1).

The benefit of standardizing is that it simplifies comparing items and understanding the meaning of weights applied to those items. The standard deviation scale makes using a simple rule of thumb based on the normal distribution easy; thinking of a standard deviation increase of 1 in each item is often easier than comparing a 35-point increase on a 100-point scale with a .012 increase in the mean of a dichotomous variable.

*Weights.* A basic starting point in constructing new scales is to give each measure in a scale equal weight. This implies that every element of the scale is equally important in arriving at a summary assessment. For many performance measures, this assumption of equal importance is at odds with both consumer and expert assessments of the measures. In previous work, we considered six options for weighting measures within scales:[21]

1. *Equal weights.* We start with equal weights as the base case since it is the option requiring the least judgment and offers a convenient method for evaluating the effect of weights on the results. All alternative weight schemes should be compared to the results on the basis of equal weights.

2. *Consumer weights.* A second option would be to ask consumers to assign weights to measures. This could be done either by surveying consumers to establish standardized weights for printed publications or by establishing an interactive mechanism that allows each individual to assign weights reflecting his or her own preferences.

3. *Expert weights.* Under this approach, experts assign weights according to their assessment of the relative importance of the measured process. Importance may be determined relative to the effect on outcomes, or it may reflect expert assessment of what is important to consumers. This is the approach used in NCQA's Diabetes Physician Recognition Program.

4. *Population weights.* Under this approach, measures are assigned a weight that reflects the proportion of the population eligible for the service represented by the measure. Importance is established on the basis of the number of people to whom the measure might be relevant.

5. *Factor weights.* If a factor-analytic approach was used to construct the reporting framework, one could use the resulting factor weights in creating aggre-

gate scales. This is the approach used by *U.S. News & World Report* for hospital performance on the technology scale.

6. *Clinical importance weights.* This approach would adopt a particular outcome (mortality, quality-adjusted life years) and develop weights that quantify the effect of the measures on the outcome. Values could be obtained from the literature or expert assessment.

## Statistical Evaluation of Differences

The final analytic consideration for public reporting is to evaluate whether results are statistically significantly different from one another. In general, ignoring statistical significance is likely to increase misinformation. The challenge is how to present the results in a way that is interpretable by users. Given that one is committed to using statistical significance to distinguish performance, some additional analytic issues must be addressed in terms of the reference point for comparison. Performance for any one entity could be compared to

- The average performance of all entities reporting the measure nationally
- The average performance of all entities reporting the measure in a market
- The average performance of the peer group in the market
- A benchmark based on actual performance (say, best result in the nation)
- A benchmark based on desired performance (best theoretical result)

There is considerable debate about the best basis for making performance comparisons among entities, although little empirical evidence exists on the extent to which these choices result in differing conclusions. Those who favor national comparison argue that it underscores the goal of having equal quality of care throughout the country. Those who favor using regional or market comparison argue that some variation nationally is unavoidable and fundamentally people can select only from local providers. Austin has shown that using peer groups for comparison affects the number of hospitals identified as mortality outliers and that the choice of comparison groups may depend on the intended use of the results.[22] Those who favor using benchmarks (rather than relative performance) prefer to emphasize the importance of a goal rather than grading on a curve. Benchmarks can be established either by observed best practices or by reference to goals (such as Healthy People 2010). These arguments often assume that the best observed performance is suboptimal. Those favoring relative performance reporting note that choices are made relative to the available options.

The choices in this area reflect beliefs about the message that a report card is intended to deliver. First, one must consider whether quality is a relative concept or absolute. In reality, there are very few absolutes in medicine (and by extension, in quality). Process quality, for example, in Donabedian's conceptualization incorporates both technical excellence (providing the right service competently) and interpersonal excellence (doing so humanely and with reference to the patient's preferences).[23] This suggests there are few interventions that are clinically appropriate and acceptable to all patients all the time. Most quality measures are designed with the idea that a higher rate of performance is desirable, but unless techniques for incorporating informed patient refusal and rare clinical contraindications are factored into the measurement method, excellent quality performance should rarely reach 100 percent.

One of the policy implications of using an absolute level of performance as the metric of comparison is that entities may be encouraged to deliver care that is either clinically inappropriate or unacceptable to patients in order to raise their level of performance. Alternatively, using relative performance as a basis of comparison could fail to establish adequate incentives to improve performance. A particular concern about using relative performance is that the best observed performance may not be very good.

The second consideration among the relative comparison options is whether to make national or regional comparisons. Using national standards establishes a policy of expecting equal excellence in delivery of health services nationally. For many measures, there is no strong rationale for expecting substantially different performance by region. We observe differences in the quality of care received by people in urban and rural areas, by racial or ethnic group, by income or insurance coverage, but in most instances there is no clinical justification for these differences. The proponents of risk or case-mix adjustment suggest that these techniques be applied to quality measurement to account for differences in performance that reflect the populations served. Using national standards may foster greater incentive for quality improvement than using regional standards. This varies with the market.

The third consideration is whether to make comparison relative to the average or best performance. Any number of cut points could be chosen within the distribution of actual performance. Reference to the average would seem to promote substantially less quality improvement activity than reference to the best. Using the best performance as an anchor may yield a conceptually clearer way of distinguishing the top and bottom performers.

Finally, it is common to use a 0.05 significance level in determining whether observed differences are statistically significant. The choice of significance level carries with it a choice about the relative importance of false negative versus false positive results. The costs of the resulting errors in classification will vary with the user of the information. Consumers would prefer to reduce the likelihood of information causing them to choose a facility or provider that was incorrectly labeled as good whereas facilities and providers would prefer to limit the chance of being falsely labeled as providing poor quality. A recent study of the implications of the choice of significance level for consumers versus hospitals in reporting mortality rate found that the optimal choice varied by user, the underlying rate of poor quality, and the size of an institution.[24]

## Summary of Methodological Issues in Reporting

This section summarizes some of the methodological choices that report card developers must make in designing public reporting. Many proprietary systems may not make their choices clear. In most instances, report card developers have made varying choices even while using the same basic data source. This has the potential to produce apparently different results and may contribute to consumers' confusion and subsequent unwillingness to use this information to guide choices. The main message, however, from this discussion is that there is no unambiguously correct way to produce public information. Since the methodological choices made affect the results, transparency of method should be highly valued.

# What Is Known About the Use of Quality Information

Evaluation of whether and how information about quality is used by audiences for making various decisions is difficult to conduct because of the complexity of the phenomenon. The studies in this area tend to be laboratory experiments or observational studies. In experiments, the elements to which an individual is exposed can be tightly controlled, allowing one to understand the relative importance of the elements in a decision process; however, the generalizability of the findings from these studies is limited. In observational studies, there is less control over a variety of factors, including the degree to which performance varies, the population is exposed to the information content, and the information is salient to the user. Observational studies often use differences in behavior as a key outcome, but they may not be able to account for the relative weight of the factor being studied in the overall decision. This section reports on the results of investigation of both types.

The general perception—supported by one prominent analysis of the literature—is that information on quality is not widely used.[25] Report cards have proliferated since that review was published, but the perception remains that information is not used by consumers.

## Consumer Use of Information

Evaluations of consumer use of information have been of three types: evaluating whether consumers are able to use information, asking consumers whether they used (or are likely to use) information for decision making, and examining whether patterns of utilization changed following release of public information.

Consumers frequently are unable to understand the content of report cards.[26] Some consumers may not have the skills necessary to use comparative information in decision making. Understanding the content is a prerequisite to using the information. Hibbard's recent work has pointed to a variety of mechanisms that can be used in displaying results to improve the usability of report cards.[27]

Consumers' reporting on their use of report cards is mixed and has been evaluated in limited markets. A study in Wisconsin found differences among groups of consumers in their exposure to a report on hospital quality ranging from 57 percent among employees (many of whom received the report directly from their employer) to 24 percent in a random household survey.[28] Consumers who were exposed to the report were significantly more likely to correctly identify high-performing hospitals than those who had not been exposed to the report both immediately following and two years after release. A substantially higher proportion were able to correctly identify poor-performing hospitals. One nationally representative study found that about one-quarter of respondents who needed hospital care had used an online tool from their health plan or provider to inform their decision. About half reported that they were reassured about going to the hospital they had selected, 37 percent did not find the information useful and it did not affect their decision, 4 percent considered changing hospitals but did not, and 12 percent changed the hospital they went to as a result of the information.[29]

Romano and Zhou found that hospitals in California that had significantly better or worse outcomes for heart attack patients did not experience any change in the number of patients obtaining care for that condition.[30] A survey of patients who underwent CABG surgery in one of four hospitals in Pennsylvania found that only 20 percent of patients were aware of the information on hospital mortality rates for that procedure; among those who were aware, less than 25 percent said the results influenced their choice of surgeon.[31] They also found that hospitals in California with a low complication rate following back surgery experienced a small increase in volume and that hospitals in New York with better and worse outcomes for CABG surgery experienced a change in volume shortly after publication of the results. They observed the strongest effects among patients enrolled in HMOs in California and among patients with Medicare in New York. An earlier quasi-experimental study of the impact of the New York State report on mortality following CABG surgery found that hospitals and physicians with better performance experienced a gain in market share and prices, although this effect diminished over time.[32]

A study of hospital mortality rates published by the federal government found that consumers were more influenced by press reports of high-profile problems at local hospitals than by the data on risk-adjusted mortality.[33] A study of New York general acute hospitals found no changes in occupancy rate after release of the federal reports on mortality rates.[34]

A study of the effect of report cards on federal employees' choice of health plans found that quality scores (based on consumer ratings of quality) significantly affected the choice of health plan, with the strongest effects seen among new employees.[35] A national survey of consumers found that most relied on family, friends, and their own doctor to make decisions about where to go for care.[36] About 40 percent of people surveyed had seen comparative information on health plans, and about one-third of those who saw the information used it (about 13 percent overall).

About half of the employees of companies in St. Louis and Denver who received health plan report cards as part of open enrollment remembered the report.[37] Among those who remembered seeing the report, 95 percent found it trustworthy, 82 percent found it helpful for learning about plan quality, 66 percent found it somewhat or very helpful in deciding whether to stay in or switch plans, and 50 percent were more confident in the decision that they made.

## Purchaser Use of Information

There is even less systematic information on use of performance data by purchasers, although they are at the forefront of efforts to increase the amount and type of information released. Purchasers are demanding that the health plans with which they contract incorporate information about performance into a variety of product offerings, including tiered provider networks that grant price differentials for patients seeking care from hospitals and physicians demonstrating better fiscal and quality performance. Experiments are under way to test the effects of paying physicians and hospitals differentially for high-quality performance. Little information is currently available on the results of either innovation.

A survey of thirty HMOs in California found that hospital contracting decisions were based primarily on accreditation status, location, and price.[38] Other factors used by some HMOs were government regulatory actions, reputation, and consumer satisfaction ratings. Those interviewed for the study expressed a variety of reservations about process and outcomes measures. A study of eleven communities where employer coalitions released hospital report cards found that in many areas multiple report cards were available in the market and that most used mortality and length-of-stay measures.[39] The authors focused primarily on whether the report cards stimulated quality improvement and concluded that most efforts were not successful from this perspective. The authors noted a number of barriers to success, among them ambiguity about the goals of public reporting (containing costs versus improving quality), conflicts about the measures being used (adequacy of risk adjustment, choice of measures, validity of results, cost of data collection), varying perceptions about the utility of public reporting, the degree of market power held by the participating employers, and lack of collaboration between purchasers and providers.

One study that conducted interviews with large purchasers in California, New York, Ohio, and Pennsylvania found that most had HEDIS data available to them; just over half used the information to select plans with which to contract.[40] A national survey of a random sample of employers with more than two hundred employees found that larger employers were more likely to use data from NCQA than smaller employers, but that a minority (11 percent) rated the information as very important.[41]

## Use by Providers

Consumers and purchasers might use performance information to make choices among providers, but providers' primary use of this information is for quality improvement. Most of the peer-reviewed studies in this area focus on hospital report cards. NCQA presented evidence from its recent report on managed care plan performance that public reporting may be associated with higher quality.[42]

One of the few studies to use an experimental design assigned hospitals to one of three conditions (public reports on quality, private reports on quality, and no reports—the control) and observed whether there were differences among the hospitals in the number of quality improvement projects initiated within nine months after the reports.[43] They found that public reporting was associated with a significantly higher rate of quality improvement projects in hospitals with public reports and low initial performance. Making reports public generated considerable negative reaction on the part of participating hospitals. A study of the long-term effects of reporting found significant improvement in performance among the public report group compared to the private report and no report groups (33 percent, 25 percent, 11 percent of hospitals demonstrating improvement, respectively).[44] There was a relationship between the number of quality improvement projects initiated and improvement in performance (average of 5.7 projects among hospitals showing significant improvement, compared to 2.6 among hospitals with no change). No significant change in market share was observed.

Two studies have been conducted on the Pennsylvania CABG surgery mortality report card. One found that whereas most cardiologists and all surgeons in the state were aware of the report, few thought it was important or discussed it with their patients.[45] Most were critical of the methods, particularly the adequacy of risk adjustment and the reliability of the data. A study of organizations in the state found that the information was a stimulus to development of marketing materials, provider monitoring, benchmarking, and collaborative improvement activities within the hospital.[46]

Five studies have been conducted on the New York cardiac reporting system. One study found considerably greater acceptance of the reports among physicians in New York than what was reported in Pennsylvania; 67 percent reported that they found the content very useful or somewhat useful, 22 percent said they routinely discussed the results with their patients, and 38 percent said the report affected referral patterns.[47] A case study in a poor-performing hospital reported that after an initial negative reaction to the report the institution used the results productively to improve collaboration and identify sources of high mortality.[48] A survey of hospital executives found that most were knowledgeable about the methods used in the New York reports and that high-mortality hospitals were more likely to be critical of the results.[49] Outcomes appear to have improved in the state following release of the information; risk-adjusted mortality rates in the state have declined from 4.17 percent to 2.45 percent.[50] This exceeded the rate of decline nationally, but some critics suggested this resulted from fewer high-risk procedures being done or from patients going out of state for care. In fact, a study found that fewer residents of New York went out of state for CABG surgery following the release, and the likelihood of having the surgery following a heart attack (one of the most high-risk reasons for surgery) increased.[51] The findings of studies conducted on other hospital report cards are similar.[52]

In its 2005 report on managed care quality, NCQA found that health plans submitting data for public release had higher performance on most measures than those submitting data not for public release.[53] NCQA previously reported accredited plans performing better than those that were not accredited, and plans reporting for public release for three consecutive years performed better than those that had not released information in all three years.[54]

# Conclusion

Despite the high level of interest in report cards on quality performance by organizations and the increased number that are being released, there are relatively few well-designed studies of the effects of public reporting on consumer, purchaser, and provider behavior. NCQA has the widest geographic reach and longest experience in producing performance reports on managed care plans. California and Minnesota have the most information available across levels in the health care system (health plans, hospitals, and medical groups). New York's program, which routinely reports risk-adjusted mortality data on one procedure, has been subject to the most extensive evaluation. Wisconsin's hospital reports benefited from the greatest attention to display issues and have been subjected to the most rigorous evaluation.

Although the evidence on use of report cards by various audiences—consumers, purchasers, providers—suggests that the information is not widely used and appears to have only a small effect on performance, the trend is clearly in the direction of releasing more information on more entities. Studies of the rate at which innovation diffuses suggest that it takes a long time for a new approach to be widely accepted.[55] The literature on making documents useful for various audiences suggests that a key problem for many of these reports may be related to poor presentation of the information.[56] We have more information on quality available today than we have ever had, but the measures available represent a small portion of the reasons people become ill or seek care—so failure to find widespread effects may be consistent with assessment of the meaningfulness or relevance of the information. Expansion of the measures available, increased attention to the methods that are used to construct report cards, better use of communication techniques that are known to be effective, and more formal evaluation of such efforts are required before we have the information necessary to draw conclusions about the utility of public reporting.

# Notes

1. Berwick, D. M., James, B., and Coye, M. J. "Connections Between Quality Measurement and Improvement." *Medical Care*, 2003, *41*(1 Suppl.), I30–I38.
2. Kohn, L. T., Corrigan, J. M., and Donaldson, M. S. (eds.). *To Err Is Human: Building a Safer Health System*. Washington, D.C.: National Academy Press, 1999.
3. McGlynn, E. A., and others. "The Quality of Health Care Delivered to Adults in the United States." *New England Journal of Medicine*, 2003, *348*, 2635–2645.
4. National Committee for Quality Assurance. *The State of Managed Care Quality*. Washington, D.C.: NCQA, 2005.
5. Crofton, C., Lubalin, J. S., and Darby, C. "Consumer Assessment of Health Plans Study (CAHPS)." (Foreword.) *Medical Care*, 1999, *37*, MS1–MS9.
6. "America's Best Health Plans." *U.S. News & World Report*, Oct. 10, 2005.
7. www.qualityindicators.ahrq.gov.
8. McGlynn, E. A., and others. *Assessing the Quality in Medical Groups: A Demonstration of the QA Tools System*. (Publication no. PM-1643-CHCF.) Santa Monica, Calif.: RAND, 2004.
9. Hibbard, J. H., Slovic, P., and Jewett, J. J. "Informing Consumer Decisions in Health Care: Implications from Decision-Making Research." *Milbank Quarterly*, 1997, *75*(3), 395–414.
10. Slovic, P. "Toward Understanding and Improving Decisions." In W. C. Howell and E. A. Fleishman (eds.), *Human Performance and Productivity. Vol. 2: Information Processing and Decision Making*. Hillsdale, N.J.: Erlbaum, 1982.

11. Hibbard, Slovic, and Jewett (1997), p. 398.
12. Hibbard, Slovic, Jewett (1997), p. 398.
13. Hibbard J. H., Slovic, P., Peters, E., and Finucane, J. L. "Strategies for Reporting Health Plan Performance Information to Consumers: Evidence from Controlled Studies." *Health Services Research*, 2002, *37*(2), 291–313.
14. Longo, D. R. "Health Care Consumer Reports: An Evaluation of Employer Perspectives." *Journal of Health Care Finance*, 2004, *30*(3), 85–92.
15. Longo, D. R., and Everett, K. D. "Health Care Consumer Reports: An Evaluation of Consumer Perspectives." *Journal of Health Care Finance*, 2003, *30*(1), 65–71.
16. Hannan, E. L., Kilburn, H., Jr., Lindsey, M. L., and Lewis, R. "Clinical Versus Administrative Data Bases for CABG Surgery: Does It Matter?" *Medical Care*, 1992, *30*(10), 892–907.
17. McGlynn, E. A. "The Outcomes Utility Index: Will Outcomes Data Tell Us What We Want to Know?" *International Journal for Quality in Health Care*, 1998, *10*(6), 485–490.
18. Zaslavsky, A. M., Zaborski, L., and Cleary, P. D. "Does the Effect of Respondent Characteristics on Consumer Assessments Vary Across Health Plans?" *Medical Care Research and Review*, 2000, *57*(3), 379-394; Elliott, M. N., and others. "Case-Mix Adjustment of the National CAHPS Benchmarking Data 1.0: A Violation of Model Assumptions?" *Health Services Research*, 2001, *36*(3), 555–573.
19. McGlynn, E. A., Adams, J., Hicks, J., and Klein, D. *Creating a Coordinated Autos/UAW Reporting System for Health Plan Performance.* (Publication no. DRU-2123-FMC.) Santa Monica, Calif.: RAND, 1999.
20. McGlynn, E. A., Adams, J., Hicks, J., and Klein, D. *Developing Health Plan Performance Reports: Responding to the BBA.* (Publication no. DRU-2122-HCFA.) Santa Monica, Calif.: RAND, 1999.
21. McGlynn, E. A., Adams, J., Hicks, J., and Klein, D. *Creating a Coordinated Autos/UAW Reporting System for Health Plan Performance.* (Publication no. DRU-2123-FMC.) Santa Monica, Calif.: RAND, 1999.
22. Austin, P. C., Alter, D. A., Anderson, G. M., and Tu, J. V. "Impact of the Choice of Benchmark on the Conclusions of Hospital Report Cards." *American Heart Journal*, 2004, *148*(6), 1041–1046.
23. Donabedian, A. *Explorations in Quality Assessment and Monitoring. Vol. I: The Definition of Quality and Approaches to Its Assessment.* Ann Arbor, Mich.: Health Administration Press, 1980.
24. Austin, P. C., and Anderson, G. M. "Optimal Statistical Decisions for Hospital Report Cards." *Medical Decision Making*, 2005, *25*, 11–19.
25. Marshall, M. M., Shekelle, P. G., Leatherman, S., and Brook, R. H. "The Public Release of Performance Data: What Do We Expect to Gain? A Review of the Evidence." *Journal of the American Medical Association*, 2000, *283*, 1866–1874.
26. Jewett, J. J., and Hibbard, J. H. "Comprehension of Quality Care Indicators: Differences Among Privately Insured, Publicly Insured, and Uninsured." *Health Care Financing Review*, 1996, *18*, 75–94.
27. Hibbard, Slovic, Peters, and Finucane (2002).
28. Hibbard, J. H., Stockard, J., and Tusler, M. "Hospital Performance Reports: Impact on Quality, Market Share, and Reputation." *Health Affairs*, 2005, *24*(4), 1150–1160.
29. "Annual Consumer Survey." WebMD Quality Services, July 2005. [www.healthshare.com/ CS/WebMD_White_Paper-Consumers_Needing Quality_Hospital_Care_Arm_Them selves_With_Quality_Data_Jul05.pdf].
30. Romano, P. S., and Zhou, H. "Do Well-Publicized Risk-Adjusted Outcomes Reports Affect Hospital Volume?" *Medical Care*, 2004, *42*(4), 367–377.

31. Schneider, E. C., and Epstein, A. M. "Use of Public Performance Reports." *Journal of the American Medical Association*, 1998, *279*, 1638–1642.

32. Mukamel, D. B., and Mushlin, A. I. "Quality of Care Information Makes a Difference." *Medical Care*, 1998, *36*, 945–954.

33. Mennemeyer, S. T., Morrisey, M. A., and Howard, L. Z. "Death and Reputation: How Consumers Acted upon HCFA Mortality Information." *Inquiry*, 1997, *34*, 117–128.

34. Vladeck, B. C., Goodwin, E. J., Myers, L. P., and Sinisi, M. "Consumers and Hospital Use: The HCFA 'Death List.'" *Health Affairs*, 1988, *7*, 122–125.

35. Wedig, G. J., and Tai-Seale, M. "The Effect of Report Cards on Consumer Choice in the Health Insurance Market." *Journal of Health Economics*, 2002, *21*, 1031–1048.

36. Robinson, S., and Brodie, M. "Understanding the Quality Challenge for Health Consumers: The Kaiser/AHCPR Survey." *Joint Commission Journal on Quality Improvement*, 1997, *23*, 239–244.

37. Fowles, J. B., Kind, E. A., Braun, B. L., and Knutson, D. J. "Consumer Responses to Health Plan Report Cards in Two Markets." *Medical Care*, 2000, *38*, 469–471.

38. Rainwater, J. A., and Romano, P. S. "What Data Do California HMOs Use to Select Hospitals for Contracting?" *American Journal of Managed Care*, 2003, *9*(8), 553–561.

39. Mehrota, A., Bodenheimer, T., and Dudley, R. A. "Employers' Efforts to Measure and Improve Hospital Quality: Determinants of Success." *Health Affairs*, 2003, *22*(2), 60–71.

40. Jewett and Hibbard (1996).

41. Hibbard, Slovic, Peters, and Finucane (2002).

42. National Committee on Quality Assurance (2005).

43. Hibbard, J. H., Stockard, J., and Tusler, M. "Does Publicizing Hospital Performance Stimulate Quality Improvement Efforts?" *Health Affairs*, 2003, *22*(2), 84–94.

44. Hibbard, J. H., Stockard, J., and Tusler, M. "Hospital Performance Reports: Impact on Quality, Market Share, and Reputation." *Health Affairs*, 2005, *24*(4), 1150–1160.

45. Schneider, E. C., and Epstein, A. M. "Influence of Cardiac-Surgery Performance Reports on Referral Practices and Access to Care." *New England Journal of Medicine*, 1996, *335*, 251–256.

46. Bentley, J. M., and Nash, D. B. "How Pennsylvania Hospitals Have Responded to Publicly Released Reports on Coronary Artery Bypass Graft Surgery." *Joint Commission Journal on Quality Improvement*, 1998, *24*, 40–49.

47. Hannan, E. L., Stone, C. C., Biddle, T. L., and DeBuono, B. A. "Public Release of Cardiac Surgery Outcomes Data in New York." *American Heart Journal*, 1997, *134*, 55–61.

48. Dziuban, S. W., McIlduff, J. B., Miller, S. J., and Dal Col, R. H. "How a New York Cardiac Surgery Program Uses Outcomes Data." *Annals of Thoracic Surgery*, 1994, *58*, 1871–1876.

49. Romano, P. S., Rainwater, J. A., and Antonius, D. M. "Grading the Graders: How Hospitals in California and New York Perceive and Interpret Their Report Cards." *Medical Care*, 1999, *37*, 295–305.

50. Hannan, E. L., and others. "Improving the Outcomes of Coronary Artery Bypass Surgery in New York State." *Journal of the American Medical Association*, 1994, *271*, 761–766.

51. Peterson, E. D., and others. "The Effects of New York's Bypass Surgery Provider Profiling on Access to Care and Patient Outcomes in the Elderly." *Journal of the American College of Cardiology*, 1998, *32*, 993–999.

52. Marshall and others (2000).

53. National Committee for Quality Assurance (2005).

54. National Committee for Quality Assurance. *The State of Managed Care Quality.* Washington, D.C.: NCQA, 1999.

55. Rogers, E. M. *Diffusion of Innovations.* New York: Free Press, 1995.

56. Hibbard and others (2002).

CHAPTER ELEVEN

# HEALTH CARE INFORMATION SYSTEMS

Jeff Luck
Paul Fu Jr.

Although information systems have long been used for administrative applications at large health care providers, payers, and government health agencies, they are now being more widely used in smaller organizations and by patients, and increasingly in clinical applications. These broader applications of information systems offer the promise of better health care system performance: improved quality, increased efficiency, and enhanced access. They must also ensure the privacy and security of personal health information stored and transmitted electronically. This chapter describes key information technology applications that are affecting the U.S. health care system and explores the benefits they are expected to produce, as well as some of the challenges concomitant with their implementation.

## Definitions

A health care *information system* comprises computerized data as well as procedures to collect, store, analyze, transfer, and retrieve that data. *Information technology* supports these systems and consists of computers, the networks and telecommunications systems that connect them, and the software that operates the computers

The authors gratefully acknowledge the assistance of Carly Panchura in the research for this chapter.

and networks. Information systems currently support a variety of administrative applications in health care, among them scheduling, financial management, and claims processing. The term *informatics* is used to describe information systems developed and implemented to support more biomedical applications, as shown in Figure 11.1. *Medical informatics* can be defined as "the scientific field that deals with biomedical information, data, and knowledge—their storage, retrieval, and optimal use for problem-solving and decision-making."[1] *Public health informatics* is the "systematic application of information and computer science and technology to public health practice, research, and learning."[2]

## The Value of Health Care Information Systems

Applications of information technology have transformed many sectors of the U.S. economy, making them more efficient, faster, and in many respects more responsive to customers.[3] This technology also offers the promise of improving the performance of the U.S. health care system, particularly by improving quality and patient safety and by increasing efficiency (especially by reducing costs).[4] In the long run, improvements in access and equity may also result.

Several analyses have delineated specific benefits that will accrue from health care information systems and called for their broader implementation:

### FIGURE 11.1. FIELDS OF BIOMEDICAL INFORMATICS AND DOMAINS OF APPLICATION.

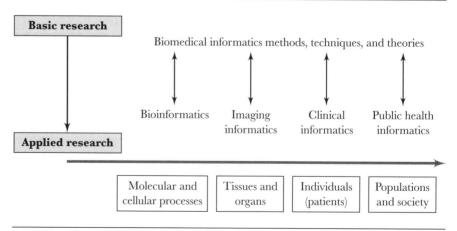

*Source:* Shortliffe, E. H. "JBI Status Report." (Editorial.) *Journal of Biomedical Informatics,* 2002, 35, 279–280.

• An influential IOM report, *Crossing the Quality Chasm,* specified use of information technology as one of the main changes needed to support redesign of the U.S. health care delivery system.[5] The Medicare Payment Advisory Commission (MedPAC) recently called for the Centers for Medicare and Medicaid Services (CMS) to accelerate adoption of health information technology (HIT), particularly to support use of pay-for-performance mechanisms to improve quality.[6]

• One analysis estimated that 75 percent adoption of seven technologies, including electronic patient-physician communication and computerized physician order entry (CPOE), could generate $2.5 billion in annual savings in Massachusetts alone.[7] Another analysis estimates a potential $78 billion annual saving based on a standardized national system for health care information exchange and interoperability among providers and payers.[8] A recent RAND analysis estimates that increased adoption of health information technology could produce a cumulative 1 percent annual increase in the productivity of the U.S. health care system[9]; annual efficiency savings from 90 percent adoption of EHRs could exceed $75 billion.[10]

• The federal government has established the Office of the National Coordinator for Information Technology (ONCHIT) to accelerate implementation of health information technology, aiming to save time, reduce duplication, and cut errors in health care delivery.[11] Sen. Hillary Clinton has sponsored legislation to provide federal funds to promote adoption of health information technology, and she has collaborated with former House Speaker Newt Gingrich to promote the initiative.[12]

Many analysts note that for the benefits of information systems to be fully realized, however, information technology must be fully incorporated into modified work processes at health care providers and payers. For example, integrated delivery systems can achieve complementary benefits from coordinated implementation of information systems and continuous quality improvement (CQI).[13]

# Applications of Information Systems by Health Care Providers

Health information technology systems have been actively deployed within U.S. health care institutions for more than four decades. The earliest health care applications emerged during the late 1960s and were enabled by two developments. First, computing power began to increase rapidly, and the advent of minicomputers made the use of technology affordable, whereas mainframes were cost-prohibitive. Second, development of health-care-specific structured programming languages made it possible to focus on the complex data environment that defined the health care encounter. MUMPS, developed by G. Octo Barnett, M.D., in the mid-1960s at Massachusetts General Hospital in Boston was a tree-structured database and programming language that was well suited to representing the medical record. It became the basis on which most successful commercial and noncommercial health care applications were created. The Veterans Administration developed a fourth-generation programming language (4GL) based on MUMPS called File Manager, which was used to develop the VistA electronic health record suite of applications.[14] From the success of VistA, the Indian Health Service and the U.S. Department of Defense adopted File Manager for development of their health information systems.

Initially, applications focused on automating administrative operations such as simple patient accounting and payroll in order to achieve the efficiency and productivity gains seen in other economic sectors. By the 1970s, there were a far greater number of administratively focused software packages available, including accounts payable and receivable, general ledger, patient accounting and billing, and resource scheduling, as well as emergence of the first clinical information systems for laboratory, radiology, and medication management.

The continued increase in microprocessor speed and power and the arrival of networking technologies transformed the ability of health care institutions to more effectively use HIT. During the 1980s and 1990s, hospital information systems were created that were designed to run the entirety of hospital operations, from admission, discharge, and transfers to patient appointments and scheduling, order control and results reporting, billing and accounts. Dumb terminals began to be replaced by desktop workstations connected to facilitywide networks, making it possible to broaden the number of individuals capable of using the system at a given time.

Practice management systems were developed; they were the physician-office counterpart to hospital information systems, combining appointment scheduling and accounting and billing in a single application specifically focused on outpatient management. Development of the first widely available personal computers during the mid-1980s (IBM PC and Apple Macintosh) significantly increased market penetration, although it was still relatively minor owing to the high cost of new technology adoption.

Clinical information systems also expanded in scope during this time. Earlier iterations focused on automating manual capture of data, such as collecting lab instrument data into a single digital location. Improvements in digital acquisition of data, as from automated laboratory instruments or CT scanners, allowed development of "silo" systems that aggregated data from multiple domain-specific subsystems. These domain-specific silo systems included laboratory, pharmacy, radiology, and emergency department information systems. It was not uncommon for early adopter health care facilities to have multiple workstations adjacent to one another, each accessing a silo system.

Over the past decade, significant developments in information technology have made it possible to collect more data than ever on the detailed encounters that make up the provider-patient care delivery process and present it more effectively to a range of users. In accordance with Moore's Law, microprocessor capacity continues to double approximately every eighteen months, with handheld personal digital assistants now having more processing power than the first supercomputers.[15] Data storage capacity is measured in terabytes and petabytes.[16] Networks have evolved from wired to wireless. The Internet has transformed how people look for information, and more important how they expect to have data and information presented.

At the micro level, clinical monitoring systems that focus on aggregation of biological signal collection (vital signs, input and output, invasive catheter readings) can transmit data continuously to upstream health information systems. At the macro level, large integrated delivery networks can consolidate data into warehouses to facilitate data mining and process improvement activities across the entire enterprise.

The ability to aggregate data and information from multiple health information systems into a single system along with a strong national focus on improving the quality and safety of health care delivery has yielded several health care applications with the potential to significantly affect the U.S. health care system.

## Clinical Decision Support Systems (CDSS)

The modern era of medicine presents three challenges for information processing and decision making. The sheer volume of clinical data produced annually, even within a single subspecialty domain, is beyond the ability of any individual clinician to master in its entirety on an ongoing basis. The National Library of Medicine indexed more than 571,000 citations during 2004.[17] Initiatives to improve the safety and quality of health care have led to development and promulgation of evidence-based clinical guidelines and best practices; research reveals that a substantial percentage (30–60 percent) of clinical decisions may change if the evidence-based recommendations are presented in context with patient data at the point of care.[18] Finally, the complexity of the care delivery process creates the potential for errors wherever there is insufficient time to fully evaluate all potential linkages.

To address these challenges, information systems that assist in the process of decision making, known as decision support systems, have been developed to use rules and straightforward representations of knowledge to assist in the decision-making process. Decision support systems that model very complex sets of rules and facts are known as expert systems.[19] Clinical decision support systems (CDSS) integrate patient-specific data along with computer-represented clinical knowledge (for example, guidelines or antibiotic resistance sensitivity) in order to frame point-of-care alerting, reporting, and order or care plan recommendations.

CDSS range in complexity and integration from simple knowledge base tools to sophisticated but passive and standalone decision aids, and to complex systems integrated into electronic medical records or computerized physician order entry systems. Simple online knowledge bases help to furnish validated or standardized clinical information for the provider; they include journal and textbook tools such as MD Consult (from an eponymous company in St. Louis) and NIH PubMed, evidence-based practice guidelines such as UpToDate (Waltham, Massachusetts) and the Cochrane Library (Oxford, United Kingdom), and reference data resources such as Micromedex (Greenwood Village, Colorado) and Medispan (Indianapolis). More sophisticated knowledge base tools such as Gideon (Los Angeles) can aid the diagnostic process by using images and decision-tree logical paths to assist with infectious disease identification. Passive CDSS require that the clinician identify the need for such a utility and secondarily to engage the system to obtain necessary feedback. Typical use of passive decision support tools is to broaden or refine a differential diagnosis or validate a decision against a clinical database.

Complex CDSS engage the user in continuous dialogue, integrating into the actual clinical workflow through intuitive human-computer interaction in a real-time fashion. Effective recommendations are patient-specific, evidence-based, and presented to the clinician consultatively, to avoid inadvertent elimination of clinical judgment. It is essential that these CDSS be integrated into the computer documentation (electronic medical and health records) and ordering (computerized physician order entry) workflow if one is to obtain the highest yield impact.[20] Active CDSS make available all six of the generic functions of clinical decision support systems: alerting, interpreting, assisting, critiquing, diagnosing, and managing decision support.[21] Using integration or messaging with underlying electronic medical record systems, the active CDSS permits continuous data surveillance, alerting clinicians when predefined rules built on clinical evidence are triggered (such as an abnormal result or adverse trend). Even though they offer the highest level of benefit to the end user, active CDSS are the most difficult to design and implement because these systems pose the greatest intrusion into the clinical decision-making workflow. However, as messaging standards evolve and the HIT industry standardizes on methods to consistently represent clinical information and knowledge across platforms, active systems will become increasingly available.

## Computerized Physician Order Entry (CPOE)

Computerized physician order entry (CPOE) systems automate the manual process by which physician orders are communicated to other health care providers, including nursing, pharmacy, and ancillary departments such as dietary, respiratory therapy, occupational therapy, and physical therapy. Basic CPOE systems achieve improvements in safety and quality by enabling entry of standardized and complete physician orders and eliminating errors that are due to illegibility or use of confusing or unfamiliar terms, expressions, or names.[22] More advanced CPOE systems integrate decision support tools into the ordering workflow, as in producing related laboratory results, local microbiologic sensitivities for appropriate antibiotic ordering, diagnosis and medication guidelines, and formulary guidance.[23]

The majority of recent emphasis has been on use of CPOE systems to improve the medication ordering process. An early study described a decrease in serious medication errors of 55 percent following CPOE introduction, with some reports ranging as high as an 80 percent effect on error prevention.[24] Other reports show significant improvement in physician prescribing practices.[25] CPOE systems have also shown a milder reduction in charges and costs.[26] Organizations as diverse as the Institute of Medicine and the Leapfrog Group (a health care buyer coalition) have identified adoption of CPOE as a recommended safety practice.[27]

However, there is a very low implementation rate, ranging between 4 and 10 percent of U.S. hospitals.[28] In addition, more recent reports suggest that CPOE systems may augment medication errors or increase mortality if not properly implemented.[29] There are also substantial barriers for adoption of CPOE systems. The significant impact on physician workflow constitutes the greatest risk for implementation failure, and yet the greatest opportunity for substantive improvement through eliminating workflow steps subject to a high rate of possible error. Perceived negative impact, such as decreased efficiency, can be used as a rallying point around which dissatisfied medical staff might effectively bring an implementation to a halt. This can be mitigated to some extent through strong administrative and medical leadership throughout the implementation, as well as extensive use of physician champions drawn from medical staff or house staff (in a teaching hospital).[30] Another possible barrier to CPOE adoption is the high cost of procurement and implementation, although more recent analysis of Leapfrog data suggests that hospital ownership may have a greater impact on the decision to commit to CPOE than positive net income or membership in a large IDN.[31]

CPOE remains an effective tool for improving patient safety if implemented appropriately. Although government and nonprofit hospitals lead the curve in adopting CPOE systems, cost and reimbursement issues need to be addressed in order to speed more widespread adoption.

## Electronic Medical Record (EMR) and Electronic Health Record (EHR)

In 2003, the electronic health record (EHR) was defined by the Institute of Medicine's Committee on Data Standards for Patient Safety as being a system that includes:

1. A longitudinal collection of electronic health information for and about persons, where health information is defined as information pertaining to the health of an individual or health care provided to an individual;
2. Immediate electronic access to person- and population-level information by authorized, and only authorized, users;
3. The provision of knowledge and decision-support that enhance the quality, safety, and efficiency of patient care; and
4. Support of efficient processes for healthcare delivery.[32]

A growing amount of data have been captured in electronic systems, ranging from clinical to administrative and financial. Typically, the data are scattered across source systems that usually span an organization. Even if they remain within a single health care delivery system, data may originate from multiple sources that do not interface with a single repository. This makes access to the complete medical "record" of any individual a challenge for all patients and providers.

The task of creating a longitudinal medical record for an individual is made more difficult as patients transition between systems of care, for financial or personal reasons. Shifting public program eligibilities (Access for Infants and Mothers, Medi-Cal and Medicaid, Healthy Families and SCHIP) may result in involuntary movement between health plans and providers. As a result, care may be disrupted and documentation scattered among providers and systems. At the traditional and safety net provider level, providers operate with thin margins and often do not have the resources to deploy or support more sophisticated electronic clinical or back office systems.

Reliable and widespread health data availability has been shown to be a key factor for the domains of clinical decision making, health system management, care process improvement, health policy analysis, and health services research.[33] However, there are additional, distinct, quantifiable benefits from use of electronic health records that can form the core business drivers initiating intraorganizational change. The IOM Committee on Data Standards for Patient Safety defined five criteria to guide identification of core EHR system functionalities that also serve as logical focus areas for assessment and planning activities.[34] There is a significant body of literature documenting the ability of clinical information systems to positively affect all of these focus areas:

1. *Improve patient safety.* The IOM noted that between forty-four thousand and ninety-eight thousand individuals die annually from preventable adverse events in the health care setting (although subsequent reviews of the report suggested that the actual magnitude may be much smaller).[35] Use of relatively simple interventions such as clinical information systems that provide physician and patient reminders, treatment planners, and patient education have been shown to be effective at preventing some adverse events, but evidence on reduction of serious medical errors needs to receive more scientifically rigorous study.[36] More sophisticated tools such as decision support systems for drug dosing and preventive care have also been shown to benefit providers and patients.[37] Clinical test results ordered by one physician may not be available to subsequent providers; this can lead to reordering of tests or missed critical values. Medication errors may also result from prescription by one provider (for instance, during an inpatient stay) and subsequent treatment (after discharge) by another where the patient is unable (or unwilling) to disclose the current active medication list.[38]

2. *Support delivery of effective patient care.* The need to access to knowledge resources, especially subspecialty topics, arises frequently during office practice. Not all information needs encountered during clinical visits are met through existing resources.[39] Lack of information can lead to lower-quality patient care. Appropriate medical care consistent with evidence-based practice guidelines are received by only 55 percent of Americans.[40] Some of these issues may be addressed through availability of online resources such as journals and texts, as well as the medical references optimized for online reference that are now increasingly accessible. Pubmed.gov makes many journals available in a full-text format. Health care systems frequently license content systemwide. Other areas, such as the effectiveness of disease management systems, show great promise but require additional study before conclusive recommendation and adoption.[41] Inefficiencies may occur from process workflow disruption. Redundant laboratory tests may be reduced if previously ordered results are made available for review during subsequent encounters.[42] Communication failures between providers (as during transition in patient care settings, or between care teams, or when moved through insurance plan coverage changes) can result in an event of omission no less adverse for a lack of malice, but systems can be implemented to standardize the exchange of information and reduce risk.[43]

3. *Facilitate management of chronic conditions.* People with chronic conditions account for more than 75 percent of all health care spending, and physicians caring

for these patients also report that the lack of care coordination leads to poor outcomes; almost half of all people with chronic medical conditions have more than one.[44] Patient education can improve control of chronic conditions.[45] Computer-based patient education has also been successful.[46] Implementation of a patient-controlled health record may allow context-sensitive delivery of patient education materials.

4. *Improve efficiency.* A General Accounting Office (GAO) study released in 2003 noted that in a 1,951 bed teaching hospital more than $8.6 million in yearly savings was accrued through replacement of paper medical charts with electronic medical records system.[47] A study released by the San Francisco-based nonprofit Health Technology Center in 2002 cited statistics showing that up to 20 percent of laboratory and X-ray tests are repeated because prior results are unavailable for review and that one in seven hospitalizations occurs because prior patient information is unavailable.[48]

5. *Feasibility of implementation.* Over the past three decades, there have been multiple efforts to coordinate these sources of data. Community health information networks were developed during the 1980s to combine services, products, and technologies that allowed data sharing by unaffiliated entities through regional databases to yield efficient delivery of community health.[49] They were not highly successful because of crippling organizational issues dealing with intraorganizational competition, data ownership and control governance, confidentiality, and high up-front costs.

However, large integrated health delivery networks have acknowledged the importance of data sharing across facilities and providers by making significant, long-term investment in health information technology. The Veterans Health Administration made an investment of $600–700 million to take a decentralized, basic hospital information system (DHCP) and transform it into VistA and CPRS, a sophisticated electronic medical records system that allows transmission and access of patient health information between regions and hospitals across the entire network and yields sources for an enterprise data warehouse used for performance management. Kaiser Permanente recently announced a multiyear, $1.8 billion investment over a decade in implementing the EpicCare (manufactured in Madison, Wisconsin) electronic medical record system. Kaiser has long been a pioneer in deploying information technology solutions to its clinicians throughout multiple regions, and this initiative is the capstone that will tie all regions together into a single EMR system.

Although there is a growing body of literature documenting distinct, quantifiable benefits from use of EHR systems within multihospital integrated delivery networks, there are an increasing number of EHR systems targeted toward the medium- and small-provider group level, and demonstrated benefits (and barriers to success) at that scale.[50] Provider associations are becoming aware of the importance of electronic documentation and are stepping up the level of involvement and interaction with members. The American Academy of Family Physicians Center for Health Information Technology is working to educate small- and medium-sized physician offices on EHR systems and to assist in acquisition and implementation of these systems.[51] The American Academy of Pediatrics has initiated a working group to assess the role of the organization in recommending specific EHR systems that appropriately support the unique health care needs of the pediatric population.[52] The "downward" push of technology into the smaller health care provider environment is enabling potential capture of even greater quantities of health care information in the near future.

## Regional Health Information Organizations (RHIO)

The need to exchange clinical information between providers and provider organizations and hospitals is not novel. Information technology has been deployed to attain this goal for decades, the earliest notable examples being the Community Health Information Networks (CHIN) implemented in the 1980s. Though the vast majority of the CHINs failed from problems with funding sustainability or technical infrastructure, there are a small handful that remain. As with most health information technology, the significant advances in computing power and networking capacity over the past fifteen years have reinvigorated the vision of fully portable clinical information.

In 2004, a presidential executive order was issued that endorsed incentives for use of HIT and formally established the Office of the National Coordinator for Health Information Technology (ONCHIT).[53] Dr. David Brailer was appointed to ONCHIT and tasked with coordinating programs and policies in order to achieve within ten years the goal of the National Health Information Infrastructure that supported access to an EHR for all Americans. The July 2004 ONCHIT report titled *The Framework for Strategic Action* stated that patient health information should be portable and accessible from all points of care, and that both deployment of electronic health record systems and EHR interoperability were mandatory for seamless flow of information from clinical setting to clinical setting. Widespread adoption of EHR systems has many challenges, but interoperability between regional collaboratives may be more achievable.

Regional health information organizations (RHIOs) are described as regional collaborations among health care entities that allow access to electronic patient health information that has been securely stored within the local community. The overall RHIO model is flexible, allowing customization of governance, technology, and policy depending on regional needs.

There have been several successful demonstration models of the RHIO concept. In 1991, the Regenstrief Institute established a data sharing network for hospital emergency departments in the greater Indianapolis region. It uses a centralized clinical repository to afford access to results and other clinical data across the city. A centralized repository model refers to a method of access to clinical information where an end user queries a single data source for clinical information. This single source is created and fed either real-time from partner entities or batch data transmission and upload. In 2004, the Indiana Health Information Exchange (IHIE) was brought into existence with the goal of broadening the Regenstrief infrastructure and involving a greater number of providers across the state.

The Santa Barbara County Care Data Exchange (SBCCDE) began in 1998 with a $10 million investment from the California HealthCare Foundation and through Carescience (now part of Quovadx), developed a national demonstration model to securely exchange patient-specific clinical information within the legal, organizational, financial, technical, and operational frameworks necessary for success. It has been described as "perhaps the best-known example of a data exchange platform for patient information" and was recently adopted as the model for the Mesa County Health Information Network in Colorado.[54] It uses a peer-to-peer approach in allowing data sharing among disparate vendor systems. Peer-to-peer refers to a method of access to clinical information where an end user client pulls down data residing on a host server operated by the data owner (the entity that generated the clinical data). A central server operated by the RHIO coordinates security and messaging but does not contain any clinical data. It is not as widely adopted as IHIE at this time, although it is rapidly gaining advocates.

Although more limited in scope, the New England Healthcare EDI Network is also an example of a success in establishing the necessary framework for exchange of data among multiple organizational entities.[55] As with SBCCDE, it focuses on a peer-to-peer approach for sharing information. In addition, there are more than one hundred community-based health information exchange projects in some stage of development in forty-five states and the District of Columbia.[56]

There are several challenges that all emerging RHIOs share.[57] Whether deployed peer-to-peer or using a central repository technical approach, successful interoperability requires both data and messaging standards and adoption of common standards by all participating parties. Patients and organizations furnishing data must be confident of the measures taken to safeguard the privacy and security of sensitive information, from source through to destination. Identifying the appropriate governance and leadership model is essential for a successful transition to operations, but this structure is likely to be highly regionalized. Without defined return-on-investment metrics for all participants, it is unclear how sufficient funding will be allocated for this effort.

## National Health Information Infrastructure (NHII) and National Health Information Network (NHIN)

The National Committee on Vital and Health Statistics (NCVHS) first described a vision and plan for the National Health Information Infrastructure (NHII) in 2001.[58] The NHII was not a specific technology solution. Rather, it was the "set of organizing principles, systems, standards, procedures, and policies" that described the framework around which to achieve the concept of complete patient-specific health information availability for patient care where and when it is needed.[59] It incorporated advances in health information technology, electronic medical and health records, and the growing number of regional health information exchange organizations to project a realistic and achievable goal. Federal initiatives surrounding public health preparedness and personal health records used the NHII as a foundation for national implementation.

Although the concept remained the same, the terminology began to evolve in 2001 with the release of the Institute of Medicine report *Crossing the Quality Chasm,* in which the need for the National Health Information Network (NHIN) was suggested.[60] The ONCHIT report *The Framework for Strategic Action* also references the NHIN; as the defining roadmap, this has set the standard terminology. Subsequent federal initiatives, such as the 2005 AHRQ funding for prototype demonstration models, have referenced the NHIN in describing the physical interoperability of regional networks and electronic health information technology systems spanning personal health, public health, and clinical medicine.

The NHIN is projected to be the infrastructure to facilitate RHIO interoperability, supplying appropriate standards and policies for execution. It is anticipated that under current assumptions RHIOs would use core toolsets (or a "common framework") in order to operationalize their systems for inter-RHIO and intra-RHIO interoperability.[61] As with the RHIO funding issue, to date there is little guidance as to the sources for capital expenditure and operating costs. One estimate places the capital expenditure cost at $156 billion, with $48 billion in annual operating costs for a model NHIN in five years, with two-thirds of estimated capital costs allocated toward achieving functionality (results reporting, CPOE, EHR, ANSI X.12 270/271, patient communication, e-prescribing) and the remaining costs for interoperability programming.[62] Current health IT spending for these functions is approximately one-eighth of the capital expenditure projection and one-tenth of the operating costs estimate. It is unlikely that this level of spending will be achieved without significant legislative support. A frequently referenced parallel is the U.S. Department of Defense Advanced Projects Research Agency (DARPA) incubation of the network that eventually became the Internet. There are several active legislative efforts in place to stimulate federal sponsorship for the NHIN.

Central to the vision of interoperable health information systems, which will allow organizations to share information easily within RHIOs or via the NHIN, are *standards* for the diverse types of clinical and administrative information generated in provision and financing of health care. *Terminology* standards, such as ICD-9 coding for medical diagnoses, common procedural terminology (CPT) codes, or the Systematized Nomenclature of Medicine (SNOMED), assign standard codes to several hundred thousand specific clinical concepts. *Messaging* standards such as Health Level 7 (HL-7) define the format of messages within which clinical or administrative data can be exchanged among information systems within an organization or across organizations. A health information standard can be created and maintained by a nonprofit consortium, such as Health Level Seven (www.hl7.org), or it may be a proprietary product such as SNOMED (owned by the College of American Pathologists). Government actions may accelerate adoption of particular standards, as occurred for example when HIPAA mandated use of several standards, including ICD-9 and CPT, or when the ONCHIT contracted for SNOMED to be made publicly available.

## Public Health Informatics

Public health informatics has been defined as systematic application of information and computer science and technology to public health practice, research, and learning.[63] It broadens the focus from the patient-clinician dyad to larger issues of how information systems can assist in analysis of data on the multiple determinants of health to improve disease prevention and population health. It differs from other biomedical informatics domains in its complex dependency on federal, state, and local government regulations. As with information systems aimed at health care delivery, the IOM has supported greater adoption of informatics tools and techniques within public health.[64]

Public health professionals have long used information technology to facilitate public health practice in areas such as communicable disease surveillance and collection and dissemination of population health information, but such systems have historically been designed and implemented in isolation.[65] Federal legislation and initiatives following the September 11, 2001, terrorist attack on the World Trade Center in New York City have led to coordination between previously separate funding and operational silos. In January 2002, $1.1 billion was allocated to enhancement of the public health infrastructure. Although the greatest attention on NHIN discussions focuses on the direct benefit to the individual patient, provider, and payer, the public health information infrastructure (PHII) component is an integral part.

The pool of data used for public health assurance activities is very broad, especially when viewed in light of a model that incorporates multiple determinants of health, such as the Evans and Stoddart health field model.[66] Clinical data are usually supplied through automated reporting of laboratory, radiology, or other ancillary test results. Trigger events, such as reportable diseases, may require follow-up manual chart review to yield necessary information. Unfortunately, where manual effort is required, clinicians may not complete the reporting process, whether mandatory or not. Electronic health records and RHIOs have the potential to greatly increase the efficacy and accuracy of public health systems by automating reporting of detailed patient information. For example, real-time emergency department chief complaint data can be obtained through messaging feeds from provider EHR systems and sent directly to decision support systems. Notably, the Health Insurance Portability and Accountability Act (HIPAA) Privacy Rule supports essential public health objectives by permitting disclosure of protected health information (PHI) for specific public health purposes, such as mandated reporting for disease prevention or control. In addition, the rule permits covered entities to make disclosures when required by laws other than those governing public health purposes.

Other sources are environmental data, which can include air quality and particulate measurements, water quality, animal deaths, and testing data (for example, West Nile virus, Lyme disease, and other tick-borne diseases); and survey data, which are critical for assessment of the health of populations. Survey datasets range from national clinical studies (National Health and Nutrition Evaluation Survey, http://www.cdc.gov/nchs/nhanes.htm) to statewide random-digit phone surveys (California Health Interview Survey, http://www.chis.ucla.edu) and to local and regional interviews (Los Angeles County Health Survey, http://lapublic health.org/ha/survey/hasurveyintro.htm).

The CDC has articulated the Public Health Information Network (PHIN) as its vision for an interoperable, multiorganizational business and technical architecture that supports public health activities and improves public health outcomes. Specifically, the PHIN spans all sources of data and targets (1) disease surveillance, (2) national health status indicators, (3) data analysis, (4) public health decision support, (5) alerting and communications, and (6) management of public health response through support for development of necessary messaging standards and common software solutions.[67] Using a group of common services (public health conceptual data model; standards for messaging and vocabulary; public health directory of people, organizations, and jurisdictions), PHIN brings together several existing programs and activities that were separately organized, including the Health Alert Network (HAN) and the National Electronic Disease Surveillance System (NEDSS); defines a new, common architecture; and sets the framework for existing application migration and future application development as part of the PHIN.

The Health Alert Network is an Internet and broadcast communications system that disseminates emergent health information, alerts, and advisories to key public health officials and first responders at the state and community levels.[68] Initiated in 1999, HAN now includes all fifty states, eight U.S. territories, the District of Columbia, and the three largest municipalities (New York City, Los Angeles County, and Chicago). The NEDSS focuses on implementation of integrated disease surveillance systems at the federal, state, and local levels.[69] NEDSS initiative goals capitalize on the movement within the health care delivery system toward electronic documentation to permit more timely and comprehensive information while not overly burdening providers. Along with HAN, it is one of the major components of the PHIN.

## Disease Registries

Chronic conditions cause significant morbidity and mortality and account for as much as 75 percent of health care spending.[70] Comprehensive disease management programs have been instituted by payers and providers so as to more effectively manage chronic ailments and provide better, safer care in a cost-effective manner. Disease registries deployed in conjunction with other care management enhancements can assist both individual patients and populations in maintaining health status. Although the first disease registries were deployed during the early 1980s at institutions such as Group Health of Puget Sound (Seattle) and Lovelace Health System (Albuquerque, New Mexico), adoption has accelerated significantly over the past decade.[71] At the micro level, disease registries track patients with chronic diseases with the goal of consolidating data from external electronic sources and manually entered records into a single repository from which the chronic condition can be more effectively managed and better preventive care delivered through reduction in omissions and gaps in care.[72] At the population level, registries can assist in identifying best practices and can generate data for reporting on the health of larger population groups, or provider performance.

Disease-specific registries are also used for program administration. However, some diseases have multiple funding streams associated with service delivery; as a result, there may be proliferation of information systems each focusing on a single aspect. For example, regarding HIV/AIDS, there are HIV registries, AIDS registries, the Ryan White program registry, and drug assistance program registries.[73] This complexity frequently leads to unnecessary data synchronization problems in reporting across multiple systems. In parallel with PHIN and federal efforts to adopt common standards, state and local agencies are starting the process of closer integration and coordination to reduce errors of omission and of commission.

## Immunization Registries

Immunization registries are databases covering population groups defined by geography or payer or provider that contain information about children and adults who receive immunization. Although focused registries were developed in the late 1980s for institutions such as Kaiser Permanente (the Kaiser Immunization Tracking System), it was not until the early 1990s that sufficient national effort and funding was focused into implementing broader immunization registries. Healthy People 2010 notes specific target immunization rates for the general population and defines the goal of having 95 percent of children age six or younger having at least two immunizations recorded in a regional registry.[74]

These registries may include decision support tools to assist in identifying needed immunizations at the point of care, analytical tools to assist in reporting rates, and care delivery tools to assist in sending electronic or paper mail reminders. Mature registries offer both process benefits (reminders and decision support) and cost benefits associated with reducing manual medical record pulls, researching past history across multiple patient documents, and overimmunizing.[75] These efficiencies are gained only if the majority of individuals within the database have up-to-date records and virtually all providers are using the system to enter immunization data. As with disease registries, the compliance rate for data completeness improves considerably if submission is automated and originates from EHR or practice management software that captures the requisite demographics and immunization and vaccine detailed information (including manufacturer, lot number, and expiration date).

# Applications of Information Systems by Health Plans and Payers

Managed care organizations (MCOs) and government health care payers (Medicare and Medicaid) have used large transaction-oriented information systems, referred to as "legacy systems," for decades.[76] The core administrative system of an MCO supports the claims adjudication process, where claims submitted by providers are approved for payment or denied on the basis of the MCO's rules and applicable contracts with providers and purchasers. These systems can be very large, handling millions of claims per month in a large MCO. The next largest database is that for members, containing demographic data as well as information about the group a member belongs to and the associated benefits for which she or he is eligible. Another database contains data about providers (such as physicians and hospitals), as well as contracted payment rates and network membership (PPO, HMO). Other information systems support premium billing and payment to providers (both capitation and fee-for-service).

These information systems contain little clinical detail and therefore have limited ability to measure and help improve population health. Other information systems that support care management activities, such as utilization management or disease management, do contain more clinical data. Because an MCO's legacy systems often operate independently, data from several of them may be extracted into a data warehouse to support reporting (such as provider profiling) and decision making (such as premium pricing).[77]

Fully electronic, and eventually real-time, interchange of information, claims, and payments between providers and MCOs would improve the efficiency of the health care system, but progress toward that goal is mixed. HIPAA mandates standards for information "transactions," but it does not require that all such transactions actually be performed electronically; furthermore, HIPAA standards do not specify all possible details of a particular transaction, such as a claim.[78] As a result, not all MCOs offer providers electronic access for preauthorization, referral, and eligibility verification, and many providers have not begun using the systems that are available.[79] Most claims are now submitted electronically, often via a clearinghouse such as WebMD.[80] However, fully automated claims adjudication is not yet the norm, and few payments to providers are made electronically.[81] In the future, widespread adoption of EHRs by providers and information sharing via RHIOs may also make clinical data for population health management more readily available to MCOs.

Changes in the health insurance market, particularly consumer-directed health plans (CDHPs), may significantly expand the scope and complexity of MCO information systems. CDHPs feature high deductibles coupled with tax-free health savings accounts (HSAs). CDHPs also offer members comparative information about the cost and quality of providers, and information about disease management. The goal of CDHPs is to reduce spending by making members more aware of the costs of care and encouraging them to choose lower-cost providers. However, the effect on spending is not yet clear, and concerns have been raised that the financial incentives of CDHPs may encourage members to underspend on preventive care.[82]

Nevertheless, significant enrollment in CDHPs would require equally significant information system changes at MCOs.[83] For example, members would need online portals to access information about providers, plus decision support systems to inform their choices. Claims systems must be coupled to financial institutions to allow payment from member HSAs. MCOs may also choose to overhaul their core systems' architecture to allow easier changes to the underlying "business rules" so that CDHP products can be customized more rapidly.

## Quality Measurement and Improvement

Quality measurement and quality improvement (QI) are core MCO activities that rely heavily on information systems. (See Chapter Eight for an overview of health care quality measurement and improvement concepts and techniques.) The most widely used set of quality indicators for MCOs is the Health Plan Employer Data and Information Set (HEDIS), a mandatory component of the National Committee for Quality Assurance (NCQA) accreditation process for MCOs.[84] HEDIS 2005 consists of approximately fifty measures describing performance dimensions, notably preventive care, member satisfaction, and service utilization.[85] Information systems that allow sharing of patient-level data greatly improve the efficiency with which an MCO can compile HEDIS measures, because much of the underlying data must be obtained from medical records.

Nevertheless, HEDIS measures only a narrow range of the spectrum of care provided to patients by MCOs. A more comprehensive set of more than four hundred specific measures of care for thirty common clinical conditions has been developed by RAND.[86] Disease-specific inclusion and exclusion criteria define which measures can be applied to a particular patient. Data to construct the measures are collected from medical records, a task that is greatly streamlined by EHRs.

Computerized clinical vignettes offer an alternative method for quality measurement.[87] Each vignette simulates a patient visit for a specified clinical condition. Physicians' responses, indicating the care they would give that patient, are then scored against explicit, disease-specific quality criteria. Because vignettes do not require the inclusion and exclusion criteria or case-mix adjustment needed by medical record-based measurement tools, they are ideally suited to quality comparison across health care systems.

Several MCOs and purchasers are initiating pay-for-performance (P4P) programs that give providers financial incentives for offering high-quality care. The largest of these is the Integrated Healthcare Association (IHA), which compiles quality indicators from medical groups contracting with MCOs in California. In its first year, IHA paid approximately $50 million in incentives.[88] At the national level, the Bridges to Excellence program sponsored by the Robert Wood Johnson Foundation creates financial incentives for groups meeting similar quality standards.[89] CMS is also developing P4P programs for Medicare.[90] Information systems are a central underpinning of P4P programs. For example, standardized electronic data collection is important for complete and cost-effective data collection by participating provider organizations. In fact, IHA uses explicit financial incentives for medical groups to make specified information technology investments.

# Emerging Medical Informatics and Bioinformatics Applications

A few key emerging areas of informatics hold significant potential to affect medical science and clinical practice: imaging, telemedicine, and bioinformatics.

## Imaging

Medical imaging can be the most IT-intensive aspect of a health care provider organization. Technology improvements are further increasing the utilization and complexity of imaging, and advances in information systems are making it easier to distribute images throughout an organization. Implementing these enhanced capabilities usually requires a large capital investment.

Images are generated and used by many medical specialties. Radiology departments have historically devoted most of their efforts to film-based, analog images such as X-rays and mammograms. However, use of other digital modalities—computed tomography (CT), magnetic resonance (MR) imaging, ultrasound, and positron emission tomography (PET) scanning—has increased dramatically in recent years.[91] Images are also central to pathology, nuclear medicine, cardiology, and other specialties.

In the traditional process, radiologists interpret images and supply reports to the referring physician in support of diagnostic decisions. Some specialists, such as orthopedists, also require direct access to the underlying images, which can be logistically cumbersome for film-based modalities. Other specialists, such as cardiologists, generate and use images (angiography, echocardiography) directly in support of their diagnostic and therapeutic decision making.

Information technology is changing how images are acquired as well as the processes by which those images are stored, distributed, and used.[92] The most comprehensive is picture archiving and control system (PACS) technology, which comprises components that allow electronic acquisition, storage, viewing, and distribution of images. PACS streamlines the radiology workflow and allows images to be easily viewed in locations outside the radiology department. However, because digital image files are so large, PACS requires a large investment in data servers, digital archiving, viewing workstations, and high-bandwidth networks, as well as IT staff.[93] Nevertheless, PACS is a relatively mature technology and implemented in a growing number of provider organizations, particularly hospitals.[94]

Integrating PACS components from multiple vendors, and with existing imaging equipment and information systems, can be challenging. Modalities such as CT and MR inherently create digital images, but they must be in a standard format if they are to be stored and accessed via PACS. The Digital Imaging and Communications in Medicine (DICOM) standard was developed to allow such image sharing.[95] X-ray or mammography images can be scanned from film generated by existing equipment, but filmless acquisition methods enable a smoother workflow and eliminate the environmental and logistical problems of film.[96] PACs must also often be integrated with an existing radiology information system (RIS) that handles patient scheduling, reporting, and other administrative functions; these systems may also incorporate sophisticated voice recognition software for radiologists to generate reports.[97]

Integrated health care provider organizations are also developing expanded capabilities that allow images from radiology as well as other specialties to be integrated with the electronic medical record and viewed at a number of facilities, and remotely.[98] These capabilities may improve efficiency and quality by enhancing physicians' ability to access images quickly,[99] but they pose even further challenges in terms of data integration and telecommunications infrastructure within an organization.[100]

Ongoing developments in imaging technology and imaging informatics offer the promise of enhanced diagnostic and therapeutic abilities in several specialties. For example, images can be used in surgical planning, and even intraoperatively.[101] Informatics developments, among them image processing, automated interpretation, and image summarization and searching, may improve the effectiveness with which images are used.[102]

## Telemedicine

Telemedicine systems use information technology and telecommunications links to enable expert clinicians to interview patients, make diagnoses, and recommend treatment at a distance.[103] The simplest telemedicine system is telephone consultation—for example, an urban physician giving advice about specific patients to rural clinic nurses. Telemedicine is most widely used in radiology and pathology, where images are transmitted from remote sites to a specialist, who then produces a written interpretation. Such applications can operate in asynchronous, or "store-and-forward," mode using plain old telephone service, or "POTS," infrastructure or the Internet. Applications are also growing in other specialties where remote interpretation of images can effectively yield diagnoses or treatment recommendations, especially dermatology, ophthalmology, and cardiology. Mental health care is an area of growing telemedicine application, allowing real-time communications between patients at remote sites and expert clinicians. However, high-bandwidth telecommunications (at least 384 kbps) are needed for such an application to be most effective.[104] Future applications, such as telesurgery, will require very complex integration of information systems, telecommunications, and robotics.[105]

Telemedicine offers a range of benefits.[106] It can greatly enhance access to specialty care for isolated populations (rural residents, prisoners, the disabled). It could be uniquely effective in military applications, for isolated bases and potentially for combat situations.[107] Telemedicine can improve quality by allowing a larger number of patients to access specialists with expertise in a particular disease. It can also increase efficiency by reducing transportation costs and taking advantage of economies of scale in use of specialized medical expertise.

Telemedicine is likely to expand for several reasons: the growing amount of health information available in electronic form via EHRs, advances in information technology, dropping telecommunications prices, ongoing cost pressures in health care, and the growth of outsourcing in many industries. Nevertheless, more sophisticated telemedicine applications require significant infrastructure.[108] To be successful, telemedicine programs require not just technology but also organizational networks within which this technology can be effectively used in clinical care.[109] Integrated health care organizations that already have organizational relationships and technical infrastructure in place are well positioned to implement telemedicine.[110] The most significant barriers to telemedicine in the United States are nontechnological: varying reimbursement standards across payers[111] and medical licensing laws that restrict consultation across state lines.

## Bioinformatics

Bioinformatics can be broadly defined as "the study of how information technologies are used to solve problems in biology."[112] A more specific definition is "conceptualizing biology in terms of molecules and applying informatics techniques to understand, and organize the information associated with these molecules, on a large scale."[113] The molecules referred to are primarily the DNA that encodes the genetic information for all organisms (the subject of genomics) and the proteins that are produced from that genetic information (and whose structure and function are the subject of proteomics).

Informatics is central to genomics and proteomics because of the vast volume of data generated and analyzed. For example, the human genome contains as many as twenty-five thousand genes encoded in more than three billion base pairs;[114] hundreds of thousands of proteins, each a complex molecule, can be produced from that genome. The development of bioinformatics was stimulated both by initiatives to map the complete genetic sequence of several organisms, notably the Human Genome Project, and concurrent spread of the Internet, which allowed researchers to share and access data rapidly.

The rapid pace of discovery in genomics and proteomics means that bioinformatics itself is evolving rapidly.[115] Broadly speaking, bioinformatics systems perform two major types of application.[116] First, large databases organize and afford access to the huge and growing amount of data about genomes, proteins, and their associated biological and medical phenomena. Second, sophisticated algorithms support tasks such as finding similarities between gene sequences or predicting the function of a protein from its amino acid sequence.

Databases of DNA and protein sequence information are the most mature bioinformatics applications, and they often incorporate sophisticated search software. For example, the National Center for Biomedical Informatics (NCBI) maintains databases of genomic and proteomic data for humans and other organisms, accessible via the Entrez search engine.[117] Swiss-Prot is a protein sequence database containing extensive annotations to related data.[118]

Bioinformatics databases and algorithms are also central to identifying the function of individual genes and the relationships between genetic variation and specific diseases.[119] For example, a researcher wishing to infer the function of a human gene from a similar gene in a mouse could use the BLAST algorithm to find regions of similarity between sequences of the two genomes.[120] The Online Mendelian Inheritance in Man (OMIM) database compiles information about human genes and elated genetic disorders.[121] New analytic techniques, particularly microarrays, are able to generate ever larger amounts of data as to how particular genes are expressed in normal and diseased tissues.[122]

Proteomics is an even more complex endeavor than genomics, entailing its own set of informatics challenges.[123] Information systems for analysis of proteomic data must also incorporate an epidemiologic understanding of the experimental conditions under which samples are collected.[124] Because analyzing the three-dimensional molecular structure of proteins is so capital- and labor-intensive, algorithms to predict the structure and function of proteins from their sequence information are promising bioinformatics applications.[125] The long-term vision of true "computational biology" is based on use of bioinformatics to understand protein interactions and predict biological processes at the cellular level.[126]

Bioinformatics will play an important role in future clinical applications of genomics and proteomics. Pharmacogenomics, which examines the relationship between genetic variation and response to drugs, will rely heavily on bioinformatics tools for drug development and clinical use.[127] As more genetic information is collected from patients and incorporated into the EHR, bioinformatics will aid clinicians in using this information effectively in clinical practice.[128]

# Privacy and Security of Electronic Health Information

As an increasing proportion of health care information is collected, stored, and transmitted in electronic rather than paper form, the risks of unauthorized use, modification, or disclosure of that information grow. For example, information about a person's medical conditions could be inappropriately disclosed to an employer supplying health insurance coverage, or personal health information could be used for marketing purposes.[129] The American public expresses ongoing concern about such risks.[130] Growth of the NHII and wider adoption of EHRs will make these risks even more salient.

Safeguarding personal health information is therefore an essential requirement of any HIS, as with those at medical groups, hospitals, MCOs, and ancillary service providers. Patients expect these organizations to protect the *privacy* of their personal health information, including detailed demographic data, medical history and conditions, and medications or treatments received. More specifically, privacy can be defined as "an individual's claim to control the circumstances in which personal information is collected, used, and transmitted."[131]

Protecting the privacy of personal health information depends on strong *security*, that is, "the technological, organizational, and administrative safety practices, policies, and procedures designed to protect data systems against unwarranted disclosure, modification, or destruction and to safeguard the system itself."[132] As will be discussed shortly, security technologies and practices have a direct impact on the design and operation of health information systems.

Individuals' concern for the privacy of their health information must be balanced against growing needs to access and aggregate health information about populations of patients.[133] For example, personal health information must be used in a public health investigation of a disease outbreak. Researchers, policy analysts, and quality improvement efforts often aggregate and analyze data about large numbers of patients. Data for these purposes can be partially deidentified (by removing addresses and replacing Social Security numbers with other identifying numbers). However, such data remain *identifiable* thanks to unique patterns in individuals' detailed demographic data and therefore must still be kept secure. Organizations that collect and hold personal health information can adopt *fair information practices* that protect privacy while allowing use of personal health information for legitimate communal purposes. Among such practices: disclosing to individuals what information is collected about them and how it is used, allowing individuals to correct the information if necessary, and allowing individuals to prevent use of their information for other purposes without their consent.[134]

At the federal level, HIPAA mandates broad privacy protection standards for health care providers and payers, and certain other organizations that receive health information from them.[135] These "covered entities" are given wide latitude to use personal health information for "treatment, payment, and health care operations," but they must obtain patients' specific authorization to use the information for marketing or other purposes. Use and disclosure of information is permitted for several activities, such as public health, law enforcement, and research.[136] Providers must allow patients access to the information in their own medical records. HIPAA preempts weaker state laws, but states are free to enact privacy protection standards more stringent than HIPAA.[137]

HIPAA also mandates security standards that covered entities must meet to protect personal health information.[138] Rather than specifying particular technologies that organizations must adopt, the standards offer guidance in several areas (administrative, physical, and technical safeguards). Within a fundamental framework of risk analysis and management, organizations have wide latitude in choosing how to implement the standards.[139] For example, they may choose to use biometric identification[140] in addition to passwords for user identification. On the other hand, they are encouraged (but not required) to use encryption when transmitting health information via the Internet.[141]

# Health Care Information Systems Challenges

Organizations must overcome several nontechnological challenges to successfully implement health information systems.[142]

## Capital Requirements and Financing

Information system implementation can require great capital investment not only for hardware and software but also for planning, project management, training, and lost efficiency during startup. These costs must be incurred before the system begins to generate financial returns, which accrue over time but whose present value must exceed the investment for the return on investment (ROI) to be favorable. The U.S. health care financing system also features limited incentives for provider organizations to invest in information systems. For example, payers seldom reward providers for the higher-quality care that may result from information system implementation, and most of the financial returns from providers' information system investments accrue to payers and purchasers.[143] It is therefore often difficult for a provider organization to make a clear business case for a specific information system. Fully integrated health care organizations such as the Veterans Health Administration can see an ROI more clearly, because long-term quality and efficiency benefits accrue to them.

Even information systems with favorable estimated ROI can be difficult to finance, because provider organizations often have limited access to capital and face many competing investment priorities, such as installing new medical technology or replacing aging facilities.[144] Providers therefore often make incremental investments; for example, a hospital may implement specific clinical applications sequentially, rather than a completely new EHR. Targeted federal funding for health information technology investments has been proposed but not yet enacted.

Physician practices face particularly significant financing challenges. Their capital is very limited, and the cost of an information system includes the time to select it and manage the implementation, as well as the extra physician time to use it; realizing a financial return requires thorough reorganization of the practice's back-office processes. Some, but not all, small practices are able to complete such an implementation successfully.[145] Larger groups are more easily able to manage the implementation process and realize a positive ROI.[146]

## Project Complexity

Information systems implementation is managerially complex and prone to failure in any industry, including health care.[147] Successful implementation requires wide-ranging modifications to work processes.[148] Nevertheless, several recommendations for success can be drawn from innovative health care organizations and other industries; as an example, senior management support and explicit attention to change management are crucial.[149] Most health care organizations buy commercial software applications rather than develop proprietary ones, and they can further reduce their implementation risk by working with experienced consultants. In any case, structured project management is essential.[150]

## Workforce Competency and Acceptance

For an information system to be successfully integrated into a modified work process, an organization's workforce must have skills to use it and the willingness to do so. This is especially challenging with respect to the clinician workforce, whose professional culture offers them substantial autonomy in how they perform their jobs. Because nurses, especially in the inpatient setting, spend a large proportion of their time planning and documenting care, they often find the benefits of information system use readily apparent. The public health workforce, however, which has historically had limited access to computers, requires substantial training to achieve adequate informatics competency.[151]

Physicians are likely to resist using a clinical information system if it significantly modifies their established work processes.[152] For example, they may need to spend more time documenting visits, or fear the added burden of responding to e-mail from patients. However, the proportion of physicians resistant to using information systems is declining; younger physicians expect to use computers routinely, and older physicians are retiring. Organizations can use a combination of mandates and incentives to facilitate information systems use among midcareer physicians. For example, the Veterans Administration offered training online and in person, and made experienced "clinical coordinators" available to encourage physicians to use the computerized patient record (CPRS) but then at a defined time mandated system use.

## Conclusions

Information technology continues to transform many sectors of the economy and society, and it is expected to have a profound effect on the U.S. health care system as well. It has already enabled mapping of the human genome and will facilitate development of more effective diagnostic and treatment technologies. Applications of information systems in clinical practice, and for sharing information across the diverse U.S. system of payers and provider organizations, are growing. The Internet enables consumers to be more informed and proactive in their own care. Large potential benefits can be realized if organizations in the U.S. health care system explicitly identify how information systems can improve quality, efficiency, and access, and then make clear and sustained commitment to implementing those systems.

## Notes

1. Shortliffe, E., and M. Blois. "The Computer Meets Medicine and Biology: Emergence of a Discipline." In E. Shortliffe and others (eds.), *Medical Informatics: Computer Applications in Health Care and Biomedicine*. New York: Springer-Verlag, 2001.

2. Yasnoff, W. A.,and others. "Public Health Informatics: Improving and Transforming Public Health in the Information Age." *Journal of Public Health Management and Practice*, 2000, *6*(6), 67–75.

3. Oliner, S. D., and Sichel, D. E. "The Resurgence of Growth in the Late 1990s: Is Information Technology the Story?" In *Finance and Economics Discussion Series*. Washington, D.C.: Federal Reserve Board, 2000.

4. The term *health information technology* (HIT) is sometimes used to describe the full range of health care information systems as described in this chapter.

5. Institute of Medicine Committee on Quality of Health Care in America. *Crossing the Quality Chasm: A New Health System for the 21st Century.* Washington, D.C.: National Academy Press, 2001.

6. Medicare Payment Advisory Commission. *Report to the Congress: Medicare Payment Policy.* Washington, D.C.: Medicare Payment Advisory Commission, 2005. [http://www.medpac.gov/publications/congressional_reports/Mar05_EntireReport.pdf].

7. First Consulting Group. *Advanced Technologies to Lower Health Care Costs and Improve Quality.* Boston: Massachusetts Technology Collaborative and New England Health Care Institute, 2003.

8. Walker, J., and others. "The Value of Health Care Information Exchange and Interoperability." Health Affairs, Web Exclusive, posted January 19, 2005.

9. Bower, A. G. *The Diffusion and Value of Health Information Technology.* Santa Monica, Calif.: RAND, 2005.

10. Hillestad, R., and others "Can Electronic Medical Record Systems Transform Health Care? Potential Health Benefits, Savings, and Costs." *Health Affairs*, 2005, *24*(5), 1103–1117.

11. "Value of HIT." Office of the National Coordinator for Health Information Technology, May 23, 2005. [http://www.os.dhhs.gov/healthit/valueHIT.html] (accessed Sept. 13, 2005).

12. McGee, M. K. "What Do Newt Gingrich and Hillary Clinton Agree on? Fed Money for Health IT." *InformationWeek*, May 11, 2005. [http://www.informationweek.com/shared/printableArticle.jhtml?articleID=163101097].

13. Narus, S. D., and Clayton, P. D. "Clinical Information Systems at Intermountain Health Care." *Imaging Economics.* February 2002. [http://www.imagingeconomics.com/issues/articles/2002-02_12.asp].

14. A fourth-generation programming language, or 4GL, is one in which the structured programming language has built-in specificity for a particular domain, such as health care; the term typically refers to languages built around database systems.

15. In 1965, Intel Corporation cofounder Gordon Moore published an article in *Electronics* whereby he postulated that the number of transistors per square inch on integrated circuit boards would double yearly for the foreseeable future. Current understanding is that data density doubles approximately every eighteen months; the expectation is that this will hold valid for approximately two decades more.

16. A bit (short for binary digit) is the smallest unit of data in a computer and is represented by a value of either 0 or 1. Computers typically store data or execute instructions in groups of eight bits; a group of eight bits is known as a byte. A kilobyte is often approximated as 1,000 bytes, but because bits are measured in binary, a kilobyte is actually 1,024 bytes (or $2^{10}$ bytes). A megabyte represents storage capacity of approximately a million bytes, or exactly $2^{20}$ (1,048,576) bytes. A gigabyte represents storage capacity of approximately a billion bytes, or exactly $2^{30}$ (1,073,741,824) bytes. A terabyte represents storage capacity of approximately a trillion bytes, or $2^{40}$ (1,099,511,627,776) bytes. A petabyte represents storage capacity of approximately a thousand trillion bytes, or $2^{50}$ (1,125,899,906,842,624) bytes. According to a University of California, Berkeley, study, "How Much Information? 2003," the entire U.S. Library of Congress print holdings would constitute approximately 136 terabytes if digitized and stored with full formatting. The World Wide Web was estimated in 2002 to contain about 170 terabytes of accessible information.

17. National Library of Medicine, National Institutes of Health. "MEDLINE Fact Sheet." June 8, 2005. [http://www.nlm.nih.gov/pubs/factsheets/medline.html] (accessed Nov. 5, 2005).

18. Pestotnik, S. L. "Expert Clinical Decision Support Systems to Enhance Antimicrobial Stewardship Programs: Insights from the Society of Infectious Diseases Pharmacists." *Pharmacotherapy*, 2005, *25*(8), 1116–1125.

19. Yasnoff, W. A., and Miller, P. L. "Decision Support and Expert Systems in Public Health." In P. W. O'Carroll and others (eds.), *Public Health Informatics and Information Systems.* New York: Springer-Verlag, 2003.

20. Pestotnik (2005).

21. Pryor, T. A. "Development of Decision Support Systems." *International Journal of Clinical Monitoring and Computing*, 1990, *7*(3), 137–146.

22. Kaushal, R., and Bates, D. W. "Computerized Physician Order Entry (CPOE) with Clinical Decision Support." In *Making Health Care Safer: A Critical Analysis of Patient Safety Practices.* Evidence Report/Technology Assessment: Number 43. AHRQ Publication No. 01-E058, July 2001. Rockville, Md.: Agency for Healthcare Research and Quality. [http://www.ahrq.gov/clinic/ptsafety/chap6.htm].

23. Evans, R. S., and others. "A Computer-Assisted Management Program for Antibiotics and Other Antiinfective Agents." *New England Journal of Medicine*, 1998, *338*(4), 232–238.

24. Bates, D. W., and others. "Effect of Computerized Physician Order Entry and a Team Intervention on Prevention of Serious Medication Errors." *Journal of the American Medical Association*, 1998, *280*(15), 1311–1316.

25. Teich, J. M., and others. "Effects of Computerized Physician Order Entry on Prescribing Practices." *Archives of Internal Medicine*, 2000, *160*(18), 2741–2747.

26. Tierney, W. M., Miller, M. E., Overhage, J. M., and McDonald, C. J. "Physician Inpatient Order Writing on Microcomputer Workstations: Effects on Resource Utilization." *Journal of the American Medical Association*, 1993, *269*(3), 379–383.

27. Adams, K., and Corrigan, J. M. (eds.). *Priority Areas for National Action: Transforming Health Care Quality.* Washington, D.C.: National Academies Press, 2003; "Leapfrog Group." [https://www.leapfroggroup.org] (accessed Oct. 2, 2005).

28. Ash, J. S., Gorman, P. N., Seshadri, V., and Hersh, W. R. "Computerized Physician Order Entry in U.S. Hospitals: Results of a 2002 Survey." *Journal of the American Medical Informatics Association*, 2004, *11*(2), 95–99.

29. Koppel, R., and others. "Role of Computerized Physician Order Entry Systems in Facilitating Medication Errors." *Journal of the American Medical Association*, 2005, *293*(10), 1197–1203; Han, Y. Y., and others. "Unexpected Increased Mortality After Implementation of a Commercially Sold Computerized Physician Order Entry System." *Pediatrics*, 2005, *116*(6), 1506–1512.

30. Poon, E. G., and others. "Overcoming Barriers to Adopting and Implementing Computerized Physician Order Entry Systems in U.S. Hospitals." *Health Affairs*, 2004, *23*(4), 184–190.

31. Group, F. C. *Computerized Physician Order Entry: Costs, Benefits, and Challenges.* Long Beach, Calif.:First Consulting Group, 2003; Cutler, D. M., Feldman, N. E., and Horwitz, J. R. "U.S. Adoption of Computerized Physician Order Entry Systems." Health Affairs, 2005, *24*(6), 1654–1663.

32. Tang, P. *Key Capabilities of an Electronic Health Record System: Letter Report.* Washington, D.C.: National Academies Press 2003.

33. Brailer, D. J., Augustinos, N., Evans, L. M., and Karp, S. *Moving Toward Electronic Health Information Exchange: Interim Report on the Santa Barbara County Data Exchange.* Oakland: California HealthCare Foundation, 2003.

34. Tang (2003).

35. Kohn, L. T., Corrigan, J. M., and Donaldson, M. S. (eds.). *To Err Is Human: Building a Safer Health System.* Washington, DC: National Academies Press, 2000; McDonald, C. J., Weiner, M., and Hui, S. L. "Deaths Due to Medical Errors Are Exaggerated in Institute of Medicine Report." *Journal of the American Medical Association,* 2000, *284*(1), 93–95; Brennan, T. A. "The Institute of Medicine Report on Medical Errors—Could It Do Harm?" *New England Journal of Medicine,* 2000, *342*(15), 1123–1125.

36. Ioannidis, J. P., and Lau, J. "Evidence on Interventions to Reduce Medical Errors: An Overview and Recommendations for Future Research." *Journal of General Internal Medicine,* 2001, *16*(5), 325–334; Balas, E. A., and others. "The Clinical Value of Computerized Information Services: A Review of 98 Randomized Clinical Trials." *Archives of Family Medicine,* 1996, *5*(5), 271–278.

37. Evans and others (1998); Hunt, D. L., Haynes, R. B., Hanna, S. E., and Smith, K. "Effects of Computer-Based Clinical Decision Support Systems on Physician Performance and Patient Outcomes: A Systematic Review." *Journal of the American Medical Association,* 1998, *280*(15), 1339–1346.

38. Parkin, D. M., Henney, C. R., Quirk, J., and Crooks, J. "Deviation from Prescribed Drug Treatment After Discharge from Hospital." *British Medical Journal,* 1976, *2*(6037), 686–688.

39. Tang, P. C., Fafchamps, D., and Shortliffe, E. H. "Traditional Medical Records as a Source of Clinical Data in the Outpatient Setting." *Proceedings of the Annual Symposium on Computing Applications in Medical Care,* 1994, 575–579; Covell, D. G., Uman, G. C., and Manning, P. R. "Information Needs in Office Practice: Are They Being Met?" *Annals of Internal Medicine,* 1985, *103*(4), 596–599.

40. McGlynn, E. A., and others. "The Quality of Health Care Delivered to Adults in the United States." *New England Journal of Medicine,* 2003, *348*(26), 2635–2645.

41. Morris, A. H. "Treatment Algorithms and Protocolized Care." *Current Opinion on Critical Care,* 2003, *9*(3), 236–240; Eccles, M., and others. "Effect of Computerised Evidence Based Guidelines on Management of Asthma and Angina in Adults in Primary Care: Cluster Randomised Controlled Trial." *British Medical Journal,* 2002, *325*(7370), 941.

42. Tierney, W. M., McDonald, C. J., Martin, D. K., and Rogers, M. P. "Computerized Display of Past Test Results: Effect on Outpatient Testing." *Annals of Internal Medicine,* 1987, *107*(4), 569–574; Stair, T. O. "Reduction of Redundant Laboratory Orders by Access to Computerized Patient Records." *Journal of Emergency Medicine,* 1998, *16*(6), 895–897.

43. Petersen, L. A., and others. "Using a Computerized Sign-out Program to Improve Continuity of Inpatient Care and Prevent Adverse Events." *Joint Commission Journal on Quality Improvement,* 1998, *24*(2), 77–87; Petersen, L. A., and others. "Does Housestaff Discontinuity of Care Increase the Risk for Preventable Adverse Events?" *Annals of Internal Medicine,* 1994, *121*(11), 866–872.

44. Solutions, P. F. *Chronic Conditions: Making the Case for Ongoing Care.* Baltimore, Md.: Johns Hopkins University, 2004.

45. Weingarten, S. R., and others. "Interventions Used in Disease Management Programmes for Patients with Chronic Illness-Which Ones Work? Meta-Analysis of Published Reports." *British Medical Journal,* 2002, *325*(7370), 925.

46. Balas (1996).

47. U.S. GAO. *Report to the Ranking Minority Member, Committee on Health, Education, Labor, and Pensions, U.S. Senate, Information Technology, Benefits Realized for Selected Health Care Functions.* Washington, D.C.: U.S. General Accounting Office, 2003.

48. Health Technology Center, and M. Phelps and Phillips, LLP. *Spending Our Money Wisely: Improving America's Healthcare System by Investing in Healthcare Information Technology.* San Francisco: Health Technology Center, 2003.

49. Dowling, A. "CHINs—The Current State." In Brennan, P. F., Schneider, S. J., and Tornquist, E. (eds.), *Information Networks for Community Health.* New York: Springer-Verlag, 1997.

50. Miller, R. H., and Sim, I. "Physicians' Use of Electronic Medical Records: Barriers and Solutions." *Health Affairs,* 2004, *23*(2), 116–126.

51. "Doctors' Office Quality—Information Technology." American Association of Family Physicians, 2004. [http://www.aafp.org/x24964.xml] (accessed Apr. 4, 2004).

52. Berkowitz, C. Personal communication. September 2004.

53. *Executive Order 13335: Incentives for the Use of Health Information Technology and Establishing the Position of the National Health Information Technology Coordinator.* Washington, D.C: Government Printing Office, 2004. [http://a257.g.akamaitech.net/7/257/2422/14mar20010800/edocket.access.gpo.gov/2004/pdf/04-10024.pdf#search=%22executive%20order%20incentives%20for%20the%20use%20of%20health%20information%20tech%22].

54. Corrigan, J. M., Greiner, A., and Erickson S. M.(eds.). *Fostering Rapid Advances in Health Care: Learning from System Demonstrations.* Washington, D.C.: National Academies Press, 2002.

55. Glaser, J. P., DeBor, G., and Stuntz, L. "The New England Healthcare EDI Network." *Journal of Healthcare Information Management,* 2003, *17*(4), 42–50.

56. Marchibroda, J., and Bordenick, J. C. *Emerging Trends and Issues in Health Information Exchange.* Washington, D.C.: eHealth Initiative, 2005.

57. Halamka, J., and others. "Exchanging Health Information: Local Distribution, National Coordination." *Health Affairs,* 2005, *24*(5), 1170–1179.

58. National Committee on Vital and Health Statistics. U.S. Department of Health and Human Services. *Information for Health: A Strategy for Building the National Health Information Infrastructure.* 2001.

59. Yasnoff, W. A., and others. "A Consensus Action Agenda for Achieving the National Health Information Infrastructure." *Journal of the American Medical Informatics Association,* 2004, *11*(4), 332–338.

60. Institute of Medicine. *Crossing the Quality Chasm: A New Health System for the 21st Century.* Washington, D.C.: National Academy Press, 2001.

61. Halamka and others (2005).

62. Kaushal, R., and others. "The Costs of a National Health Information Network." *Annals of Internal Medicine,* 2005, *143*(3), 165–173.

63. Yasnoff, W. A., and others. "Public Health Informatics: Improving and Transforming Public Health in the Information Age." *Journal of Public Health Management Practice,* 2000, *6*(6), 67–75.

64. Gebbie, K. M., Rosenstock, L., and Hernandez, L. M. (eds.). *Who Will Keep the Public Healthy? Educating Public Health Professionals for the 21st Century.* Washington, D.C.: National Academies Press, 2003.

65. Friede, A., and O'Carroll, P. W. "CDC and ATSDR Electronic Information Resources for Health Officers." *Journal of Public Health Management Practice,* 1996, *2*(3), 10–24.

66. Evans, R. G., and Stoddart, G. L. "Producing Health, Consuming Health Care." *Social Science & Medicine,* 1990, *31*(12), 1347–1363.

67. "PHIN: Overview." Centers for Disease Control and Prevention. [http://www.cdc.gov/phin/overview.html] (accessed Sept. 12, 2005).

68. "Health Alert Network." Centers for Disease Control and Prevention. [http://www.phppo.cdc.gov/han] (accessed Nov. 24, 2005).

69. "National Electronic Disease Surveillance System." Centers for Disease Control and Prevention. [http://www.cdc.gov/nedss] (accessed Dec. 16, 2005).

70. Metzger, J. *Using Computerized Registries in Chronic Disease Care.* Oakland: California Healthcare Foundation, 2004.

71. Metzger (2004).

72. Kilo, C. M. "Transforming Care: Medical Practice Design and Information Technology: How One Innovative Medical Practice Has Eliminated Many Office Visits and Improved Continuity of Care for Patients with Chronic Conditions." *Health Affairs*, 2005, *24*(5), 1296–1301.

73. Lumpkin, J. R., and Richards, M. S. "Transforming the Public Health Information Infrastructure." *Health Affairs*, 2002, *21*(6), 45–56.

74. Saarlas, K. N., Edwards, K., Wild, E., and Richmond. P. "Developing Performance Measures for Immunization Registries." *Journal of Public Health Management Practice*, 2003, *9*(1), 47–57.

75. Horne, P. R., Saarlas, K. N., and Hinman, A. R. "Costs of Immunization Registries: Experiences from the All Kids Count II Projects." *American Journal of Preventive Medicine*, 2000, *19*(2), 94–98.

76. Malec, B. T. "Managed Care Applications." In C. J. Austin and S. B. Boxerman (eds.), *Information Systems for Health Services Administration*. Chicago: Health Administration Press, 1998; Slubowski, J. S. "Information Systems in Managed Health Care Plans." In P. R. Kongstvedt (ed.), *The Managed Health Care Handbook*. Gaithersburg, Md.: Aspen, 2001.

77. Kongstvedt, P. R. "Using Data and Provider Profiling in Medical Management." In P. R. Kongstvedt (ed.), *The Managed Health Care Handbook*. Gaithersburg, Md.: Aspen, 2001.

78. Goedert, J. "Electronic Transactions: Standards Aren't Common." *Health Data Management*, 2003, *11*(11), 36–40, 42.

79. Gillespie, G. "Uncertainty Clouds Online, Real-Time World." *Health Data Management*, 2004, *12*(5), 50–52, 54.

80. Goedert, J. "Claims Automation in a New Environment." *Health Data Management*, 2005, *13*(3), 30–31.

81. Featherly, K. "Healthcare Moves to Close Payment Loop Automatically." *Healthcare Informatics*, 2004, *21*(1), 12.

82. Buntin, M. B., and others. *"Consumer-Driven" Health Plans: Implications for Health Care Quality and Cost.* Santa Monica, Calif.: RAND, 2005; Davis, K. "Consumer-Directed Health Care: Will It Improve Health System Performance?" *Health Services Research*, 2004, *39*(4 Pt. 2), 1219–1234.

83. Gillespie, G. "Managed Care Applications Evolve." *Health Data Management*, 2002, *10*(6), 56–60, 62–63; Margolis, J. H., "Managed Care: The Health Plan of Tomorrow." *Health Management Technology*, 2004, *25*(1), 32–34, 36–37; O'Dell, S., and Hansen, J. "The Next-Generation Health Plan: Not If, But When and How." *Healthplan*, 2003, *44*(2), 54–58.

84. "MCO Accreditation Information." [http://www.ncqa.org/Programs/HEDIS] (accessed Sept. 13, 2005).

85. "The Health Plan Employer Data and Information Set (HEDIS)." [http://www.ncqa.org/Programs/HEDIS] (accessed Sept. 13, 2005).

86. McGlynn and others (2003).

87. Peabody, J. W., and others. "Measuring the Quality of Physician Practice by Using Clinical Vignettes: A Prospective Validation Study." *Annals of Internal Medicine*, 2004, *141*(10), 771–780.

88. "IHA Projects: Pay for Performance." [http://www.iha.org/Ihaproj.htm] (accessed Sept. 13, 2005).

89. "Bridges to Excellence: Rewarding Quality Across the Health Care System." [http://www.bridgestoexcellence.org/bte/index.html] (accessed Sept. 13, 2005).

90. "Medicare 'Pay for Performance (P4p)' Initiatives." [http://www.cms.hhs.gov/media/press/release.asp?Counter=1343] (accessed Sept. 13, 2005).

91. Beinfeld, M. T., and Gazelle, G. S. "Diagnostic Imaging Costs: Are They Driving up the Costs of Hospital Care?" *Radiology*, 2005, *235*(3), 934–939.

92. Greenes, R., and Brinkley, J. "Imaging Systems." In E. Shortliffe and others (eds.), *Medical Informatics: Computer Applications in Health Care and Biomedicine.* New York: Springer-Verlag, 2001.

93. Cao, X., and Huang, H. K. "Current Status and Future Advances of Digital Radiography and PACS." *IEEE Engineering in Medicine and Biology*, 2000, *19*(5), 80–88; Carrino, J. A., "Digital Imaging Overview." *Seminars in Roentgenology*, 2003, *38*(3), 200–215.

94. Hagland, M. "Integrating PACS." *Healthcare Informatics*, 2005, *22*(2), 50, 52, 54.

95. "DICOM: Digital Imaging and Communications in Medicine." [http://medical.nema.org] (accessed Aug. 15, 2005).

96. Cao and Huang (2000); Pisano, E. D., and Yaffe, M. J. "Digital Mammography." *Radiology*, 2005, *234*(2), 353–362.

97. Samei, E., and others. "AAPM/RSNA Tutorial on Equipment Selection: PACS Equipment Overview: General Guidelines for Purchasing and Acceptance Testing of PACS Equipment." *Radiographics*, 2004, *24*(1), 313–334.

98. Bui, A. A., and others. "Effect of an Imaging-Based Streamlined Electronic Healthcare Process on Quality and Costs." *Academic Radiology*, 2004, *11*(1), 13–20.

99. Avrin, D., Wiggins, R. H., III, and Bahr, C. "Beyond PACS: Getting Images to Referring Physicians." *Seminars in Ultrasound CT and MR*, 2003, *24*(6), 428–433.

100. Briggs, B. "Diagnostic Images Flowing Among Clinicians." *Health Data Management*, 2004, *12*(11), 42–44, 46, 48 passim.

101. Greenes and Brinkley (2001).

102. Sinha, U., and others. "A Review of Medical Imaging Informatics." *Annals of the New York Academy of Sciences*, 2002, *980*(1), 168–197.

103. Craig, J., and Patterson, V. "Introduction to the Practice of Telemedicine." *Journal of Telemedicine and Telecare*, 2005, *11*(1), 3–9; Field, M. J. (ed.). *Telemedicine: A Guide to Assessing Telecommunications in Health Care.* Washington, D.C.: National Academy Press, 1996.

104. Krupinski, E., and others. "Telemedicine/Telehealth: An International Perspective. Clinical Applications in Telemedicine/Telehealth." *Telemedicine Journal and E-Health*, 2002, *8*(1), 13–34.

105. American Telemedicine Association. [http://www.atmeda.org/news/newres.htm] (accessed Aug. 18, 2005).

106. Craig and Patterson (2005); Bashshur, R. L. "Telemedicine/Telehealth: An International Perspective. Telemedicine and Health Care." *Telemedicine Journal and E-Health*, 2002, *8*(1), 5–12.

107. Lam, D. "TATRC U.S. Army Telemedicine and Advanced Technology Research Center." *Military Medical Technology Online,* 2004, *8*(4). [http://www.military-medical-technology.com/linkto.cfm?DocID=480].

108. Ackerman, M., and others. "Telemedicine/Telehealth: An International Perspective. Telemedicine Technology." *Telemedicine Journal and E-Health*, 2002, 8(1), 71–78.

109. Krasnow, D., and Rodrigues, R. J. "International Perspectives." In S. F. Viegas and K. Dunn (eds.), *Telemedicine: Practicing in the Information Age*. Philadelphia: Lippincott-Raven, 1998; Shannon, G., and others. "Telemedicine/Telehealth: An International Perspective. Organizational Models of Telemedicine and Regional Telemedicine Networks." *Telemedicine Journal and E-Health*, 2002, *8*(1), 61–70.

110. Jossi, F. "Telehealth." *Healthcare Informatics*, 2005, *22*(2), 66, 68.

111. "Report on Reimbursement." [http://www.atmeda.org/news/Reiumburement%20 White%20paperfinal.pdf] (accessed Aug. 18, 2005).

112. Altman, R. B. "Bioinformatics in Support of Molecular Medicine." *Proceedings of AMIA Symposium*, 1998, 53–61.

113. Luscombe, N. M., Greenbaum, D., and Gerstein, M. "What Is Bioinformatics? A Proposed Definition and Overview of the Field." *Methods of Information in Medicine*, 2001, *40*(4), 346–358.

114. "The Science Behind the Human Genome Project: Basic Genetics, Genome Draft Sequence, and Post-Genome Science." [http://www.ornl.gov/sci/techresources/Human_ Genome/project/info.shtml] (accessed Aug. 22, 2005).

115. Kanehisa, M., and Bork, P. "Bioinformatics in the Post-Sequence Era." *Nature Genetics*, 2003, *33*(Suppl.), 305–310.

116. "A Science Primer: Bioinformatics." 2004. [http://www.ncbi.nlm.nih.gov/About/primer/ bioinformatics.html] (accessed Aug. 23, 2005); Altman, R. "Bioinformatics." In E. Shortliffe and others (eds.), *Medical Informatics: Computer Applications in Health Care and Biomedicine*. New York: Springer-Verlag, 2001.

117. "Entrez, The Life Sciences Search Engine." [http://www.ncbi.nlm.nih.gov/gquery/ gquery.fcgi] (accessed Aug. 23, 2005).

118. "Swiss-Prot Protein Knowledgebase." [http://us.expasy.org/sprot] (accessed Aug. 23, 2005).

119. "Gene Gateway—Exploring Genes and Genetic Disorders." [http://www.ornl.gov/sci/ techresources/Human_Genome/posters/chromosome] (accessed Aug. 23, 2005).

120. "Basic Local Alignment Search Tool (BLAST)." [http://www.ncbi.nlm.nih.gov/BLAST] (accessed Aug. 23, 2005).

121. "Online Mendelian Inheritance in Man (OMIM) Database." [http://www.ncbi.nlm.nih. gov/entrez/query.fcgi?db=OMIM] (accessed Aug. 23, 2005).

122. Miller, P. L. "Opportunities at the Intersection of Bioinformatics and Health Informatics: A Case Study." *Journal of the American Medical Informatics Association*, 2000, *7*(5), 431–438.

123. Patterson, S. D., and Aebersold, R. H. "Proteomics: The First Decade and Beyond." *Nature Genetics*, 2003, *33*(Suppl.), 311–323; Tyers, M., and Mann, M. "From Genomics to Proteomics." *Nature*, 2003, *422*(6928), 193–197.

124. Boguski, M. S., and McIntosh, M. W. "Biomedical Informatics for Proteomics." *Nature*, 2003, *422*(6928), 233–237.

125. Altman (2001); Thornton, J. "Structural Genomics Takes off." *Trends in Biochemical Science*, 2001, *26*(2), 88–89.

126. Kanehisa and Bork (2003); Altman, R. B., and Klein, T. E. "Challenges for Biomedical Informatics and Pharmacogenomics." *Annual Review of Pharmacology and Toxicology*, 2002, *42*, 113–133.

127. "Medicine and the New Genetics." [http://www.ornl.gov/sci/techresources/Human_ Genome/medicine/medicine.shtml] (accessed Aug. 23, 2005).

128. "Medical Privacy Stories." 2003. [http://www.healthprivacy.org/usr_doc/Storiesupd.pdf] (accessed Aug. 11, 2005).

129. "Medical Privacy Stories" (2003).

130. Westin, A. "How the Public Views Health Privacy: Survey Findings from 1978 to 2005." 2005. [http://www.pandab.org] (accessed Aug. 11, 2005).

131. Gostin, L. O. "Personal Privacy in the Health Care System: Employer-Sponsored Insurance, Managed Care, and Integrated Delivery Systems." *Kennedy Institute of Ethics Journal,* 1997, *7*(4), 361–376.

132. Gostin (1997).

133. Hodge, J. G., Jr., Gostin, L. O., and Jacobson, P. D. "Legal Issues Concerning Electronic Health Information: Privacy, Quality, and Liability." *Journal of the American Medical Association,* 1999, *282*(15), 1466–1471.

134. "A Review of the Fair Information Principles: The Foundation of Privacy Public Policy." 2004. [http://www.privacyrights.org/ar/fairinfo.htm] (accessed Aug. 11, 2005).

135. "Protecting the Privacy of Patients' Health Information." 2003. [http://www.hhs.gov/news/facts/privacy.html] (accessed Aug. 11, 2005).

136. "Summary of the HIPAA Privacy Rule." 2003. [http://www.hhs.gov/ocr/privacysummary.pdf] (accessed Aug. 11, 2005).

137. "The State of Health Privacy." 2002. [http://www.healthprivacy.org/info-url_nocat2304/info-url_nocat.htm] (accessed Aug. 11, 2005).

138. "Security 101 for Covered Entities." 2004. [http://www.cms.hhs.gov/hipaa/hipaa2/education/Security percent20101_Cleared.pdf] (accessed Aug. 11, 2005).

139. Grove, T. "Summary Analysis: The Final HIPAA Security Rule." 2003. [http://www.hipaadvisory.com/regs/finalsecurity/summaryanalysis.htm] (accessed Aug. 11, 2005).

140. Liu, S., and Silverman, M. "A Practical Guide to Biometric Security Technology." *IT Professional,* 2001, *3*(1), 27–32.

141. Kelly, G., and McKenzie, B. "Security, Privacy, and Confidentiality Issues on the Internet." *Journal of Medical Internet Research,* 2002, *4*(2), E12.

142. Hersh, W. "Health Care Information Technology: Progress and Barriers." *Journal of the American Medical Association,* 2004, *292*(18), 2273–2274; Shortliffe, E. H. "Strategic Action in Health Information Technology: Why the Obvious Has Taken So Long." *Health Affairs,* 2005, *24*(5), 1222–1233.

143. Hillestad and others (2005); Middleton, B., and others. "Accelerating U.S. EHR Adoption: How to Get There from Here. Recommendations Based on the 2004 ACMI Retreat." *Journal of the American Medical Informatics Association,* 2005, *12*(1), 13–19.

144. Haugh, R. "Cost Drivers: Credit." *Hospital Health Network,* 2004, *78*(6), 48, 57.

145. Miller, R. H., and others. "The Value of Electronic Health Records in Solo or Small Group Practices." *Health Affairs,* 2005, *24*(5), 1127–1137.

146. Audet, A. M., and others. "Information Technologies: When Will They Make It into Physicians' Black Bags?" *MedGenMed,* 2004, *6*(4), 2.

147. Standish Group. *The CHAOS Report.* West Yarmouth, Mass.: Standish Group, 1995.

148. Walker, J. M. "Electronic Medical Records and Health Care Transformation." *Health Affairs,* 2005, *24*(5), 1118–1120.

149. DeLuca, J. M., and Enmark, R. *The CEO's Guide to Health Information Systems* (2nd ed.). San Francisco: Jossey-Bass, 2002; Wager, K. A., Lee, F. W., and Glaser, J. P. *Managing Health Care Information Systems: A Practical Approach for Health Care Executives.* San Francisco: Jossey-Bass, 2005.

150. "Project Management Institute." [http://www.pmi.org/info/default.asp] (accessed Sept. 15, 2005).

151. Richards, J. "Core Competencies in Public Health Informatics." In P. W. O'Carroll and others (eds.), *Public Health Informatics and Information Systems*. New York: Springer-Verlag, 2003.

152. McDonald, C. J., and others. "Physicians, Information Technology, and Health Care Systems: A Journey, Not a Destination." *Journal of the American Medical Informatics Association*, 2004, *11*(2), 121–124.

CHAPTER TWELVE

# PERFORMANCE MEASUREMENT OF NURSING CARE

Jack Needleman
Ellen T. Kurtzman
Kenneth W. Kizer

More than 1.3 million nurses, or 59 percent of all U.S. nurses, work in America's short-term (49 percent), long-term (3.6 percent), psychiatric (1.5 percent), federal government (2.9 percent), or otherwise classified (2.1 percent) hospitals.[1] Although nurses represent the single largest provider of inpatient care, little is known about their contribution to provision of care that is safe, beneficial, patient-centered, timely, efficient, and equitable.[2] Recent scientific studies and media coverage have focused on the extent to which the health care system has major lapses in quality that result in diminished patient safety and health care outcomes.[3] As a result, the degree to which the availability of nurses, the organization of the nursing workforce, and the work environment in which nurses practice contribute to the growing health care quality chasm has gained increased attention from providers, researchers, payers, consumer organizations, and the public. As evidence, consider the following:

• Because of hospital mergers and the process of care restructuring directed at lowering costs in the 1990s, many registered nurses (RNs) report that they are working harder than ever, spending less time taking care of increasingly ill patients, and consequently seeing the safety and quality of patient care deteriorating.[4] Moreover, efforts to restructure the delivery of hospital patient care to lower the costs of care have resulted in claims that total nursing staff is being reduced and licensed practical nurses (LPNs) and assistive personnel are being substituted for RNs.[5]

• There is a growing and compelling body of evidence that the size of the nursing workforce, mix of RNs and other staff, and nurses' work environment influence patient safety and complication rates. This evidence includes studies at the hospital and unit level, and surveys of staff nurses.

• There is some evidence that nurse staffing per day in hospitals increased in the 1990s. Buerhaus and colleagues report that the ratio of RNs to hospital beds increased from 0.651 in 1983 to 1.115 in 1996, while the ratio of LPNs per bed decreased steadily and the ratio of aides per bed fluctuated over this same time.[6] Kovner and colleagues report similar findings.[7] In a study of California hospitals, Spetz found an increase in the number of hours worked by nursing personnel from 1977 to 1996, which was attributed to falling length of stay (LOS) and rising patient acuity.[8] Similar findings are reported by Anderson and Kohn.[9]

• While staffing has increased, in light of increased patient acuity some speculate that staffing may not have increased enough. Aiken and colleagues found, after adjusting for case mix, that hospital nurse staffing fell 7.3 percent between 1981 and 1993, and they question whether hospitals have reduced staffing to an unsafe level.[10] Similarly, Minnick and Pabst found in a study of seventy-seven nursing units that acuity-adjusted nursing hours per patient day had decreased.[11]

Nurses' dissatisfaction with current working conditions has contributed to a substantial shortage of nurses in hospitals. The vacancy rate in a 2001 survey of hospitals was estimated at 13 percent nationally, with 15 percent of hospitals reporting a vacancy rate of more than 20 percent.[12] Paralleling this immediate vacancy problem is the argument that nursing has become a less attractive profession for those who traditionally entered it. Women graduating from high school in the 1990s were 35 percent less likely to enroll in a nursing education program than women born in the 1970s. Researchers estimate that if there is no change in enrollment trends, with the aging of the baby boom generation the United States may have a shortage of four hundred thousand nurses in 2020, a shortfall of 20 percent.[13]

Dissatisfaction with current working conditions has also encouraged some nursing unions to press for legislated or regulatory changes to mandate minimum staffing levels or restrict mandatory overtime. The California Nurses Association successfully pressed for such legislation in its home state; proposed regulations to implement the legislation have been published. Legislation is pending in other states.

Together, the concerns about nurse staffing in hospitals, nursing's influence on patient safety and health care outcomes, and the condition of the nursing workforce have led to increased interest in measuring and reporting nursing's performance. It is possible to identify multiple interrelated goals or purposes for such measurement and reporting:

- To quantify nursing's influence on patient safety and health care outcomes, with a special focus on promoting the highest level of quality in acute care hospitals
- To enhance the clinical practice of nursing personnel and nursing-related quality improvement projects
- To promote provider accountability to the public, including but not limited to public reporting and financial incentives
- To identify levels of staffing—including appropriate standards—and approaches to organizing nursing in hospitals to be implemented by hospitals and supported by payers and other public and private parties
- To facilitate identification of priority areas for research needed in measuring nursing-sensitive care
- To address the need to educate and train the current and future workforce
- To support benchmarking and sharing of best practice
- To promote translation of the state of science of nursing care into delivery of nursing care

This chapter reviews recent efforts and issues involved in identifying a set of nursing-sensitive performance measures.[14] It examines the scope of nursing's contribution to hospital care, priorities for measuring nursing care, current systems and initiatives to implement or develop systems for measuring nursing care (with special emphasis on the National Quality Forum's endorsement of national voluntary consensus standards[15]), and challenges and future considerations.

# The Scope of Nursing's Contribution to Inpatient Hospital Care

Establishing the scope—or boundaries—of nursing practice is a critical step in both understanding nursing's contribution to patient safety and health care outcomes and measuring those aspects of practice that are most relevant to inpatient hospital quality.

## Nurses' Work

To measure nursing performance, it is useful to begin with an understanding of the work that nurses do. How nurses' work should be conceptualized and classified has been subject to extensive debate for some time, as nurses attempt to define the spheres of practice that are autonomous to nursing or collaborative with other health professions (most notably physicians) and in which nurses attempt to integrate models of nursing as a scientific discipline and as an art.[16]

The variety of alternative descriptions of nurses' work can make it difficult for nurses to talk to one another about their work, to develop computerized nursing information systems (since that requires choices to be made on frameworks and concepts), and to communicate with policy makers and the public about nursing.[17] A range of activities have sought to standardize the language used to define nursing diagnosis, interventions, and outcomes. An early effort to define a standard structure for nursing diagnosis was put forward in 1973 by the North American Nursing Diagnosis Association (NANDA), and that system has been updated on an ongoing basis.[18] Separately, the Center for Nursing Classification in the University of Iowa Nursing School developed systems of classifying nursing interventions[19] and nursing outcomes.[20] Since 1994, NANDA and researchers at the University of Iowa have been working jointly to refine, integrate, and extend these systems.[21] This may be the basis for a standard classification system for the United States.

Three alternative systems of classifying nurses' work suggest the range of activities involved in nursing. The Omaha system, described by Martin and Scheet, puts nurses' activities into four broad categories: (1) health teaching, guidance, and counseling; (2) treatments and procedures; (3) case management; and (4) surveillance.[22] Specific activities or nursing interventions are assigned to each category.

Another classification, by Hendrickson and colleagues, divides nurses' activities into patient care activities at the bedside and other patient care.[23] *Bedside activities* include feeding, bathing, cleaning, dressing, procedure therapies, medications, education and support of the patient, education and support of the family, assessment and rounds, and transfers and mobility. *Nonbedside patient care* includes charting, orders, other documentation, interaction with others on the telephone or in person, coordination at shift changes, and preparing therapies. This list of activities adds concreteness to the conceptual categories in the Omaha system. The list can be nested within the Omaha system, although not unambiguously. Assessment and rounds, for example, might fall into both case management and surveillance, an example that underscores the multitasking implicit in nurses' work. The list also illustrates the significant amount of time required for nonbedside patient care and nonpatient care activities. Hendrickson and colleagues found in their study that only 31 percent of nurses' time was spent with patients.

A third classification system, by Irvine, Sidani, and Hall, classifies nurses' roles into independent, dependent, and interdependent functions.[24] They define nurses' independent roles as assessment, diagnosis, intervention, and follow-up care, while their dependent functions include execution of medical orders and physician-initiated treatments. Interdependent functions—those that nurses engage in that are partially or totally dependent on the functions of other health care providers—include communication, case management, coordination of care, continuity and monitoring, and reporting.

All classifications underscore the important work of nurses outside of carrying out treatments or procedures ordered by others, and their active role in monitoring patient condition, managing and coordinating care, and educating patients and preparing them and their families to care for themselves. To be fully effective, performance systems should capture the impact of nurses' work in each of these domains.

As patients in hospitals become more acutely ill, and as hospitals attempt to redesign how nurses' work is carried out, the mix of activities conducted by nurses has shifted. Table 12.1 presents an illustration of the shift over a three-year period in the top ten activities of nurses at a large community hospital in Pennsylvania as work was redesigned. Notable among these changes was the increase in professional judgment, patient education, and assessing data on patients, as well as the reduction in time spent bathing and turning patients and intake and output—that is, a shift to tasks requiring more training and judgment.

## TABLE 12.1. COMPARISON OF CHANGES IN TOP TEN RN ACTIVITIES DURING THREE YEARS OF WORK REDESIGN.

| Activity | 1993 | | 1994 | | 1995 | |
|---|---|---|---|---|---|---|
| | Rank | Percent | Rank | Percent | Rank | Percent |
| Charting | 1 | 7.9 | 2 | 8.7 | 4 | 7.6 |
| Patient assessment | 2 | 7.3 | 3 | 7.9 | 1 | 10.3 |
| Medication administration | 3 | 6.9 | 1 | 8.8 | 3 | 8.5 |
| Bathing | 4 | 6.7 | 4 | 6.7 | | |
| Report | 5 | 4.9 | 5 | 5.2 | 5 | 5.1 |
| Respond to patient's requests | 6 | 3.9 | 6 | 4.5 | 7 | 3.3 |
| Close observation | 7 | 3.4 | 7 | 4.4 | 6 | 4.6 |
| Vital signs | 8 | 3.2 | 8 | 3.1 | 8 | 3.3 |
| Turning | 9 | 3.0 | 9 | 2.9 | | |
| Intake and output | 10 | 2.7 | 10 | 2.9 | | |
| Professional judgment | | | | | 2 | 9.5 |
| Patient education | | | | | 9 | 2.9 |
| Assessing patient data | | | | | 10 | 2.5 |
| Percentage of time captured | | 50 | | 55 | | 58 |

*Source:* Anne Pederson. "A Data-Driven Approach to Work Redesign in Nursing Units." *Journal of Nursing Administration,* 1997, *27*(4), 49–54.

## Organizing to Accomplish Nurses' Work

Hospitals organize their nursing functions in a variety of ways, and the approaches may vary over time and across units within a hospital. Using a modified Delphi technique, Brennan and colleagues have identified eleven dimensions along which nursing models vary.[25] Among the models that have been defined:

- *Team.* Under the leadership of a professional nurse, a group of staff work together to carry out the full functions of professional nurses for a group of patients. The team consists of an RN and unlicensed assistive personnel and may include a licensed practical nurse.
- *Primary.* One primary nurse is assigned to care for all of the patient's needs for the duration of the patient's hospital stay. Responsibility is for twenty-four hours.
- *Functional.* A task-oriented method in which a function is assigned to a staff member. One nurse is responsible for administering medications and another for treatments.
- *Case management.* Care coordinated by a case manager who may or may not provide the nursing care. A care map or pathway is used to guide care.
- *Total patient care.* Provision of patient care whereby each nursing staff member is assigned to give complete care to a group of patients during a given shift.
- *Patient-centered (focused) care.* Organization for provision of as many elements of patient care as possible by caregivers closest to the patient. Implementation of patient-focused care includes developing multiskilled workers through extensive cross-training of caregivers.

These definitions have overlapping elements and are not always used consistently. Minnick has found, for example, that when nurse managers were asked about the specific practice behaviors of nurses on their units, there was little correspondence to the goals of the stated "nursing model" and concludes that a questionnaire identifying specific practices rather than asking about models may be necessary to accurately capture information on the organization of nursing in a hospital.

# Issues in Constructing Nursing-Sensitive Performance Measures

In addition to the scope of nursing practice, the characteristics of performance measures needs to be defined before identifying candidate measures. It should be recognized that not all candidate measures deserve equal consideration, particularly given the pressing need for measures in this area and the undeveloped state of nursing care performance measurement among hospitals.

## Conceptual Frameworks for Performance Systems: Structure, Process, and Outcome Measures

The classic Donabedian model of quality measurement identifies structure, process, and outcome as three dimensions along which quality can be analyzed. Generally, existing nursing performance measurement systems have adopted a mix of measures from the structure-process-outcome dimensions. The American Nursing Association indicators, for example, include registered nursing hours per patient day (a structural measure), nurse satisfaction (a process measure), and nosocomial infection (an outcome measure). Outcome measures are frequently preferred for measuring system performance, but because many factors can influence outcomes besides nursing care, correctly interpreting outcome measures requires appropriate controls for these other factors, controls that can be difficult to implement. At the other end of the spectrum, structural measures are often viewed as too rigid; because many processes can affect how structure influences outcomes, this is seen as an imperfect proxy for how the system is performing. Process measures, like structural measures, are often easier to measure, but their connection to patient outcomes must be validated.

## Linkage to Nursing Care

There are a substantial number of quality or performance measures in health care that are clear and clearly documented. Did the patient receive beta blockers after a heart attack if there were no contraindications? Did the patient receive prophylactic antibiotics within a fixed time before surgery? Was the wrong drug administered, or administered at the wrong dose? For some nursing care, problems or lapses in performance should also be observable in charts—failure to give a drug on time, for example. Other lapses in care may not be documented; inadequate or rushed catheter care will not be charted.

Where lapses in care cannot be charted, it is impossible to tie specific outcomes to inadequate nursing. A urinary tract infection or a stress-induced upper gastrointestinal bleed may not be clearly linkable to nursing because of such documentation gaps. Establishing links between nursing care and many outcomes depends on an understanding of the likely etiology of the adverse event or complication rather than direct evidence abstracted from a chart.

## Measuring at the Unit or Hospital Level

Studies of nursing have been conducted at the nursing unit and hospital levels. The nursing unit is a natural one at which to conduct measurement and assess performance. Nursing is organized and delivered within units. The count of patients and count of nurses is precise, while at the hospital level there are issues of averaging across varying units and inpatient and outpatient activities. Nurse staffing and performance can vary across units within a hospital. Indeed, in some cases there is more variability in nursing or patients within a hospital than across them.[26] It is at this level that the ANA has organized its principal data collection.

There are several drawbacks to measurement at the unit level, however. First, it is expensive, requiring either special data collection or chart abstracting. Hospital-level data can be collected in the same way, but hospital-level analysis is often conducted using administrative data such as hospital discharge datasets, American Hospital Association survey data, or Medicare cost reports. Because administrative data are relatively inexpensive compared to unit-level customized data, the number of hospitals from which data can be collected and analyzed and whose performance can be compared is much larger. Second, over the course of an admission patients may move among units. In these cases, attributing complications or adverse outcomes to care in a specific unit may be difficult.

In addition, confidentiality and privacy for both patients and nurses may diminish the usefulness of unit-level reporting. For example, in the event that the number of nurses or patients on a unit is so few as to enable identification and use of results for punitive purposes, hospital-level reporting offers some protections. There are clear trade-offs among scope, cost, precision, and privacy that must be addressed in defining a nursing performance system.

### Availability and Comparability+ Data

The issue of using administrative datasets or custom datasets is one of cost, but two other issues also emerge in making a choice among alternative sources of data. The first is that nursing records are generally not available through administrative datasets. Discharge data are abstracted from physician notes, and nurses' notes are not used for diagnosis or procedures. Second, the data systems for nursing diagnosis, intervention, and outcomes that nurses have developed are not standardized. Lack of standardization and lack of automation discourage use of nursing data from patient charts. As patient records are standardized and nursing informatics becomes more strongly established,[27] this problem may be reduced. An issue in developing a nursing performance system is whether to anticipate these developments or plan for the immediate future assuming their absence.

## Measuring Nursing Performance

Nursing performance measurement is an emerging "enterprise." Florence Nightingale, the legendary architect of professional nursing, is quoted as saying, "To understand God's thoughts, we must study statistics, for these are the measure of His purpose,"[28] but it is a relatively recent phenomenon to measure, analyze, and report nursing's impact on care.

## An Overview of Factors Believed to Influence Nursing's Performance

A range of factors have been put forward as influencing the performance of nursing. These factors fall into four broad categories: nurse training and competencies, physical plant and structure, nursing organization, and work environment and culture.

Nurse training and competencies reflect the skills individual nurses bring to the hospital and the bedside. Formal training—level of education, advanced practice training, knowledge of specific equipment and patient conditions—are a part of this factor. Research on factors influencing successful nurse decision making add additional competencies that are provided partly by training and partly by experience. The models put forward vary, but they have included such factors as clinical skills, knowledge and understanding, interpersonal skills, problem-solving skills, clinical judgment, and moral sensibility.[29]

Physical plant and structure can influence workload, but they can also contribute to performance. Computerization can reduce errors in order entry and retrieval and charting. Nursing unit layout can influence the ability to quickly respond to patient needs or obtain needed supplies or drugs quickly and without error. Standardization in design of patient rooms and equipment may also contribute to reduced errors on the part of nurses.[30]

The presence of some types of equipment can also reduce the risk of drug errors or of a nurse injuring herself or himself. The U.S. nursing workforce is aging,[31] and as it ages ergonomic considerations become more important in ensuring that older nurses can do their work accurately and effectively.

Nursing organization should influence nursing performance, but its precise impact is not well established. Direct comparison is rare in the literature, and the absence of consistently applied definitions and rigor in the design of research makes it hard to draw strong conclusions. Thomas and Bond report several studies that suggest primary nursing produces better outcomes, but the designs are weak and none examines the factors influencing why hospitals select specific models.[32] Studies that focus on the proportion of RNs in the nursing workforce in hospitals, without regard to the specific model used to organize nursing, consistently find a positive impact of a higher mix of RNs on a range of patient outcomes.

The impact of nursing work environment and culture has been more widely studied, using a variety of instruments and alternative datasets. Many of these studies focus on nurse satisfaction with their work, but others examine the association of patient outcomes with various aspects of work environment and culture, either individually or collectively. Aiken's work on magnet hospitals and hospital mortality is an example of such studies.[33] Among the factors that have been associated with good nursing performance are flattening of organizational structures, increased professional status for staff nurses associated with shared governance and increased autonomy over practice and the practice environment, and effective communication among nurses, physicians, and administrators.[34]

## Recent Activities and Efforts to Measure Nursing Care Performance

A range of activities relate directly or indirectly to measurement of nursing performance in hospitals.

***ANA Nursing Safety and Quality Initiative.*** In 1994, the ANA began its Nursing Safety and Quality Initiative.[35] This initiative involved development of hospital quality indicators, recruitment of nurses and hospitals to collect data on staffing and the indicators in six states (California, Texas, Arizona, Virginia, North Dakota, and Minnesota), and pooling of the data for future analysis in a repository, the National Database of Nursing Quality Indicators (NDNQI).[36] The ten initial indicators selected included a mix of patient outcomes, process measures, and measures of nurse staffing, which can be viewed as structure measures. The *outcome measures* included

- Nosocomial infection rate (bacteremia)
- Patient injury rate
- Patient satisfaction with nursing care
- Patient satisfaction with pain management
- Patient satisfaction with educational information
- Patient satisfaction with care

*Process of care measures* were

- Maintenance of skin integrity (patients with pressure ulcers)
- Nurse staff satisfaction

- *Nursing measures* included

- Proportion of nursing care hours provided by registered nurses
- Total nursing care hours per patient day

Parallel to this activity, ANA also contracted for a study using patient discharge abstracts of the association of nurse staffing with four outcomes: pressure ulcers, pneumonia, urinary tract infections, and postoperative infections. The study found an association of these four outcomes with the proportion of licensed nursing hours provided by registered nurses, and it also found an association of licensed hours per day with pressure ulcers, postoperative infections, and length of stay.[37]

***Federal Efforts.*** In 1996, the Institute of Medicine issued a report that found a "serious paucity of recent research" on nurse staffing and quality.[38] In response to that report, four federal agencies—the Health Resources and Services Administration, Health Care Financing Administration (now the Centers for Medicare and Medicaid Services), Agency for Healthcare Research and Quality (AHRQ), and National Institute for Nursing Research—developed a research agenda and jointly and individually funded a range of research projects intended to fill this gap.[39] One study from this group was published in 2001 by the federal government,[40] and more recently the results were presented in the *New England Journal of Medicine*.[41] The study tested associations between nurse staffing and eleven patient outcomes in medical patients and fourteen in surgical patients.

***Institute of Medicine.*** In response to mounting concern about the adverse effects of poor or inadequate nurse staffing, the IOM released a report in 1996 titled *Nursing Staff in Hospitals and Nursing Homes*.[42] Fourteen recommendations resulted from the study, largely focused on increasing the nursing labor market and the readiness of that market (nurse staffing, staffing mix, work-related injuries). Additionally, under contract with AHRQ the IOM undertook a recent study of the work environment for nurses and patient safety. This report, *Keeping Patients Safe: Transforming the Work Environment of Nurses* (2004), reviews the working conditions of nurses and their relationship to patient safety.[43]

***American Nurses Credentialing Center—Magnet Hospitals.*** An alternate approach to defining measures of interest associated with nursing and testing their association is to identify hospitals that have a reputation for good nursing and success in recruiting and retaining nurses, and then look at their characteristics. This is the approach taken in identifying magnet hospitals.[44] A substantial body of research has examined the nature of the nursing systems in magnet hospitals, and nurses' satisfaction with these hospitals. Key attributes of the magnet hospitals were the visibility and seniority of the nurse administrators in the hospital hierarchy, flat organization of the nursing service with few supervisory layers, decision making decentralized to the nursing unit, substantial nurse autonomy coupled to a primary nursing model, collaborative nurse-physician relationships, high proportion of the nursing staff being RNs, and high RN-to-patient ratio.[45] There is less research on the association of patient outcomes and magnet hospital status, but in separate studies Aiken and colleagues found magnet hospital status associated with lower Medicare mortality[46] and higher patient satisfaction among AIDS patients.[47]

The magnet hospital concept has evolved into a formal accreditation process, directed by the American Nurses Credentialing Center within the ANA. The characteristics that described magnet hospitals have become criteria for designation within the Magnet Nursing Services Recognition Program,[48] and as such they may represent a series of process measures for nursing system performance.

*Patient Satisfaction Measurement.* Still another approach to identifying high-performing nursing systems is to systematically assess patient satisfaction with dimensions of nursing care that are associated with nursing. One such system is the ANA Nursing Indicators, discussed earlier, which uses as its survey form the Patient Satisfaction Instrument.[49] Another survey, not targeted to nursing but applicable to domains in which nurses work, is the Picker Institute Patient Satisfaction Survey. A well-validated instrument, it seeks information from patients about their experience with care. It asks questions in six domains, summarized in Table 12.2. Items with direct relation to nursing are in italics.

The Picker Institute in the United States ceased independent operation, but the survey has been taken over by HBS International.[50] It is accepted by the Joint Commission on Accreditation of Healthcare Organizations (JCAHO) as a measure of hospital performance in meeting patient needs for education, self-care, and expectations of care.

The federal government has recently initiated an effort to develop a standardized public domain instrument to measure patient perspectives on care. This instrument, the Hospital Consumer Assessment of Health Plans Survey (HCAHPS), includes items regarding patient perception of the quality of communication with nursing staff. HCAHPS is currently undergoing consensus review through the National Quality Forum.

### *Joint Commission on Accreditation of Healthcare Organizations (JCAHO).*
JCAHO accredits more than sixteen thousand health care organizations in the United States, including some five thousand hospitals. Over the past decade, it has substantially expanded its accreditation process to require more process and outcome measures.[51] In a recent action, it created a new standard for accreditation: "The organization uses data on clinical/service screening indicators in combination with human resource screening indicators to assess staffing effectiveness."

Under this standard, the organization is required to select two clinical or service indicators and correlate them with two human resource indicators. One of the clinical or service indicators and one of the human resource indicators must be drawn from a JCAHO-specified list. The indicators must be examined longitudinally.

## TABLE 12.2. PICKER INSTITUTE SURVEY DOMAINS AND ILLUSTRATIONS OF INFORMATION SOUGHT.

**Respect for patients' values, preferences, and expressed needs**

Having enough say about one's treatment

*Being treated with respect and dignity*

*People not talking in front of you as if you weren't there*

**Coordination of care**

*How organized the hospital was*

Wait time to go to room

Tests performed on time

**Information and education**

*Getting understandable answers to important questions*

*Given explanations for delays*

*Getting enough information about condition and treatment*

**Physical comfort**

*Feeling that staff did everything they could to control pain*

*Appropriate call button response time*

**Emotional support**

*Having confidence and trust in the doctors and nurses*

*Doctors and nurses discussed your anxieties and fears about condition*

Involvement of family and friends

Having enough opportunity to talk to doctors

Getting enough information needed to help in patient's recovery

**Continuity and transition**

Given clear explanations of purpose of medications

Told about side effects, danger signals, when to resume usual activities

*Note:* Italicized items have a direct relationship to nursing.

*Source:* University of Arkansas Medical Sciences [http://www.uams.edu/gme/patient.htm] (accessed June 19, 2002).

***American Hospital Association.*** The issue of hospital workforce and its perfor-mance has also become the focus of activity at the American Hospital Associa-tion. Its Commission on Workforce for Hospitals and Health Systems recently released the report *In Our Hands: How Hospital Leaders Can Build a Thriving Workforce.*[52] In the report, the commission trumpeted the need to transform "hospitals into modern day organizations in which all aspects of the work are designed around patients and the needs of staff to care for and support them" and to "improve the workplace partnership by creating a culture in which hospital staff . . . are valued, have sustained voice in shaping institutional policies, and receive appropriate rewards and recognition for their efforts." The report calls for changes that would bring workload and staffing into better balance and assure staff of more time with patients, and specific mechanism for introducing new technologies and redesigning work and work processes. Enhanced systems that measure the performance of nursing would potentially allow hospitals to assess whether they are moving closer to or further from these goals.

***California Nursing Outcomes Coalition (CalNOC).*** CalNOC is a collaborative project of ANA/California, the Association of California Nurse Leaders, and the CalNOC Steering Committee. Under this collaborative, a California statewide nursing quality outcomes database has been constructed with more than 130 active hospital participants. Measures include the ANA/NDNQI measures as well as a number that are unique to CalNOC participants (for example, contract labor, staffing ratios, restraint prevalence). Additionally, CalNOC is pilot testing additional measures as well as existing measures with unique populations for future use (catheter associated blood stream infections, pediatric hospitals). The Veterans Health Administration (VHA) and the Department of Defense (DOD) are in the process of establishing nursing outcomes databases modeled after the CalNOC database.

***Institute for Healthcare Improvement.*** IHI has engaged nearly one hundred organizations as members of its Impact Network. Members use a collaborative approach to learning and improvement on one of five topics, among them workforce development. As part of the collaborative method, participating members select measures that can be used to gauge progress. Currently, nearly thirty hospitals are dealing with workforce development issues collecting personnel measures, including nursing, in some of these areas: turnover, vacancy, retention, recruitment, loyalty and staff satisfaction, patient satisfaction, and staff costs.

***Health Plans, Hospitals, and Multihospital Systems.*** A number of hospitals, hospital systems, and health plans have also initiated nursing performance measurement efforts. What follows are merely examples of efforts to better understand nursing's contribution to hospital outcomes and patient safety.

Kaiser Permanente initiated the Inpatient Nursing Quality Indicator Project (INQIP). Under this project, more than seventy indicators of inpatient nursing care are collected and analyzed at the unit, hospital, and regional levels. A smaller subset of these measures are analyzed nationally. INQIP measures are generated from eleven unique data collection instruments within three "families": patient education, pain management (labor and delivery, medical and surgical and critical care, neonatal intensive care unit or NICU, pediatrics, and postpartum), and specialty indicators (breast feeding, critical care sedation and safety, NICU developmental care, pediatric immunizations, functional mobility). Observational and survey data from the instruments are used to derive measures generally related to nursing assessment and evaluation, patient perception of care, patient learning, and nurse-provided education.

VHA Inc., which represents more than twenty-two hundred community-based hospitals (24 percent of all U.S. hospitals), also has several national and regional workforce initiatives that include nursing-related measurement. Specifically, under VHA Inc.'s "Tomorrow's Workforce," thirty-nine hospital systems are collecting six human resource metrics and staff satisfaction. Another fifty to sixty hospitals are participating in regional-level measurement activities based on these same measures. The focus of these efforts is not nursing-specific, but data are analyzed in subcategories that include RNs and advance practice nurses along with LPNs and aides.

# Measuring Nursing Performance: The State of the Science

Given the imperative to better understand nursing's influence on patient outcomes, a growing body of empirical research has been undertaken to quantify nursing performance and its impact. This emerging research has focused primarily on examining the association between measures of the process and structure of nursing care and patient outcomes.

## Research on Outcomes Influenced by Nursing

Outcome measurement is one of the cornerstones of performance measurement, and to that end a range of outcomes have been tested for an association with nursing. There is substantial evidence of an association of nurse staffing and a range of hospital-acquired infections, including pneumonia and urinary tract infection (although not sepsis). There is evidence of an association of nurse staffing and other adverse outcomes, including falls, medication errors, pain management, shock and cardiac arrest, upper gastrointestinal bleeding, and length of stay (which may influence costs of care). The evidence of an effect of nurse staffing on overall hospital mortality is mixed, and we conclude that the association has not yet been fully demonstrated. There is evidence for an effect of nurse staffing on a subset of deaths, those among patients who have a life-threatening complication whose course might be influenced by early detection and intervention ("failure to rescue"). Evidence for other outcomes, most notably pressure ulcers and deep vein thrombosis, is mixed. Additionally, RN hours as a proportion of all nursing staff hours are associated more strongly, and with more outcomes, than RN hours per patient day.[53]

Typically, as shown in Table 12.3, rates of adverse events are 3–9 percent lower in hospitals with RN staffing at the 75th percentile of the distribution of hospitals compared to hospitals at the 25th percentile.

## Issues in Measuring Outcomes

Collectively, this research finds a variety of outcomes associated with nurse staffing. What should we make of the failure to consistently find an association with nursing and mortality or other outcomes that one might expect to be associated with it? There are several possible explanations, and they have implications for the design of nursing performance systems.

### TABLE 12.3. SUMMARY OF ASSOCIATION OF LOWER NURSE STAFFING AND PATIENT OUTCOMES.

| Patient Pool | Outcome | Higher Rate for Outcome Is Associated with: | | Difference in Rate Between Low- and High-RN hospitals (%) |
| --- | --- | --- | --- | --- |
| | | Lower Proportion of RNs | Fewer RN Hours Per Day | |
| Medical patients | Length of stay | X | X | 3.5–5.2 |
| | Urinary tract infection | X | X | 3.6–9.0 |
| | Upper gastrointestinal bleeding | X | X | 5.1–5.2 |
| | Pneumonia | X | | 6.4 |
| | Shock or cardiac arrest | X | | 9.4 |
| | Failure to rescue | X | | 2.5 |
| Surgical patients | Urinary tract infection | X | | 4.9 |
| | Failure to rescue | | X | 5.9 |

*Note:* The column "Difference in rate between low- and high-RN hospitals" is an estimate of the reduction in adverse events that would be realized if RN staffing were that of a hospital at the 75th percentile of the distribution rather than the 25th percentile.

*Source:* Derived from Needleman, J., and others. Nurse Staffing and Patient Outcomes in Hospitals. Boston: Harvard School of Public Health, Feb. 28, 2001. Report no.: Final Report submitted under contract 230-99-0021 [http://bhpr.hrsa.gov/nursing/staffstudy.htm].

*Are the Data Captured and Retrieved?* To associate an outcome with nursing, or to use an outcome as an indicator, one must have confidence that the outcome is reported in the dataset used with sufficient frequency and regularity that the rate is a good measure of nursing's performance. For unit-based studies, with data collection in real time from charts on the floor, with staff sensitized to identify and record specific events, data capture and retrieval may not be an issue. For studies in which these conditions are not met, problems in the data-generating process may undercut the confidence that can be placed in measures. As noted in a study of the implementation of ANA indicators in one medical center, "the extent to which databases are in place to capture any of these indicator data reduces the need for labor-intensive chart abstraction and thus enhances the ease of retrievability."[54]

*How Specific and Linkable Is the Outcome to Nursing?* Many factors may contribute to an outcome, of which nursing is only one and perhaps not the most important. Variations in rate unrelated to nursing add noise to the data and make observing an association more difficult. Variations due to other factors associated with nursing can also make statistical inference difficult. For example, Jennings and colleagues question the use of bacteremia as a nursing-related infection, noting that "nosocomial infections may be less relevant if the focus remains on bacteremia from central lines. Physicians usually insert these lines, and the possibility of contamination on insertion cannot be discounted."[55]

*Infrequent Events.* There are two problems in demonstrating that infrequently occurring events are associated with nursing in statistical analysis. First, the power of the analysis is reduced. Second, a substantial number of hospitals will have no cases of infrequent events—even if nurse staffing is low and nursing is associated with the event—simply because most hospitals are small and the pool of patients in which the complication can occur is small. A large number of hospitals with no events also reduces the power of the analysis. If one believes in the link between a specific complication and nurse staffing on the basis of clinical judgments, then one can use it, but one should not expect such events to be validated in cross-sectional statistical analyses of hospital experience.

*Risk Adjustment.* Risk adjustment is critical for comparing the rate of adverse events across hospitals. Inadequate risk adjustment may have weakened results in some studies, and it could be especially difficult to do in unit-level analyses.[56] Thus there are a range of reasons no association might have been observed in these studies, and the reasons influence the design of a nursing performance system. There is a need for continued efforts to refine and improve measures and data used to generate them.

## Issues in Measuring Processes of Care and Structural Proxies

In examining measures of process and structure, one needs to question whether the nurse staffing is adequate relative to patient needs and whether other organizational factors amenable to change influence nursing performance. Several measurement problems stand in the way of finding answers to these two questions: variations in nursing case mix, differences in physical plant, differences in organization and culture across nursing units or hospitals, and counting nurses within the hospital.

*Patient-Level Adjustment: Nursing Case Mix.* Case mix makes a difference in the adequacy of nurse staffing on a unit or in a hospital. Frailer patients, bed-bound patients, and those requiring closer monitoring all require more nursing time. One hospital may be adequately staffed for its patient acuity at six hours per patient day while another is short-staffed. Adjustment is necessary if comparisons are to be made across hospitals or over time.

The adjustment should be made on the basis of nursing need, not general patient acuity or need for all services. A number of studies have used the average diagnosis-related group (DRG) case-mix index for the hospital to adjust estimates of nursing hours or nursing FTEs per patient day.[57] There are many advantages to using the DRG case-mix index (it is a standardized measure that can be calculated from the discharge abstract data and has been widely used in prior research), but it has a number of weaknesses. Most significant, studies show that DRGs are poorly correlated with patient nursing need.[58]

An alternative measure would be the staffing projection that emerges from nursing workload or nurse staffing systems such as Medicus system of Quadramed and GRASP Workload Management System. All accredited hospitals are supposed to have such systems, although approximately half of U.S. hospitals use a system developed at that hospital. In principle, the staffing that emerges from these systems is adjusted to the physical plant and nursing model used at the hospital. One potential performance measure would be the ratio of actual-to-projected staffing, as estimated from the system.

There are several important limitations of these systems as they currently exist. Because there are so many hospital-specific systems, systems are not comparable across hospitals and there is no gold standard for measuring staffing. Systems differ in the staffing need they would project in the same case mix in the same hospital.[59] Systems require validating, updating, and recalibration if the estimates are to remain valid.[60] Hospitals may also adjust their projection system to staff tightly or generously. Though the potential to use data from these systems in performance measurement is high, these issues need to be addressed before comparison across hospitals can be viewed as reliable.

For studies that attempt to compare outcomes and staffing across hospitals or acuity-adjusted staffing over time, systems that are codable in administrative datasets are needed, but no such systems currently exist. As has been noted, DRG case-mix indexes are poorly correlated with needed nurse staffing. Several researchers have, however, used the DRG patient classification framework to construct patient nursing acuity measures. One approach has been to group DRGs into clusters according to anticipated nursing needs, or to divide DRGs into more homogeneous categories relative to nursing levels, using measures such as number of secondary diagnoses or number of MDCs into which secondary diagnoses fall.[61] Another approach is to estimate the nursing workload for each DRG and construct a nursing case mix from this DRG weight.[62]

***Physical Plant Impacts on Nurse Staffing Needs and Organization.*** Research has found a range of factors that influence the efficiency with which nurses can carry out their work, notably physical layout, communications systems,[63] and computerization.[64] The physical layout of a hospital nursing unit can influence nurse staffing needs and the ability of nursing staff to observe patients closely.[65]

Physical layout, communications systems, and computerization all vary widely among hospitals, and systems to measure adequacy of nursing must take such differences into account. In theory, creation of hospital-specific staff projection systems, or customization of commercial systems such as Quadramed's Medicus or GRASP, should take such differences into account. Data to incorporate such information into hospital-level monitoring systems, or to adjust staffing per patient day from hospital-level measurement, are currently not available.

***Impact of Work Organization on Nursing Need.*** The least-studied dimension of factors that influence need for nursing and nursing effectiveness are those associated with work organization. These include characteristics of the nurses themselves, the composition of the nursing team, scheduling and coordination, and culture and work environment.[66] Studies have demonstrated that they all have an impact on nursing performance and outcomes.[67]

Minnick and Pabst found that there was a tendency in hospitals to underassign nurses on units in which the suggested hours of care from the acuity or workload system were high.[68] These units have high staffing, but not as high as needed. They note that if adjustment for acuity is not adequate in analysis, it will appear that higher nurse staffing is associated with poorer outcomes. They also suggest that if nurse administrators assign more experienced staff to these understaffed units, the greater experience might offset some of the increased risk of poor outcomes due to insufficient staffing.

Since nursing models are likely to be chosen in response to the mix of staff and staff skills available (and, in turn, hospitals are likely to hire staff that fit their nursing model), knowing the nursing model in use should yield information about the staff structure in a hospital. Unfortunately, as noted earlier, definitions of models are not always used consistently. This is another issue that must be addressed in designing performance measurement systems.

Organizational culture, particularly elements related to nurse autonomy, ability to exercise professional judgment and participate in nursing unit decision making, social support, and stress, have all been found to be associated with nurse satisfaction and nursing performance. Many studies use direct surveys of staff nurses to obtain information about organization and culture. A number of instruments have been used, among them the Nursing Work Index,[69] Insel and Moos's Work Environment Scale (WES),[70] McCloskey/Mueller Satisfaction Scale (MMSS),[71] and Job Content Questionnaire (JCQ).[72] Surveys are expensive to undertake, and overworked nurses may resist responding to requests to participate. The domains and focus of the instruments differ, and one must decide for what dimensions of the work environment it is most important to obtain information.

***Counting Nurses.*** Counting the size and composition of the nursing staff in a hospital would appear to be straightforward, but this proves not to be the case conceptually or operationally. One issue is whom to count. Are nursing managers part of the nursing staff for purposes of counting nurses? If it is a unit study, how should staff that work in several units be counted?[73] Interest is usually in productive hours of care to inpatients in all nursing categories, but data systems do not furnish the information needed to construct these measures with great precision. Nursing staff are often reported in full-time equivalents (FTEs), but nursing hours and shifts vary across hospitals, making the translation of FTEs into hours of care imprecise. Aide data are absent in national databases; they have never been collected by Medicare and were dropped from the American Hospital Association annual survey in 1994. Agency and contract staff are incompletely reported in staffing surveys. Inpatient nurse staffing (with the exception of a few state datasets) must be estimated from hospital-level staffing, which is always imprecise. Information on overtime—an emerging issue in nurse staffing—is available from only a few state datasets.

How nursing hours per day is interpreted is also influenced by the scope of nurses' work in the hospital and the impact on nursing of nonnurse direct patient care providers. Nurses operate in teams within nursing units and in coordination with other services (transport, pharmacy, phlebotomy, dietary). There are no good measures in most systems of labor in these areas, only overall staffing. Analysis of the adequacy of nurse staffing and nursing performance needs to take into account the availability of support services in these other areas.

# NQF's Endorsed National Voluntary Consensus Standards for Nursing-Sensitive Care

In February 2003, the National Quality Forum (NQF)[74] undertook a fourteen-month project to study the relationship between nursing personnel and quality and degree to which national voluntary consensus standards for nursing-sensitive care could be established. Recognizing the nature of the emerging evidence base and the degree to which significant challenges exist in standardizing nursing measurement, the project surveyed the field to identify the range of measures in use and critically assessed the evidence base supporting the measures. NQF's process involved a large and highly diverse group of stakeholders in a structured process directed at endorsing a set of national nursing-sensitive performance measures.

NQF relied on two key processes to drive the endorsement of nursing-sensitive consensus standards: its unique Consensus Development Process (CDP) and the Measure Evaluation Process. The Consensus Development Process is the formal approach taken by NQF to endorse standards, including performance measures, quality indicators, preferred practices, and reporting guidelines. The Measure Evaluation Process was used as the primary mechanism to achieve standard development, the first step in the consensus process. This process involved establishing a purpose for the standards, developing a conceptual framework for measurement, devising a scope and set of priorities to guide measure selection, evaluating candidate measures on the basis of standard measure evaluation criteria, and recommending proposed consensus standards. A summary of the purpose statement, framework for measurement, scope and priorities, and measure evaluation criteria can be found in the final report of this project.[75]

NQF sought measures that reflected the contribution of nursing personnel to providing quality care. To this end, a unique assessment of "nursing sensitivity" was conducted. Specifically, measures that were recommended as proposed consensus standards represent structural, process, and outcome measures that are linked by evidence to nursing variables. To be designated as a nursing-sensitive consensus standard, the measure had to directly measure some element of nurse staffing that has been associated with better quality care or be quantifiably influenced by nursing personnel, although the relationship did not need to be shown to be causal or exclusive to nursing. The culmination of this effort was the endorsement by the NQF board of directors in April 2004 of fifteen national voluntary consensus standards for nursing-sensitive care (Table 12.4) and eleven related research and implementation recommendations (Table 12.5).

## TABLE 12.4. NQF-ENDORSED NATIONAL VOLUNTARY CONSENSUS STANDARDS FOR NURSING-SENSITIVE CARE.

| Framework Category | Measure | Description |
|---|---|---|
| Patient-centered outcome measures | Death among surgical inpatients with treatable serious complications (failure to rescue) | Percentage of major surgical inpatients who experience a hospital-acquired complication (sepsis, pneumonia, gastrointestinal bleeding, shock or cardiac arrest, deep vein thrombosis or pulmonary embolism) and die |
| | Pressure ulcer prevalence | Percentage of inpatients who have a hospital-acquired pressure ulcer (stage 2 or greater) |
| | Falls prevalence[a] | Number of inpatient falls per inpatient days |
| | Falls with injury | Number of inpatient falls with injuries per inpatient days |
| | Restraint prevalence (vest and limb only) | Percentage of inpatients who have a vest or limb restraint |
| | Urinary catheter-associated UTI for intensive care unit (ICU) patients[a] | Rate of UTI associated with use of urinary catheters for ICU patients |
| | Central line catheter-associated blood stream infection rate for ICU and high-risk nursery (HRN) patients[a] | Rate of blood stream infections associated with use of central line catheters for ICU and HRN patients |
| | Ventilator-associated pneumonia for ICU and HRN patients[a] | Rate of pneumonia associated with use of ventilators for ICU patients and HRN patients |
| Nursing-centered intervention measure | Smoking cessation counseling for acute myocardial infarction (AMI)[a] | Percentage of AMI inpatients with history of smoking within the past year who received smoking cessation advice or counseling during hospitalization |
| | Smoking cessation counseling for heart failure (HF)[a] | Percentage of HF inpatients with history of smoking within the past year who received smoking cessation advice or counseling during hospitalization |
| | Smoking cessation counseling for pneumonia[a] | Percentage of pneumonia inpatients with history of smoking within the past year who received smoking cessation advice or counseling during hospitalization |

## TABLE 12.4. NQF-ENDORSED NATIONAL VOLUNTARY CONSENSUS STANDARDS FOR NURSING-SENSITIVE CARE, Cont'd.

| Framework Category | Measure | Description |
|---|---|---|
| System-centered measures | Skill mix (RN, LPN, UAP, and contract) | • Percentage of registered nursing (RN) care hours of total nursing care hours<br>• Percentage of licensed vocational or practical nursing (LVN/LPN) care hours of total nursing care hours<br>• Percentage of unlicensed assistive personnel (UAP) care hours of total nursing care hours<br>• Percentage of contract hours (RN, LVN or LPN, and UAP) of total nursing care hours |
| | Nursing care hours per patient day (RN, LPN, and UAP) | • Number of RN care hours per patient day<br>• Number of nursing staff hours (RN, LVN or LPN, UAP) per patient day |
| | Practice Environment Scale—Nursing Work Index (composite and five subscales) | Composite score and mean presence scores for subscales derived from PES-NWI:<br>• Nurse participation in hospital affairs<br>• Nursing foundations for quality of care<br>• Nurse manager ability, leadership, and support of nurses<br>• Staffing and resource adequacy<br>• Collegial nurse-physician relations |
| | Voluntary turnover | Number of voluntary uncontrolled separations during the month for RNs and advanced practice nurses, LPNs, and nurse assistants or aides |

*Note:* [a] These measures have been previously endorsed as National Voluntary Consensus Standards for Hospital Care. See National Quality Forum. *National Voluntary Consensus Standards for Hospital Care: An Initial Performance Measure Set.* Washington, D.C.: National Quality Forum, 2003.

## TABLE 12.5. NQF-ENDORSED RECOMMENDATIONS FOR RESEARCH AND IMPLEMENTATION.

| Research Recommendation | General Description |
| --- | --- |
| Development of workforce measures and empirical base to support them | Research should be undertaken on the relationshipbetween nursing variables and patient outcomes. |
| Development of pain assessment and management measures | Research should be undertaken to identify measures that specifically explore nursing's contribution to assessment and management of pain. |
| Development of nurse-centered intervention process measures | Research should be undertaken to determine the relationship between patient outcomes and process measures. |
| Sufficiency of measures against evaluation criteria | Research should be initiated that investigates and documents each measure's adequacy against the NQF evaluation criteria. |
| Development of measures where gaps in consensus exist | Additional research should be undertaken to address a broad range of important areas for which no measures exist. |
| **Implementation Recommendation** | **General Description** |
| Recommendation related to data issues | Providers, researchers, and information system vendors need to develop better data systems to support nursing care monitoring functions. |
| Use for Quality Improvement | Measures should be collected and analyzed by providers at the hospital unit level. |
| Implementation | The readiness of provider organizations to implement these consensus standards is an overall indication of their commitment to quality. |
| Scope of consensus standards | The NQF-endorsed consensus standards for nursing-sensitive performance should be viewed by health care stakeholders as a constellation of measures (measure set). |
| Improving the set | Review of the initial set of voluntary consensus standards for nursing-sensitive care should be conducted regularly. |

*Source:* National Quality Forum. *National Voluntary Consensus Standards for Hospital Care: An Initial Performance Measure Set.* Washington, D.C.: National Quality Forum, 2004.

In the course of this work, NQF found that confidence in many proposed or previously used measures was limited by an inadequate research base or absence of validating studies, issues of data reliability, or questions about how closely the measure was associated with nursing and nursing care. As a result, most of the measures included in the dataset require primary data collection or chart abstraction—activities involving significant effort or cost. The research and implementation recommendations call for efforts to broaden the range of available measures, conduct validation studies for existing measures for which the evidence base is limited, systematize data collection, and incorporate collection and construction of measures into ongoing systems to reduce the cost of measuring nursing and nursing related work.

## Conclusions

Measuring the performance of hospital nursing care is becoming increasingly important in an attempt to monitor the impact of nurse staffing levels in hospitals and to support hospital nursing-related quality improvement activities. Developing effective performance measurement systems enables health care stakeholders to better understand and monitor the degree to which nursing care influences patient safety and health care quality. NQF's work builds on a growing body of research and an expanding number of initiatives intended for this purpose. To date, several health systems, government agencies, and accreditation organizations have committed to implementing the NQF endorsed set of nursing-sensitive consensus standards. However, these commitments represent early adoption of standards that are intended for widespread, national use.

Clearly, even though NQF's work to endorse a set of national voluntary consensus standards for nursing-sensitive care is a first step in gaining consensus on measures for this purpose, much work remains to be done. A fully functional system of nursing-sensitive performance measurement requires developing measures that address all the domains of nursing that should be monitored and all the aspects of health care quality (care that is safe, beneficial, efficient, patient-centered, timely, and equitable), addressing technical issues needed to effectively analyze the impact of nursing (risk adjustment and other hospital-to-hospital and longitudinal variations), developing data systems that yield the information needed to implement the model system, regularly improving the set of endorsed standards so that they reflect the most current science and empirical evidence, and persuading all health care stakeholders (consumers, purchasers, providers, and so on) that measurement and reporting nursing-sensitive standards make a difference in the care and quality that are delivered. Each of these tasks requires substantial development work and construction and maintenance of the infrastructure to sustain the performance measurement efforts.

# Notes

1. U.S. Department of Health and Human Services, Health Resources and Services Administration, Bureau of Health Professions, Division of Nursing. "The Registered Nurse Population: Findings from the National Sample Survey of Registered Nurses, March 2000." ftp://ftp.hrsa.gov/bhpr/rnsurvey2000/rnsurvey00.pdf (accessed Feb. 14, 2005).

2. In *Crossing the Quality Chasm,* the Institute of Medicine identifies six aims of the health care quality system: safe, effective, efficient, timely, patient-centered, and equitable. In October 2000, the NQF board of directors adopted a purpose statement that largely mirrors the IOM aims but states that another aim should be "beneficial," which encompasses but also goes beyond effectiveness.

3. Institute of Medicine, Committee on the Quality of Health Care in America. *Crossing the Quality Chasm: A New Health System for the 21st Century.* Washington, D.C.: National Academy Press, 2001; Committee on the Work Environment for Nurses and Patient Safety. *Keeping Patients Safe: Transforming the Work Environment of Nurses.* (A. Page, ed.) Washington, D.C.: National Academies Press, 2004.

4. Greiner, A. *Cost and Quality Matters: Workplace Innovations in Health Care Industry.* Washington, D.C.: Economics Policy Institute, 1995; Wunderlich, and others. (Institute of Medicine, Committee on the Adequacy of Nurse Staffing in, and Homes Nursing.) *Nursing Staff in Hospitals and Nursing Homes: Is It Adequate?* Washington, D.C.: National Academy Press, 1996; Shindul-Rothschild, J. "Patient Care: How Good Is It Where You Work?" *American Journal of Nursing,* 1996, *96*(3), 22–24; Peter D. Hart Research Associates. *Health Professionals' View of Quality: A National Survey.* Washington, D.C.: Peter D. Hart Research Associates, 1997; Advisory Commission on Consumer Protection and Quality in the Health Care Industry. *Engaging the Health Care Workforce.* Washington, D.C.: Advisory Commission on Consumer Protection and Quality in the Health Care Industry, 1997; Schultz, M., and van Servellen, G. "A Critical Review of Research on Hospital Mortality Among Medical-Surgical and Acute Myocardial Infarction Patients." *Nursing and Health Sciences,* 2000, *2*(2), 103–112; Aiken, L., and others. "Nurses' Reports on Hospital Care in Five Countries." *Health Affairs,* 2001, *20*(3), 43–53.

5. Barter, M., McLaughlin, F. E., and Thomas, S. A. "Use of Unlicensed Assistive Personnel by Hospitals." *Nursing Economics,* 1994, *12*(2), 82–87; Bernreuter, M., and Cardona, S. "Survey and Critique of Studies Related to Unlicensed Assistive Personnel from 1975 to 1997, Part 2." *Journal of Nursing Administration,* 1997, *27*(7/8), 49–55; Brider, P. "Morale Skidding with Restructuring." *American Journal of Nursing,* 1996 *96*(2), 62–64; Gilliland, M. "Workforce Reductions: Low Morale, Reduced Quality Care." *Nursing Economics,* 1997,*15*(6), 320–322; McCloskey, J. C., Bulecheck, G. M., Moorhead, S., and Daly, J. "Nurses' Use and Delegation of Indirect Care Interventions." *Nursing Economics,* 1996, *14*(1), 22–33; O'Neil, E., and Riley, T. "Health Workforce and Education Issues During System Transition." *Health Affairs,* 1996, *15*(1), 105–112.

6. Buerhaus, P. I., and Staiger, D. O. "Managed Care and the Nurse Workforce." *Journal of the American Medical Association,* 1996, *276*(18), 1487–1493; Buerhaus, P. I., and Auerbach, D. "Slow Growth in the United States of the Number of Minorities in the RN Workforce." *Image: Journal of Nursing Scholarship,* 1999, *31*(2), 179–183.

7. Kovner, C. T., Jones, C. B., and Gergen, P. J. "Nurse Staffing in Acute Care Hospitals, 1990-1996." *Policy, Politics, and Nursing Practice,* 2000, *1*(3), 194–204; Kovner, C., and others. "Nurse Staffing and Post-Surgical Adverse Events: An Analysis of Administrative Data from a Sample of U.S. Hospitals, 1990-1996." *Health Services Research,* 2002, *37*(3), 611–629.

8. Spetz, J. "Hospital Employment of Nursing Personnel: Has There Really Been a Decline?" *Journal of Nursing Administration,* 1998, *28*(3), 20–27.

9. Anderson, G., and Kohn, L. "Employment Trends in Hospitals, 1981-1993." *Inquiry,* 1996, *33*(1), 79–84.

10. Aiken, L. H., Sochalski, J., and Anderson, G. F. "Downsizing the Hospital Nursing Workforce." *Health Affairs,* 1996, *15*(4), 88–92.

11. Minnick, A. F., and Pabst, M. K. "Improving the Ability to Detect the Impact of Labor on Patient Outcomes." *Journal of Nursing Administration,* 1998, *28*(12), 17–21.

12. First Consulting Group. *The Healthcare Workforce Shortage and Its Implications for America's Hospitals.* Long Beach, Calif.: First Consulting Group, 2001.

13. Buerhaus, P. I., and Needleman, J. "Policy Implications of Research on Nurse Staffing and Quality of Patient Care." *Policy, Politics, and Nursing Practice,* 2000, *1*(1), 5–15.

14. Nursing-sensitive performance measures are processes and outcomes—and structural proxies for these processes and outcomes (such as skill mix, nurse staffing hours)—that are affected, provided, or influenced by nursing personnel—but for which nursing is not exclusively responsible. Nursing-sensitive measures must be quantifiably influenced by nursing personnel, but the relationship is not necessarily causal.

15. *Voluntary consensus standards* are defined as "common and repeated use of rules, conditions, guidelines or characteristics for products or related processes and production methods, and related management systems practices; the definition of terms; classification of components; delineation of procedures; specification of dimensions, materials, performance, designs, or operations; measurement of quality and quantity in describing materials, processes, products, systems, services, or practices; test methods and sampling procedures; or descriptions of fit and measurements of size or strength." U.S. Office of Management and Budget, Revised Circular A-119, *Federal Participation in the Development and Use of Voluntary Consensus Standards and in Conformity Assessment Activities,* Feb. 10, 1998.

16. Snyder, M., Egan, E. C., and Nojima, Y. "Defining Nursing Interventions." *Image: The Journal of Nursing Scholarship,* 1996, *28*(2), 137–141; Timpson, J. "Nursing Theory: Everything the Artist Spits Is Art?" *Journal of Advanced Nursing,* 1996, *23*(5), 1030–1036; Hilton, P. A. "Theoretical Perspectives of Nursing: A Review of the Literature." *Journal of Advanced Nursing,* 1997, *26*(6), 1211–1220.

17. Snyder, Egan, and Nojima (1996).

18. North American Nursing Diagnosis Association. *Nursing Diagnoses: Definitions and Classification, 1999-2000* (3rd ed.). Philadelphia: North American Nursing Diagnosis Association, 1999.

19. McCloskey, J. C., and Bulecheck, G. M. (eds.). *Nursing Interventions Classification (NIC): Iowa Intervention Project* (3rd ed.). St. Louis: Mosby, 2000.

20. Johnson, M., Maas, M., and Moorhead, S. (eds.). *Nursing Outcomes Classification (NOC)* (2nd ed.). St. Louis: Mosby, 2000.

21. Aquilino, M. L., and Keenan, G. "Having Our Say: Nursing's Standardized Nomenclatures." *American Journal of Nursing,* 2000, *100*(7), 33–38.

22. Martin, K. S., and Scheet, N. J. *The Omaha System: Applications for Community Health Nursing.* Philadelphia: Saunders, 1992.

23. Hendrickson, G. T., Doddato, M., and Kovner, C. T. "How Do Nurses Use Their Time?" *Journal of Nursing Administration,* 1990, *20*(3), 31–37.

24. Irvine, D., Sidani, S., and Hall, L. M. "Linking Outcomes to Nurses' Roles in Health Care." *Nursing Economics,* 1998, *16*, 58–87.

25. Brennan, P. F., Anthony, M., Jones, J., and Kahana, E. "Nursing Practice Models: Implications for Information System Design." *Journal of Nursing Administration,* Oct. 1998, *28*(10), 26–31.

26. Minnick, A. F., and others. "What Influences Patients' Reports of Three Aspects of Hospital Services?" *Medical Care,* 1997, *35*(4), 399–409.

27. Henry, S. B. "Nursing Informatics: State of the Science." *Journal of Advanced Nursing,* 1995, *22*(6), 1182–1192; Coenen, A., and others. "Toward Comparable Nursing Data: American Nurses Association Criteria for Data Sets, Classification Systems, and Nomenclatures." *Computers in Nursing,* 2001, *19*(6), 240–248; Goossen, W. T., and others. "A Comparison of Nursing Minimal Data Sets." *Journal of the American Medical Informatics Association,* 1998, *5*(2), 152–163.

28. Salsburg, D. *The Lady Tasting Tea: How Statistics Revolutionized Science in the Twentieth Century* (1st ed.). New York: Freeman, 2001.

29. Yura, H., and Walsh, M. *The Nursing Process: Assessing, Planning, Implementing, Evaluating.* Norwalk, Conn.: Appleton Century Crofts, 1967; Norman, G. R. "Defining Competence: A Methodological Review." In V. R. Neufeld and G. R. Norman (eds.), *Assessing Clinical Competence.* New York: Springer, 1985; Taylor, C. "Rethinking Nursing's Basic Competencies." *Journal of Nursing Care Quality,* 1995, *9*(4), 1–13.

30. Reiling, J., and others. "Facility Designing Around Patient Safety and Its Effect on Nursing." *Nursing Economics,* 2003, *21*(3), 143–147.

31. Buerhaus, P. I., Staiger, D. O., and Auerbach, D. I. "Implications of an Aging Registered Nurse Workforce." *Journal of the American Medical Association,* 2000, *283*(22), 2948–2954.

32. Thomas, L. H., and Bond, S. "The Effectiveness of Nursing: A Review." *Journal of Clinical Nursing,* 1995, *4*(3), 143–151.

33. Aiken, L. H., Smith, H. L., and Lake, E. T. "Lower Medicare Mortality Among a Set of Hospitals Known for Good Nursing Care." *Medical Care,* 1994, *32* (8), 771–787.

34. Avallone, I., and Gibbon, B. "Nurses' Perceptions of Their Work Environment in a Nursing Development Unit." *Journal of Advanced Nursing,* 1998, *27*(6), 1193–1201; Havens, D. S., and Aiken, L. H. "Shaping Systems to Promote Desired Outcomes: The Magnet Hospital Model." *Journal of Nursing Administration,* 1999, *29*(2), 14–20; Robinson, C. A. "Magnet Nursing Services Recognition: Transforming the Critical Care Environment." *AACN Clinical Issues,* 2001, *12*(3), 411–423.

35. Rowell, P. A., and Milholland, D. K. "Nursing and Threats to Patient and Nurse Safety and Quality of Patient Care." *Journal of Nursing Care Quality,* 1998, *12*(4), 9–13; Burtt, K. "State Nurses Associations Work to Prove Nursing Quality." *American Journal of Nursing,* 1998, *98*(5), 58–60.

36. Burtt (1998); Blecke, J., and Decker, S. "ANA Quality Indicators: Meaningful Measurement." *Michigan Nurse,* 1997, *70*(9), 9–10.

37. Network, Inc. *Nurse Staffing and Patient Outcomes in the Inpatient Hospital Setting.* Baltimore: American Nurses Association, 2000.

38. Wunderlich, G. S., Sloan F. A., and Davis C. K. (eds.). *Nursing Staff in Hospitals and Nursing Homes.* (Institute of Medicine.) Washington, D.C.: National Academy Press, 1996.

39. Buerhaus and Needleman (2000).

40. Needleman, J., and others. *Nurse Staffing and Patient Outcomes in Hospitals.* Boston: Harvard School of Public Health, 2001.

41. Needleman, J., and others. "Nurse-Staffing Levels and the Quality of Care in Hospitals." *New England Journal of Medicine,* 2002, *346*(22), 1715–1722.

42. Wunderlich, Sloan and Davis (1996).

43. Institute of Medicine (U.S.). Committee on the Work Environment for Nurses and Patient Safety. *Keeping Patients Safe: Transforming the Work Environment of Nurses.* Washington, D.C.: National Academies Press, 2003, p. A.

44. McClure, M. L., and Hinshaw, A. S. *Magnet Hospitals Revisited: Attraction and Retention of Professional Nurses.* (American Academy of Nursing.) Washington, D.C.: American Nurses, 2002.

45. Scott, J. G., Sochalski, J., and Aiken, L. "Review of Magnet Hospital Research: Findings and Implications for Professional Nursing Practice." *Journal of Nursing Administration,* 1999,*29*(1), 9–19; Havens and Aiken (1999).

46. Aiken, Smith, and Lake (1994).

47. Aiken, L. H., and others. "Organization and Outcomes of Inpatient AIDS Care." *Medical Care,* 1999, *37*, 760–772.

48. Robinson (2001).

49. Hinshaw, A. S., and Atwood, J. R. "A Patient Satisfaction Instrument: Precision by Replication." *Nursing Research,* 1982, *31*(3), 170–175, 191.

50. "Integrated System Links Cost Data, Patient Satisfaction Scores for the First Time." *Data Strategy Benchmarks,* 1999, *3*(10), 153–157, 145.

51. McGreevey, C., Nadzam, D., and Corbin, L. "The Joint Commission on Accreditation of Healthcare Organizations' Indicator Measurement System: Health Care Outcomes Database." *Computers in Nursing,* 1997, *15*(2 Suppl.), S87–S94.

52. AHA Commission on Workforce for Hospitals and Health Systems. *In Our Hands: How Hospital Leaders Can Build a Thriving Workforce.* Chicago: American Hospital Association, 2002.

53. For a detailed review of the literature, see Needleman, J. N., Kurtzman, E. T., and Kizer, K. W. *Performance Measurement of Nursing Care: State of the Science and Consensus Development* (prepared for Robert Wood Johnson Foundation), Washington, D.C.: National Quality Forum, Feb. 25, 2005.

54. Jennings, B. M., and others. "Lessons Learned While Collecting ANA Indicator Data." *Journal of Nursing Administration,* 2001, *31*(3), 121–129.

55. Jennings and others (2001).

56. Petryshen, P., O'Brien-Pallas, L. L., and Shamian, J. "Outcomes Monitoring: Adjusting for Risk Factors, Severity of Illness, and Complexity of Care." *Journal of the American Medical Informatics Association,* 1995, *2*(4), 243–249.

57. Aiken, Sochalski, and Anderson (1996); Anderson and Kohn (1996).

58. Halloran, E. J. "Nursing Workload, Medical Diagnosis Related Groups, and Nursing Diagnoses." *Research in Nursing and Health,* 1985, *8*(4), 421–433; Halloran, E. J., and Kiley, M. "Nursing Dependency, Diagnosis-Related Groups, and Length of Hospital Stay." *Health Care Financing Review,* 1987, *8*(3), 27–36; O'Brien-Pallas, L., Irvine, D., Peereboom, E., and Murray, M. "Measuring Nursing Workload: Understanding the Variability." *Nursing Economics,* 1997, *15*(4), 171–182.

59. O'Brien-Pallas, L., Cockerill, R., and Leatt, P. "Different Systems, Different Costs? An Examination of the Comparability of Workload Measurement Systems." *Journal of Nursing Administration,* 1992, *22*(12), 17–22; Carr-Hill, R. A., and Jenkins-Clarke, S. "Measurement Systems in Principle and in Practice: The Example of Nursing Workload." *Journal of Advanced Nursing,* 1995, *22*, 221–225.

60. Hernandez, C. A., and O'Brien-Pallas, L. L. "Validity and Reliability of Nursing Workload Measurement Systems: Strategies for Nursing Administrators." *Canadian Journal of Nursing Administration,* 1996 *9*(4) 33–52.

61. Trofino, J. "JCAHO Nursing Standards: Nursing Care Hours and LOS per DRG—Part I." *Nursing Management,* 1989, *20*(1), 29–32; Prescott, P. A., and others. "The Patient Intensity for Nursing Index: A Validity Assessment." *Research in Nursing and Health,* 1991, *14*(3), 213–221; Soeken, K. L., and Prescott, P. A. "Patient Intensity for Nursing Index: The Measurement

Model." *Research in Nursing and Health*, 1991, *14*(4), 297–304; Diers, D., and Bozzo, J. "Nursing Resource Definition in DRGs: RIMS/Nursing Acuity Project Group." *Nursing Economics*, 1997 *15*(3) 124–130, 137.

62. Ballard, K. A., Gray, R. F., Knauf, R. A., and Uppal, P. "Measuring Variations in Nursing Care per DRG." *Nursing Management*, 1993, *24*(4), 33–36; Lichtig, L. K., Knauf, R. A., and Milholland, D. K. "Some Impacts of Nursing on Acute Care Hospital Outcomes." *Journal of Nursing Administration*, 1999, *29*, 25–33.

63. Minnick, A., Pischke-Winn, K., and Sterk, M. B. "Introducing a Two-Way Wireless Communication System." *Nursing Management*, 1994, *25*(7), 42–47.

64. Kovner, C. T. "Computers in Nursing: From the Pencil to the PC." *Journal of the New York State Nurses Association*, 1995, *26*(1), 30–31; Marr, P., and others. "Bedside Terminals and Quality of Nursing Documentation." *Computers in Nursing*, 1993, *11*(4), 176–182; Pabst, M. K., Scherubel, J. C., and Minnick, A. F. "The Impact of Computerized Documentation on Nurses' Use of Time." *Computers in Nursing*, 1996, *14*(1), 25–30; Shamian, J., Hagen, B., Hu, T., and Fogarty, T. E. "Nursing Resource Requirement and Support Services." *Nursing Economics*, 1992, *10*(2), 110–115.

65. Seelye, A. "Hospital Ward Layout and Nurse Staffing." *Journal of Advanced Nursing*, 1982, *7*(3), 195–201; Olsen, R. V. "Cluster-Designed Nursing Unit Improves Job Performance." *Hospitals*, 1983, *57*(24), 48–50.

66. O'Brien-Pallas, Irvine, Peereboom, and Murray (1997).

67. Carr-Hill and Jenkins-Clarke (1995).

68. Minnick and Pabst (1998).

69. Aiken, L. H., and Patrician, P. A. "Measuring Organizational Traits of Hospitals: The Revised Nursing Work Index." *Nursing Research*, 2000, *49*(3), 146–153.

70. Avallone and Gibbon (1998).

71. Anonymous. "10 ANA Quality Indicators for Acute Care Settings." (American Nurses Association.) *Healthcare Benchmarks*, 1999, *6*(12), 138–139; Jennings and others (2001).

72. Karasek, R. A. *The Job Content Questionnaire and User's Guide. Version 1.1.* Los Angeles: Department of Industrial and Systems Engineering, University of Southern California, 1985; Landsbergis, P. "Occupational Stress Among Health Care Workers: A Test of the Job Demands-Control Model." *Journal of Organizational Behavior*, 1988, *9*, 217–239; McNeely, E. *In the Shadow of the Organization: Work and Well-Being on the Front Line—A Comparative Analysis of the Psychosocial Milieu in Hospitals and Its Effect on Employee Health.* Waltham, Mass.: Brandeis University; 1995; Seago, J. A., and Faucett, J. "Job Strain Among Registered Nurses and Other Hospital Workers." *Journal of Nursing Administration*, 1997, *27*(5), 19–25.

73. Jennings and others (2001).

74. The National Quality Forum (NQF) was created in 1999 in response to the President's Advisory Commission on Consumer Protection and Quality in the Health Care Industry. NQF's mission is to develop and implement a national strategy for health care quality measurement and reporting. Established as a unique public-private partnership, the NQF is a private, not-for-profit public benefit corporation with broad participation from more than three hundred member organizations representing all sectors of the health care industry, including consumers, employers, insurers, providers, and other critical stakeholders.

75. National Quality Forum. *National Voluntary Consensus Standards for Nursing-Sensitive Care: An Initial Performance Measure Set.* Washington, D.C.: National Quality Forum, 2004.

PART FOUR

## SPECIAL POPULATIONS

CHAPTER THIRTEEN

# LONG-TERM CARE AND THE ELDERLY POPULATION

Steven P. Wallace
Emily K. Abel
Nadereh Pourat
Linda Delp

As the population ages, long-term care becomes a critical issue.[1] Reduction in infectious diseases has contributed to a historic increase in life expectancy, from 47 years in 1900 to 77.3 years in 2002.[2] Because the birthrate has also fallen, elderly people constitute a growing segment of the population. By 2030, when most baby boomers will have aged, one in five Americans (sixty-seven million people) will be age sixty-five or over.[3] Because the rate of disability increases with age, the growth of the "oldest old" is especially important. Adults aged eighty-five and older are more than five times as likely as those sixty-five to seventy-four to need assistance with daily activities (17.7 percent versus 3.1 percent respectively).[4]

Long-term care is the set of health and social services delivered over a sustained period to people who have lost (or never acquired) some capacity for personal care; ideally, it enables recipients to live with as much independence and dignity as possible.[5] Provided in institutional, community, and home settings, long-term care encompasses an array of services ranging from high-tech care to assistance with such daily activities as walking, bathing, cooking, and managing money. It can be furnished by paid providers (formal care) or unpaid family and friends (informal care), or by a combination of the two. Long-term care differs from most topics discussed in this volume because it includes social as well as medical services.

This chapter reviews the recent literature on long-term care, showing how financial considerations have framed the dominant policy debate and research agenda. Policy makers frequently view the nursing home as a low-cost alternative to the hospital and consider community services and family care as less expensive substitutes for a nursing home, making quality-of-life issues a secondary priority. Both policy makers and researchers also tend to overlook the diversity among older Americans, as well as the problems faced by low-income women who serve as caregivers (whether paid or unpaid).

## Institutional Care

The most well-known type of long-term care institution is the nursing home. Nursing homes are facilities with nursing and other medical services that care for people with short-term recovery, end-of-life, or long-term chronic care needs. About one-third of persons are discharged from a nursing home because they stabilize or recover. Nursing homes include those that provide posthospital "subacute" care (medical care at an intensity just below that in the hospital), rehabilitation, and long-term medical care for those with chronic and disabling conditions. Of the one-quarter who die in a nursing home, almost half were in the facility for less than three months and one-third were there for over a year.[6] The other major type of long-term care institution is assisted living. These facilities have become popular during the past ten to fifteen years because they offer assistance to people who do not need continuous nursing or medical care but do require some assistance with daily activities.

Public policy first encouraged establishment of private long-term care institutions when Old Age Assistance (public aid for low-income elderly) was established in 1935 and specifically barred residents of public facilities from receiving this aid. The program allowed local governments to close their unpopular almshouses for the poor and ill, transferring the care of the ill and dependent elderly to private facilities and shifting the costs to the states and federal government.[7] The federal government gave funds directly for construction of nursing homes in the 1950s to solve a shortage of hospital beds and to save money by discharging hospital patients to a less-intensive level of care.

Public funding of nursing homes expanded dramatically after the passage of Medicare and Medicaid in 1965, fueling a rapid growth in the number of facilities. Both programs defined nursing homes as predominantly medical institutions, emphasizing the nursing over the home.[8] Prospective payment for hospital care using Diagnosis-Related Groups (DRGs), starting in 1984, furnished strong incentives to hospitals to reduce the length of hospital stay and discharge patients sooner to nursing homes. In response, some nursing homes increased their emphasis on medical services so they could capture more Medicare funding from posthospital patients. The Balanced Budget Act (BBA) of 1997 introduced prospective payment for Medicare nursing homes and slowed the shift from hospital to nursing home care.[9] The reimbursement formula for nursing home care in general encourages for-profit enterprises; more than two-thirds of nursing home residents are in for-profit facilities.[10]

Although most older people assume that Medicare covers nursing home stays, it accounts for only 12 percent of the $111 billion spent annually on nursing homes. Medicare pays for one hundred days of posthospital recovery care ("post-acute care") in a nursing home, but it offers no coverage for custodial care. Medicaid, by contrast, pays for custodial as well as skilled nursing care and therefore pays for 46 percent of all nursing home costs. The second largest source of funds for nursing homes is private out-of-pocket payment, which accounts for 28 percent of costs. Although two-fifths of nursing home users enter facilities paying privately, many of them become eligible for Medicaid after "spending down" or depleting their resources. A year in a nursing home typically costs $50,000 or more,[11] a sum that exceeds the income of about two-thirds of all families headed by an older person.[12] Nursing home spend-down has attracted policy attention because those who do so account for a significant proportion of Medicaid nursing home expenditures, and because the phenomenon is a demonstration of the catastrophic costs of long-term care.[13]

Nursing homes dominate long-term care spending for the elderly, consuming two-thirds of all long-term care spending.[14] Research has distinguished two types of nursing home user: (1) someone with a short stay, typical of posthospital use; and (2) someone with a longer stay, typical of more custodial use.[15] The long-stay residents consume most nursing home funds.[16] Research in this area has been used extensively in developing private long-term care insurance.[17] Because supply tends to drive the use of nursing homes, most states limit construction of new facilities as a way to limit Medicaid costs.[18]

Alternative reimbursement methods have been found to influence access and quality of nursing home care.[19] Studies suggest that although various techniques, especially prospective payment, have slowed the increase in costs, they also have reduced access for Medicaid patients and limited the supply of beds below the needed level in some areas.[20] To discourage nursing homes from taking only the least disabled (and least expensive) Medicaid patients, some states have tried reimbursement formulae that pay more for the care of the most disabled. But this system may have the unintended consequence of reducing access for those needing only custodial care. One group of researchers concluded that the reimbursement rate often reflects the state budget balance and overall state resources more than the actual costs of providing nursing home care or improving quality.[21]

Although economic issues dominate research and policy, widespread concern about the treatment of nursing home residents (especially after highly publicized scandals) has kept some attention on quality-of-care issues.[22] Studies documenting high use of chemical and physical restraints, inadequate supervision of care by physicians and professional nurses, and the poor quality of life in many institutions helped inform detailed language on nursing home quality in the federal 1987 Omnibus Budget Reconciliation Act (OBRA). Quality has improved since that time, but researchers continue to document how nursing homes can achieve further reductions in urinary incontinence, pressure sores, malnutrition, and pain.[23] Others have examined quality differences between for-profit and not-for-profit nursing homes, finding that the latter generally provide better care.[24] Almost all of the research on nursing home quality of care has focused on medical outcomes, with little work addressing the quality of life in facilities from the older person's perspective.[25]

One tool used to monitor nursing home quality is the federally mandated "minimum data set" (MDS), which compiles information on every resident of a facility. The MDS contains individual assessment items covering seventeen areas, such as mood and behavior, physical functioning, and skin conditions. The data are used to identify potential quality-of-care problems when indicators such as the rate of pressure sores or weight loss are higher than average. In addition to quality oversight, some state Medicaid programs and Medicare use MDS data to adjust nursing home payments to reflect the expected resource needs of their residents, referred to as case-mix adjustments.[26] Introduction of this monitoring system contributed to an improvement in quality of care, although much room for quality improvement remains.[27] Because research shows a direct relationship between staffing level and quality of care, many states have mandated minimum staffing levels for nursing homes above the federal standard.[28]

Public policies seek to improve nursing home quality through market mechanisms in addition to regulatory means. Websites such as www.medicare.gov/NhCompare/ have information on quality of care including MDS data, staffing levels, and complaints. This approach assumes that searching for long-term care is like shopping for a TV and that families act as knowledgeable, rational consumers who can use this complex data to balance cost, quality, distance, and other relevant nursing home characteristics to make good decisions. Research suggests this is unfortunately not often the case.[29]

The 1999 U.S. Supreme Court decision in *Olmstead* v. *L.C.* may also have a profound policy impact on long-term care. The court ruled that the Americans with Disabilities Act (ADA) applied to public programs and that states had to administer their Medicaid (and other) programs in a way that offers assistance in the least restrictive setting possible when desired by recipients. This has given states and the federal government a push to prioritize home and community services over nursing homes,[30] although tight state budgets have kept most action at the planning level with limited program innovation.[31]

Increasingly popular alternatives to nursing homes are assisted living facilities (ALF), known in some states as residential care facilities for the elderly (RCF-E) or board and care facilities. ALFs were inspired by the social care model of group-housing facilities started in Scandinavia. The first ALFs in the United States were established in the 1980s as a less medicalized alternative to nursing homes for older people with disabilities who did not need medical care. The construction boom in the 1990s was followed by a period of consolidation. Today, almost one million people reside in ALFs; one-third of all licensed beds are in California, Florida, and Pennsylvania.[32] The facilities typically offer twenty-four-hour staff for basic functional and medication assistance as needed, two to three meals per day, light housekeeping, social activities, and some transportation.[33] Although forty-two states have provisions for Medicaid home care services to ALF residents, in most states even Medicaid-eligible residents must pay privately for the room-and-board component of care. Government regulation and market oversight tend to be much looser than with nursing homes because they are regulated solely by state licensing laws. Many consumers have difficulty obtaining necessary information before entry.[34]

## Community-Based Services

For many, long-term care conjures up the image of bedridden elderly residents in nursing homes. But most older people with functional limitations remain at home, often receiving assistance from family and friends as well as community agencies. Community-based services include an array of services such as home care, adult day care, transportation, and congregate meals. Home care includes high-tech equipment, home-delivered meals, visiting nurses, home health aides with some training who can give basic personal care such as help with bathing, and home-makers or untrained workers who assist with housecleaning and some personal care. We refer to both in-home and out-of-home services as community-based services in this chapter.

Medicare pays for limited community-based care because it emphasizes medically oriented, post-acute home care, not the ongoing social support services many people need to live independently in the community. Recipients must be home-bound, under the care of a physician, and in need of part-time or intermittent skilled nursing or physical or speech therapy.[35] How these rules were interpreted was loosened in the early 1990s, resulting in rapid growth in Medicare expenditures for home health care. In reaction, Congress severely restricted reimbursements in 1997, leading to a 45 percent drop in expenditures the following year and little growth thereafter.[36]

An exception to Medicare's community-based care restrictions is the Program for All-Inclusive Care of the Elderly (PACE), which was added as a permanent Medicare benefit in 1997. This program combines Medicare and Medicaid funding in a capitated program that provides all the acute and long-term care services for low-income older persons who are disabled enough to qualify for Medicaid nursing home care. The integrated delivery model offers a continuum of community-based care and medical services, usually built around extensive use of adult day care, to maintain nursing-home-eligible elders in their own homes. Yet a number of barriers, including the requirement that disabled elders must leave their personal physician and switch to the program's physician panel, have limited this program to serving only ten thousand elders nationally.[37]

Unlike Medicare, Medicaid does not limit community-based services to posthospital care. The government's concern with reducing Medicaid nursing home spending encouraged expansion of Medicaid coverage of community-based services. Legislation passed in 1981 gave states the option of applying for waivers from existing Medicaid rules in order to supply case management, personal care, respite care, and adult day care—as long as total spending did not increase as a result of the added services.[38] The growth in the availability and popularity of home and community services has led Medicaid funding for these services to grow from $5.8 billion in 1992 to $22 billion in 2001, when it served 2.1 million disabled persons of all ages.[39] States have wide discretion in enacting policies to cap community-based long-term care "waiver program" costs, including limiting the number of persons who can receive services. As a result, more than 150,000 people were on waiting lists for these services in 2002.[40]

Another major federal program that funds services for elderly people in the community is the Older Americans Act (OAA). Title III of the OAA spent $1.1 billion in 2005 for supportive services such as transportation and information or referral (32 percent of funds), congregate meals in locations such as senior centers (35 percent), home-delivered meals (17 percent), preventive health programs (2 percent), and caregiver support programs (14 percent).[41] The OAA also funds a nursing home ombudsman program that places trained volunteers in willing facilities to act as advocates for patients in those facilities.[42] The OAA receives a fixed allocation of funds each year, in contrast to Medicaid and Medicare funding, which are formula-driven budgets based on use and charges. The cap on OAA spending and its relatively unchanged budget from year to year create a situation where some services run out of money before the end of the year and refuse to accept new clients. Moreover, the amount of assistance for each recipient tends to be even lower than that furnished by Medicaid programs.[43]

The policy focus on cost containment has shaped the direction of research on community care. Community-based services are usually cheaper than nursing home care for a single individual[44] and services can delay institutionalization,[45] but total costs tend to be higher because more people are served by community-based care than would have been served by nursing homes.[46] These findings, coupled with rising Medicaid costs, have stimulated research on identifying clients at imminent risk of institutionalization or those inappropriately placed in nursing homes so that community services can be targeted to them alone.[47] Drawing primarily on the Andersen model of health services utilization,[48] researchers have identified characteristics of elderly people that increase the probability of nursing home placement: advanced age, poorer health status, increased functional impairment, being white, living alone, and not owning a home.[49] One limitation of targeting Medicaid home care eligibility to a high disability level and high institutionalization risk is that functional decline often develops gradually and the need for home care exists along a continuum. Thus people who would benefit from moderate help remain ineligible, and those who need substantial help bump up against arbitrary dollar or hour limits that exist primarily to reduce home care costs. A more client-focused paradigm makes all disabled persons eligible for some home care, with the quantity of care varying continuously according to need.[50]

Another body of research addresses the policy concern that publicly funded care not substitute for care provided "free" by family and friends. Such a concern is based on the premise that formal (paid) and informal (unpaid) services are interchangeable and that an hour of paid care results in one less hour of care by family members. Most studies of the intersection of formal and informal services focus exclusively on allocating tasks between family caregivers and formal providers. Family members, however, typically conceptualize caregiving as a complex relationship, not simply as a set of discrete tasks. If a paid homemaker assumes the task of bathing a disabled parent, the caregiving children or child is likely to continue to express concern for the parent though other supportive actions. It is thus not surprising that researchers consistently find that formal services supplement rather than supplant informal care.[51]

A similar line of research arises from the fear that a large number of elderly people will come out of the woodwork to use new services because community-based services such as household cleaning, unlike nursing homes, are believed to be universally desired at a high level of service. This fear too appears to be misdirected. Some elderly people postpone assistance until they are extremely disabled in order to maintain for as long as possible a sense of independence.[52] Having absorbed a value system that glorifies self-sufficiency, they may be unable to rely on others even when very needy. Some elderly people also cling to housekeeping chores as a way of separating themselves from their more severely impaired counterparts. As Alan Sager comments, "The notion of a horde of greedy old people and lazy family members anxious to soak up new public benefits appears to be more a projection by a few wealthy legislators accustomed to domestic and hotel and restaurant service than it is a realistic image of our nation's elderly citizens."[53]

Moreover, one person's "latent demand" is another's "unmet need."[54] Those who fear that expansion of community services will generate additional demand implicitly acknowledge that the elderly are drastically underserved. Less than half of the 5.6 million functionally impaired older people who receive ADL or IADL assistance in the community receive any formal care. The key policy questions involve determining the minimum adequate level of long-term care that should be available to all older persons and then identifying how to finance the needed increment above current services.[55]

Policy on the quality of existing community-based care is at least fifteen years behind similar nursing home policy. Methods have been developed to monitor and guide quality improvement in Medicare home health agencies,[56] but little work has been conducted on determining appropriate quality indicators for non-medical home care.

## Informal Care

Research offers overwhelming evidence to refute the enduring myth that families abandon their elderly relatives. Shanas was one of the first scholars to show that elderly people remain in close contact with surviving kin,[57] and more recent studies demonstrate that this contact translates into assistance during times of crisis. Families and friends deliver 70–80 percent of the services disabled elderly people receive.[58] It is estimated that 13.5 million households contain at least one caregiver for a person age sixty-five or older who lives in the same house or a different one.[59]

Informal care continues to be allocated on the basis of gender. Women account for about three-quarters of those caring for an older person. Compared with men caregivers, women caregivers are older, married, and the primary caregiver. Women furnish more intensive and complex care, are more likely to report difficulty with care provision and balancing caregiving with other family and employment responsibilities, and are more likely than men to suffer from poor emotional health secondary to caregiving.[60] Daughters are more likely than sons to live with dependent parents and serve as the primary caregiver.[61]

Research on informal care typically focuses on the burden it imposes. Studies have found that caregivers experience a range of physical, emotional, social, and financial problems. In many cases, caregiving responsibilities reignite family conflict, impose financial strain, and encroach on both paid employment and leisure activity.[62]

Despite the many reports of caregiver burden, limited assistance is available. The dominant concern of policy makers is that caregivers will unload responsibilities on the state. As a result, policy makers support social services and financial assistance for caregivers only insofar as they serve to postpone or prevent institutionalization. The major demand of many caregivers is respite services, which afford temporary relief from care.[63] Although most states have established respite programs, they tend to be underfunded and able to serve only a small number of families, as well as offering very few hours of care.[64] State programs to reimburse caregivers for their services typically limit payment to those caring for patients deemed most vulnerable to institutionalization. Stringent eligibility criteria often exclude caregivers who are spouses, children over the age of eighteen, relatives who live apart from the care receiver, and relatives with income over a certain amount. The level of reimbursement tends to be low.[65]

The policy response to the conflict between wage work and family care has also been limited. The Family and Medical Leave Act (FMLA), passed with widespread acclaim in 1993, covers leave of no more than twelve weeks, includes no wage replacement, excludes part-time and contingent workers and those employed in small firms, and defines family narrowly. Workers who are white, middle-class, and married are most likely to be able to take advantage of the act.[66] One study found more than three-quarters of workers who qualified for FMLA leaves did not take them because they could not afford to go without pay.[67] Most state programs have similar restrictions. California recently became one of the few states to have paid family leave. The state partially covers such leave through the short-term disability system.[68]

Somewhat more substantial than the FMLA is the National Caregiver Support Program (NCSP). This program was established in 2000 through the Older Americans Act (OAA), which uses a social services model to provide services to all persons over age sixty (and now their caregivers as well) with no required means test. The most common NCSP service is information and referral. Limited funding for this program restricts its ability to make available more costly services such as respite care to many caregivers.[69] Future funding decisions will determine if the program remains largely symbolic or if it grows into a significant source of support for caregivers nationwide.

Unlike respite services, financial compensation, and workplace reforms, programs enhancing the ability of caregivers to adapt to their responsibility enjoy enthusiastic support. The low cost of such programs partly explains their appeal. It is far cheaper to establish a ten-week course of lectures for caregivers than to give them the services of homemakers and home health aides over a period of months or even years. In addition, many caregivers attest to the benefit of such programs. Support groups alleviate the intense isolation surrounding caregiving. Educational programs that dispense information about the disease process or new equipment dispatched to the home boost competence and confidence. Counseling services help caregivers disentangle unresolved emotional issues from the process of delivering care.[70] We believe that a major disadvantage of these programs is that they reinforce the belief that our primary goal should be to help caregivers adjust to their unavoidable burden rather than to make care for the dependent population more just and humane.

## Variations in the Need for Formal Services

As the previous two sections have shown, the research and policy focus on financial considerations has overshadowed other public health concerns such as equity, adequacy, and quality. Understanding variations by race, ethnicity, gender, and class can help identify critical research and policy issues that hitherto received inadequate attention.[71]

A high immigration rate, increasing life expectancy, and aging of the population have led to an elderly population that is becoming increasingly African American, Latino, Native American, and Asian American. These groups constituted approximately 17.5 percent of the elderly population in 2000 and are expected to represent about 39 percent by 2050.[72] Elderly African Americans have the highest rate of death and disability, caused in part by high incidence of hypertension, diabetes, circulatory problems, and arthritis. Elderly African Americans also are more likely to assess their health as fair or poor.[73] Older Latinos have a generally favorable mortality pattern but become disabled earlier and more often than non-Latino whites. For a large number of elderly Latino immigrants, obtaining long-term care is complicated by limited English proficiency and fewer years of experience with the U.S. health care system.[74] The health status of Asian American elderly generally is similar to that of white elderly. Aggregate data, however, mask the increasing diversity within Asian American communities, many of whom are immigrants with limited English proficiency. Some Asian Americans groups, especially those with many recent immigrants, have long-term care needs differing dramatically from those of whites.[75] Thus, programs aimed at the types and levels of functional disability of elderly whites may be less appropriate.

Long-term care needs also differ by gender. Women constitute 58 percent of the elderly population and 70 percent of those eighty-five and over.[76] Women at every age experience more functional limitations than men. They also have a disproportionate need for formal long-term care because they frequently survive their partners and subsequently live alone without sufficient social support. Men are thus more likely to receive informal support from co-resident spouses and while women rely more on children who are not co-resident, and they therefore receive fewer hours of assistance. The total amount of formal, paid care extended to men and women is similar, leaving women with less assistance overall.[77]

Class also influences the need for long-term care. Research on aging in the United States generally focuses on income (which is a point-in-time measure of cash flow) rather than class (which is a long-term position in the economic stratification system that also includes assets and occupational position). Research outside the United States suggests that class position has a direct impact on health status, independent of access to health care. A Swedish study reported that manual workers were more than three times as likely as white collar workers to have a mobility limitation, a class disparity that begins early in life and persists into old age.[78] In the United States, functional limitations are highest among elderly people with lower wealth, independent of income. Lower assets and not owning a home are stronger predictors of functional limitation than income and education until age eighty-five.[79] Although assets are a better indicator of class than income, more research is needed to understand the relationship between class and disability over the life course.

Race and ethnicity, gender, and class interact, intensifying the need for long-term care and aggravating access barriers. The disability rate is highest among older African American women, being about 50 percent higher than for older white males.[80] Those with the greatest need for long-term care have the least ability to pay for it. The poverty rate for all elderly in 2002 was 10.4 percent, but it was 23.8 percent for African Americans and 21.4 percent for Latinos. The rate is higher for older women than men (12.4 percent versus 7.7 percent), and for those living alone compared to those in married couple families (19.2 percent versus 5.1 percent). Among older women living alone, 47.1 percent of Latinas and 40.6 percent of African Americans are in poverty. Differences by race in wealth (home equity, stocks, other investments) are even larger, with the median net worth of households headed by an older white person being five times higher than one headed by an older African American ($205,000 versus $41,000).[81] Inequality in resources helps to explain why more than 60 percent of African American and Latinos who enter a nursing home are on Medicaid, compared to 37 percent of whites. In contrast, 28 percent of whites who enter a nursing home pay privately, compared to 5 percent of African Americans.[82] The term *multiple jeopardy* has been used to describe this cumulative disadvantage of age, race, gender, and class in regard to health and income.[83]

## Variations in Using Long-Term Care

Characteristics such as gender, race, ethnicity, and class exert a significant influence on the use of LTC services. As a result, there is more unmet need for long-term care by women, minorities, and the poor.

*Gender.* Women are much more likely to enter a nursing home than men; 70 percent of nursing home residents are women, and women are twice as likely as men to use a nursing home at some point in their lives.[84] Yet after a lifetime of caring for others, many women are bereft of essential support at home when they are most in need.[85] Policy makers and researchers rarely address the social and economic policies responsible for the predominance of women in nursing homes. The extent to which women enter nursing homes because of the inadequacy of community services is unknown.

*Race and Ethnicity.* African Americans have historically used nursing homes less than whites. In 1973, older whites were about twice as likely as older African Americans to be in a nursing home. Since that time, the white utilization rate has dropped about 30 percent, while the African American rate has nearly doubled, resulting in higher nursing home use for African Americans than whites.[86] Two factors help to explain this dramatic shift. First, the growth in assisted living is concentrated among the middle-class white population that can afford to pay privately.[87] Whereas 1.5 million persons live in nursing homes, many of the more than 750,000 in assisted living might have had to use a nursing home ten years earlier.[88] Second, since disability among African Americans is higher than for whites, it is possible that the growth in moderate- (versus high-) intensity home-care services has enabled more whites than African Americans to remain at home.

There has been less research on the relationship between race and ethnicity and use of community services. Some studies report that minority elderly use community-based care at the same rate as whites (or more frequently) after controlling for need and resources.[89] Other studies find that African Americans and Latinos are less likely to use community services.[90] The variation in findings appears to be related to the populations studied. If only community-dwelling elderly are in the sample, long-term care use does not vary often by race. But if both institutional and community elders are analyzed together, racial differences remain. Because African American and white elders have dissimilar patterns and locations of care, it is important to understand racial and ethnic patterns in the entire continuum of care.

Several reasons could account for racial and ethnic differences in long-term care utilization.[91] Some studies suggest that minority elderly people are less knowledgeable than whites about the types and functions of many community-based services. Others suggest that nursing homes have discriminatory admission policies, that health professionals are less likely to refer minority elderly people to formal services, or that family structure and earlier inception of parenthood results in contrasting use patterns.[92] This racial and ethnic variation is typically overlooked by policy makers, who design programs for the "average" elder who is white and middle-class.[93]

*Class.* Some observers argue that social policy for older people in the United States creates a two-class system. Low-income elderly rely on Medicaid and other poverty programs, while those who are better off benefit from tax preferences, employment-based retiree benefits, and privately purchased Medicare supplemental policies. Poverty programs are most vulnerable to cuts because their constituency lacks political and economic clout.[94]

Specific research on class factors in long-term care is sparse and primarily deals with the problems faced by Medicaid recipients. The quality of life of Medicaid nursing home residents appears to be especially poor. Medicaid recipients tend to be relegated to institutions that, according to some measures, offer the worst-quality care.[95]

Even within a facility, residents relying on Medicaid sometimes receive less care than private-pay residents. Medicaid also does not pay for "incidentals" such as laundering personal clothing or making a phone call. All such expenses must come from the $30–70 per month (varying by state) that Medicaid recipients are allowed to keep;[96] the federally mandated minimum has not risen since 1988.[97]

Class also affects distribution of community-based services. Because most people who receive such care pay privately—only the poorest elders qualify for Medicaid services—utilization varies directly with income.[98] Older persons who receive privately paid home care receive almost 50 percent more hours than those who receive care from public programs.[99]

Although Medicaid increases access to community-based services, 71 percent of noninstitutionalized older people with a poverty-level income do not receive Medicaid.[100] Other elderly, called "tweeners," have income just above the poverty level and therefore do not quality for Medicaid but are too poor to pay privately for services.[101]

There is a class bias of noninstitutional care, especially home health care. First, the deregulation and cost-containment measures of the 1980s eased Medicare restrictions on proprietary home health agencies. In 2000, about one-third of home health patients were being served by a for-profit agency.[102] These agencies seek out the best-paying (privately insured) patients, leaving others for non-profit and government agencies. Second, large multihospital systems looking for a relatively inexpensive way to expand have been eager to acquire home health agencies.[103] Third, for-profit chains have expanded. Currently, 81.6 percent of the thirty-eight largest home care organizations are members of for-profit chains.[104] These changes have increased the competitiveness of the home health care market, putting agencies under growing pressure to generate revenue by focusing on the most remunerative patients and the best-paid services and thus decreasing access for those whose care is less profitable.[105] Little research has attempted to determine if the quality of care varies by type of payment or ownership or affiliation of the home health agency.

The greatest difference by class may lie in services furnished outside the bounds of established organizations. Although most studies ignore the vast network of helpers recruited through ad hoc, informal arrangements, some evidence suggests that disabled elderly people rely disproportionately on this type of assistance.[106] Abel's study of fifty-one predominantly white, middle-class women caring for elderly parents found that just fifteen used services from a community agency, but twenty-eight hired helpers who were unaffiliated with a formal agency. Nine of the unaffiliated home care aides worked forty hours a week, and sixteen offered around-the-clock care.[107] A national survey found 30 percent of all caregivers had received paid help from a hired housekeeper in the past year, with whites and high-income caregivers the most likely to have this assistance.[108] The help from such workers typically is not included in government statistics; however, it constitutes a major source of assistance to the affluent that is not available to others.

## Private Sector Financing Initiatives

The inequities in long-term care may become even more apparent if initiatives to rely more on private sector financing win increased support. Such initiatives take two forms. Some, such as home equity conversion and individual medical accounts, seek to promote private saving, which can then be used to finance long-term care. Others attempt to bring individuals together to pool the risks of paying for long-term care; these mechanisms include private long-term care insurance and continuing-care retirement communities.[109]

Advocates of such programs argue that the growing segment of the elderly population that is sufficiently well off to be able to pay for long-term care should not rely on limited government funds.[110] Critics charge that expansion of the private sector would sharpen the divide between rich and poor. Most private-sector approaches are beyond the reach of low- and middle-income elderly people. Many elderly have neither enough equity in their home to pay for extended long-term care nor enough income to pay for comprehensive private long-term care insurance.[111] In 2005, a policy paying $150 a day for a nursing home and $112 a day for home care for up to five years cost an average annual premium of $3,333 at sixty and $6,178 at seventy.[112] Policies with coverage for assisted living, increased length of coverage, and inflation-indexed benefits are being offered.[113] Examination of individuals with private long-term care insurance reveals a well-informed population who use the benefits and are satisfied with their policies.[114]

Entry fees for continuing-care retirement communities can be as high as $440,000 for a two-bedroom house for a couple, with monthly fees of $4,267. Increased private financing may also dissolve whatever popular support public programs currently enjoy. Walter Leutz writes: "This could clearly lead to a two-class system of care, which would be rationalized by arguments that blame elderly victims for not insuring. It would not be uncommon to hear the argument that those who don't plan for the future don't deserve such a generous program, and so on into the all-too-familiar pattern."[115]

## Workers in the Long-Term Care System

Paid as well as unpaid caregivers suffer from the failure to fund long-term care adequately. Nursing homes, home health agencies, budget-strapped state and local governments, and the elderly themselves seek to save money by keeping wages low. In 1999 the median annual wage of a home care aide was $9,000; nursing home aides earned just $3,000 more. Not surprisingly, the families of nearly half of those workers lived in or near poverty (under 200 percent of the poverty level).[116] The job has other disadvantages as well. Disabling injuries are common and the incidence for both nursing home aides and home care aides is far higher than for hospital workers and private-sector workers in other industries.[117] Stress is another occupational hazard. Some stress stems from the fiscal constraints and bureaucratic rules that often prevent workers from providing what they consider high-quality care. Discrimination and abuse easily emanate from the racial, ethnic, gender, and class differences between workers on the one hand and administrators and patients on the other. Home care aides who live in have little ability to control their schedule, are often on call twenty-four seven, and find themselves treated "like maids."[118]

Unionization has produced significant reform in California. Until the mid-1990s the state in-home supportive services program offered minimum-wage jobs with no benefits. Although 8 percent of the workers still receive the state minimum wage of $6.75 per hour, approximately 25 percent now earn at least $9.50 and have access to health, dental, and vision care.[119] The union also enabled workers to join consumer advocacy groups to lobby against budget cuts and for program improvements. An Oakland home care worker commented, "I used to think this work was degrading. But since joining the union I see how it has given us respect."[120] New York City's Cooperative Home Care Associates and the Wellspring model of nursing home care also give workers more voice in home care and nursing home policies.[121]

## Conclusion

The rapid growth of the older population will put new strains on our long-term care system, especially when the baby boom generation reaches age eighty-five beginning around 2030. We can confidently predict that this cohort will, disproportionately, be widowed women with high rates of disability and poverty; many will be members of racial and ethnic minorities.

Although the priority in both policy and research is typically on cost containment, the most critical issue is how we can provide adequate and high-quality long-term care services equitably to this growing and diverse population. The limited financial resources of many older people create a need for a universal Medicare type of social insurance for long-term care. But current policies seek to reduce public funding, not increase it. Unfortunately, the underlying long-term care needs will not disappear simply because policy makers fail to address them.

# Notes

1. Spector, W. D., and Fleishman, J. A. *The Characteristics of Long-Term Care Users.* Rockville, Md.: Agency for Health Care Research and Quality, Sept. 2000. (AHRQ pub. no. 00-0049.)

2. U.S. National Center for Health Statistics. *National Vital Statistics Reports.* Hyattsville, Md.: U.S. National Center for Health Statistics, Nov. 10, 2004.

3. U.S. Census Bureau. "U.S. Interim Projections by Age, Sex, Race, and Hispanic Origin." Mar. 18, 2004. [http://www.census.gov/ipc/www/usinterimproj] (accessed June 30, 2005).

4. U.S. National Center for Health Statistics. "Early Release of Selected Estimates Based on Data from the January-September 2004 National Health Interview Survey." Mar. 23, 2005. [http://www.cdc.gov/nchs/data/nhis/earlyrelease/200503_12.pdf] (accessed July 10, 2005).

5. Kane, R. A., Kane, R. L., and Ladd, R. C. *The Heart of Long-Term Care.* New York: Oxford University Press, 1998.

6. Jones, A. "The National Nursing Home Survey: 1999 Summary." *Vital Health Statistics,* 2002, *13*(152).

7. Quadagno, J. *The Transformation of Old Age Security: Class and Politics in the American Welfare State.* Chicago: University of Chicago Press, 1988.

8. Institute of Medicine. *Improving the Quality of Care in Nursing Homes.* Washington, D.C.: National Academy Press, 1986.

9. Dalton, K., and Howard, H. A. "Market Entry and Exit in Long-Term Care: 1985–2000." *Health Care Financing Review,* Winter 2002, *24*(2), 17–32.

10. Jones (2002).

11. Allen, K. G. *Long-Term Care Financing: Growing Demand and Cost of Services Are Straining Federal and State Budgets.* Washington, D.C.: U.S. Government Accountability Office, Apr. 27 2005. (GAO-05-564T.)

12. U.S. Census Bureau. "Age of Reference Person, by Total Money Income in 2003, Type of Family, Race and Hispanic Origin of Reference Person." (Table FINC-02.) *Current Population Survey, 2004 Annual Social and Economic Supplement.* Mar. 25, 2004. [http://pubdb3.census.gov/macro/032004/faminc/new02_001.htm] (accessed July 14, 2005).

13. Allen (2005); Adams, E. K., Meiners, M. R., and Burwell, B. O. "Asset Spend-Down in Nursing Homes." *Medical Care,* 1993, 31, 1–23.

14. Freiman, M. P. *A New Look at U.S. Expenditures for Long-Term Care and Independent Living Services, Settings, and Technologies for the Year 2000.* Washington, D.C.: AARP Public Policy Institute, Apr. 2005. (2005-04.)

15. Liu, K., McBride, T., and Coughlin, T. "Risk of Entering Nursing Homes for Long Versus Short Stays." *Medical Care,* 1994, *32*, 315–327.

16. Kemper, P., Spillman, B. C., and Murtaugh, C. M. "A Lifetime Perspective on Proposals for Financing Nursing Home Care." *Inquiry,* 1991, *28,* 333–334.

17. Cohen, M. A., Kumar, N., and Wallack, S. S. "Long-Term Care Insurance and Medicaid." *Health Affairs,* 1994, *13,* 127–139.

18. Harrington, C., and others. "Trends in State Certificate of Need and Moratoria Programs for Long Term Care Providers." *Journal of Health and Social Policy,* 2004, *19*(2), 31–58.

19. Grabowski, D. C., Feng, Z., Intrator, O., and Mor, V. "Recent Trends in State Nursing Home Payment Policies." *Health Affairs,* Jan.-June 2004 (Suppl. Web exclusives), W4-363-373.

20. Davis, M. A., Freeman, J. W., and Kirby, E. C. "Nursing Home Performance Under Case-Mix Reimbursement: Responding to Heavy-Care Incentives and Market Changes." *Health Services Research,* 1998, *33*(4), 815–834.

21. U.S. General Accounting Office. *California Nursing Homes: Federal and State Oversight Inadequate to Protect Residents in Homes with Serious Care Violations.* Washington, D.C.: U.S. General Accounting Office, 1998. (GAO/T-HEHS-98-219.)

22. Wunderlich, G. S., and Kohler, P. O. (eds.). *Improving the Quality of Long-Term Care.* Washington, D.C.: Institute of Medicine, National Academy Press, 2001.

23. Zimmerman, S., and others. "Assisted Living and Nursing Homes: Apples and Oranges?" *Gerontologist,* Apr. 2003, *43*(spec. no. 2), 107–117.

24. Hillmer, M. P., and others. "Nursing Home Profit Status and Quality of Care: Is There Any Evidence of an Association?" *Medical Care Research Review,* 2005, *62*(2), 139–166.

25. For an exception, see Kane, R. L., and Kane, R. A. "What Older People Want from Long-Term Care, and How They Can Get It." *Health Affairs,* Nov. 1, 2001, *20*(6), 114–127.

26. U.S. General Accounting Office. *Nursing Homes: Federal Efforts to Monitor Resident Assessment Data Should Complement State Activities.* Washington, D.C.: U.S. General Accounting Office, Feb. 2002. (GAO-02-279.)

27. Wunderlich and Kohler (2001).

28. Harrington, C. "Nurse Staffing in Nursing Homes in the United States." *Journal of Gerontological Nursing,* 2005, *31*(2), 18–23.

29. Ryan, A. A., and Scullion, H. F. "Nursing Home Placement: An Exploration of the Experiences of Family Carers." *Journal of Advanced Nursing,* 2000, *32*(5), 1187–1195; Hikoyeda, N., and Wallace, S. P. "Do Ethnic-Specific Long Term Care Facilities Improve Resident Quality of Life? Findings from the Japanese American Community." *Journal of Gerontological Social Work,* 2001, *36*(1/2), 83–106.

30. Teitelbaum, J., Burke, T., and Rosenbaum, S., "Olmstead V.L.C. and the Americans with Disabilities Act: Implications for Public Health Policy and Practice." *Public Health Reports,* May-June 2004, *119*(3), 371–374.

31. Fox-Grage, W., Coleman, B., and Folkemer, D. *The States' Response to the Olmstead Decision: A 2003 Update.* Washington, D.C.: National Conference of State Legislatures, 2004.

32. Mollica, R. *State Assisted Living Policy.* Portland, Me.: National Academy for State Health Policy, November 2002. (LTC15.)

33. "Assisted Living: How Much Assistance Can You Really Count on?" *Consumer Reports,* July 2005, *70*(7), 28–34.

34. U.S. General Accounting Office. *Assisted Living: Examples of State Efforts to Improve Consumer Protections.* Washington, D.C.: U.S. GAO, Apr. 2004. (GAO-04-684.)

35. U.S. Department of Health and Human Services. *Medicare and You 2005.* Baltimore: Center for Medicare and Medicaid Services, Jan. 2005. (CMS-10050.)

36. Pear, R. "Medicare Spending for Care at Home Plunges by 45%." *New York Times,* Apr. 21, 2000, A1.

37. Gross, D. L., Temkin-Greener, H., Kunitz, S., and Mukamel, D. B. "The Growing Pains of Integrated Health Care for the Elderly: Lessons from the Expansion of PACE." *Milbank Quarterly,* 2004, *82*(2), 257–282.

38. U.S. General Accounting Office. *Long-Term Care Case Management: State Experiences and Implications for Federal Policy.* Washington, D.C.: U.S. General Accounting Office, 1993. (GAO/HRD-93-52.)

39. Kitchener, M., Ng, T., Miller, N., and Harrington, C. "Medicaid Home and Community-Based Services: National Program Trends." *Health Affairs,* Jan.-Feb. 2005, *24*(1), 206–212.

40. Kitchener, Ng, Miller, and Harrington (2005).

41. U.S. Administration on Aging. "Title III—Grants for State and Community Programs on Aging, FY 2005 Annual Allocation." *U.S. Administration on Aging.* [http://www.aoa.gov/about/legbudg/current_budg/state_allocations/T3_2005.pdf] (accessed July 22, 2005).

42. Estes, C. L., Zulman, D. M., Goldberg, S. C., and Ogawa, D. D. "State Long Term Care Ombudsman Programs: Factors Associated with Perceived Effectiveness." *Gerontologist,* Feb. 1, 2004, *44*(1), 104–115.

43. Wallace, S. P. "The No Care Zone: Availability, Accessibility, and Acceptability in Community-Based Long-Term Care." *Gerontologist,* 1990, *30*, 254–261; Estes, C. L., Swan, J. H., and Associates. *The Long-Term Care Crisis: Elders Trapped in the No-Care Zone.* Thousand Oaks, Calif.: Sage, 1993.

44. Chappell, N. L., and others. "Comparative Costs of Home Care and Residential Care." *Gerontologist,* June 2004, *44*(3), 389–400.

45. Gaugler, J. E., Kane, R. L., Kane, R. A., and Newcomer, R. "Early Community-Based Service Utilization and Its Effects on Institutionalization in Dementia Caregiving." *Gerontologist,* Apr. 1, 2005, *45*(2), 177–185.

46. Weissert, W., Chernew, M., and Hirth, R. "Titrating Versus Targeting Home Care Services to Frail Elderly Clients: An Application of Agency Theory and Cost-Benefit Analysis to Home Care Policy." *Journal of Aging and Health,* Feb. 2003, *15*(1), 99–123.

47. Safran, D. G., Graham, J. D., and Osberg, J. S. "Social Supports as a Determinant of Community-Based Care Utilization Among Rehabilitation Patients." *Health Services Research,* 1994, *28*, 729–750.

48. Andersen, R. M. "Revisiting the Behavioral Model and Access to Medical Care: Does It Matter?" *Journal of Health and Social Behavior,* 1995, *36*, 1–10.

49. Wallace, S. P., Levy-Storms, L., Kington, R. S., and Andersen, R. M. "The Persistence of Race and Ethnicity in the Use of Long-Term Care." *Journals of Gerontology, Series B, Psychological Sciences and Social Sciences,* 1998, *53*(2), S104-S112; Kersting, R. C. "Impact of Social Support, Diversity, and Poverty on Nursing Home Utilization in a Nationally Representative Sample of Older Americans." *Social Work in Health Care,* 2001, *33*(2), 67–87.

50. Weissert, Chernew, and Hirth (2003).

51. Jette, A. M., Tennstedt, S., and Crawford, S. "How Does Formal and Informal Community Care Affect Nursing Home Use?" *Journals of Gerontology, Social Sciences,* 1995, 50B, S4-S12; Muramatsu, N., and Campbell, R. T. "State Expenditures on Home and Community Based Services and Use of Formal and Informal Personal Assistance: A Multilevel Analysis." *Journal of Health and Social Behavior,* Mar. 2002, *43*(1), 107–124.

52. Kane, Kane, and Ladd (1998); Wallace (1990).

53. Sager, A. "A Proposal for Promoting More Adequate Long-Term Care for the Elderly." *Gerontologist,* 1983, *23*, 13–17.

54. Feldblum, C. R. "Home Health Care for the Elderly: Programs, Problems, and Potentials." *Harvard Journal on Legislation,* 1985, *22*, 193–254.

55. Harrington, C., and others. "A National Long-term Care Program for the United States— A Caring Vision." *Journal of the American Medical Association*, 1991, *266*, 3023–2029.

56. Shaughnessy, P. W., and others. "Improving Patient Outcomes of Home Health Care: Findings from Two Demonstration Trials of Outcome-Based Quality Improvement." *Journal of the American Geriatrics Society*, 2002, *50*(8), 1354–1364.

57. Shanas, E. "The Family as a Social Support System in Old Age." *Gerontologist*, 1979, *19*, 169–174.

58. Abel, E. K. *Who Cares for the Elderly? Public Policy and the Experiences of Adult Daughters*. Philadelphia: Temple University Press, 1991.

59. Barrett, L. L. *Caregiving in the U.S*. Washington, D.C.: National Alliance for Caregiving and AARP, Apr. 2004.

60. Navaie-Waliser, M., Spriggs, A., and Feldman, P. H. "Informal Caregiving Differential Experiences by Gender." *Medical Care*, 2002, *40*(12), 1249–1259.

61. Robinson, K. M. "Family Caregiving: Who Provides the Care, and at What Cost?" *Nursing Economics*, 1997, *15*(5), 243–247.

62. Abel (1991).

63. Gonyea, J. *Feminist Perspectives on Family Care: Policies for Gender Justice*. Thousand Oaks, Calif.: Sage, 1995.

64. Gonyea (1995).

65. Burwell, B. O. *Shared Obligations: Public Policy Influences on Family Care for the Elderly*. Washington, D.C.: Health Care Financing Administration, 1986.

66. Hudson, R. B., and Gonyea, J. G. "Time Not Yet Money: The Politics and Promise of the Family Medical Leave Act." *Journal of Aging and Social Policy*, 2000, *11*(2–3), 189–200.

67. Green, M. "Taking Leave: California's New Paid Family Medical Leave Act Could Be Copied in Other States." *Best's Review*, Feb. 2005, *105*(10), 27–32.

68. Green (2005).

69. Administration on Aging. *The Older Americans Act National Family Caregiver Support Program*. Washington, D.C.: U.S. Department of Health and Human Services, June 2004.

70. Abel (1991).

71. Estes, C. L. "Political Economy of Aging." In C. L. Estes and Associates (eds.), *Social Policy and Aging*. Thousand Oaks, Calif.: Sage, 2001.

72. Federal Interagency Forum on Aging Related Statistics. *Older Americans 2004: Key Indicators of Well-Being*. Washington, D.C.: U.S. Government Printing Office, Nov. 2004.

73. Rooks, R. N, Whitfield, K. E. "Health Disparities Among Older African Americans: Past, Present, and Future Perspectives." In K. E. Whitfield (ed.), *Closing the Gap: Improving the Health of Minority Elders in the New Millennium*. Washington, D.C.: Gerontological Society of America, 2004.

74. Wallace, S. P., and Villa, V. M. "Equitable Health Systems: Cultural and Structural Issues for Latino Elders." *American Journal of Law and Medicine*, Summer-Fall 2003, *29*(2–3), 247–267.

75. Park-Tanjasiri, S., Wallace, S. P., and Kazue, S. "Picture Imperfect: Hidden Problems Among Asian Pacific Islander Elderly." *Gerontologist*, Dec. 1995, *35*(6), 753–760.

76. U.S. National Center for Health Statistics. *Health, United States, 2004*. Hyattsville, Md.: U.S. National Center for Health Statistics, 2004.

77. Katz, S. J., Kabeto, M., and Langa, K. M. "Gender Disparities in the Receipt of Home Care for Elderly People with Disability in the United States." *Journal of the American Medical Association*, Dec. 20, 2000, *284*(23), 3022–3027.

78. Ahacic, K., Parker, M. G., and Thorslund, M. "Mobility Limitations 1974–1991: Period Changes Explaining Improvement in the Population." *Social Science and Medicine*, 2003, *57*(12), 2411–2422.

79. Robert, S., and House, J. S. "SES Differentials in Health by Age and Alternative Indicators of SES." *Journal of Aging and Health*, Aug. 1996, *8*(3), 359–388.

80. Federal Interagency Forum on Aging Related Statistics (2004).

81. Federal Interagency Forum on Aging Related Statistics (2004).

82. Jones (2002).

83. Markides, K. S. "Minority Aging." In M. W. Riley, B. B. Hess, and K. Bond (eds.), *Aging in Society: Selected Reviews of Recent Research.* Hillsdale, N.J.: Erlbaum, 1983.

84. Laditka, S. B. "Modeling Lifetime Nursing Home Use Under Assumptions of Better Health." *Journals of Gerontology, Series B: Psychological Sciences and Social Sciences*, 1998, *53*(4), S177–S187.

85. Navaie-Waliser, Spriggs, and Feldman (2002).

86. Ness, J., Ahmed, A., and Aronow, W. S. "Demographics and Payment Characteristics of Nursing Home Residents in the United States: A 23-Year Trend." *Journals of Gerontology, Series A: Biological Sciences and Medical Sciences*, 2004, *59A*(11):, 1213–1217.

87. Howard, D. L., and others. "Distribution of African Americans in Residential Care/Assisted Living and Nursing Homes: More Evidence of Racial Disparity?" *American Journal of Public Health*, Aug. 2002, *92*(8), 1272–1277.

88. Golant, S. M. "Do Impaired Older Persons with Health Care Needs Occupy U.S. Assisted Living Facilities? An Analysis of Six National Studies." *Journals of Gerontology, Series B: Social Sciences*, 2004, *59B*(2), S68–S79.

89. Wallace, S. P., Levy-Storms, L., and Ferguson, L. R. "Access to Paid In-Home Assistance Among Disabled Elderly People: Do Latinos Differ from Non-Latino Whites?" *American Journal of Public Health*, 1995, *85*, 970–975; White-Means, S. I., and Rubin, R. M. "Is There Equity in the Home Health Care Market? Understanding Racial Patterns in the Use of Formal Home Health Care." *Journals of Gerontology, Series B, Psychological Sciences and Social Sciences*, July 1, 2004, *59*(4), S220–S229.

90. Wallace, Levy-Storms, Kington, and Andersen (1998); Borrayo, E. A., Salmon, J. R., Polivka, L., and Dunlop, B. D. "Utilization Across the Continuum of Long-Term Care Services." *Gerontologist*, Oct. 1, 2002, *42*(5), 603–612; Cagney, K. A., and Agree, E. M. "Racial Differences in Skilled Nursing Care and Home Health Use: The Mediating Effects of Family Structure and Social Class." *Journals of Gerontology, Series B, Psychological Sciences and Social Sciences*, 1999 *54*(4), S223–S236.

91. Barresi, C. M., and Menon, G. "Diversity in Black Family Caregiving." In Z. Harel and M. Williams (eds.), *Black Aged: Understanding Diversity and Service Needs.* Thousand Oaks, Calif.: Sage, 1990; Spence, S. A., and Atherton, C. R. "The Black Elderly and the Social Service Delivery System: A Study of Factors Influencing the Use of Community-Based Services." *Journal of Gerontological Social Work*, 1991, *16*, 19–35.

92. Cagney and Agree (1999); Falcone, D., and Broyles, R. "Access to Long-Term Care: Race as a Barrier." *Journal of Health Politics, Policy, and Law*, 1995, *19*, 583–595; Wallace, S. P. "The Political Economy of Health Care for Elderly Blacks." *International Journal of Health Services*, 1990, *20*, 665–680; Pourat, N., Andersen, R., and Wallace S. "Postadmission Disparities in Nursing Home Stays of Whites and Minority Elderly." *Journal of Health Care for the Poor and Underserved*, Aug. 2001, *12*(3), 352–366; Cagney, K. A., and Agree, E. M. "Racial Differences in Formal Long-Term Care: Does the Timing of Parenthood Play a Role?" *Journals of Gerontology, Series B: Psychological Sciences and Social Sciences*, May 1, 2005, *60*(3), S137–S145.

93. Wallace, S. P., Enriquez-Haass, V., and Markides, K. "The Consequences of Color-Blind Health Policy for Older Racial and Ethnic Minorities." *Stanford Law and Policy Review*, 1998, *9*(2), 329–346.

94. Estes (2001).

95. Cohen, J. W., and Spector, W. D. "The Effect of Medicaid Reimbursement of Quality of Care in Nursing Homes." *Journal of Health Economics,* 1996, *15*(1), 23–48; Mor, V., and others. "Driver to Tiers: Socioeconomic and Racial Disparities in the Quality of Nursing Home Care." *Milbank Quarterly,* 2004, *82*(2), 227–256.

96. Meyer, M. H. "Gender, Race, and the Distribution of Social Assistance: Medicaid Use Among the Frail Elderly." *Gender and Society,* 1994, *8,* 8–28.

97. U.S. Center for Medicare and Medicaid Services (CMS). "Medicaid Manual, Part 03—Eligibility, Section 3703.2." CMS, Sept. 16, 2004. [http://www.cms.hhs.gov/manuals/45_smm/sm_03_3_3700_to_3714.2.asp#_toc490889347] (accessed July 15, 2005).

98. Langa, K. M., Chernew, M. E., Kabeto, M. U., and Katz, S. J. "The Explosion in Paid Home Health Care in the 1990s: Who Received the Additional Services?" *Medical Care,* Feb. 2001, *39*(2), 147–157.

99. Liu, K., Manton, K. G., and Aragon, C. "Changes in Home Care Use by Disabled Elderly Persons: 1982–1994." *Journals of Gerontology, Series B: Psychological Sciences and Social Sciences,* 2000, *55B*(4), S245–S253.

100. U.S. Select Committee on Aging. *Aging America: Trends and Projections.* Washington, D.C.: U.S. Department of Health and Human Services, 1991.

101. Knickman, J. R., and others. "Wealth Patterns Among Elderly Americans: Implications for Health Care Affordability." *Health Affairs,* May 1, 2003, *22*(3), 168–174.

102. "Current Home Health Care Patients." National Center for Health Statistics, Feb. 2004. [http://www.cdc.gov/nchs/data/nhhcsd/curhomecare00.pdf] (accessed July 15, 2005).

103. Estes, Swan, and Associates (1993); Hoechst Marion Roussel. *Care Digest Series.* Kansas City, Mo.: Hoechst Marion Roussel, 1999.

104. Nyman, J. A. "Continuing Care Retirement Communities and Efficiency in the Financing of Long-Term Care." *Journal of Aging and Social Policy,* 2000, *11*(2–3), 89–98.

105. Leutz, W. N. "Long-Term Care for the Elderly: Public Dreams and Private Realities." *Inquiry,* 1986, *23,* 134–140.

106. Wallace, Levy-Storms, Kington, and Andersen (1998).

107. Abel (1991).

108. Barrett (2004).

109. U.S. General Accounting Office. *Baby Boom Generation Presents Financing Challenges.* Washington, D.C.: U.S. General Accounting Office; 1998. (GAO/T-HEHS-98-107.)

110. Kane, Kane, and Ladd (1998).

111. Leutz (1986).

112. U.S. Government Accountability Office. *Long-Term Care Insurance.* Washington, D.C.: U.S. Government Accountability Office, 2006. (GAO-06-401.)

113. Cohen, M. A. "Private Long-Term Care Insurance: A Look Ahead." *Journal of Aging and Health,* Feb. 2003, *15*(1), 74–98.

114. Cohen, M. A., Miller, J., and Weinrobe, M. "Patterns of Informal and Formal Caregiving Among Elders with Private Long-Term Care Insurance." *Gerontologist,* Apr. 2001, *41*(2), 180–187.

115. Leutz (1986).

116. Yamada, Y. "Profile of Home Care Aides, Nursing Home Aides, and Hospital Aides: Historical Changes and Data Recommendations." *Gerontologist,* 2002, *42*(2), 199–206.

117. Baron, S., and Habes, D. J. *NIOSH Health Hazard Evaluation Report.* Cincinnati: Alameda County Public Authority for In-Home Support Services, 2004. (HETA no. 2001-0139-2930); Meyer, J. D., and Muntaner, C. "Injuries in Home Health Care Workers: An Analysis

of Occupational Morbidity from a State Compensation Database." *American Journal of Industrial Medicine,* 1999, *35*(3), 295–301.

118. Benjamin, A. E., and Matthias, R. E. "Work-Life Differences and Outcomes for Agency and Consumer-Directed Home-Care Workers." *Gerontologist,* 2004, *44*(4), 479–488.

119. Howes, C. "Upgrading California's Home Care Workforce: The Impact of Political Action and Unionization." In R. Milkman (ed.), *The State of California Labor.* Los Angeles: Institute for Labor and Employment, University of California, 2004.

120. Delp, L., and Quan, K. "Homecare Worker Organizing in California: An Analysis of a Successful Strategy." *Labor Studies Journal,* 2002, *27*(1), 1–23.

121. Stone, R. I. "The Direct Care Worker: The Third Rail of Home Care Policy." *Annual Review of Public Health,* 2004, *25*, 521–537.

CHAPTER FOURTEEN

# AIDS IN THE TWENTY-FIRST CENTURY

## Challenges for Health Services and Public Health

David S. Zingmond
William E. Cunningham

The epidemic of acquired immune deficiency syndrome (AIDS) presents to the health care system myriad challenges, which have changed over time. In the 1980s and early 1990s, there were few highly effective treatments. However, advancements in the treatment of HIV disease have demonstrated longer survival and improved quality of life for people with HIV disease. New treatments have demonstrated reduced morbidity and mortality associated with HIV infection.[1] Even so, frequent side effects, the evolution of drug-resistant HIV, and the unknown durability of the suppressive action of antiretroviral regimens render uncertain their long-term effects on quality of life and survival.[2] Furthermore, HIV infection remains contagious, often disabling, and potentially fatal. Of particular concern is evidence of a lack of equity in the treatment of HIV disease among minorities, women, the uninsured and Medicaid-insured, and heterosexual and injection drug users, compared to other groups.[3] Such challenges increasingly force health care policy makers, planners, and administrators to reevaluate the organization, delivery, and financing of AIDS health services.

Health services providers and researchers must understand the needs of people infected with HIV, as well as accessibility to care, cost of care, and quality of services. First, important characteristics of the changing epidemiology and treatment patterns of AIDS should be understood in the context of real-life health care delivery. Second, providers and managers must integrate emerging data on the accessibility, costs, and quality of services in this era of more effective AIDS treatments. At the same time, the unique problems of diverse subpopulations and service systems should be addressed more rigorously. Third, these issues have to be examined not only within the arena of formal medical services but more broadly within the continuum of care, from prevention to ambulatory medical and psychosocial services to hospital and long-term care. Fourth, the implications and research needs for policy, planning and program administration in health services should be considered. Developing an approach for addressing the various agendas within the context of national and local health policy for HIV, as well as other chronic diseases, is paramount.

In this chapter, existing knowledge about critical issues of HIV/AIDS is discussed. The purpose is to provide the necessary background for addressing the challenges of the disease and for developing health policy, planning, and program implementation. Approaches to critical policy problems are suggested, and crucial areas for new investigation are identified to guide future HIV/AIDS health policy.

## The Changing Epidemiology and Clinical Treatment of HIV/AIDS

AIDS is a chronic infection, characterized by progressive failure of the immune system and development of opportunistic infections or cancers. HIV is an unusual type of virus (known as a retrovirus) that causes immune suppression leading to AIDS. Individuals infected with HIV develop antibodies within a short period of time and may exhibit no symptoms for many years. Typically, the immune system weakens gradually and the blood level of CD4 cells (a type of white blood cell known as a T-helper or inducer lymphocyte) declines from a normal level of 1,200–1,400 cells/mm$^3$. People with few CD4 cells are prone to opportunistic infections and certain cancers. Symptoms such as persistent fever, night sweats, and weight loss begin to occur more frequently once the CD4 count drops below 500 cells/mm$^3$. It is unclear whether everyone with asymptomatic HIV infection and CD4 count greater than 200 will eventually go on to develop AIDS; a small proportion of those infected have shown no sign of immune failure after more than a decade.[4] In addition to the CD4 count, the most powerful predictor of survival is the quantity of HIV RNA per ml of serum (known as viral load).[5] The natural history of progression to AIDS has been estimated at eleven years from time of HIV infection.[6] Newer HIV treatment regimens have significantly improved survival; for those individuals under care, HIV has become a chronic disease like heart disease or diabetes, which are generally not fatal or disabling when appropriately managed. New treatments such as integrase inhibitors, fusion inhibitors, and immune modulators are available, leading to additional hope and additional challenges.[7] Side effects of medications contribute to multiple medical comorbidities.[8]

## Epidemiology

By 2003, worldwide 34.6 million to 42.3 million people were living with HIV infection, and more than 20 million had died of AIDS. It is estimated that in the single year 2003, 4.8 million people became infected with HIV, and 2.9 million died of AIDS.[9] In the United States, an estimated 1.5 million Americans are living with HIV infection, including a growing number of women and persons of color.[10] By the end of 2003, 929,985 people were diagnosed with AIDS (Table 14.1), and there have been 524,060 deaths from AIDS, for a case fatality rate of 56 percent (Table 14.2). Each year, there are some 40,000 new cases of AIDS reported in the United States.[11] The rate of new cases of AIDS decreased among whites but rose among blacks and Latinos between 1999 and 2003.[12] For the overall adult population, HIV has not been in the list of the leading causes of death since 1997; since 1995, there have been seven consecutive years of decrease in the adjusted death rate due to HIV.[13] Although the overall number of annual deaths has dropped by more than 50 percent from a high of 49,897 in 1995 to 18,017 in 2003, women and persons of color account for an increasing proportion of AIDS-related deaths relative to earlier years (Table 14.2).[14] Reduction in mortality is thought to be due to improvements in treatment, although they have not improved health as much for women as for men, nor for persons of color compared to whites. Further evidence of the overall improvement of the health of persons with HIV in the United States is the reduction in age-adjusted mortality for HIV (5.9 per 100,000 in 1997 compared to 15.6 per 100,000 in 1995) and the 30 percent decline in hospitalizations for HIV between 1995 and 1997.[15] As discussed in this chapter, an inequitable distribution of treatment to persons of colors, women, and other disadvantaged groups probably accounts for the corresponding disparities in health improvements for these groups.

Widely recognized risk factors for transmission of HIV are male-to-male sexual contact, male-to-female sexual contact, injection drug use (IDU), blood product exposure, and perinatal transmission from mother to infant (during pregnancy, delivery, or possibly breast feeding). Frequently, individuals are exposed through multiple infection routes, and so the actual mode of HIV transmission may be unclear. A substantial portion of HIV-infected persons are unaware of their underlying HIV infection. Many cases of HIV infection remain underreported in the United States, because they may not meet the Centers for Disease Control (CDC) definition of AIDS and some states have no reporting requirements for HIV infection; the accuracy of diagnosing and reporting HIV/AIDS also varies by geographic location and affected population. The growth of the HIV/AIDS epidemic is, however, in large part due to changes in the modes of transmission and the sociodemographic characteristics of the groups in which the epidemic is growing fastest.[16] Unlike the early epidemic, the rate of increase in HIV transmission is

## TABLE 14.1.  CUMULATIVE AIDS CASES
## IN THE UNITED STATES THROUGH DECEMBER 2003[a].

|  | N | Percentage |
|---|---|---|
| Age at diagnosis (years) |  |  |
| <13 | 9,419 | 1 |
| 13–14 | 891 | 0 |
| 15–24 | 37,599 | 4 |
| 25–34 | 311,137 | 33 |
| 35–44 | 365,432 | 39 |
| 45–54 | 148,347 | 16 |
| 55–64 | 43,451 | 5 |
| >65 | 13,711 | 1 |
| Race and ethnicity |  |  |
| White, not Hispanic | 376,834 | 41 |
| Black, not Hispanic | 368,169 | 40 |
| Hispanic | 172,993 | 19 |
| Asian and Pacific Islander | 7,166 | 1 |
| American Indian and Alaska Native | 3,026 | 0 |
| Transmission category |  |  |
| Male adult or adolescent[e] |  |  |
| Male-to-male sexual contact | 440,887 | 59 |
| Injection drug use | 175,988 | 23 |
| Male-to-male sexual contact and injection drug use | 62,418 | 8 |
| Heterosexual contact | 56,403 | 8 |
| Other[b] | 14,191 | 2 |
| Subtotal | 749,887 | 81 |
| Female adult or adolescent[e] |  |  |
| Injection drug use | 70,558 | 41 |
| Heterosexual contact | 93,586 | 55 |
| Other[b] | 6,535 | 4 |
| Subtotal | 170,679 | 18 |
| Child(<13 years at diagnosis)[e] |  |  |
| Perinatal | 8,749 | 93 |
| Other[c] | 670 | 7 |
| Subtotal | 9,419 | 1 |
| Region of residence |  |  |
| Northeast | 285,040 | 31 |
| Midwest | 91,926 | 10 |
| South | 337,409 | 36 |
| West | 186,100 | 20 |
| U.S. dependencies, possessions, and associated nations | 29,511 | 3 |
| Total[d] | 929,985 | 100 |

## TABLE 14.1. CUMULATIVE AIDS CASES
## IN THE UNITED STATES THROUGH DECEMBER 2003,[a] Cont'd.

*Notes:*

[a] Includes persons with a diagnosis of AIDS from the beginning of the epidemic through 2003.

[b] Includes hemophilia, blood transfusion, perinatal, and risk factor not reported or not identified.

[c] Includes hemophilia, blood transfusion, and risk factor not reported or not identified.

[d] Includes persons of unknown race or multiple races and persons of unknown sex. Cumulative total includes 1,796 persons of unknown race or multiple races and 1 person of unknown sex. Because column totals were calculated independently of the values for the subpopulations, the values in each column may not sum to the column total.

[e] Percentages are calculated for within-group comparisons. Sub-total percentage calculated relative to the total cases.

*Source*: Data for this table taken from U.S. Centers for Disease Control and Prevention *HIV AIDS Surveillance Report 15* (2005). These numbers do not represent reported case counts. Rather, they are point estimates, which result from adjustments of reported case counts. The reported case counts are adjusted for reporting delays and for redistribution of cases in persons initially reported without an identified risk factor. The estimates do not include adjustment for incomplete reporting.

slower among whites and men who have sex with men (MSM) than communities of color and heterosexuals.

## Treatment

The main type of treatment is medication to combat loss of immune function and to prevent specific disease complications. The most widely used drugs are antiretrovirals (ARVs), which slow the progress of HIV infection and boost immune function. The earliest developed antiretrovirals used to treat HIV disease were in the class of drugs known as nucleoside reverse transcriptase inhibitors (NRTI), including zidovudine (ZDV/AZT), didanosine (ddI), and zalcitabine or dideoxycitidine (ddC). Newer generations of antiretrovirals, protease inhibitors (PI) and non-nucleoside reverse transcriptase inhibitors (NNRTI), are frequently key ingredients in combinations that often include three or more medications. Such combinations, or "cocktails," constitute what has become known as highly active antiretroviral therapy (HAART). Accumulating data from clinical and pathogenesis studies support institution of combination antiretroviral therapy for patients with HIV infection and evidence of declining immune function.[17] Current clinical guidelines support initiation of HAART for individuals with AIDS or those HIV-infected individuals without AIDS but with a CD4 count less than 350 cells/mm$^3$.[18] Delay in diagnosis of HIV or institution of therapy is thought to represent poor access or poor quality of care. Difficulties with adherence to medication regimens have been eased with the introduction of simplified dosing regimens. Despite gains

## TABLE 14.2. ESTIMATED DEATHS OF PERSONS WITH AIDS IN THE UNITED STATES, 1998 TO 2003.[a]

| | Year Of Death | | | | | Percentage Change 1999/2000 vs. 2002/2003 |
| --- | --- | --- | --- | --- | --- | --- |
| | 1999 | 2000 | 2001 | 2002 | 2003 | |
| **Age at death (years)** | | | | | | |
| < 13 | 97 | 51 | 48 | 35 | 29 | −131 |
| 13–14 | 18 | 8 | 4 | 11 | 8 | −37 |
| 15–24 | 232 | 216 | 270 | 199 | 229 | −5 |
| 25–34 | 3,258 | 2,823 | 2,512 | 2,143 | 1,928 | −49 |
| 35–44 | 7,706 | 7,138 | 7,525 | 6,896 | 6,970 | −7 |
| 45–54 | 4,994 | 5,203 | 5,548 | 5,737 | 5,964 | 13 |
| 55–64 | 1,556 | 1,631 | 1,873 | 1,840 | 2,146 | 20 |
| > 65 | 630 | 670 | 743 | 696 | 741 | 10 |
| **Race and ethnicity** | | | | | | |
| White, not Hispanic | 5,834 | 5,559 | 5,524 | 5,128 | 4,767 | −15 |
| Black, not Hispanic | 9,106 | 8,832 | 9,345 | 8,923 | 9,048 | 0 |
| Hispanic | 3,341 | 3,162 | 3,435 | 3,274 | 3,915 | 10 |
| Asian and Pacific Islander | 113 | 103 | 108 | 94 | 85 | −21 |
| American Indian and Alaska Native | 79 | 67 | 83 | 79 | 78 | 7 |
| **Transmission category** | | | | | | |
| Male adult or adolescent[b] | | | | | | |
| Male-to-male sexual contact | 6,703 | 6,316 | 6,479 | 6,012 | 6,015 | −8 |
| Injection drug use | 4,425 | 4,182 | 4,298 | 4,126 | 4,166 | −4 |
| Male-to-male sexual contact and injection drug use | 1,335 | 1,334 | 1,396 | 1,285 | 1,233 | −6 |
| Heterosexual contact | 1,403 | 1,417 | 1,585 | 1,526 | 1,644 | 11 |

| | | | | | |
|---|---|---|---|---|---|
| Other[b] | 194 | 204 | 174 | 166 | 140 | −30 |
| Subtotal | 14,061 | 13,454 | 13,932 | 13,116 | 13,198 | −5 |
| Female adult or adolescent[c] | | | | | | |
| Injection drug use | 2,051 | 1,925 | 1,985 | 1,956 | 2,056 | 1 |
| Heterosexual contact | 2,157 | 2,192 | 2,444 | 2,335 | 2,584 | 12 |
| Other | 97 | 92 | 92 | 89 | 95 | −3 |
| Subtotal | 4,305 | 4,209 | 4,521 | 4,379 | 4,736 | 7 |
| Region of residence | | | | | | |
| Northeast | 5,698 | 5,294 | 5,344 | 5,015 | 6,140 | 1 |
| Midwest | 1,712 | 1,685 | 1,839 | 1,550 | 1,343 | −17 |
| South | 7,406 | 7,352 | 7,624 | 7,526 | 7,068 | −1 |
| West | 2,952 | 2,681 | 2,817 | 2,520 | 2,588 | −10 |
| U.S. dependencies, possessions, and associated nations | 723 | 729 | 900 | 947 | 877 | 20 |
| Total[d] | 18,491 | 17,741 | 18,524 | 17,557 | 18,017 | −2 |

Notes:
[a] Includes persons who died with AIDS, from the beginning of the epidemic through 2003.

[b] Includes hemophilia, blood transfusion, and risk factor not reported or not identified.

[c] Includes hemophilia, blood transfusion, perinatal, and risk factor not reported or not identified.

[d] Includes persons of unknown race or multiple races and persons of unknown sex. Cumulative total includes 640 persons of unknown race or multiple races. Because column totals were calculated independently of the values for the subpopulations, the values in each column may not sum to the column total.

Source: Data for this table taken from U.S. Centers for Disease Control and Prevention, HIV AIDS Surveillance Report 15 (2005). These numbers do not represent reported case counts. Rather, they are point estimates, which result from adjustments of reported case counts. The reported case counts are adjusted for reporting delays and for redistribution of cases in persons initially reported without an identified risk factor. The estimates do not include adjustment for incomplete reporting.

in development of HAART medications and regimens, problems continue. Bothersome side effects and complications often affect persons taking these medications, which may influence adherence. More important, HIV sometimes develops resistance to antiretroviral medications, creating circumstances of (1) potential treatment failure and (2) development of HIV that is resistant to current medications.[19] An increasing rate of HIV resistant to current medications, especially among those newly infected, may be the next crisis in the treatment of HIV infection.

Antibiotics are used to prevent or to treat a common pneumonia (pneumocystis carinii or PCP) or other opportunistic infections that develops in persons with AIDS.[20] Introduction of HAART has changed the need for prophylactic treatment in many patients. Primary and secondary prophylaxis of opportunistic infections (for example, against PCP and mycobacterium avium complex or MAC) may be discontinued for patients with restored immune function as a result of receiving combination antiretroviral therapy.[21]

Most clinical services are directed toward monitoring for immune function decline, development of specific HIV complications (PCP, infectious diarrhea, or central nervous system infection), and reduction of treatment side effects. This monitoring involves use of the full range of medical services from physical examination to radiology to laboratory tests. Ongoing monitoring is also important because concomitant infectious diseases (for example, tuberculosis and hepatitis) and metabolic complications of treatment (diabetes, lipid disorders) remain common problems. Laboratory testing of infecting HIV specimen for resistance to various treatments has become an large part of clinical care for HIV-infected persons.[22] In the absence of a complete cure from traditional medical treatment, some people with HIV/AIDS may also resort to alternative medicine. Alternative therapies fall into four primary groups: nonconventional drug treatment, nutrition and diet modification (vitamins, minerals, and herbs), acupuncture and chiropractic, and psychospiritual intervention. Estimates of the incidence of alternative therapy usage range from 29 percent to 42 percent of AIDS patients surveyed.[23]

Investigators are beginning to shed light on important patterns in utilization of health served by persons with HIV/AIDS. Available information on population and system characteristics and how they determine access to medical care, costs, and quality of services are important considerations. Nationally representative data from the HIV Costs and Services Utilization Study (HCSUS) filled many critical gaps in information on these topics and represent a major source of information for this chapter.

***Access to Regular Medical Care and Delays in Care.*** Having a regular source of medical care is recognized as important for the general population, as well as for those with various chronic diseases. Problems in access to care for people with

HIV may be reflected in the degree to which they are in regular care. The HCSUS estimated that about half (between 36 and 63 percent) of all nonmilitary, nonincarcerated adults in the contiguous United States with known or unknown HIV infection see a provider outside of an emergency room at least every six months.[24] More than three months elapsed from the initial HIV positive test until first medical care for HIV in nearly one-third of the HCSUS national sample of HIV-infected persons in regular care. The median duration of this delay was one year.[25] In a progressive infection such as HIV, such a lengthy delay is alarming from personal and public health standpoints alike.[26] Opportunities for education about the disease, transmission to others, and social support may be missed during such delays.

***Public Benefits, Income, and Health Insurance.*** As HIV disease progresses, many people experience disability and unemployment and rely on public entitlements and private disability programs for income maintenance and health care benefits. These include Social Security Disability Income (SSDI) and Supplemental Security Income (SSI) administered by the Social Security Administration. Medicaid and Medicare become primary payers for health care with the onset of disability and depletion of personal funds.

Overall, much of the HIV-infected population is covered by public insurance.[27] It is estimated that 29 percent of the population in care is covered by Medicaid alone, and 19 percent is covered by Medicare with or without other insurance coverage. Private insurance covers 32 percent of the population, while 20 percent of persons with HIV disease have no health insurance coverage. Public insurance also finances the majority of HIV-related care.[28] Although public insurance covers about half of the HIV population, it accounts for 62 percent of HIV-related costs. Private insurance accounts for only 28 percent of HIV-related costs, while the uninsured account for 11 percent of HIV-related costs.[29]

As with other costly chronic conditions, insurance companies have sometimes denied benefits to HIV-positive individuals on the basis of preexisting conditions. Insurance companies sometimes require HIV antibody testing of insurance applicants and deny policies to those testing positive. Litigation has been one common avenue to resolve eligibility for health insurance benefits.[30]

***Barriers to Care.*** Lack of insurance and underinsurance represent formidable financial barriers to HIV/AIDS.[31] Persons with HIV/AIDS are more likely than the general population to be uninsured or to have Medicaid insurance.[32] Although evidence suggests that access to care for the uninsured and Medicaid populations increased between 1996 and 1998, it remains suboptimal.[33] Compared to those with private insurance, the uninsured and those with Medicaid are less likely to receive protease inhibitor therapy and more likely to never receive any antiretro-viral medication.[34] Even among the insured, substantial disparities in access per-sist because of other barriers to care such as competing subsistence needs. For example, HCSUS found that more than one-third of people went without or post-poned medical care because of one or more subsistence needs, and that minorities, women, and drug users were most likely to report these problems. Going without or postponing care for one of the four subsistence needs was associated with sig-nificantly greater multivariate odds of never receiving ARVs and having low over-all access to care.[35] Competing caregiver responsibilities may also prevent persons with HIV disease from receiving timely medical care. About 16 percent of HIV-infected patients with children delay seeking medical care, while 14 percent of those living with another HIV-positive individual also delay seeking medical care in HCSUS. Generally, women are more likely to report putting off care than men because they are more likely to be caring for someone else.[36] Thus studies of the HCSUS sample have shown that addressing social needs may actually compete (in terms of time, energy, and money) with obtaining medical care. Other barriers may include disability from HIV/AIDS disease, loss of employment, and social stigma resulting in the loss of private insurance coverage or moving to less gen-erous coverage.[37] Others may be reluctant to use their private insurance because of concern about confidentiality and threats to employment.

Lack of insurance, poverty, and underutilization of ambulatory services often coincide within the groups in which the epidemic is spreading most rapidly. For example, research early in the epidemic found that disadvantaged groups (mi-norities, women, injection drug users) often lack insurance, have difficulty with access to continuity care, and do not receive needed treatment.[38] Research con-ducted since the advent of HAART has found that blacks, Latinos, and women continue to have trouble accessing important HIV treatment.[39] Compared to whites, blacks were more likely to have poor access to outpatient care and less likely to receive protease inhibitors.[40] In addition, female injection drug users were less likely to receive HAART compared to homosexual men.[41] Similar findings were seen in the Florida Medicaid population.[42] However, the investigators could not control for HIV/AIDS stage.

Understanding the reasons behind nonreceipt of antiretroviral therapy is im-portant. An investigation into potential reasons for not receiving HAART at one community center showed that 31 percent (twenty-eight of eighty-eight) individ-uals did not receive HAART.[43] Among these twenty-eight patients not receiving HAART, for three patients the provider never discussed it; for six, the provider discussed HAART but did not recommend it; sixteen patients declined HAART despite their provider's recommendation; and three accepted their provider's rec-ommendation but never started HAART. Patients cited not being ready for strict adherence to a complex treatment regimen and fear of side effects as reasons for refusing HAART. In contrast, providers did not recommend HAART to individuals with active drug use, lack of engagement with care, and homelessness, depression, and feeling well without HAART.

The high costs associated with newly developed AIDS medications (not all of which are covered by insurance) may also serve as a barrier to treatment for disadvantaged groups. Studies of the diffusion of AIDS treatments such as zidovudine show that when new AIDS treatments are developed they take time to diffuse through the population but often do so unevenly.[44] A similar pattern has been observed in more recent studies of protease inhibitors.[45] Big gaps tend to be found between advantaged and disadvantaged groups in the use of new treatments, particularly a short time after they are introduced into the population, but the gap tends to converge over time, though not disappear.[46] One reason blacks and other disadvantaged groups have delayed access to the newest, most effective treatments may be that they are less likely to participate in clinical trials because of access barriers, mistrust, or poorer health status.[47]

Stability and continuity of care are particularly important for persons with HIV infection. However, discontinuity in HIV care has been identified as a problem in obtaining appropriate access to care.[48] A cohort study in one low socioeconomic urban population found that failure to suppress viral load with HAART was associated with higher rates of missed clinic appointments, nonwhite ethnicity, and drug use.[49] Similar findings were found in a second cohort, which also demonstrated a clinical consequence: men with longer interruption and HAART[50] discontinuers had a significantly higher rate of HIV RNA and lower CD4 cell counts.[51] From a health services standpoint, a potential consequence of discontinuity is greater use of the emergency department for nonemergency medical services. Inadequate access is often cited as the reason for inappropriate ER use.[52] HCSUS found that people with suboptimal access to care also overuse emergency room care.[53] In the Women's Interagency HIV Study, HIV-positive HAART users (without AIDS) had emergency room and hospitalization use patterns similar to those of HIV-negative women, but discontinuation of HAART resulted in a relative increase in hospital use.[54] In addition to continuity, comprehensiveness of care is important to ensure optimal care. For example, evidence suggests that access to a broad range of services is associated with better outcomes in that poor access to comprehensive general medical care has been shown to result in poor access to needed PCP prophylaxis.[55]

Other nonfinancial barriers to access to care are language barriers, cultural competence, and illiteracy. For example, one study found that Latinos had poorer survival compared to whites, even after controlling for insurance status, socioeconomic status, and having a regular source of care. These findings suggest that Latinos may face access barriers related to language and culture that result in suboptimal treatment and worse outcomes.[56]

Access to care may also be related to costs of HIV care, prevention, and health outcomes. In a study of hospitalized HIV patients in Southern California, better access to comprehensive community-based services was associated with fewer hospitalizations for HIV disease, which suggests that costs may be reduced with adequate access to care.[57] In this sample of patients, better access to general medical care was also associated with greater use of prehospital HIV testing and counseling.[58] Other research on persons with symptomatic HIV disease found that better access to care predicted improved health-related quality of life (HRQOL) outcomes.[59] State policies toward providing care through state Medicaid and drug assistance programs contribute to reducing differences in access to care and the mortality rate.[60] California and New York have more generous policies than Texas and Florida, and they have seen disparities in mortality outcomes decrease more since introduction of HAART than Texas and Florida.[61] Thus improving access to care may prevent spread of the disease and improve outcomes without excessive costs.

## Costs

Current federal funding for HIV/AIDS in fiscal year 2005 is estimated to total $19.7 billion, with 59 percent for care, 15 percent for research, 9 percent for cash and housing assistance, 4 percent for prevention, and 12 percent for combating the international epidemic.[62] About 46 percent of these costs are for hospitalization and 40 percent for medications.[63] Total pharmaceutical costs in 1997 were about $9,000 per person per year, $7,000 of which was for antiretroviral medications.[64] Since the beginning of the epidemic, the largest category of direct AIDS care costs has been for hospital utilization. However, there has been an overall reduction since the advent of HAART medications: a 30 percent reduction in the number of hospitalizations and a 40 percent reduction in the number of days hospitalized.[65] Thus AIDS costs are not as great as feared earlier in the epidemic, and there is little reason to expect that AIDS costs will become disproportionate to other chronic diseases and threaten the financing system. The $6.7 billion in annual expenditures that HIV care consumed is less than 1 percent of the more than $700 billion spent on health care in 1996. This may be considered relatively small in relation to the 7 percent of total potential years lost owing to HIV in the United States—an amount more than pneumonia, influenza, chronic obstructive pulmonary disease, diabetes mellitus, and chronic liver disease combined.[66] However, costs vary greatly as a function of the population served, the type of provider, and the region of the country.[67] Because it is known that sicker patients costs more regardless of the disease, there is concern that much of this variation is related to the adequacy of outpatient care provided to various populations. Inadequate outpatient care could result in delayed initiation of HAART treatment or treatment with less effective medications and result in higher morbidity and mortality, development of preventable opportunistic infections, and more rapid progression of the disease. Available data suggest that HIV/AIDS patients from groups with lower socioeconomic status and less access to care (minorities, drug users, women) use costlier sources of care (such as emergency rooms and hospitals) for longer duration, raising the concern that these variations in cost are due to variations in provider quality. Hence the costs of HIV/AIDS care should be examined in the context of the quality of care as well.

## Quality of Care

The emphasis of HIV/AIDS quality of care assessment centers on whether persons with HIV/AIDS receive appropriate clinical treatment specific to their stage of HIV disease.

*Underuse of Therapy.* Despite available clinical guidelines to inform HIV providers, certain subpopulations are less likely to receive these treatments. In HCSUS, blacks and women were less likely to receive HAART therapy, compared to whites and white men, respectively.[68] In addition, blacks and Hispanics were less likely to receive appropriate PCP and MAC prophylactic therapies, compared to whites.[69] Other research found that public insurance (compared to private insurance) may be associated with poorer level of quality, or inappropriate care.[70]

*Hospital and Physician Experience and Specialization.* Experience in treating HIV disease is another important predictor of better quality of care. Studies have found that hospitals and staffs with greater experience in treating HIV/AIDS have lower inpatient mortality.[71] Greater physician experience in treating HIV/AIDS also predicts longer survival.[72] The preponderance of evidence in AIDS indicates that the critical factor in producing better quality care is experience with a sufficient volume of patients with AIDS, rather than specialty certification in infectious disease, immunology, or oncology.[73] Although experience fosters the knowledge to provide quality care, physician attitude toward patients (for instance, regarding perceived reliability to follow treatment regimens) do influence optimal prescribing of HAART for patients.[74]

*Patient Satisfaction.* Satisfaction is also an important indicator of the quality of care and adequacy of services for persons with HIV disease. Patient dissatisfaction has been shown in the general population to predict utilization, continuity of care, switching providers, adherence to treatment, delays in obtaining treatment, and health outcomes.[75] In a study of persons with AIDS, Stein and colleagues found that IDUs, the uninsured, and public hospital patients were less satisfied with the technical and interpersonal care they received, as well as with their access to care.[76] Similarly, in a study in Boston, blacks and drug users had lower patient satisfaction in multivariate analysis.[77] In another cohort of HIV-infected persons, higher physical health-related quality of life was associated with greater satisfaction with the care that they received.[78] Individuals receiving care in public clinics for tuberculosis had much higher satisfaction with care than individuals with HIV receiving care in the private sector, suggesting that greater coordination in the public sector for HIV would improve patient satisfaction.[79]

***Adherence to Treatment.*** Adherence is essential for successful treatment of persons with HIV because inadequate dosing of antiretroviral medications may not suppress viral replication and may allow HIV to form new genetic variants of the virus. These variants can be resistant to entire classes of drugs, rendering certain combinations of drugs ineffective. Drug-resistant strains of HIV are also transmittable to others, creating an alarming public health threat.[80] The reasons for nonadherence are multifaceted, but they must be understood in order to develop effective interventions.[81] Long-term adherence to treatment with antiretroviral regimens is critical to survival with HIV infection, but problems in adhering are commonly reported. In HCSUS, only 57 percent of those who were taking antiretroviral medications reported that they actually took all their medications as they were prescribed.[82] Blacks, Hispanics, women, and heavy alcohol and drug users were the groups least likely to adhere to treatment. Surprisingly, adherence was not necessarily worse if there were more pills to take, but it was better when persons were aware that the medications are effective and that nonadherence could lead to viral resistance. Other factors associated with poor adherence were adverse side effects, traveling, forgetfulness, emotional distress, lack of social support, poor-quality relationship with one's provider, low education, and low health literacy.[83]

***Health-Related Quality of Life Outcomes.*** The goal of providing medical care is to improve outcomes. Thus outcomes are a marker of quality of care. One important outcome of HIV care is health-related quality of life. HRQOL is increasingly recognized as an important facet of health status and health service delivery for those with HIV disease, one that consists of physical and mental functioning and well-being from the perspective of individuals. HRQOL is perhaps one of the most important health outcomes to examine in HIV disease because of the disease's bothersome symptomatology, high mortality, and the resultant need for regular and urgent medical services. Various drug treatments for HIV may also affect HRQOL differently than they affect disease progression and physiologic markers of outcomes.

Both clinical trials and observational studies of HIV disease now commonly include generic measures of HRQOL outcomes to evaluate the simultaneous effects of clinical interventions, treatment side effects, and disease impact over time.[84] HRQOL measures have been shown to be associated with CD4 count, symptom severity, length of hospital stay, and disease progression (from asymptomatic HIV infection to symptomatic infection, to AIDS).[85] The associations between HRQOL and the clinical indicators of health status of patients support the hope that aggressive diagnostic evaluation and targeted treatment of abnormalities may improve function and patients' sense of well-being. Although there are associations between HRQOL and clinical and utilization measures, one study found that only 12–33 percent of the variability in HRQOL was accounted for by the clinical, utilization, and demographic variables examined,[86] suggesting that HRQOL measures tap aspects of health that extend beyond physiologic parameters. HRQOL measures can thus be useful tools for assessing both the physical and the mental health outcomes of HIV disease within inpatient and outpatient settings. The associations between HRQOL and the clinical indicators of health status of patients support the hope that astute diagnostic evaluation and targeted treatment of abnormalities may improve function and patients' sense of well-being.

## Toward a Comprehensive Continuum of Care

Persons with HIV/AIDS often present themselves to health care delivery systems in need of immediate, acute care services. However, the course of the illness is now more commonly characterized by a gradual decline in physical, cognitive, and emotional function and well-being, which may require primary care, supportive care, housing, supervised living, home health care, and hospice services.[87] Intermittent episodes of severe complications sometimes represent specific disease complications or less definitive symptoms. Longer periods of relative quiescence sometimes give way to subtle decline in functioning and loss of ability to perform usual daily activities without assistance.[88] As a result, people living with AIDS often need an array of personal and social services to support community-based living in the least restrictive setting.[89]

Providing a continuum of care is the ideal. What the continuum consists of is open to debate and is shaped by the availability of financial resources supporting various programs. In general, the continuum can encompass prevention services, public benefits and insurance counseling, primary care, dental care, mental and substance abuse, physical and occupational therapy, coordination of long-term care, social services, and secondary and tertiary health care. Combining medical and supportive social services may be the best approach to furnishing a continuum of care at the community level. As public and private payers search for cost-effective ways to provide quality care, the focus has shifted from hospital care to integrating key services such as prevention, primary care, mental health and substance abuse treatment, social services, and dental services.

## Prevention and Education

Controlling the AIDS epidemic depends on education and public health strategies to reduce high-risk behaviors. Groups with increasing incidence are targeted for intervention: men who have sex with men (increasing after a drop in the 1990s), IDUs, women who have partners with risk factors, adolescents, and minority ethnic groups. Education and outreach have been major approaches to risk reduction. However, controversy continues around condom education in schools and needle-exchange programs. Such controversy has prevented implementation of these programs throughout the United States. Recent research estimates that only 2.2 percent of U.S. high schools offer condom education programs, while syringe distribution is illegal in all but four states.[90] Syringe exchange programs do appear to be increasing in number, supported through private and local funding.[91] The potential use of abstinence-only programs for teenagers has become highly politicized, despite these programs' success in other countries.[92] As the author points out, the main message of these programs—"abstinence until marriage"—has little meaning to young gay men for whom same-sex marriage is not currently a legal option in the United States.[93] Other approaches for this population may be more effective.

Despite lay concerns that condom education and needle exchange programs promote increased sexual activity and injection drug use, recent empirical research found no justification for these concerns.[94] Condom education programs have not been associated with increased sexual activity in adolescents. Rather, research demonstrates that condom education programs have increased condom use among young people who choose to lead a sexually active lifestyle.[95] Similarly, rather than promote further injection drug use, needle exchange programs have reduced HIV infection by increasing the availability of clean needles for those who choose to use injection drugs.[96]

Testing and counseling services are considered vital to monitoring HIV/AIDS, but these practices are often underused. It is estimated that fewer than 40 percent of people in the United States with HIV risk factors have been tested for HIV.[97] Periodic screening in the general population appears to be cost-effective, strengthening the policy argument for testing.[98] Confidentiality concerns affect HIV testing and care-seeking behavior.[99] A substantial proportion of untested individuals say they would be tested if their results could not be identified.[100] Furthermore, people tested anonymously sought testing and medical care earlier in the course of HIV disease than did those tested confidentially.[101]

There are many licensed tests for clinical diagnosis of HIV infection, but historically the most common is the enzyme-linked immunosorbent assay (ELISA) test. In recent years, rapid HIV tests (as with saliva) have been approved by the FDA and are likely to revolutionize testing for HIV infection.[102] Rapid testing has been shown to be feasible in the setting of labor and delivery, clinics, and prisons.[103] These studies showed that rapid testing resulted in a high rate of receiving subsequent care for HIV infection. Rapid testing has opened the door for potential self-testing for HIV infection;[104] the public health ramifications may be dramatic. Studies have shown that access to continuous medical care is associated with timely receipt of HIV testing and counseling services.[105] Introduction of self-testing may shift the balance away from the doctor's office and opportunities to provide counseling and early prevention before the positive test.

Because of recent breakthroughs in antiretroviral therapy, the use of postexposure prophylaxis (PEP) as a risk-reduction method has recently been given more attention. PEP is introduction of antiretroviral therapy after possible exposure to HIV through sexual contact or injection drug use. Although the CDC recommends use of PEP for health care professionals occupationally exposed to HIV, health care workers are increasingly receiving inquiries from the public about PEP following nonoccupational high-risk HIV exposure (that is, sex or injection drug use). Although somewhat limited, recent research suggests it would be reasonable to use PEP after exposure to HIV through sex and injection drug use, only if the probability of exposure to HIV (through these behaviors) is of the same order of magnitude as percutaneous occupational exposures.[106] For individuals with continuing or low-risk exposure, more traditional state-of-the-art risk-reduction programs (education and outreach) are suggested.

Partner notification of people with HIV, though potentially beneficial in promoting risk reduction and prevention of HIV, is not systematically used across states. Because of confidentiality concerns, most states have voluntary programs and are not required to reveal the identity of the person infected. Additionally, notification is not possible if the index case has had anonymous sex partners, and it may be inefficient in populations with high prevalence of HIV infection.

## Mental Health and Drug Use

In the beginning of the AIDS epidemic, many community-based organizations, such as the Shanti Foundation, were created to help with the grief associated with death and dying from AIDS. As more people with HIV became long-term survivors, mental health services and formal and informal support networks became more important for the individual coping with the illness.

The prevalence of psychiatric disorders (major depression, dysthymia, generalized anxiety disorders, and panic attacks) and substance abuse is disproportionately high among people with HIV disease.[107] Similar to the general population, psychiatric and substance abuse disorders within the HIV population may impair quality of life, adversely affect access to appropriate health care, and compromise adherence with complicated medication regimens.[108] Psychiatric and substance abuse disorders may also be associated with sexual behavior and drug-using activity that endangers others with the risk of HIV infection.[109] Concurrent psychiatric disease may result in prolonged hospitalization, possibility from the need for case management, but it does not appear to affect receipt of antiretrovirals in people under care in one state Medicaid program.[110]

Consequently, there is substantial need for drug and alcohol abuse treatment. Reducing substance abuse can improve HIV prevention, as well as appropriate use of services and disorders. Many HIV-infected people need treatment for psychiatric disorders, with or without concomitant treatment for HIV. To the extent that mental health, substance abuse, and medical services are all needed, patients would benefit from coordination of these services—for example through sharing of medical records, streamlining assessment of benefits eligibility, and providing the services in close proximity to reduce transportation barriers and inconvenience.

## Oral Health and Dental Services

Oral manifestations, such as candida, mouth ulcers, and gum disease, are common in HIV disease. The occurrence of oral lesions is important for prognosis and affects quality of life. There is a broad consensus that people with HIV should see a dentist regularly.[111] However, HCSUS findings suggest that many of these individuals do not use dental care regularly.[112] Specific characteristics were associated with lower use of dental services: not having a regular source of care, not having health insurance, lower educational attainment, female gender, and black ethnicity. The source of care also influenced dental care utilization. Patients whose usual source of care was a VA clinic were most likely to use dental services, suggesting that comprehensive delivery systems (the VA, for instance) may facilitate use of dental services.

HIV-infected patients have substantial dental care needs. It is estimated that 52 percent of HIV patients have a regular need for ongoing dental care; IUDs and low-income patients were more likely to perceive a need for dental care.[113] Despite high need for dental services, dentists have not been universally receptive to caring for people with HIV.[114] It can be very difficult to find a dentist willing to treat an HIV patient. Dentists have seen themselves at considerable risk from HIV infection. Their attitude may result in less disclosure by HIV patients to the dentist. One previous study found that only 53 percent of patients had told their dentist of their infection.[115] Women may be particularly at risk of poor access to dental care.[116]

Dental and medical services also have interrelated roles in management of HIV. Oral health problems associated with HIV are often more complicated and resistant to treatment than those in the general population and require the attention of both medical and dental personnel. Without early and adequate access to dental and medical care, periodontal disease in the immunocompromised patient can lead to life-threatening infection. HCSUS found that more than 58,000 persons under treatment for HIV in the United States had unmet medical or dental needs. Unmet dental needs were more than twice as prevalent as unmet medical needs; 11,576 people were estimated to have both unmet dental and medical needs. Low income was most likely to report unmet needs for both dental and medical care. Of particular policy concern, the uninsured and those insured by Medicaid without dental benefits had more than three times the odds of unmet needs for both types of care than the privately insured.[117]

## Informal Social Support

Social support from family and friends has been shown to benefit HRQOL.[118] In HIV populations, the perceived availability of social support has been shown to be related to lowered hopelessness and depression and to increased feelings of psychological well-being.[119] Social resources are also important in affecting service use. People with more social services available to them were less likely to use formal mental health services.[120] Social support can be the key in facilitating access to necessary services by helping to overcome disruption that is due to loss of employment and financial problems.

*Formal Supportive Services.* Few studies have assessed the need for supportive health-related and social services. These services have been traditionally provided by AIDS service organizations (ASOs) such as Gay Men's Health Care Crisis in New York, AIDS Project Los Angeles, and San Francisco AIDS Foundation. Supportive services can include meals, food banks or pantries, residential facilities, buddies, transportation, child care, public benefits counseling, and respite care. In HCSUS, a high level of unmet need (16-40 percent) was identified for a variety of supportive services: benefits advocacy, substance abuse treatment, emotional counseling, home health care, and housing services. Unmet needs were highest for the first three. Nonwhites had higher unmet needs for any one of the five services. Compared to nongraduates of high school, participants with some college had less unmet need for substance abuse treatment and any unmet need; participants who were college graduates had less unmet need for emotional counseling and any unmet need. Being unstably housed was associated with higher unmet need for benefits advocacy and home health care.[121]

*Caregivers.* The number of people who provide home care to those with HIV/AIDS has increased. This trend suggests the need to focus on developing more home and community-based services. In HCSUS, 21 percent of the HIV-positive used home care services. Use of home care services was concentrated among persons with AIDS: 39.5 percent received home care, compared to 9.5 percent of those at earlier disease stages.[122] It is not clear under what circumstances home care services may substitute for or complement more expensive inpatient services, although there is some evidence that its use decreases overall costs.[123] As the population with HIV changes, however, the availability of informal home care (furnished by friends and family) may decrease, threatening the adequacy of the formal home care system.

# Organizing Comprehensive Care and Services

The organization of care for individuals living with HIV infection requires that payers and policy makers ensure access to primary care providers, coordination with specialty providers, and access to necessary medications.

## Providers

Up to three-quarters of primary care physicians in the United States have cared for an HIV-positive patient, but national data on the distribution of current providers and the amount of care they provide are lacking. Understanding current HIV care requires understanding both the sites and types of providers. Costs, access, and quality of care depend on patient characteristics and those of the providers. Data from HCSUS indicate that racial concordance affects receipt of care; African American patients with white physicians had delayed receipt of HAART compared to African American patients with African American physicians. White patients were not affected.[124] Physician attitude toward intravenous drug users and beliefs regarding adherence appear to account for relatively later use of protease inhibitor use among intravenous drug users, Latinos, women, and the poor.[125] As the HIV epidemic spreads into new populations, addressing physician attitudes will be critically important in providing timely and appropriate care.

## Managed Care

HIV/AIDS treatment is offered in an increasingly wide array of settings, including those that incorporate managed care practices. Although the majority of Americans receive their health coverage through private insurance companies and managed care organizations, the number of persons with AIDS covered by private plans has decreased over time.[126] Private insurers have reduced their exposure to HIV-infected people, because of the fear of high-risk individuals and partially as a result of highly inflated estimates of the average cost of an AIDS case.[127] People with HIV may therefore find it difficult to purchase an individual policy. Strategies to reduce provider risk also include tighter underwriting guidelines, use of HIV testing for enrollment, and denying insurance to those with a history of sexually transmitted disease.

Some states are experimenting with capitated arrangements and managed care as a way to promote better access to care for Medicaid recipients. Medicaid traditionally has paid for care of the HIV-infected through fee-for-service (FFS) arrangements, but over the past decade a managed care (HMO) approach has been adopted that includes care of HIV-infected beneficiaries. By 1999, forty-four states enrolled HIV-infected Medicaid beneficiaries in risk-based managed care plans.[128] Nationwide, Medicaid managed care programs have had to address adequacy of reimbursement for care, access to HIV medication, and access to experienced HIV providers.[129] Although clinical needs and associated costs are fairly constant, program design and reimbursements vary widely.[130] Primary components of these programs beyond standard managed care packages include higher capitation rate, a separate FFS HIV drug benefit, and allowance of HIV specialists to be primary care providers for HIV-infected patients.[131] These components are intended to meet the challenge of developing a system that ensures efficient and high-quality care with incentives and rules to satisfy the needs of patients, physicians, payers, and organizations in a balanced way. Very little is known about the impact on costs and quality of care when reimbursement for AIDS is capitated. In the California Medicaid program, AIDS patients in managed care appear to have similar mortality and hospitalization rates at three years, but lower use of HAART as individuals in traditional FFS Medicaid.[132]

## Case Management

Addressing problems of access, cost, and quality of HIV/AIDS care in medical and community-based settings has highlighted the importance of reducing service fragmentation and developing more comprehensive approaches to delivery. Case management has often been suggested as a strategy for coordinating care.

There are many definitions of *case management*, but most approaches include "core activities": intake and assessment; a comprehensive, multidisciplinary care plan; referrals to social and medical services; monitoring of care; modification of care plans on the basis of current problems; and client advocacy.[133] For many, case management may offer community-based alternatives to hospitalization, which may be more cost-effective and humane. Use of home services, such as intravenous antibiotics and total parenteral nutrition, may save 30–50 percent of hospital costs.[134]

Case management has been found to contribute to longevity between HIV diagnosis and death and between first hospitalization and death.[135] Findings from the HCSUS showed that case management was associated with decreased unmet needs.[136] In longitudinal analysis, having a case-manager predicted receipt of combination antiretroviral therapy.[137]

## Policy Implications and Research Needs for Management, Planning, and AIDS Policy

The HIV/AIDS epidemic has spread out from its initial geographic epicenters to much broader communities of the socially and economically disadvantaged. Concurrently, the range of medical treatments for HIV and AIDS complications has grown more effective, as well as more complex. The settings in which these treatments are administered are increasingly diverse, including those that incorporate managed care principles, such as public as well as private health maintenance organizations. Despite these developments, public policy decisions related to HIV/AIDS have thus far relied primarily on studies that use convenience samples of the earliest affected cohort—mostly white males with male-to-male sexual contact as the identified mode of exposure. Using this information to guide public policy and other decisions concerning HIV/AIDS is potentially misguiding.

HIV/AIDS is only one of many public health problems and social issues that confront the United States as it begins the twenty-first century. The initial impetus for action has waned as the epidemic enters its third decade and the populations most affected by AIDS change. Within the HIV/AIDS community, allocation of scarce resources is politically charged. Should more funds be directed toward prevention, or should treatment take priority? How can research funds have the greatest impact: through a return to basic science, or expanded access to new treatments and accelerated clinical trials? What is the appropriate funding relationship between medical services and social services? Similarly vexing questions plagued the debate about proper allocation of resources between AIDS and other diseases. Certainly no easy answers exist for these questions, and powerful interest groups can be found on every side. A debate about priorities is healthy, but there is potential for conflict that may do a disservice to people living with HIV infection. Developing partnerships and networks to effectively organize and deliver health and social services is paramount.

## Health Policy Issues and Options

As HIV infection increases in communities of color and among the poor, the financial burden on public payers and health care providers will inevitably increase. Reliance on Medicaid has profound implications for people with HIV/AIDS as public support for Medicaid wanes. In addition, new federal eligibility mandates of the 1990s have increased the cost of Medicaid to states. As a result, many state legislatures are searching for ways to effectively control the costs of the program. Rate setting of provider payments is one way states have attempted to control their Medicaid costs. Moving persons into managed Medicaid health plans has also become common. In many states, the reimbursement level has not kept up with inflation; Medicaid generally pays providers less than their cost of care. As providers limit the number of Medicaid patients they serve, access to care may deteriorate for those dependent on Medicaid.

Medicare currently pays for a smaller portion of AIDS expenditures than Medicaid because of the twenty-nine-month waiting period from the onset date of disability. One policy alternative is to significantly reduce or entirely eliminate this waiting period.[138] The proportion on Medicare has increased greatly since the 1990s, probably because people are living longer with the infection. The Congressional Budget Office estimated that a reduced AIDS-specific waiting period would cost the federal government $3 billion over five years, while it would generate $550 million in Medicaid savings to the states.[139] Medicare administrators may be unwilling to support another disease-specific expansion of the program, given the agency's experience with end-stage renal disease (ESRD), wherein costs ballooned since implementation. It is important to note that Medicare eligibility is only a partial solution for persons with AIDS because Medicare has no outpatient prescription drug benefit and most treatments for HIV disease are pharmacologically based.

Expansion of employer-based insurance is highly unlikely with the demise of the Clinton administration's 1993 Health Security Act and its employer mandate provision. Policy attention should be directed toward maintenance of private health insurance for those living with HIV infection. Some states have programs that pay private health insurance and Consolidated Omnibus Budget Reconciliation Act (COBRA) premiums of persons with AIDS and other high-cost illnesses; California and New York are the largest examples. These programs represent a win-win situation for persons with AIDS and public agencies. People with AIDS are able to remain with their current health care providers and maintain continuity of care. At the same time, public providers and payers are relieved of a substantial portion of the burden of care and treatment by shifting it to the private sector.

A large number of federal agencies and offices have responsibility for AIDS health services and health policy, among them the Department of Health and Human Services Office of HIV/AIDS policy, the White House Office of AIDS Health Policy, the Agency for Health Research and Quality (AHRQ), the Health Resources and Services Administration (HRSA), numerous branches of the CDC, and numerous institutes within the NIH. Better coordination is needed for the activities of these agencies and offices, and as well as the many private, state, and local organizations involved in AIDS health services and policy. Such coordination may improve the ability of these organizations to deliver HIV-related health services efficiently and effectively.

## Ryan White CARE Act and ADAP Programs

The Ryan White Comprehensive AIDS Resource Emergency Act (CARE) was originally signed in 1990, as a federal program designed to improve the quality and availability of care for persons with HIV/AIDS and their families. Under title I of the Care Act, a variety of medical and supportive services were covered: primary health care, case management, home health, food services, hospice care, housing, transportation, and prevention and education services.[140] The main target populations for these services were the poor and the uninsured.

Under Title I, cities qualifying for Title I funds are defined as Eligible Metropolitan Areas (EMAs). Appropriation of Title I funds is awarded by two methods: (1) formula (based on cumulative AIDS cases and cumulative AIDS incidence) and (2) supplemental applications among the EMAs. These supplemental plans must include a plan for additional funds based on needs not met by the formula grants, a high incidence of AIDS, and proof of existing commitment of area resources. In these additional applications, the needs of infants, children, women, and families are also to be addressed.

Within each EMA, the priorities for spending Title I funds must be established by HIV Health Services Planning Councils. Many EMAs have designated planning councils by expanding existing HIV-AIDS planning bodies. Examples of the type of organization represented on planning councils are housing, drug treatment providers, the American National Red Cross, the United Way, the Department of Veterans Affairs, and private foundations. The CARE Act also requires that people with HIV/AIDS be voting members of HIV Health Services Planning Councils.

Research suggests that the CARE act has been successful in improving access to some Title I services (such as basic medical care) for low-income populations.[141] A study of CARE and non-CARE clients in San Francisco found no difference in utilization of physician visits, hospitalizations, or emergency rooms, after adjusting for sociodemographic characteristics and health status.[142] However, the study also found high unmet need for dental care, home health care, and alternative therapies—suggesting that further strategies are required to increase access to care for low-income HIV-infected populations.

Pharmacy support, through the ADAP (AIDS Drug Assistance Program), is a new but increasingly important component of the CARE act.[143] Under the ADAP, uninsured and underinsured persons with HIV disease can access newly developed treatment medications (for example, protease inhibitors). Although expensive, ADAP does appear to have economic benefits through offsetting higher hospitalization costs.[144] Although the CARE act has been successful in increasing availability of medical and nonmedical services for persons with HIV disease, concern has arisen whether CARE act funding spent on newly developed medications is too high (HAART). Although timely use of newly developed treatment medications is important to manage HIV disease, many who use these drugs often become disabled and also need supportive services. Thus policy makers are faced with a dilemma because CARE funding spent on expensive medications may reduce funding for available supportive services, thereby possibly exacerbating unmet needs for supportive services.

## Needs of Special Populations

Certain special populations deserve attention: HIV-positive women, children, adolescents, certain ethnic groups, drug dependent individuals, and those suffering from psychiatric disorders. These groups may face additional barriers to early intervention and access to care.

***Women.*** In 2003, 11,498 women were diagnosed with AIDS, nearly a 10 percent increase from the previous year.[145] AIDS is the fourth leading cause of death for twenty-to-forty-year-old women. African American and Latina women account for more than 75 percent of infected women dying with AIDS (Table 14.2) and 80 percent of the AIDS cases reported for women in 2003.[146] The course of clinical care differs somewhat from men; women present to the medical care system at more advanced stages of the disease than do men, and they develop some unique complications (for instance, cervical cancer). Women also use services differently,[147] and ensuring primary care at the site of HIV care may decrease potential adverse outcomes of gynecological abnormalities such as cervical cancer.[148] Some studies indicate that differences between men and women in their use of services such as the emergency room and inpatient and outpatient sites may be explained by factors of insurance status, stage of illness, and transmission risk.[149]

Obstetric and gynecological conditions and procedures may contribute substantially to the health service use of women.[150] The availability of obstetric and gynecological services, licensing and funding for trained health care providers, shortages of obstetricians, and the limited HIV experience of health care providers with HIV-infected women may influence health service access and use. About 25 percent of women receiving care in the United States have dependent children under the age of eighteen.[151] The competing responsibilities of care giving for children or other HIV-infected people in the household often act as barriers to receipt of timely care.[152] Other gender-specific factors that may influence utilization are misdiagnosis or undiagnosed HIV-related conditions, sexual or domestic violence, and commercial sex work.[153]

**Children.**  In thirty-three areas with confidential name-based HIV infection reporting, there were 2,614 children (up to twelve years old) with HIV/AIDS.[154] According to national AIDS case reporting, by December 2003 1.0 percent (n = 9,419) of AIDS cases had been reported in children less than thirteen years old; 59 percent of childhood AIDS cases are African American and 23 percent are Hispanic. Infection in children is generally acquired perinatally, and almost 91 percent have mothers with (or with known risk for) HIV infection.[155] More than one-half of mothers of perinatally infected children were IDUs or had a sexual partner who injected drugs. As many as 25 percent of children born to HIV-positive mothers are infected.[156] Although HCSUS found that only 4 percent of children of women who were HIV-positive tested positive for HIV, this figure may be considered a lower bound, because nearly half (42 percent) of HIV-positive women with children had not been tested.[157]

The costs of pediatric AIDS are higher than the costs of adult AIDS, largely due to higher hospital costs. They are estimated at about $35,000-$37,000 per year, which includes inpatient care, outpatient care, home health, and pharmacy service.[158] Medicaid has been the primary payer for both hospital and community-based services for pediatric AIDS.[159] Contributing to the high costs are complications of medical management through the absence, disability, or death of one or both parents from AIDS or drug use, urban poverty, and complex social conditions.[160]

**Adolescents.**  AIDS is the seventh leading cause of death in people ages fifteen to twenty-four and contributes to premature mortality of those who are supposed to be healthy, productive, and expected to live a normal life span. Nearly three times as many males compared to females between fifteen and twenty-four are reported to have AIDS. This population is of particular concern because of the number of sexual contacts and behaviors that contribute to increased risk and likelihood of infection. However, reporting needs to be improved: risk is not given by adolescents with AIDS for more than one-third of male patients and one-half of females.[161] Although adolescents are more aware of HIV transmission and AIDS, many have misperceptions about sexual activity, drug use, and prevention measures. Despite adequate knowledge, most adolescents continue to participate in unprotected sex.[162]

***Ethnic Groups.*** HIV/AIDS disproportionately affects certain ethnic groups; African Americans and Hispanics are most likely to be HIV-infected. Furthermore, African Americans are less likely to receive HAART than whites for a variety of reasons, among them lack of insurance, lack of regular care, and competing needs for food, clothing, and housing, as well as attitudes and beliefs such as distrust of doctors. These same groups more often experience barriers to both access and outreach. Many may not be aware of the benefits of receiving early treatment. Hispanics exposed to HIV by drug use and heterosexual sex tend not to have a usual source of care at HIV diagnosis.[163] Hispanic men and Hispanic patients exposed to HIV by drug use and heterosexual sex are likely to require special attention when one considers interventions to improve access to care for Hispanic patients who are HIV-infected. Geographic barriers to care may pose access concerns. Female immigrants from sub-Saharan Africa appear to be at higher risk of being infected with HIV than other individuals seen at regional STD clinics, suggesting that this population needs focused intervention for HIV prevention.[164] Sites of care for HIV/AIDS may not be in familiar neighborhood settings. Agencies may not be prepared to deal with the special cultural needs of racial and ethnic minorities.[165] For example, blacks in one urban area were much more likely to receive information through their church.[166] Health organizations working collaboratively with religious organizations and health care providers might be more effective in developing AIDS prevention strategies in these populations.

These issues may exacerbate the vulnerability already experienced by people with HIV/AIDS in receiving the full range of health care services that are needed and available.

***Drug Dependent Individuals and Those with Psychiatric Disorders.*** The prevalence of drug dependence and psychiatric disorders remains disproportionately high in HIV populations. This has important clinical and public health implications. The availability of effective, albeit complicated, treatments for HIV requires infected persons to access care, use services appropriately, and adhere strictly to medication regimens. Failure to adhere closely to treatment may facilitate development of medication-resistant viral strains that can render antiretroviral medications ineffective and increase the likelihood of transmission of resistant strains. Psychiatric disorders, drug use, and drug dependence are likely to limit adherence to treatment as well as access to appropriate comprehensive medical and mental health care and substance abuse treatment. High prevalence of these disorders points to the importance of integrating mental health and substance abuse treatment into the ongoing clinical care of people with HIV infection.

## Future Issues in HIV/AIDS Health Services Research

Ideally, policy and planning options are based on evidence of the effectiveness of treatment and acceptable level of cost in delivering such treatment. The completion of the landmark HCSUS study vastly improved policy-relevant AIDS health services data. This study has made available data relevant on a range of issues pertinent to HIV policy, notably costs and utilization, access and barriers to care, adherence, quality of life, social support services, mental health, dental health, and quality of care. New research efforts must continue to include the changing clinical profile of the epidemic. In addition, research efforts must yield insights into national trends, such as regional variation in the patterns of HIV-related disease complications. Changes in treatment patterns and in the price of medication over time make prediction of future costs even more difficult. The many nonmedical costs of HIV/AIDS should be examined: direct costs of transportation, informed support, and housing as well as indirect costs of disability days from work resulting from treatment or deteriorating health. In response to these needs, in 2004 the Centers for Disease Control and Prevention funded a new HIV/AIDS surveillance project, the "Morbidity Monitoring Project" (MMP). This ongoing project will recruit each year a nationwide representative sample of more than ten thousand HIV-infected individuals receiving medical care (viral load test, CD4+ counts, or antiretroviral treatment in the past twelve months) for medical record abstraction and patient interview.

Studies of special populations will also be needed: women, children, adolescents, IDUs, persons in rural communities, and the racial and ethnic minorities who constitute a growing proportion of the HIV-infected population. Data collected on cost and utilization will enable policy makers to compare current patterns of cost and utilization across the spectrum of HIV disease, across geographical areas, across the range of institutional and individual providers (including managed care settings), and for both insured and uninsured populations, as well as variations in financing and provider arrangements.

Given that side effects are likely to be associated with medications used to treat HIV disease, further research is needed to develop and evaluate interventions to improve adherence with treatment regimens. Such research takes on greater salience with the widespread use of HAART medications. Particular populations of interest for future adherence research include those with mental disorders, substance abusers, or both.

Lack of insurance, poverty, and underuse of ambulatory treatment likely will continue within the groups in which the epidemic is spreading most rapidly. Disadvantaged groups (minorities, women, IDUs, and the poor) experience difficulty more often in obtaining access to outpatient care. In addition, they may not receive appropriate treatment, which can account for greater mortality in those populations. People with impaired access to health services often use costlier sources of medical care and use them for a longer duration. Furthermore, variations in the quality of AIDS care by geographic region, sociodemographic group, and type of provider likely reflect poor-quality care for certain individuals.

In view of these concerns, the important characteristics of the changing epidemiology of AIDS and clinical treatment patterns need to be constantly under review in order to address problems in access, cost, and quality. Health service delivery systems must be developed to address the emerging needs of diverse population groups affected by HIV/AIDS. Additionally, it is important that Ryan White CARE programs also address the emerging needs of diverse population groups affected by HIV/AIDS. Neither the arena of formal medical services nor supportive services can be overlooked. Developing finance and delivery systems within the context of long-range planning and evaluation is paramount. Existing knowledge and critical gaps in information about HIV/AIDS have been reviewed to constitute a basis for addressing the current and future challenges that HIV/AIDS presents for development of relevant health policy and health and social services planning and program implementation.

# Notes

1. Palella, F. J. Jr., and others. "Declining Morbidity and Mortality Among Patients with Advanced Human Immunodeficiency Virus Infection: HIV Outpatient Study Investigators." *New England Journal of Medicine*, 1998, *338*(13), 853–860; Hogg, R. S., and others. "Improved Survival Among HIV-Infected Individuals Following Initiation of Antiretroviral Therapy." *Journal of the American Medical Association*, 1998, *279*(6), 450–454.

2. Wainberg, M. A., and Friedland, G. "Public Health Implications of Antiretroviral Therapy and HIV Drug Resistance." *Journal of the American Medical Association*, 1998, *279*(24), 1977–1983; Cohen, O. J., and Fauci, A. S. "HIV/AIDS in 1998—Gaining the Upper Hand?" *Journal of the American Medical Association*, 1998, *280*(1), 87–88.

3. Shapiro, M. F., and others. "Variations in the Care of HIV-Infected Adults in the United States: Results from the HIV Cost and Services Utilization Study." *Journal of the American Medical Association*, 1999, *281*(24), 2305–2315; Andersen, R., and others. "Access of Vulnerable

Groups to Antiretroviral Therapy Among Persons in Care for HIV Disease in the United States." HCSUS Consortium. HIV Cost and Services Utilization Study. *Health Services Research*, 2000, *35*(2), 389–416.

4. Kirchhoff, F., and others. "Brief Report: Absence of Intact NEF Sequences in a Long-Term Survivor with Nonprogressive HIV-1 Infection." *New England Journal of Medicine*, 1995, *332*(4), 228–232; Pantaleo, and others. "Studies in Subjects with Long-Term Nonprogressive Human Immunodeficiency Virus Infection." *New England Journal of Medicine*, 1995, *332*(4), 209–216.

5. Mellors, J. W., and others. "Prognosis in HIV-1 Infection Predicted by the Quantity of Virus in Plasma." Science, 1996, *272*(5265), 1167–1170; O'Brien, and others. "Changes in Plasma HIV-1 RNA and CD4+ Lymphocyte Counts and the Risk of Progression to AIDS." (Veterans Affairs Cooperative Study Group on AIDS.) *New England Journal of Medicine*, 1996, *334*(7), 426–431; O'Brien, W. A., and others. "Changes in Plasma HIV RNA Levels and CD4+ Lymphocyte Counts Predict Both Response to Antiretroviral Therapy and Therapeutic Failure." (VA Cooperative Study Group on AIDS.) *Annals of Internal Medicine*, 1997, *126*(12), 939–945.

6. Pantaleo and others (1995).

7. Hong, H., and others. "Identification of HIV-1 Integrase Inhibitors Based on a Four-Point Pharmacophore." *Antiviral Chemistry and Chemotherapy*, 1998, *9*(6), 461–472; Kovacs, J. A., and others. "Increases in CD4 T Lymphocytes with Intermittent Courses of Interleukin-2 in Patients with Human Immunodeficiency Virus Infection: A Preliminary Study." *New England Journal of Medicine*, 1995, *332*(9), 567–575.

8. Currier, J. S., and Havlir, D. V. "Complications of HIV Disease and Antiretroviral Therapy." *Topics in HIV Medicine*, 2005, *13*(1), 16–23; Currier, J., "Top Stories of 2004: HAART and the Heart." *AIDS Clinical Care*, 2005, *17*(1), 2; Currier, J. S., and Havlir, D. V. "Complications of HIV Disease and Antiretroviral Therapy: Highlights of the 11th Conference on Retroviruses and Opportunistic Infections," Feb. 8–11, 2004, San Francisco. *Topics in HIV Medicine*, 2004, *12*(1), 31–45; Havlir, D. V., and Currier, J. S. "Complications of HIV Infection and Antiretroviral Therapy." *Topics in HIV Medicine*, 2003, *11*(3), 86–91.

9. Steinbrook, R., "The AIDS Epidemic in 2004." *New England Journal of Medicine*, 2004, *351*(2), 115–117.

10. Centers for Disease Control and Prevention (CDC). *HIV/AIDS Surveillance Report 15*, Atlanta: Department of Health and Human Services, Centers for Disease Control and Prevention, 2004.

11. National Center for Health Statistics. "Acquired Immunodeficiency Syndrome (AIDS) Cases, According to Age at Diagnosis, Sex, Detailed Race, and Hispanic Origin: United States, Selected Years 1985–2003." In *Health, United States, 2004 with Chartbook on Trends in the Health of Americans.* Hyattsville, Md.: National Center for Health Statistics, 2004.

12. CDC (2004).

13. Kochanek, K., Murphy, S., Anderson, R., and Scott, C. "Deaths: Final Data for 2002." *National Vital Statistics Reports, 53*(5), 2004.

14. CDC (2004).

15. National Center for Health Statistics. "Decreasing Hospital Use for HIV." In *NCHS Health E-Stats.* Hyattsville, Md.: National Center for Health Statistics, 2005.

16. CDC (2004).

17. Carpenter, C. C., and others. "Antiretroviral Therapy in Adults: Updated Recommendations of the International AIDS Society-USA Panel." *Journal of the American Medical Association*, 2000, *283*(3), 381–390; Carpenter, C. C., and others. "Antiretroviral Therapy for HIV

Infection in 1998: Updated Recommendations of the International AIDS Society-USA Panel." *Journal of the American Medical Association*, 1998, *280*(1), 78–86.

18. Hirsch, M. S., and others. "Antiretroviral Drug Resistance Testing in Adults Infected with Human Immunodeficiency Virus Type 1: 2003 Recommendations of an International AIDS Society-USA Panel." *Clinical Infectious Diseases*, 2003, *37*(1), 113–128; Yeni, P. G., and others. "Antiretroviral Treatment for Adult HIV Infection in 2002: Updated Recommendations of the International AIDS Society-USA Panel." *Journal of the American Medical Association*, 2002, *288*(2), 222–235.

19. Clavel, F., and Hance, A. J. "HIV Drug Resistance." *New England Journal of Medicine*, 2004, *350*(10), 1023–1035; Little, S. J., and others. "Antiretroviral-Drug Resistance Among Patients Recently Infected with HIV." *New England Journal of Medicine*, 2002, *347*(6), 385–394.

20. Pradier, C., and others. "Reducing the Incidence of Pneumocystis Carinii Pneumonia: A Persisting Challenge." *AIDS*, 1997, *11*(6), 832–833.

21. Zellweger, C., and others. "Long-Term Safety of Discontinuation of Secondary Prophylaxis Against Pneumocystis Pneumonia: Prospective Multicentre Study." *AIDS*, 2004, *18*(15), 2047–2053; Goldman, M., and others. "Safety of Discontinuation of Maintenance Therapy for Disseminated Histoplasmosis After Immunologic Response to Antiretroviral Therapy." *Clinical Infectious Diseases*, 2004, *38*(10), 1485–1489; Vibhagool, A., and others. "Discontinuation of Secondary Prophylaxis for Cryptococcal Meningitis in Human Immunodeficiency Virus-Infected Patients Treated with Highly Active Antiretroviral Therapy: A Prospective, Multicenter, Randomized Study." *Clinical Infectious Diseases*, 2003, *36*(10), 1329–1331; Mussini, C., and others. "Discontinuation of Secondary Prophylaxis for Pneumocystis Carinii Pneumonia in Human Immunodeficiency Virus-Infected Patients: A Randomized Trial by the CIOP Study Group." *Clinical Infectious Diseases*, 2003, *36*(5), 645–651; Shafran, S. D., and others. "Successful Discontinuation of Therapy for Disseminated Mycobacterium Avium Complex Infection After Effective Antiretroviral Therapy." *Annals of Internal Medicine*, 2002, *137*(9), 734–737; Furrer, H., and others. "Discontinuation of Primary Prophylaxis Against Pneumocystis Carinii Pneumonia in HIV-1-Infected Adults Treated with Combination Antiretroviral Therapy: Swiss HIV Cohort Study." *New England Journal of Medicine*, 1999, *340*(17), 1301–1306.

22. Yeni, P. G., and others. "Treatment for Adult HIV Infection: 2004 Recommendations of the International AIDS Society-USA Panel." *Journal of the American Medical Association*, 2004, *292*(2), 251–265.

23. Abrams, D. I., "Alternative Therapies in HIV Infection." *AIDS*, 1990, *4*(12), 1179–1187; Greenblatt, R. M., Hollander, H., McMaster, J. R., and Henke, C. J. "Polypharmacy Among Patients Attending an AIDS Clinic: Utilization of Prescribed, Unorthodox, and Investigational Treatments." *Journal of Acquired Immune Deficiency Syndrome*, 1991, *4*(2), 136–143; Hsiao, A. F., and others. "Complementary and Alternative Medicine Use and Substitution for Conventional Therapy by HIV-Infected Patients." *Journal of Acquired Immune Deficiency Syndrome*, 2003, *33*(2), 157–165.

24. Bozzette, S. A., and others. "The Care of HIV-Infected Adults in the United States: HIV Cost and Services Utilization Study Consortium." *New England Journal of Medicine*, 1998, *339*(26), 1897–1904.

25. Turner, B. J., and others. "Delayed Medical Care After Diagnosis in a U.S. National Probability Sample of Persons Infected with Human Immunodeficiency Virus." *Archives of Internal Medicine*, 2000, *160*(17), 2614–2622.

26. Samet, J. H., and others. "Trillion Virion Delay: Time from Testing Positive for HIV to Presentation for Primary Care." *Archives of Internal Medicine*, 1998, *158*(7), 734–740.

27. Bozzette and others (1998).

28. Fleishman, J. A., and Mor, V. "Insurance Status Among People with AIDS: Relationships with Sociodemographic Characteristics and Service Use." *Inquiry,* 1993, *30*(2), 180–188.

29. Bozzette and others (1998).

30. Senak, M. S., *HIV, AIDS, and the Law: A Guide to Our Rights and Challenges.* New York: Insight Books, 1996.

31. Shapiro and others (1999); Andersen and others (2000); Katz, M. H., and others. "Health Insurance and Use of Medical Services by Men Infected with HIV." *Journal of Acquired Immune Deficiency Syndromes and Human Retrovirology,* 1995, *8*(1), 58–63.

32. Green, J., and Arno, P. S. "The 'Medicaidization' of AIDS: Trends in the Financing of HIV-Related Medical Care." *Journal of the American Medical Association,* 1990, *264*(10), 1261–1266.

33. Shapiro and others (1999).

34. Shapiro and others (1999).

35. Cunningham, W. E., and others. "The Impact of Competing Subsistence Needs and Barriers on Access to Medical Care for Persons with Human Immunodeficiency Virus Receiving Care in the United States." *Medical Care,* 1999, *37*(12), 1270–1281.

36. Stein, M. D., and others. "Delays in Seeking HIV Care Due to Competing Caregiver Responsibilities." *American Journal of Public Health,* 2000, *90*(7), 1138–1140.

37. Crawford, A., "Stigma Associated with AIDS: A Meta-Analysis." *Journal of Applied Social Psychology,* 1996, *26*(5), 398–416; Rotheram-Borus, M. J., Draimin, B. H., Reid, H. M., and Murphy, D. A. "The Impact of Illness Disclosure and Custody Plans on Adolescents Whose Parents Live with AIDS." *AIDS,* 1997, *11*(9), 1159–1164; Kass, N. E., and others. "Changes in Employment, Insurance, and Income in Relation to HIV Status and Disease Progression: The Multicenter AIDS Cohort Study." *Journal of Acquired Immune Deficiency Syndrome,* 1994, *7*(1), 86–91.

38. Stein, M. D., and others. "Differences in Access to Zidovudine (AZT) Among Symptomatic HIV-Infected Persons." *General Internal Medicine,* 1991, *6*(1), 35–40; Moore, R. D., Stanton, D., Gopalan, R., and Chaisson, R. E. "Racial Differences in the Use of Drug Therapy for HIV Disease in an Urban Community." *New England Journal of Medicine,* 1994, *330*(11), 763–768; Mor, V., and others. "Variation in Health Service Use Among HIV-Infected Patients." *Medical Care,* 1992, *30*(1), 17–29; Fleishman, J. A., Hsia, D. C., and Hellinger, F. J. "Correlates of Medical Service Utilization Among People with HIV Infection." *Health Services Research,* 1994, *29*(5), 527–548.

39. Shapiro and others (1999).

40. Shapiro and others (1999); Andersen and others (2000); Bing, E. G., and others. "Protease Inhibitor Use Among a Community Sample of People with HIV Disease." *Journal of Acquired Immune Deficiency Syndromes and Human Retrovirology,* 1999, *20*(5), 474–480.

41. Cunningham, W. E., and others. "Prevalence and Predictors of Highly Active Antiretroviral Therapy Use in Patients with HIV Infection in the United States. HCSUS Consortium: HIV Cost and Services Utilization." *Journal of Acquired Immune Deficiency Syndrome,* 2000, *25*(2), 115–123.

42. Anderson, K. H., and Mitchell, J. M. "Differential Access in the Receipt of Antiretroviral Drugs for the Treatment of AIDS and Its Implications for Survival." *Archives of Internal Medicine,* 2000, *160*(20), 3114–3120.

43. Maisels, L., Steinberg, J., and Tobias, C. "An Investigation of Why Eligible Patients Do Not Receive HAART." *AIDS Patient Care and STDs,* 2001, *15*(4), 185–191.

44. Crystal, S., Sambamoorthi, U., and Merzel, C. "The Diffusion of Innovation in AIDS Treatment: Zidovudine Use in Two New Jersey Cohorts." *Health Services Research*, 1995, *30*(4), 593–614.

45. Palella and others (1998); Shapiro and others (1999); Sambamoorthi, U., Moynihan, P. J., McSpiritt, E., and Crystal, S. "Use of Protease Inhibitors and Non-Nucleoside Reverse Transcriptase Inhibitors Among Medicaid Beneficiaries with AIDS." *American Journal of Public Health*, 2001, *91*(9), 1474–1481.

46. Cunningham and others (2000).

47. Diaz, T., and others. "Differences in Participation in Experimental Drug Trials Among Persons with AIDS." *Journal of Acquired Immune Deficiency Syndromes and Human Retrovirology*, 1995, *10*(5), 562–568; Lynn, L. A., "AIDS Clinical Trials: Is There Access for All?" *Journal of General Internal Medicine*, 1997, *12*(3), 198–199; Stone, V. E., and others. "Race, Gender, Drug Use, and Participation in AIDS Clinical Trials: Lessons from a Municipal Hospital Cohort." *Journal of General Internal Medicine*, 1997, *12*(3), 150–157; Cunningham, W. E., and others. "Comparison of Health-Related Quality of Life in Clinical Trial and Nonclinical Trial Human Immunodeficiency Virus-Infected Cohorts." *Medical Care*, 1995, *33*(4 Suppl.), AS15–AS25; Gifford, A. L., and others. "Participation in Research and Access to Experimental Treatments by HIV-Infected Patients." *New England Journal of Medicine*, 2002, *346*(18), 1373–1382.

48. Kissinger, P., and others. "Compliance with Public Sector HIV Medical Care." *Journal of the National Medical Association*, 1995, *87*(1), 19–24.

49. Lucas, G. M., Chaisson, R. E., and Moore, R. D. "Highly Active Antiretroviral Therapy in a Large Urban Clinic: Risk Factors for Virologic Failure and Adverse Drug Reactions." *Annals of Internal Medicine*, 1999, *131*(2), 81–87; Valdez, H., and others. "Human Immunodeficiency Virus 1 Protease Inhibitors in Clinical Practice: Predictors of Virological Outcome." *Archives of Internal Medicine*, 1999, *159*(15), 1771–1776.

50. Kates, J., and Leggoe, A. W. *HIV/AIDS Policy Fact Sheet: The HIV/AIDS Epidemic in the United States*. Menlo Park, Calif. : Kaiser Family Foundation, 2005.

51. Li, X., and others. "Interruption and Discontinuation of Highly Active Antiretroviral Therapy in the Multicenter AIDS Cohort Study." *Journal of Acquired Immune Deficiency Syndrome*, 2005, *38*(3), 320–328.

52. Schoenbaum, E. E., and Webber, M. P. "The Underrecognition of HIV Infection in Women in an Inner-City Emergency Room." *American Journal of Public Health*, 1993, *83*(3), 363–368; Markson, L. E., Houchens, R., Fanning, T. R., and Turner, B. J. "Repeated Emergency Department Use by HIV-Infected Persons: Effect of Clinic Accessibility and Expertise in HIV Care." *Journal of Acquired Immune Deficiency Syndromes and Human Retrovirology*, 1998, *17*(1), 35–41; Kelen, G. D., and others. "Profile of Patients with Human Immunodeficiency Virus Infection Presenting to an Inner-City Emergency Department: Preliminary Report." Annals of Emergency Medicine, 1990, *19*(9), 963–969; Kelen, G. D., and others. "Human Immunodeficiency Virus Infection in Emergency Department Patients: Epidemiology, Clinical Presentations, and Risk to Health Care Workers—The Johns Hopkins Experience." *Journal of the American Medical Association*, 1989, *262*(4), 516–522.

53. Shapiro and others (1999).

54. Palacio, H., and others. "Healthcare Use by Varied Highly Active Antiretroviral Therapy (HAART) Strata: HAART Use, Discontinuation, and Naivety." *AIDS*, 2004, *18*(4), 621–630.

55. Turner, B. J., and others. "Clinic HIV-Focused Features and Prevention of Pneumocystis Carinii Pneumonia." *Journal of General Internal Medicine*, 1998, *13*(1), 16–23.

56. Cunningham and others (2000); Kalichman, S. C., Ramachandran, B., and Catz, S. "Adherence to Combination Antiretroviral Therapies in HIV Patients of Low Health Literacy." *Journal of General Internal Medicine*, 1999, *14*(5), 267–273.

57. Cunningham, W. E., and others. "Access to Community-Based Medical Services and Number of Hospitalizations Among Patients with HIV Disease: Are They Related?" *Journal of Acquired Immune Deficiency Syndromes and Human Retrovirology*, 1996, *13*(4), 327–335.

58. Mosen, D. M., and others. "Is Access to Medical Care Associated with Receipt of HIV Testing and Counselling?" *AIDS Care*, 1998, *10*(5), 617–628.

59. Cunningham and others (1995); Cunningham, W. E., and others. "The Prospective Effect of Access to Medical Care on Health-Related Quality-of-Life Outcomes in Patients with Symptomatic HIV Disease." *Medical Care*, 1998, *36*(3), 295–306.

60. Morin, S. F., and others. "Responding to Racial and Ethnic Disparities in Use of HIV Drugs: Analysis of State Policies." *Public Health Reports*, 2002, *117*(3), 263–272.

61. Morin and others (2002).

62. Kates and Leggoe (2005).

63. Bozzette and others (1998).

64. Bozzette, S. A., and others. "Expenditures for the Care of HIV-Infected Patients in the Era of Highly Active Antiretroviral Therapy." *New England Journal of Medicine*, 2001, *344*(11), 817–823.

65. National Center for Health Statistics (2005).

66. Fingerhut, L., and Warner, M. *Injury Chartbook: Health, United States 1996–1997*. Hyattsville, Md.: National Center for Health Statistics, 1997; Pamuk, E., and others. *Socioeconomic Status and Health Chartbook: Health, United States, 1998*. Hyattsville, Md.: National Center for Health Statistics, 1998.

67. Bozzette and others (2001).

68. Andersen and others (2000).

69. Asch, S. M., and others. "Underuse of Primary Mycobacterium Avium Complex and Pneumocystis Carinii Prophylaxis in the United States." *Journal of Acquired Immune Deficiency Syndrome*, 2001, *28*(4), 340–344.

70. Bennett, C. L., and others. "Relation Between Hospital Experience and In-Hospital Mortality for Patients with AIDS-Related Pneumocystis Carinii Pneumonia: Experience from 3,126 Cases in New York City in 1987." *Journal of Acquired Immune Deficiency Syndrome*, 1992, *5*(9), 856–864.

71. Bennett and others (1992); Cunningham, W. E., and others. "The Effect of Hospital Experience on Mortality Among Patients Hospitalized with Acquired Immunodeficiency Syndrome in California." *American Journal of Medicine*, 1999, *107*(2), 137–143; Stone, V. E., Seage, G. R. 3rd, Hertz, T., and Epstein, A. M. "The Relation Between Hospital Experience and Mortality for Patients with AIDS." *Journal of the American Medical Association*, 1992, *268*(19), 2655–2661; Bennett, C. L., and others. "The Relation Between Hospital Experience and In-Hospital Mortality for Patients with AIDS-Related PCP." *Journal of the American Medical Association*, 1989, *261*(20), 2975–2979.

72. Kitahata, M. M., and others. "Physicians' Experience with the Acquired Immunodeficiency Syndrome as a Factor in Patients' Survival." *New England Journal of Medicine*, 1996, *334*(11), 701–706.

73. Hecht, F. M., and others. "Optimizing Care for Persons with HIV Infection: Society of General Internal Medicine AIDS Task Force." *Annals of Internal Medicine*, 1999, *131*(2), 136–143; Lewis, C. E., "Management of Patients with HIV/AIDS: Who Should Care?"

*Journal of the American Medical Association,* 1997, *278*(14), 1133–1134; Holmes, W. C., "Quality in HIV/AIDS Care: Specialty-Related or Experience-Related?" *Journal of General Internal Medicine,* 1997, *12*(3), 195–197; Landon, B. E., and others. "Physician Specialization and Antiretroviral Therapy for HIV." *Journal of General Internal Medicine,* 2003, *18*(4), 233–241; Landon, B. E., and others. "Physician Specialization and the Quality of Care for Human Immunodeficiency Virus Infection." *Archives of Internal Medicine,* 2005, *165*(10), 1133–1139.

74. Wong, M. D., and others. "Racial and Ethnic Differences in Patients' Preferences for Initial Care by Specialists." *American Journal of Medicine,* 2004, *116*(9), 613–620; King, W. D., and others. "Does Racial Concordance Between HIV-Positive Patients and Their Physicians Affect the Time to Receipt of Protease Inhibitors?" *Journal of General Internal Medicine,* 2004, *19*(11), 1146–1153; Ding, L., and others. "Predictors and Consequences of Negative Physician Attitudes Toward HIV-Infected Injection Drug Users." *Archives of Internal Medicine,* 2005, *165*(6), 618–623.

75. Marquis, M. S., Davies, A. R., and Ware, J. E., Jr., "Patient Satisfaction and Change in Medical Care Provider: A Longitudinal Study." *Medical Care,* 1983, *21*(8), 821–829; Pascoe, G. C., "Patient Satisfaction in Primary Health Care: A Literature Review and Analysis." *Evaluation and Program Planning,* 1983, *6*(3–4), 185–210; O'Brien, M. K., Petrie, K., and Raeburn, J. "Adherence to Medication Regimens: Updating a Complex Medical Issue." *Medical Care Review,* 1992, *49*(4), 435–454; Marshall, G. N., Hays, R. D., and Mazel, R. "Health Status and Satisfaction with Health Care: Results from the Medical Outcomes Study." *Journal of Consulting and Clinical Psychology,* 1996, *64*(2), 380–390.

76. Stein, M. D., Fleishman, J., Mor, V., and Dresser, M. "Factors Associated with Patient Satisfaction Among Symptomatic HIV-Infected Persons." *Medical Care,* 1993, *31*(2), 182–188.

77. Stone, V. E., Weissman, J. S., and Cleary, P. D. "Satisfaction with Ambulatory Care of Persons with AIDS: Predictors of Patient Ratings of Quality." *Journal of General Internal Medicine,* 1995, *10*(5), 239–245.

78. Preau, M., and others. "Health-Related Quality of Life and Patient-Provider Relationships in HIV-Infected Patients During the First Three Years After Starting PI-Containing Antiretroviral Treatment." AIDS Care, 2004, *16*(5), 649–661.

79. Solorio, M. R., Asch, S. M., Globe, D., and Cunningham, W. E. "The Association of Access to Medical Care with Regular Source of Care and Sociodemographic Characteristics in Patients with HIV and Tuberculosis." *Journal of the National Medical Association,* 2002, *94*(7), 581–589.

80. Wainberg and Friedland (1998); Hecht, F. M., and others. "Sexual Transmission of an HIV-1 Variant Resistant to Multiple Reverse-Transcriptase and Protease Inhibitors." *New England Journal of Medicine,* 1998, *339*(5), 307–311.

81. Mehta, S., Moore, R. D., and Graham, N. M. "Potential Factors Affecting Adherence with HIV Therapy." *AIDS,* 1997, *11*(14), 1665–1670.

82. Wenger, N., and others. "Patient Characteristics and Attitudes Associated with Antiretroviral Adherence." In 6th Conference on Retroviruses and Opportunistic Infections, Chicago, Jan. 31–Feb. 4, 1999.

83. Kalichman, Ramachandran, and Catz (1999); Mehta, Moore, and Graham (1997).

84. Hays, R. D., and others. "Health-Related Quality of Life in Patients with Human Immunodeficiency Virus Infection in the United States: Results from the HIV Cost and Services Utilization Study." *American Journal of Medicine,* 2000, *108*(9), 714–722; Bozzette, S. A., and others. "Derivation and Properties of a Brief Health Status Assessment Instrument for

Use in HIV Disease." *Journal of Acquired Immune Deficiency Syndromes and Human Retrovirology,* 1995, *8*(3), 253–265; Hays, R. D., and Shapiro, M. F. "An Overview of Generic Health-Related Quality of Life Measures for HIV Research." *Quality of Life Research,* 1992, *1*(2), 91–97; Wachtel, T., and others. "Quality of Life in Persons with Human Immunodeficiency Virus Infection: Measurement by the Medical Outcomes Study Instrument." *Annals of Internal Medicine,* 1992, *116*(2), 129–137; Wu, A. W., and others. "The Effect of Mode of Administration on Medical Outcomes Study Health Ratings and EuroQol Scores in AIDS." *Quality of Life Research,* 1997, *6*(1), 3–10; Copfer, A. E., and others. "The Use of Two Measures of Health-Related Quality of Life in HIV-Infected Individuals: A Cross-Sectional Comparison." *Quality of Life Research,* 1996, *5*(2), 281–286; Revicki, D. A., Wu, A. W., and Murray, M. I. "Change in Clinical Status, Health Status, and Health Utility Outcomes in HIV-Infected Patients." *Medical Care,* 1995, *33*(4 Suppl.), AS173–AS182; Stanton, D. L., and others. "Functional Status of Persons with HIV Infection in an Ambulatory Setting." *Journal of Acquired Immune Deficiency Syndrome,* 1994, *7*(10), 1050–1056; Wu, A. W., and others. "Functional Status and Well-Being in a Placebo-Controlled Trial of Zidovudine in Early Symptomatic HIV Infection." *Journal of Acquired Immune Deficiency Syndrome,* 1993, *6*(5), 452–458.

85. Globe, D. R., Hays, R. D., and Cunningham, W. E. "Associations of Clinical Parameters with Health-Related Quality of Life in Hospitalized Persons with HIV Disease." *AIDS Care,* 1999, *11*(1), 71–86; Wilson, I. B., and Cleary, P. D. "Clinical Predictors of Functioning in Persons with Acquired Immunodeficiency Syndrome." *Medical Care,* 1996, *34*(6), 610–623; Wu, A. W., and others. "A Health Status Questionnaire Using 30 Items from the Medical Outcomes Study: Preliminary Validation in Persons with Early HIV Infection." *Medical Care,* 1991, *29*(8), 786–798; Burgess, A., and Riccio, M. "Cognitive Impairment and Dementia in HIV-1 Infection." *Baillieres Clinical Neurology,* 1992, *1*(1), 155–174; Lubeck, D. P., and Fries, J. F. "Health Status Among Persons Infected with Human Immunodeficiency Virus: A Community-Based Study." *Medical Care,* 1993, *31*(3), 269–276; Bozzette, S. A., Hays, R. D., Berry, S. H., and Kanouse, D. E. "A Perceived Health Index for Use in Persons with Advanced HIV Disease: Derivation, Reliability, and Validity." *Medical Care,* 1994, *32*(7), 716–731; Ganz, P. A., and others. "Describing the Health-Related Quality of Life Impact of HIV Infection: Findings from a Study Using the HIV Overview of Problems—Evaluation System (HOPES)." *Quality of Life Research,* 1993, *2*(2), 109–119; Tsevat, J., and others. "Health Values of Patients Infected with Human Immunodeficiency Virus: Relationship to Mental Health and Physical Functioning." *Medical Care,* 1996, *34*(1), 44–57; Kaplan, R. M., and others. "The Quality of Well-Being Scale: Applications in AIDS, Cystic Fibrosis, and Arthritis." *Medical Care,* 1989, *27*(3 Suppl.), S27–S43; Wu, A. W., and others. "Quality of Life in a Placebo-Controlled Trial of Zidovudine in Patients with AIDS and AIDS-Related Complex." *Journal of Acquired Immune Deficiency Syndrome,* 1990, *3*(7), 683–690.

86. Globe, Hays, and Cunningham (1999).

87. Hays and Shapiro (1992); Hays, R., and others. "Health Related Quality of Life in HIV Disease." *Assessment,* 1995, *2*(4), 363–380; Wu, A., and Rubin, H. "Measuring Health Status and Quality of Life in HIV and AIDS." *Psychology and Health,* 1992, *6*, 251–264.

88. Lubeck, D. P., and Fries, J. F. "Changes in Quality of Life Among Persons with HIV Infection." *Quality of Life Research,* 1992, *1*(6), 359–366.

89. Marx, R., Katz, M. H., Park, M. S., and Gurley, R. J. "Meeting the Service Needs of HIV-Infected Persons: Is the Ryan White Care Act Succeeding?" *Journal of Acquired Immune Deficiency Syndromes and Human Retrovirology,* 1997, *14*(1), 44–55; Katz, M. H., and others.

"Prevalence and Predictors of Unmet Need for Supportive Services Among HIV-Infected Persons: Impact of Case Management." *Medical Care,* 2000, *38*(1), 58–69.

90. Schuster, M. A., Bell, R. M., Berry, S. H., and Kanouse, D. E. "Students' Acquisition and Use of School Condoms in a High School Condom Availability Program." *Pediatrics,* 1997, *100*(4), 689–694; Schuster, M. A., Bell, R. M., Berry, S. H., and Kanouse, D. E. "Impact of a High School Condom Availability Program on Sexual Attitudes and Behaviors." *Family Planning Perspectives,* 1998, *30*(2), 67–72, 88; Burris, S., Finucane, D., Gallagher, H., and Grace, J. "The Legal Strategies Used in Operating Syringe Exchange Programs in the United States." *American Journal of Public Health,* 1996, *86*(8 Pt. 1), 1161–1166; Kirby, D. B., and Brown, N. L. "Condom Availability Programs in U. S. Schools." *Family Planning Perspectives,* 1996, *28*(5), 196–202.

91. Des Jarlais, D. C., McKnight, C., and Milliken, J. "Public Funding of U. S. Syringe Exchange Programs." *Journal of Urban Health,* 2004, *81*(1), 118–121; Vlahov, D., and others. "Needle Exchange Programs for the Prevention of Human Immunodeficiency Virus Infection: Epidemiology and Policy." *American Journal of Epidemiology,* 2001, *154*(12), 70S-77.

92. Jaffe, H., "Public Health: Enhanced: Whatever Happened to the U.S. AIDS Epidemic?" *Science,* 2004, *305*(5688), 1243–1244.

93. Jaffe (2004).

94. Schuster and others (1998); Longshore, D., Annon, J., and Anglin, M. D. "Long-Term Trends in Self-Reported HIV Risk Behavior: Injection Drug Users in Los Angeles, 1987 Through 1995." *Journal of Acquired Immune Deficiency Syndromes and Human Retrovirology,,* 1998, *18*(1), 64–72.

95. Schuster and others (1997); Schuster and others (1998).

96. Heimer, R., "Syringe Exchange Programs: Lowering the Transmission of Syringe-Borne Diseases and Beyond." *Public Health Reports,* 1998, *113* (Suppl 1. ), 67–74.

97. Phillips, K. A., Coates, T. J., and Catania, J. A. "Predictors of Follow-Through on Plans to Be Tested for HIV." *American Journal of Preventive Medicine,* 1997, *13*(3), 193–198.

98. Sanders, G. D., and others. "Cost-Effectiveness of Screening for HIV in the Era of Highly Active Antiretroviral Therapy." *New England Journal of Medicine,* 2005, *352*(6), 570–585.

99. Bindman, A. B., and others. "Multistate Evaluation of Anonymous HIV Testing and Access to Medical Care: Multistate Evaluation of Surveillance of HIV (MESH) Study Group." *Journal of the American Medical Association,* 1998, *280*(16), 1416–1420.

100. Phillips, Coates, and Catania (1997); Phillips, K. A., and Coates, T. J. "HIV Counselling and Testing: Research and Policy Issues." *AIDS Care,* 1995, *7*(2), 115–124.

101. Bindman and others (1998).

102. Keenan, P. A., Keenan, J. M., and Branson, B. M. "Rapid HIV Testing: Wait Time Reduced from Days to Minutes." *Postgraduate Medicine,* 2005, *117*(3), 47–52.

103. Kendrick, S. R., Kroc, K. A., Withum, D., Rydman, R. J., and others. "Outcomes of Offering Rapid Point-of-Care HIV Testing in a Sexually Transmitted Disease Clinic." *Journal of Acquired Immune Deficiency Syndromes,* 2005, *38*(2), 142–146; Bulterys, M., and others. "Rapid HIV-1 Testing During Labor: A Multicenter Study." *Journal of the American Medical Association,* 2004, *292*(2), 219–223; "Rapid Point-of-Care Testing for HIV-1 During Labor and Delivery—Chicago, Illinois, 2002." *Morbidity and Mortality Weekly Report,* 2003, *52*(36), 866–868; Kendrick, S. R., Kroc, K. A., Couture, E., and Weinstein, R. A. "Comparison of Point-of-Care Rapid HIV Testing in Three Clinical Venues." *AIDS,* 2004, *18*(16), 2208–2210.

104. Spielberg, F., Levine, R. O., and Weaver, M. "Self-Testing for HIV: A New Option for HIV Prevention?" *Lancet Infectious Diseases,* 2004, *4*(10), 640–646.

105. Mosen and others (1998); Phillips and Coates (1995).

106. Lurie, P., and others. "Postexposure Prophylaxis After Nonoccupational HIV Exposure: Clinical, Ethical, and Policy Considerations." *Journal of the American Medical Association*, 1998, *280*(20), 1769–1773; Gerberding, J. L., and Katz, M. H. "Post-Exposure Prophylaxis for HIV." *Advances in Experimental Medicine and Biology*, 1999, *458*, 213–222.

107. Brown, G. R., and others. "Prevalence of Psychiatric Disorders in Early Stages of HIV Infection." *Psychosomatic Medicine*, 1992, *54*(5), 588–601; Williams, J. B., and others. "Multidisciplinary Baseline Assessment of Homosexual Men with and Without Human Immunodeficiency Virus Infection. II. Standardized Clinical Assessment of Current and Lifetime Psychopathology." *Archives of General Psychiatry*, 1991, *48*(2), 124–130; Blazer, D. G., Kessler, R. C., McGonagle, K. A., and Swartz, M. S. "The Prevalence and Distribution of Major Depression in a National Community Sample: The National Comorbidity Survey." *American Journal of Psychiatry*, 1994, *151*(7), 979–986; Kessler, R. C., and others. "Lifetime and 12-Month Prevalence of DSM-III-R Psychiatric Disorders in the United States: Results from the National Comorbidity Survey." *Archives of General Psychiatry*, 1994, *51*(1), 8–19.

108. Wells, K. B., and others. "The Functioning and Well-Being of Depressed Patients: Results from the Medical Outcomes Study." *Journal of the American Medical Association*, 1989, *262*(7), 914–919; Wells, K. B., "Depression in General Medical Settings: Implications of Three Health Policy Studies for Consultation-Liaison Psychiatry." *Psychosomatics*, 1994, *35*(3), 279–296; Sherbourne, C. D., Wells, K. B., and Judd, L. L. "Functioning and Well-Being of Patients with Panic Disorder." *American Journal of Psychiatry*, 1996, *153*(2), 213–218.

109. Darrow, W. W., and others. "Risk Factors for Human Immunodeficiency Virus (HIV) Infections in Homosexual Men." *American Journal of Public Health*, 1987, *77*(4), 479–483.

110. Walkup, J. T., Sambamoorthi, U., and Crystal, S. "Use of Newer Antiretroviral Treatments Among HIV-Infected Medicaid Beneficiaries with Serious Mental Illness." *Journal of Clinical Psychiatry*, 2004, *65*(9), 1180–1189; Hoover, D. R., Sambamoorthi, U., Walkup, J. T., and Crystal, S. "Mental Illness and Length of Inpatient Stay for Medicaid Recipients with AIDS." *Health Services Research*, 2004, *39*(5), 1319–1339.

111. Weinert, M., Grimes, R. M., and Lynch, D. P. "Oral Manifestations of HIV Infection." *Annals of Internal Medicine*, 1996, *125*(6), 485–496.

112. Coulter, I. D., and others. "Associations of Self-Reported Oral Health with Physical and Mental Health in a Nationally Representative Sample of HIV Persons Receiving Medical Care." *Quality of Life Research*, 2002, *11*(1), 57–70.

113. Capilouto, E. I., Piette, J., White, B. A., and Fleishman, J. "Perceived Need for Dental Care Among Persons Living with Acquired Immunodeficiency Syndrome." *Medical Care*, 1991, *29*(8), 745–754.

114. Gerbert, B., Maguire, B. T., and Spitzer, S. "Patients' Attitudes Toward Dentistry and AIDS." *Journal of the American Dental Association*, 1989 (Suppl.), 16S-21S; Hazelkorn, H. M., "The Reaction of Dentists to Members of Groups at Risk of AIDS." *Journal of the American Dental Association*, 1989, *119*(5), 611–619; Davis, M., "Dentistry and AIDS: An Ethical Opinion." *Journal of the American Dental Association*, 1989 (Suppl.), 9S-11S; Scheutz, F., "HIV Infection and Dental Care: Views and Experiences Among HIV-Seropositive Patients." *AIDS Care*, 1990, *2*(1), 37–42; Weyant, R. J., Bennett, M. E., Simon, M., and Palaisa, J. "Desire to Treat HIV-Infected Patients: Similarities and Differences Across Health-Care Professions." *AIDS*, 1994, *8*(1), 117–121.

115. Perry, S. W., and others. "Self-Disclosure of HIV Infection to Dentists and Physicians." *Journal of the American Dental Association*, 1993, *124*(9), 51–54.

116. Shiboski, C. H., Palacio, H., Neuhaus, J. M., and Greenblatt, R. M. "Dental Care Access and Use Among HIV-Infected Women." *American Journal of Public Health*, 1999, *89*(6), 834–839.

117. Heslin, K. C., and others. "A Comparison of Unmet Needs for Dental and Medical Care Among Persons with HIV Infection Receiving Care in the United States." *Journal of Public Health Dentistry*, 2001, *61*(1), 14–21.

118. Sherbourne, C. D., Meredith, L. S., Rogers, W., and Ware, J. E., Jr. "Social Support and Stressful Life Events: Age Differences in Their Effects on Health-Related Quality of Life Among the Chronically Ill." *Quality of Life Research*, 1992, 1(4), 235–246.

119. Zich, J., and Temoshok, L. "Perceptions of Social Support in Men with AIDS and ARC: Relationships with Distress and Hardiness." *Journal of Applied Social Psychology*, 1987, *17*(3), 193–215; Hays, R., Chauncey, S., and Tobey, L. "The Social Support Networks of Gay Men with AIDS." *Journal of Community Psychology*, 1990, *18*, 374–385.

120. Sherbourne, C. D., "The Role of Social Support and Life Stress Events in Use of Mental Health Services." *Social Science and Medicine*, 1988, *27*(12), 1393–1400.

121. Katz and others (2000).

122. Landon and others (2005).

123. Schur, C., and others. *Measuring Utilization and Costs of AIDS Health Care Services, Final Report.* Rockville, Md.: Health Resources and Services Administration, 1991; Widman, M., Light, D. W., and Platt, J. J. "Barriers to Out-of-Hospital Care for AIDS Patients." *AIDS Care*, 1994, *6*(1), 59–67.

124. King and others (2004).

125. Ding (2005); Wong, M. D., and others. "Disparities in HIV Treatment and Physician Attitudes About Delaying Protease Inhibitors for Nonadherent Patients." *Journal of General Internal Medicine*, 2004, *19*(4), 366–374.

126. Office of Technology Assessment. *AIDS and Health Insurance: An OTA Survey (Staff Paper).* Washington, D.C.: OTA, 1988.

127. Green, J., Oppenheimer, G. M., and Wintfeld, N. "The $147,000 Misunderstanding: Repercussions of Overestimating the Cost of AIDS." *Journal of Health Politics, Policy, and Law*, 1994, *19*(1), 69–90.

128. Rawlings-Sekunda, J., *Trends in Serving People with HIV/AIDS Through Medicaid Managed Care.* Portland, Me.: National Academy for State Health Policy, 1999.

129. Rawlings-Sekunda, J., and Kaye, N. *Emerging Practices and Policy in Medicaid Managed Care for People with HIV/AIDS: Case Studies of Six Programs.* Portland, Me.: National Academy for State Health Policy, 1998.

130. Rawlings-Sekunda and Kaye (1998); Bartlett, J. G., "HIV/AIDS Managed Care Program." *Transactions of the American Clinical Climatology Association*, 2000, *111*, 112–120.

131. Rawlings-Sekunda (1999); Rawlings-Sekunda and Kaye (1998); Bartlett, J. G., and Moore, R. "A Comprehensive Plan for Managed Care of Patients Infected with Human Immunodeficiency Virus." *Clinical Infectious Disease*, 1999, *29*(1), 50–55; Conviser, R., Gamliel, S., and Honberg, L. "Health-Based Payment for HIV/AIDS in Medicaid Managed Care Programs." *Health Care Financing Review*, 1998, *19*(3), 63–82.

132. Zingmond, D., Ettner, S., and Cunningham, W. "The Impact of Managed Care on Access to Highly Active Anti-Retroviral Therapy and on Outcomes Among Medicaid Beneficiaries with AIDS." *Medical Care Research and Review*, forthcoming.

133. Mor and others (1992).

134. Hart, J. S., and Redding, K. L. "A Physician's Perspective on the Advantages of Home Medical Care: The Other Side of Case Management." *Texas Medicine*, 1994, 90(2), 50–54.

135. Sowell, R. L., and others. "Impact of Case Management on Hospital Charges of PWAs in Georgia." *Journal of the Association of Nurses in AIDS Care,* 1992, *3*(2), 24–31.

136. Katz and others (2000).

137. Katz and others (2000).

138. Makadon, H. J., Seage, G. R. 3rd, Thorpe, K. E., and Fineberg, H. V. "Paying the Medical Cost of the HIV Epidemic: A Review of Policy Options." *Journal of Acquired Immune Deficiency Syndromes,* 1990, *3*(2), 123–133.

139. Congressional Budget Office. *Cost Estimates.* U.S. House of Representatives, 1987.

140. Bowen, G. S., and others. "First Year of AIDS Services Delivery Under Title I of the Ryan White Care Act." *Public Health Reports,* 1992, *107*(5), 491–499; Thurman, S. L., "The Ryan White Care Act." *Journal of the Association of Nurses in AIDS Care,* 1993, *4*(4), 45–49.

141. Marx and others (1997); Marx, R., Chang, S. W., Park, M. S., and Katz, M. H. "Reducing Financial Barriers to HIV-Related Medical Care: Does the Ryan White Care Act Make a Difference?" *AIDS Care,* 1998, *10*(5), 611–616.

142. Marx and others (1998).

143. Buchanan, R. J., and Smith, S. R. "State Implementation of the AIDS Drug Assistance Programs." *Health Care Financing Review,* 1998, *19*(3), 39–62.

144. Goldman, D. P., and others. "The Impact of State Policy on the Costs of HIV Infection." *Medical Care Research and Review,* 2001, *58*(1), 31–53.

145. CDC (2004).

146. CDC (2004).

147. Hellinger, F. J., "The Use of Health Services by Women with HIV Infection." *Health Services Research,* 1993, *28*(5), 543–561; Palacio, H., and others. "Access to and Utilization of Primary Care Services Among HIV-Infected Women." *Journal of Acquired Immune Deficiency Syndromes,* 1999, *21*(4), 293–300.

148. Stein, M. D., and others. "Screening for Cervical Cancer in HIV-Infected Women Receiving Care in the United States." *Journal of Acquired Immune Deficiency Syndromes,* 2001, *27*(5), 463–466.

149. Mor and others (1992).

150. Carpenter, C. C., and others. "Human Immunodeficiency Virus Infection in North American Women: Experience with 200 Cases and a Review of the Literature." *Medicine,* 1991, *70*(5), 307–325.

151. Schuster, M. A., and others. "HIV-Infected Parents and Their Children in the United States." *American Journal of Public Health,* 2000, *90*(7), 1074–1081.

152. Stein and others (2000).

153. Zierler, S., and others. "Violence Victimization After HIV Infection in a U. S. Probability Sample of Adult Patients in Primary Care." *American Journal of Public Health,* 2000, *90*(2), 208–215.

154. CDC (2004).

155. Scott, G., and Parks, W. *Pediatric AIDS.* Philadelphia: Lippincott, 1994; Hogart, D., Kochanek, K., and Murphy, S. "Deaths: Final Data for 1997." *National Vital Statistics Reports, 47*(19). Hyattsville, Maryland: National Center for Health Statistics, 1999. *HIV/AIDS Surveillance Report, Third Quarter.* Atlanta: Centers for Disease Control and Prevention, U.S. Department of Health and Human Services, 1993.

156. CDC (1993).

157. Schuster and others (2000).

158. Hsia, D. C., Fleishman, J. A., East, J. A., and Hellinger, F. J. "Pediatric Human Immunodeficiency Virus Infection: Recent Evidence on the Utilization and Costs of Health Services." *Archives of Pediatric and Adolescent Medicine*, 1995, *149*(5), 489–496; Conviser, R., Grant, C. M., and Coye, M. J. "Pediatric Acquired Immunodeficiency Syndrome Hospitalizations in New Jersey." *Pediatrics*, 1991, *87*(5), 642–653.

159. Ball, J., and Thaul, S. *Pediatric AIDS-Related Discharges in a Sample of U.S. Hospitals: Demographics, Diagnoses and Resource Use.* Rockville, Md.: Agency for Health Care Policy and Research, U.S. Department of Health and Human Services, 1992.

160. Birn, A., Santelli, J., and Burwell, L. "Pediatric AIDS in the United States: Epidemiological Reality Versus Government Policy." *International Journal of Health Policy*, 1991, *20*, 617–630.

161. CDC (2004); Hein, K., "'Getting Real' About HIV in Adolescents." *American Journal of Public Health*, 1993, *83*(4), 492–494.

162. Katz, M. H., McFarland, W., Guillin, V., Fenstersheib, M., and others. "Continuing High Prevalence of HIV and Risk Behaviors Among Young Men Who Have Sex with Men: The Young Men's Survey in the San Francisco Bay Area in 1992 to 1993 and in 1994 to 1995." *Journal of Acquired Immune Deficiency Syndromes and Human Retrovirology*, 1998, *19*(2), 178–181; Koniak-Griffin, D., and Brecht, M. L. "AIDS Risk Behaviors, Knowledge, and Attitudes Among Pregnant Adolescents and Young Mothers." *Health Education and Behavior*, 1997, *24*(5), 613–624; Anderson, J. E., and others. "HIV Risk Behavior, Street Outreach, and Condom Use in Eight High-Risk Populations." AIDS *Education and* Prevention, 1996, *8*(3), 191–204; Rotheram-Borus, M. J., Koopman, C., Haignere, C., and Davies, M. "Reducing HIV Sexual Risk Behaviors Among Runaway Adolescents." *Journal of the American Medical Association*, 1991, *266*(9), 1237–1241.

163. Morales, L. S., and others. "Sociodemographic Differences in Access to Care Among Hispanic Patients Who Are HIV Infected in the United States." *American Journal of Public Health*, 2004, *94*(7), 1119–1121.

164. Harawa, N. T., and others. "HIV Prevalence Among Foreign- and US-Born Clients of Public STD Clinics." *American Journal of Public Health*, 2002, *92*(12), 1958–1963.

165. U.S. Department of Health and Human Services. *HIV/AIDS Work Group on Health Care Issues for Hispanic Americans.* Rockville, Md.: U. S. Department of Health and Human Services, 1991.

166. Cunningham, W. E., Davidson, P. L., Nakazono, T. T., and Andersen, R. M. "Do Black and White Adults Use the Same Sources of Information About AIDS Prevention?" *Health Education and Behavior*, 1999, *26*(5), 703–713.

# CHAPTER FIFTEEN

# HEALTH REFORM FOR CHILDREN AND FAMILIES

Moira Inkelas
Neal Halfon
David Lee Wood
Mark A. Schuster

Throughout the past century, expert panels and government commissions have highlighted the importance of certain basic principles for children's health care. Over the past decade, the Maternal and Child Health Bureau's (MCHB) Bright Futures Project has reiterated that health care for children should be comprehensive, continuous, coordinated, and accountable. Despite great technical advances and development of important programs that have improved the health and changed the lives of many children, the system of care for children in the United States has yet to embody the principles of Bright Futures and the recommendations of these expert panels. Many children lack insurance and experience numerous barriers to receiving appropriate care. The medical, developmental, and environmental threats to children have changed in nature and complexity, and the system of care that has evolved to meet these changing needs is fragmented, disorganized, and difficult to navigate.

As the health care marketplace continues to change, attention should be directed toward how these changes affect the availability and quality of essential child health services. The changing marketplace poses its own set of challenges, but significant changes in organization and payment of health services create new opportunities to construct a child health system that is more responsive to current and emerging health needs of children and better able to overcome deficiencies in the current system. Unfortunately, many of the specific services that should be included in a higher-performing system of children's health care might not meet the narrower financial goals of many managed care organizations. How can development of a better quality child health system be supported—a system that permits home visitation for families at risk, early intervention services for children with potential developmental delay, preventive mental health services for children who are abused and neglected, and comprehensive services to children with special medical needs? How can these and other services be ensured when they may not be profitable to the health care industry?

Whether ongoing marketplace changes and complementary federal and state health financing policies improve the organization of children's health services and children's health status overall depends on the extent to which these and other questions are addressed. How do children fare under a health system restructuring that is driven primarily by cost considerations? How will access and quality of child health services be affected by financing changes in the public and private sectors? Can current access barriers to comprehensive, coordinated health services be resolved? How can the principles outlined in Bright Futures guide transformation of children's health services? By what standard should we evaluate the effectiveness of new organizational approaches to delivering child health services?

This chapter examines the key issues underlying the incongruity between the needs of children and families and the current and evolving structure of health services in the United States. We describe the unique health needs of children and the rationale for a child standard of care to ensure that emerging systems can meet these needs. Next, we examine characteristics of the U.S. health care system that influence children's access to care, including the disjointed organization of health services, and financial and structural barriers to health care. In the context of proliferating state-based initiatives and sweeping market-based reforms in the health system, we present several options for accommodating the special needs of children. Finally, we describe how emerging models of care can be modified to provide more effective, organized, and family-centered health services for children.

# Special Health Needs of Children

The 2004 Institute of Medicine (IOM) report *Children's Health, the Nation's Wealth*[1] defined health as "the extent to which individual children or groups of children are able or enabled to (a) develop and realize their potential, (b) satisfy their needs, and (c) develop the capacities that allow them to interact successfully with their biological, physical, and social environments."

The committee went on to specify the domains of health that policies and services are designed to influence: "Health conditions, which capture disorders or illnesses of the body systems; functioning, which focuses on the manifestations of health on an individual's daily life; and health potential, which captures the development of assets and positive aspects of health, such as competence, capacity and developmental potential."

Implicit in this definition and the strategies that IOM proposes for addressing children's health needs is an understanding that children's health needs and risks differ fundamentally from those of adults and thus require special consideration in structuring, organizing, and delivering health services.[2] Among the unique characteristics of childhood that have important implications for health system design are a child's developmental vulnerability, dependency, and differential patterns of morbidity and mortality.

## Developmental Vulnerability

Developmental vulnerability refers to rapid and cumulative physical and emotional changes that characterize childhood, and the potential impact that illness, injury, or untoward family and social circumstances can have on a child's life-course trajectory. Physical health conditions (such as low birthweight or asthma) as well as the child's social environment (severe poverty, unstable family, environmental exposures such as lead) can harm the developmental process.[3] The Life Course Health Development model has been used to elucidate the dynamic relationships between factors that can promote or adversely affect children's capacity to achieve their physical, emotional, and cognitive potential.[4] Studies demonstrate two phenomena: the substantial, cumulative impact of early exposures and adverse social conditions on health status throughout the life course; and the role of critical developmental periods in which early insults cause long-term consequences by programming physiological pathways to function in a manner that is harmful over the short run (during childhood) or the entire life span.[5] The brain science revolution and comparable advances in genetics also make clear the role of gene-environment interaction early in life, and the potential to intervene early to minimize disparities and optimize outcomes. Research linking the impact of various risks and insults to developmental pathways supports broader conceptualization of health determinants and of health services.

The potential to alter the life-course trajectory is illustrated by studies that demonstrate the effectiveness of timely intervention in modifying adverse biological and social conditions that may harm a child's development. For example, cognitive development and behavioral competence at preschool age is greater when low-birthweight children receive supportive family and educational services.[6] For the estimated 5–17 percent of children with dyslexia—a neurological disorder that typically impairs reading ability and school performance and achievement—intervening early can have a dramatic impact on a child's learning trajectories.[7]

Such studies support the notion that timely and appropriately organized services can prevent loss of developmental potential; they highlight the mutability of various risks and their life-course effects.[8]

Children's developmental vulnerability also implies that interventions must be sustained over time to appropriately address periodic, recurrent, and ongoing biological and environmental threats. For example, although comprehensive early childhood intervention programs that serve socially disadvantaged children have improved young children's cognitive abilities, postintervention exposure to ongoing social disadvantage may offset earlier gains.[9] Discontinuities in health care and interrupted eligibility for early childhood intervention programs are examples of modifiable threats to sustained developmental improvement for at-risk children.

Health disparities have an important connection with developmental vulnerability. Eliminating health disparities has become a major national health policy goal. More than ever, it is recognized that many health disparities in adults and the elderly have their origin in childhood. Disparities linked to dietary pattern, health behavior, and environmental exposure begin in childhood and are compounded over the life span. This brings greater attention to how protective and health-promoting factors in childhood can lead to enhancement of long-term health capacity and functioning and how risks and the absence of health-promoting assets can lead to significant health disparities.

## New and Differential Morbidities

The declining prevalence in the United States of nutritional and infectious disease and the changing patterns of childhood risk have increased the prominence of other causes of morbidity and mortality.[10] Children are affected by a broad and complex array of conditions termed "new morbidities": drug and alcohol use, family and neighborhood violence, emotional disorders, learning problems, and so on. These new morbidities originate in complex family or socioeconomic conditions rather than an exclusively biological etiology and cannot be adequately addressed by traditional medical services.[11] Instead, such conditions require a continuum of comprehensive services that include multidisciplinary assessment, treatment, and rehabilitation as well as community-based prevention strategies to sustain positive outcomes.[12] Such multidisciplinary approaches often incorporate and integrate public and private sector services. For example, early intervention, family preservation, and violence prevention programs involve broad-based, multisector approaches that transcend agency and service sector boundaries.[13]

The types and patterns of condition for children are changing, and patterns of morbidity and the manifestation of medical conditions in children fundamentally differ in their pathophysiology and treatment relative to adults.[14] Serious, chronic medical conditions are less prevalent in children and usually are related to birth or congenital anomalies, rather than the degenerative conditions that affect adults. Age-specific drug metabolism, disease expression, and health status assessments differentiate children from adults. For example, in children cardiac conditions may result from any number of distinct congenital malformations, whereas in adults they are dominated by a single degenerative disorder (atherosclerotic heart disease). These differences explain why pediatric specialists are more prepared to diagnose and treat many children's chronic and severe conditions. Age-related differences in disease prevalence, expression, and management have important implications for issues such as ensuring appropriate access to care, developing age-specific quality assessment measures, guaranteeing availability of adequately trained providers, and furthering regional distribution of pediatric health professionals and services.[15]

## Dependency

Children also have complex and changing dependency relationships that affect their development and their use of health services. Children depend on their parents or other caregivers to recognize and respond to their health needs, organize their care and authorize treatment, and comply with recommended treatment regimens. The importance of this dependency for children's access to health care is illustrated by studies comparing maternal utilization of health services with children's use of care. Studies find that maternal and child use of care is highly correlated, irrespective of the level of health status.[16] Recent reports such as those by the National Commission on Children and the Carnegie Commission on Early Childhood further address the interdependency of family and social environments and their impact on children's health and development.[17]

# Health Service Delivery for U.S. Children

Although the principle that children's health services should be organized into a comprehensive, coordinated, continuous, and accessible system of health services is broadly supported, it is not clear how evolution in the health care marketplace and restructuring of the delivery system advance these principles for all children. Using a conceptual framework depicted in Figure 15.1, *Children's Health, the Nation's Wealth* suggests that effectively addressing health conditions, health functioning, and health potential requires health services that achieve the following:[18]

• *Modify pre-disease pathways* by minimizing risk of exposure before it occurs and by actively promoting development of health capacities. For example, young children at risk for poor language development whose parents receive counseling and assistance from pediatric clinicians can have clinically meaningful improvement in language.[19]

• *Reduce exposure to health compromising events.* For example, counseling parents on infant sleep position through the national Back to Sleep campaign in 1992 was accompanied by a 50 percent decline in the incidence of sudden infant death syndrome (SIDS).[20]

• *Modify the relationship between exposure and the onset of disease,* once the child has been exposed, to alter the exposure-outcome pathway. For example, meningitis can be avoided in children who are exposed but receive prophylactic antibiotics in a timely fashion.

• *Modify the disease course and reduce impact* through appropriate diagnostic, treatment, rehabilitation, and habilitation services. For example, children with cystic fibrosis who are diagnosed early and given an integrated care management program have dramatically increased life span and functional capacity.[21]

Children's health care therefore encompasses health promotion and disease prevention services; diagnostic, treatment, and rehabilitation services; health education programs, and other supportive social services. To offer this array in a directed and integrated fashion, health care delivery strategies are necessarily broad and specify multisector service delivery pathways that integrate medical, public health, educational, and social services. For example, to identify developmental

## FIGURE 15.1. WHERE SERVICES CAN EFFECT CHANGE IN HEALTHY DEVELOPMENT.

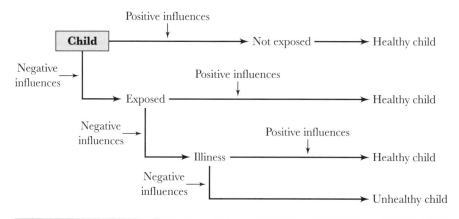

*Source:* National Research Council and Institute of Medicine. *Children's Health, the Nation's Wealth: Assessing and Improving Child Health.* (Committee on Evaluation of Children's Health. Board of Children, Youth, and Families, Division of Behavioral and Social Sciences and Education.) Washington, D.C.: National Academies Press, 2004.

delays as early as possible, population monitoring can take place in a child care center or Head Start site, while screening may take place at a pediatric office. Diagnostic evaluation and ultimately services for such delays may take place in a variety of settings depending on financing, availability, and how a particular state or region has organized publicly funded services for outreach, diagnosis, and treatment. Given this complexity, achieving the systems outcome of timely identification requires having more defined pathways, multiple types of settings for identification, and collaboration among multiple community agencies and programs. The array of programs and financing streams makes it challenging to consolidate personal medical care services and other services heretofore delivered by the community health sector into vertically integrated delivery systems that follow a medical model. Managed care arrangements can effectively organize primary and specialty medical services for healthy populations and for acute conditions. However, the newer morbidities have complex socioeconomic and environmental determinants that often require intense, sustained, and coordinated health services that neither the current system nor the emerging managed care arrangements are structured to provide.[22]

## Child Health Service Sectors

The U.S. child health system has been characterized as a patchwork of disconnected programs, each with its own eligibility, administrative, and funding criteria.[23] The three distinct yet interdependent sectors that constitute child health services—the personal medical and preventive services sector; the population-based, community health services sector; and the health-related support services sector—have unique histories, mandates, organizational characteristics and constraints, and funding streams.[24]

***Personal Medical and Preventive Services.*** Personal medical and preventive health services for children include primary and specialty medical services, which are generally delivered in private and public medical offices, hospitals, and laboratories. Restructuring the organization of the personal health service care sector, where the majority of health care dollars are spent, is the major focus of current health system reform and improvement efforts. Personal medical services are principally funded through private health insurance, by the federal Medicaid program and State Children's Health Insurance Program (SCHIP), and by out-of-pocket payments from families.[25]

***Population-Based Community Health Services.*** The second sector of child health services includes population-based health promotion and disease prevention services, such as immunization delivery and monitoring programs, lead screening and abatement programs, and child abuse prevention. This sector is also home to the growing array of early childhood disease prevention, health promotion, and developmental optimization programs that states and communities are putting in place to promote early learning and health development.[26] Other community health services are special child abuse treatment programs and rehabilitative services for children with complex congenital conditions or other chronic debilitating diseases. Community-based programs often have outreach responsibilities for children's health services, such as early intervention and monitoring programs for infants at risk for developmental disability and case management and financing for children with serious chronic diseases. Funding for this sector comes from federal programs such as Medicaid's Early Periodic Screening, Diagnosis, and Treatment program (EPSDT), Title V (Maternal and Child Health) of the Social Security Act, and many other categorical programs.[27]

***Health-Related Support Services.*** The third sector of the child health system comprises health-related support services, such as nutrition education, early intervention, rehabilitation, and family support programs. Among the services in this sector are parent education and skill building in families with infants at risk for developmental delay that is due to physiological (low birthweight) or social (very low income) risks, or special education and psychotherapy for children with HIV. Funding for these services comes from diverse agencies, among them the U.S. Department of Agriculture (funding the Supplemental Food Program for Women, Infants, and Children, or WIC) and the Department of Education (providing outreach and services through the Individuals with Disabilities Education Act, or IDEA).

## Fragmented Delivery System

These three child health sectors have evolved separately,[28] and the patchwork nature of the programs that make up each sector poses real challenges to forging a continuum of integrated services. Incremental federal and state funding for children's health programs has produced this array of categorical, condition-specific, means-tested programs that are not well integrated within or between the child health service sectors. Many of these programs were developed to fill a gap or address an emerging need (child abuse, HIV, mental health problems, lead toxicity), yet there is often little coordination within federal, state, and local governing authorities, nor any attempt to link with private sector efforts. Program administrative mandates and categorical or block grant criteria often determine the number of children who can be served.

Some states have moved to establish omnibus coordinating agencies or administrative councils for children and family services. These include children's cabinets, which have been set up by many governors in recent years.[29] The MCHB is the single federal agency charged with improving the health status and organization of service systems for children at the federal level. Some have argued that this lone federal agency has neither the authority nor sufficient funding to accomplish this ambitious mission, but this pivotal entity has been successful in launching many important initiatives to improve coordination and integration of existing health services.[30] Strategic objectives of the MCHB include ensuring a "medical home" for all children, improving early and ongoing identification of health and developmental concerns, insuring all children, organizing community systems of services that are easy for families to use, promoting family-centered care, and transitioning adolescents with special health care needs successfully into adult systems of care. In 2003 MCHB launched the State Early Childhood Comprehensive Systems initiative to assist state health departments focus their efforts on improving healthy development and early learning for young children, by coordinating the efforts of state and local level health, mental health, early care and education, family support, and education services.

## Integrating Services

Achieving better health outcomes for the growing number of children afflicted with multiple and complex problems requires coordinated health and health-related services that may include primary and specialty medical care, case management, early intervention, and special education.[31] Recent efforts to rationalize the organization and allocation of child health services are exemplified by the infant and toddler portion of the IDEA legislation. The 1986 amendments to this legislation mandate interagency collaboration and regional service integration as part of a state planning process for early childhood intervention services. In many states, this has resulted in organized comprehensive and coordinated assessment and treatment services for infants and young children at risk for development disabilities owing to a variety of adverse perinatal outcomes or environmental factors.

Other examples of integrated delivery models developed for children at risk demonstrate efficiency in providing coordinated, multisectoral services for children. The National Institute of Mental Health created the Child and Adolescent Service System Program initiative to increase states' capacity to create coordinated systems of care in mental health for children and youth.[32] An example of such a mental health service integration model, developed in Ventura County, California, involves the collaboration of health, juvenile justice, mental health, and education agencies for the purpose of coordinating service delivery to children and reducing out-of-home placement for children with severe mental health conditions. Evaluations of the Ventura Model demonstrated improved mental health outcomes in children and lower frequency of out-of-home placement.[33]

Innovative models, designed to facilitate service coordination by decategorizing funding streams and creating flexible funding pools, include a series of ongoing demonstration projects that have taken place in communities in the United States over the past decade.[34] These projects illustrate some of the strategies used to integrate services and increase children's access to appropriate services, by rationalizing provision of public funds.

Part of the difficulty in integrating health services comes from the sheer volume of categorical programs, as well as the scope of eligibility and financial constraints that inhibit greater coordination.[35] Table 15.1 illustrates part of this challenge. A comprehensive approach to providing preventive, diagnostic, treatment, and rehabilitative services across the physical, emotional, cognitive, and social domains would require integration of many programs and funding sources. The MCHB launched the State Early Childhood Comprehensive Systems initiative in 2002 to address state-level policy issues that create complexity and undermine alignment of public programs affecting early childhood, including Medicaid, early care and education, mental health, and family support.

# Financing Children's Health Care

Intimately linked to structure and organization of health services is how these services are financed. A range of funding streams currently fund parts of the full continuum of services that children need. However, health insurance remains a principal determinant of children's access to medical care. Financial barriers to medical care result primarily from lack of insurance for primary care services (such as well-child care and immunizations) or specialty child health services (such as mental health services and rehabilitative therapy).

## Uninsured Children

Public child health insurance eligibility has expanded as studies continue to document significant differential access to health care for uninsured children. Children without health insurance are less likely to have routine doctor visits or receive care for injuries, and more likely to delay seeking care.[36] In the 1997 National Health Interview Survey (NHIS), parents of uninsured children reported a higher rate of unmet medical, dental, medication, and vision needs than did parents of

## TABLE 15.1. PUBLIC PROGRAMS IN
## CHILD HEALTH SERVICE AND HEALTH NEED DOMAINS.

| Health Service | Health Need | | | | |
|---|---|---|---|---|---|
| | **Physical** | **Emotional** | **Cognitive** | **Family** | **Social** |
| Prevention | Title XIX<br>Title XXI<br>Title V<br>Title X<br>WIC<br>MCH block grant | Title X<br>PL 99–457 | Title XIX<br>Title X<br>PL 99–457<br>Head Start | Title X<br>Head Start<br>TANF<br>PL 99–457 | Title IV<br>HUD<br>TANF |
| Early identification | Title XIX<br>Title XXI<br>Title V<br>Title X<br>WIC<br>MCH block grant | Title XIX<br>PL 99–457 | Title XIX<br>PL 99–457 | Title XX<br>Title IV | Title IV |
| Diagnosis | Title XIX<br>Title XXI<br>Title V<br>PL 99–457 | Title XIX<br>PL 99–457 | Title XIX<br>PL 99–457 | Title XX<br>Title IV<br>PL 99–457 | Title IV |
| Treatment | Title XIX<br>Title XXI<br>Title V<br>PL 99–457 | Title XIX<br>PL 99–457 | Title XIX<br>PL 99–457 | | Title IV |

*Source:* Halfon, N., and Berkowitz, G. "Health Care Entitlements for Children: Providing Health Services As If Children Really Mattered." In M. A. Jensen and S. G. Goffin (eds.), *Visions of Entitlement: The Care and Education of America's Children.* Albany, N.Y.: SUNY Press, 1993.

privately insured children.[37] Delay in care for common childhood conditions that have potentially disabling effects (such as ear infection leading to hearing loss) has been attributed to families' lack of health coverage for the child.[38] Uninsured preschoolers have less immunization coverage and receive fewer recommended well-child visits.[39] Uninsured families are also more likely to rely on the emergency room to be their regular source of care.[40] Lack of health insurance can as well result in families restricting their children's participation in sports and other activities because of concern about their ability to pay for care in the event of injury.[41]

Unmet needs for medical care during the year are substantially higher not only for uninsured children (with 12.6 percent having an unmet need) but for children insured for part of the year (13.4 percent) in comparison to full-year-insured children with public insurance (1.4 percent) or private insurance (0.7 percent).[42]

The proportion of uninsured children in the United States rose 40 percent between 1977 and 1987,[43] and by 1989 13.3 percent of children were uninsured.[44] The percentage of children covered by employer-based insurance dropped steadily for more than a decade. The decline in private insurance coverage for children resulted from elimination of dependent coverage on the part of some employers, rising cost to employees of optional dependent coverage, and an economic shift toward service jobs without health benefits. The percentage of children with employer-based coverage declined from 60.7 percent in 1987 to 56.2 percent in 1992, accounting for nearly three million children losing coverage.[45] The rate has not increased, remaining at 56.8 percent in 2003.[46]

Expansion of the Medicaid program in the mid-1990s partially compensated for this erosion in employer-based insurance.[47] The number of children covered by Medicaid rose by approximately half, from 13.6 percent of U.S. children in 1989 (8.9 million children) to 19.9 percent in 1993 (13.7 million).[48] By 2003 more than one-quarter of children (25.8 percent) were covered by Medicaid.[49] Although Medicaid extends coverage to children in the lowest-income families, about three-quarters of uninsured children (77.1 percent) live in families with income above the poverty level.[50] In 2003, 17.4 percent of children with family income of 100–199 percent of the federal poverty level were uninsured.[51] About 82 percent of uninsured children lived in families with one or more parents working full-time, and nearly all (96.2 percent) are U.S. citizens.[52] Enactment of the federal State Children's Health Insurance Program (SCHIP) also compensated for the decline in private coverage for children. Between 1998 and 2003, the number of uninsured children dropped from about 10.7 million children (15 percent) to 8.4 million children (11.5 percent).[53] About 70.1 percent of uninsured children in 2003 were eligible for Medicaid or SCHIP coverage but were unenrolled.[54]

***Medicaid Participation.*** Medicaid participation has been hampered by eligibility rules that cause discontinuities in children's enrollment.[55] Complex Medicaid eligibility criteria and fluctuations in family income result in significant turnover in enrollees each year. In the 1990s the General Accounting Office (renamed the Government Accountability Office in 2004) estimated that 40 percent of Medicaid TANF (Temporary Assistance for Needy Families) enrollees lose Medicaid coverage each year.[56] Duration of enrollment is a critical Medicaid program issue for children. This not only undermines access to care but limits the ability of states to measure quality of care for these children; a recent study found that only 39 percent of two-year-olds in Medicaid managed care health plans met the twelve-month continuous enrollment criteria for inclusion in the National Committee for Quality Assurance HEDIS measurement.[57]

A significant proportion of children who are Medicaid-eligible remain unenrolled. This is particularly true for Latino children.[58] Eligibility expansion has extended coverage, but eligible children still do not participate for reasons of the delinking of Medicaid from cash assistance, limited outreach[59] and parent knowledge,[60] and complex rules that are difficult for eligibility workers to administer.[61] In 1993, an estimated 2.3 million uninsured children were Medicaid-eligible.[62] By 2003, the estimate was 4.1 million.[63] The 1994–95 NHIS showed that unenrolled Medicaid-eligible children have poorer access to health care than enrolled children with greater unmet need (17.9 vs. 6.2 percent) and a higher incidence of lacking regular source of care (23.0 vs. 5.6 percent).[64]

***State Children's Health Insurance Program.*** Enactment of the State Children's Health Insurance Program in 1997 as Title XXI of the Social Security Act extended health insurance to children who had not been eligible for Medicaid or private, employer-based coverage. SCHIP extended coverage to approximately one-third of the eleven million uninsured children[65] living in families with income between the existing Medicaid eligibility threshold and 200 percent of the federal poverty level. Initially authorized for 1997 through 2001, SCHIP included provisions to prevent children who otherwise could be enrolled in private employer-based insurance from participating in SCHIP.[66] Specific provisions of the SCHIP legislation addressed some historical limitations of Medicaid.[67] States were required to implement outreach programs and ensure that children found not to be eligible for SCHIP would be referred to or enrolled in Medicaid if eligible. States also were permitted to extend twelve months of eligibility to a child once Medicaid eligibility was established so that eligibility losses caused by month-to-month income fluctuations could be reduced. By 1999, SCHIP had achieved a 45 percent participation rate among eligible children.[68] Recent studies show that state policy choices in SCHIP influence program outcomes. For example, adoption of a six-month waiting period to enroll, use of asset testing, premium requirements, prohibiting self-declaration of income, and lack of a presumptive eligibility policy during the application period are all associated with lower enrollment in states that implement these policies.[69] State variation in participation, ranging from about 35 to 60 percent in a survey sample, shows the importance of these policies for achieving high participation.[70]

***Private Insurance.*** Children with employment-based health coverage also are at risk for loss of insurance and disruption of care. Health insurance for children covered under their parents' employment is jeopardized with job loss or job change. As the economy shifts from high-paying, benefit-rich manufacturing jobs to lower-paying, benefit-poor service jobs, dependent coverage is less ensured. For example, 25 percent of children from thirteen to eighteen months old in a large health maintenance organization had experienced some disruption of coverage during the previous five-month period.[71] Uninsurance among workers and their families who could receive employer-based insurance but are not enrolled also has been studied.[72]

Even those children and families with health insurance frequently are underinsured for essential primary medical care, including well-child care, immunizations, and specialty care. In 1992, 50 percent of indemnity insurance health plans covered well-child care and 65 percent of preferred provider organizations (PPOs) covered immunizations.[73] Children with special health care needs caused by a congenital condition, chronic illness, or injury may lack adequate private medical coverage, especially for speech therapy, behavioral therapy, physical therapy, and other essential services.[74] About 58.1 percent of parents self-report that private health insurance adequately covers the service benefits needed by their child with special needs.[75] Moreover, despite the demonstrated efficacy of nonmedical social services for health and developmental outcomes, services such as home visitation and health-related consultation are rarely benefits for privately insured children. In contrast, Medicaid generally covers these services.

*Cost Sharing.*  Nearly all health plans apply cost-sharing mechanisms to minimize unnecessary use of medical services and thereby limit expenditures. The RAND Health Insurance Experiment found that placing cost-sharing requirements on families for primary and preventive care services reduced children's use of these discretionary services.[76] Although short-term adverse outcomes from reduced use of medical care were not detected in the RAND study, the sensitivity of children's basic ambulatory medical services to cost sharing was demonstrated.[77] With the expansion of managed care, more preventive services such as immunization and well-child care are routinely covered, and administration fees, deductibles, co-payments, and other cost-sharing mechanisms are less often applied for preventive and primary care visits. In contrast, cost sharing continues to be applied to acute and chronic care services. For many poor, near-poor, and even middle-income families, even nominal cost sharing poses a significant barrier to care.

## Nonfinancial Barriers to Care

Children's access to medical care traditionally has been measured by analyzing utilization patterns for specific provider services (such as number of annual physician visits), designated populations (adolescents, children in foster care), children with specific conditions (for instance, those with asthma), or specific services (immunization, prenatal care, and so on).[78] Such analyses have identified many factors that impede use of care and that appear to account for differential usage (as by ethnicity, income, and residence) when controlling for health need (as measured by health status indicators and number and type of conditions).[79] Nonfinancial barriers to care include structural, environmental, and personal impediments such as bureaucratic complexity in the organization of child health services, cultural barriers based on ethnicity or language, and provider distribution or shortage, among others.[80]

***Race and Ethnicity.*** In addition to income, differential access has been consistently documented on the basis of race and ethnicity. Differential access and use associated with race and ethnicity may result from varying modes of utilization, insurance barriers, and the cultural competency of providers. Nonwhite children and adolescents have fewer physician visits and are less likely to have continuity of care.[81] Studies of access to care of Latino children have also indicated a high rate of uninsurance and differential patterns of use that are based on parental immigration status.[82] Recent surveys show that the quality of care received by Latino children is often lower, with parents reporting receiving less counseling on health promotion topics and having more difficulty obtaining the information they need when their child has a chronic health condition.[83] Problems of care and health outcomes for African American children improve when targeted interventions can overcome organizational barriers.[84] A study of African American women receiving prenatal care in an environment that potentially equalizes access to care (a U.S. Army base) detected a lower infant mortality rate and underscores the important role that special barriers have in poor health outcomes for children.[85]

***Regular Sources of Care.*** As Barbara Starfield has demonstrated in numerous reviews of access to care, having a regular source of primary care is particularly important for children.[86] Children with a regular source of care are more likely to receive needed medical services and immunizations, resulting in a higher level of satisfaction reported by the family.[87] Having a regular source of care is principally determined by insurance status, and the insurance effect on access is often mediated by having a regular provider.[88] In several studies, the type and characteristics of the regular care provider have their own independent effect on use, irrespective of type of insurance coverage. Therefore, considering the type of a usual source of care is important in analyzing differences in access among children. It is a key indicator of the success of insurance expansions such as SCHIP.[89]

***Provider Training.***  Emerging patterns of morbidity in children, including complex risks, health conditions, and social problems, pose new challenges to health care providers and delivery systems.[90] Surveys and anecdotal reports document inadequacies in clinical training for health professionals and their inability to identify, treat, or refer children suffering from complex medical conditions, mental disorders, developmental problems, complex psychosocial problems, and abuse and neglect.[91] In one study, physicians' assessments identified fewer than 50 percent of emotional problems of the children who were screened.[92] These inadequacies are a function of provider training and knowledge, systemic undervaluing of assessment for new morbidities, and a shortage of community-based treatment resources for these problems.[93] Physicians report in national surveys that knowledge about complex, means-tested public programs for children, the time involved, and their familiarity with screening tools are all barriers to children being identified and referred for developmental concerns.[94]

***Distribution of Providers.***  Geographic access barriers pose problems for both insured and uninsured poor families. Travel time for a family in an underserved urban area or rural location may be substantial[95] and result in reduced use of care.[96] For poor children, a limited supply of local physicians is associated with reduced access to preventive care services[97] and routine emergency room use for nonemergent sick care.[98] Although the overall number of pediatricians has risen over the past two decades, the geographic distribution of pediatricians relative to the child population has not improved significantly.[99] The shortage of local primary care providers for poor children has been further compromised in recent years. The number of office-based physicians delivering primary care services in low-income areas declined by 45.1 percent between 1963 and 1980.[100] Low reimbursement and administrative requirements of the Medicaid program are also associated with low participation of physicians in this important program for children. Pediatrician participation in Medicaid is substantially higher in states with higher reimbursement, less use of capitation, and fewer physician-perceived administrative barriers to participation such as paperwork requirements.[101]

Children who receive care in an office-based setting are more likely to receive continuity of care and coordination of services. One effect of the shortage in office-based primary care providers has been a high, and often inappropriate, rate of emergency department utilization.[102] People who identify their regular provider of care as a hospital outpatient department, rather than a medical office, are significantly less likely to see the same provider on a subsequent visit,[103] and young children receive less preventive care, including immunizations, in these settings.[104] In recent years, the outpatient department of a hospital has grown as the site of the regular source of care for poor children in lieu of the office of a private physician.[105]

# Improving the Child Health System

The task of integrating personal medical services with complementary community-based health, social, and educational services demands substantial coordination as well as financial incentives. Achieving health system objectives for children requires greater access to health insurance, integration of services, quality measurement, public and community monitoring of performance (including data systems, involvement of communities, and new measures of how well community systems are performing), and tailoring managed care delivery systems to meet the developmental needs of all children and the special needs of vulnerable child populations.[106]

## Health Insurance

In the early 1990s, it seemed that national health care reform might make available universal coverage and usher in a more organized system. Instead, state-initiated health insurance expansions for children took center stage. Some states obtained Medicaid demonstration waivers and used this flexibility to convert to managed care systems and expand coverage for previously uninsured groups.[107] Other states embarked on health insurance expansion for children using state funding (such as Pennsylvania's Child Health Insurance Program, or CHIP), or developed programs that combine public and private revenues (such as Colorado's Child Health Plan). Another form of child health insurance expansion was the Blue Cross and Blue Shield Caring Program for Children.[108] Such privately funded programs primarily covered well-child services and care for acute and chronic illness, but not hospitalization. Thus, program costs were relatively modest.

Enactment of SCHIP in 1997 further strengthened the role of states in administering unique, state-based health insurance programs for children. State options to determine benefit package, cost sharing, and enrollment mechanisms in SCHIP have contributed to the difference in insurance eligibility and program structure across states.[109] Past experience with children's incomplete participation in Medicaid and their failure to be covered by employer-based insurance when it is available has produced a challenge for SCHIP.[110]

## Health System Integration

Expansion of health insurance coverage and system reorganization on the basis of managed care cannot guarantee children's access to a system of health care that is comprehensive and coordinated. Structural and organizational characteristics of the current health system must be addressed to improve allocation and quality of health services for children and families.[111]

The principles of comprehensive, continuous, and coordinated care originally embodied in Medicaid's EPSDT program, and reinforced in 1989 amendments to Title XIX, recognize that access to basic ambulatory medical care does not suffice to meet the needs of children with complex health conditions and environmental risks. For such children, screening, diagnostic, and treatment services must be supplemented with a constellation of supportive services, including outreach, comprehensive case management home visiting, and family counseling services.[112] Several authors have suggested that services should address existing health conditions but should also be sensitive to the functional and developmental capacities of the child as well as to the family's needs and the community environment.[113] This implies a systematic focus on strategically optimizing investment in children's health development.

Programs designed to reduce health risks and promote protective factors have been tested for children at risk of adverse developmental or other outcomes. In a cost-conscious era, initiatives to broaden and integrate child health services and develop linkage across sectors must demonstrate both effectiveness (improved health outcomes, in an applied setting) and efficiency (cost impact).[114] Home visiting and other early intervention programs targeted to at-risk families have proven cost-effective in improving children's health status, cognitive functioning, and academic performance, while decreasing dependence on public assistance.[115] Until recently, few of these successful demonstration and local community projects were implemented statewide. North Carolina's SmartStart, California's Children and Family First Act, and Vermont's Success by Six all report new statewide efforts targeting the health and development of all young children. These are broad, population-based health promotion and disease prevention programs, where the medical sector plays a key role. It is not clear to what degree these new population-based initiatives will become comprehensive and integrated with traditional children's medical services.

The potential of integrated service programs, such as early intervention or school-linked health services, is uncertain in the current managed care marketplace. They are not likely to reduce the short-term costs of a managed care organization by reducing hospitalization or other high-cost medical expenditure. Instead, the savings from these programs may be realized in a lower incidence of special education participation, enhanced family functioning, and lower welfare outlays.[116] Savings are likely to accrue to the education, mental health, juvenile justice, and other business sectors, rather than to the organization that provided the care. It may be more difficult for states to continue to support integrated cross-sector delivery efforts such as early intervention programs, school-based clinics, or many public health safety net programs. Over the past decade, many of these services were paid for (in the case of early intervention and school-based clinics) or heavily subsidized (in the case of public clinics and hospitals) with Medicaid funds. As Medicaid funds are diverted into commercial managed care contracts, the ability of the state or local community to use these funds for community health programs and health-related support services may be reduced. Continued development of integrated continuums poses a fundamental challenge to states and localities that choose not to earmark some portion of their Medicaid funds or identify new revenues for this purpose (as California and North Carolina have done).

Although direct control over Medicaid funds may decline, the range of mechanisms that states are implementing (combined or separate medical and mental health managed systems, service exclusions, and so on) presents an opportunity to test what types of public-private arrangement prove effective. The infrastructure of the managed care organization may create new opportunities for coordination, if not integration.[117] Greater attention to early childhood development, coupled with the need for Medicaid (and SCHIP) managed care contractors to forge relationships with existing public programs for children, could spur enhanced integration. For example, statewide population-based early childhood health and development promotion programs in California, North Carolina, and Vermont are already being linked with initiatives on the part of local health care providers and managed care organizations. There is a tremendous opportunity to understand which managed care mechanisms serve as barriers or facilitators to quality health care, to identify measures that capture the unique objectives of children's health care, and to use state intervention in Medicaid and SCHIP as a research laboratory.

## Measures of Health Care Quality for Children

Government agencies, medical professional organizations, and multidisciplinary expert working groups have all developed normative definitions of comprehensive primary care.[118] For example, standards have been issued by the federal MCHB and the American Academy of Pediatrics for children's medical care, and by the Child Welfare League of America for the health needs of children in foster care.[119] The Bright Futures recommendations, originally funded by the MCHB in the mid-1990s, presents a comprehensive set of standards for the content of well-child services.[120] The principles embodied in Bright Futures reaffirm the need for an integrated health care system that is comprehensive, continuous, accessible, coordinated, and accountable. Other research and health care organizations are developing practice guidelines for particular services or medical conditions on the basis of evidence or the consensus of an expert panel.[121]

In the private sector, the NCQA developed the Health Employer Data Information Set (HEDIS), which compares commercial health plan performance on quality indicators of effectiveness of care, access, and utilization. HEDIS and other quality assurance systems based on administrative data do not capture all domains of quality that are of interest for children's health care. Family satisfaction information collected from patients can supplement utilization and administrative data, particularly for difficult-to-measure constructs such as perceived access. The Consumer Assessment of Health Plans (CAHPS) consumer satisfaction surveys ask parents about their child's health care and have a supplemental survey for parents of children with special health care needs (CSHCN). The Child and Adolescent Health Measurement Initiative (CAHMI) has developed quality care measures that specifically address the health care needs of children. For example, the CAHMI Promoting Healthy Development Survey (PHDS) examines provision of developmentally relevant services to children from birth to three. Although the CSHCN supplement and the PHDS have not yet been adopted as required CAHPS components for NCQA certification, and though the CSHCN supplement has been adopted voluntarily by a number of states, the PHDS has been fielded by only a few states, notably Vermont and Washington.

There are a number of reasons that developing performance measures and standards of care for children and families is a unique and challenging undertaking.[122] Because children are constantly developing, it is difficult to attribute positive or negative characteristics of their health care to their functioning and future outcomes. The complexity of some constructs that define quality care for children (comprehensive, family-centered, integrated) makes it difficult to create valid quality indicators that can be used for performance comparison. Additionally, the relatively small number and heterogeneity within a group of children with a particular kind of complex medical condition is a methodological challenge in creating standards and performance measures associated with those standards.

## Public Accountability and Monitoring

Public accountability for ensuring that all children have access to comprehensive health care has not been part of U.S. child health policy. In the European nations that maintain population-based service delivery models and use public health nurses and other providers to track and monitor infants through the preschool years, compliance with immunization schedules and age-appropriate preventive care visits is substantially higher than in the United States.[123] A combination of universal access to preventive care and integrated health information systems permits such population-based assurance.

Despite recent advances in health information systems, data systems currently are not structured or capable of producing child-focused information on encounters with the broader child health system, including the public health, nutrition, and school-based health sectors. Some efforts are under way across the United States to introduce model systems that can be used to ensure delivery of the most basic of medical services for children. An example is the Robert Wood Johnson Foundation's All Kids Count initiative, which supports demonstrations of state and local immunization information and monitoring systems.[124] Detailed information on quality of care and health outcomes has also been limited.[125] National surveys such as NHIS and its supplements on children and on individuals with disabilities, and the Medical Expenditure Panel Survey, have produced much of the national data on children's access, use, and costs of health care. Since 2000 the National Center for Health Statistics has fielded three new surveys designed to address this information gap: the National Survey on Early Childhood Health, the National Survey of Children with Special Health Care Needs, and the National Survey of Children's Health.

Community performance monitoring is also important for children's systems of care.[126] Because children's health services are delivered in multiple sectors, a community rather than a specific public program or commercial managed care organization may have the most to gain or lose from investing in its children's health. Such a monitoring process would include evaluating which aspects of the system facilitate or hinder access, using information about best practices to make improvements where necessary, and examining improvement by monitoring children's outcomes.

Ideally, community systems should be organized to respond to the determinants of children's health, in terms of availability of services, providers, and programs.[127] Normative standards for children's health care have identified the need for coordination across programs and organizations. To capture the potential contribution to children's health from the sectors responsible for their care, performance should thus be measured at the community level. Consideration of standards of care for children should not neglect administrative and community-level attributes that promote or undermine quality. For example, measures of service and system integration can be applied to evaluate performance within and among the child health service sectors. Defining the critical pathways by which coordination (when successful) takes place constitutes an initial step in developing the measures and the infrastructure for community performance monitoring.[128] Linking the results to specific organizational attributes would then make it possible to improve those system attributes that affect quality. Monitoring these attributes is important for policy and planning purposes.[129] For example, a number of communities are devising population-based report cards on determinants of children's health that, when linked to a monitoring system, can be used to mobilize change.[130] These initiatives may be an initial step toward the population-based accountability that has been lacking for children and families.

## Managed Care for Children

Historically, many Medicaid-insured children received medical care in safety-net public health facilities, where provider continuity and comprehensive health care were not always available.[131] Past difficulties in access and fragmentation of the delivery system, coupled with rapidly rising costs, helped spur the transition in the 1990s from fee-for-service to managed care Medicaid programs. By 2004, 61.3 percent of Medicaid beneficiaries nationally were enrolled in managed care delivery systems, with managed care the predominant arrangement in forty states and only three states maintaining traditional fee-for-service programs.[132] Many SCHIP programs also turned to managed care arrangements, and children covered by commercial health insurance are affected by these trends. Approximately six of every ten enrollees in managed care were in a for-profit health plan by 1995.[133] The effectiveness and improvement of managed care as a delivery system is an important policy question for both publicly and privately insured children.[134]

In early studies, managed care organizations demonstrated marginally higher preventive care utilization for maternal and child health services.[135] In a unique study that randomized families to managed care or to fee-for-service arrangements, managed care plans successfully reduced emergency room use and ambulatory visits for nonsevere conditions but did not appear to reduce medical services for children with acute needs. The authors concluded that managed care can rationalize care without inappropriate rationing of care.[136] Other studies comparing access and use under fee-for-service or managed care arrangements have produced mixed results.[137]

There is concern that managed care organizations' lack of experience with comprehensive delivery systems for children, and their tendency to control rather than coordinate services, could jeopardize care for children with chronic illness.[138] Managed care arrangements are largely untested in terms of their ability to cost-effectively manage the care of vulnerable children. Many children with special health needs (such as serious medical conditions) or with special circumstances (foster children, homeless children) have been excluded from previous studies of health outcomes, use, or costs. Even when included in such studies, they often make up such a small proportion of the study sample that evaluation of the impact of managed care on their health outcomes is impossible. In addition, Medicaid beneficiaries (and often commercial insurance enrollees as well) in most states were initially offered a choice between fee-for-service and managed care. Several studies show that children electing not to enroll in managed care are more likely to have certain medical diagnoses or higher health care utilization than children who do enroll.[139] It is thus difficult to compare the experiences of children who elect to enroll and those who do not, particularly without detailed information about their health care needs.

Several studies suggest the kinds of access barriers that children with special health needs might confront within a managed care organization. A survey of pediatricians participating in managed care plans revealed a high rate of denied referral to a specialist for children.[140] Early studies of managed care for children with special health care needs suggested that managed care plans limit mental health and related services, as well as access to specialists.[141] Another survey of administrators from twenty-two managed care plans found that few plans made a special effort to ensure inclusion of pediatric providers in the network.[142]

As managed care expands in the U.S. marketplace, research on the outcomes and effectiveness in such systems is important.[143] However, it is not only differences between enrolled populations that make comparison difficult for children. Variation in managed care structures, benefits, and implementation across regions makes it difficult to generalize experience within one region or study to other localities. For example, a 1998 survey of state Medicaid programs showed a variety of mixed financing arrangements affecting children's services, including medical and behavioral health contracts, service exclusion, and diagnosis exclusion.[144] In the absence of generalizable findings about managed care impact, certain important focus areas have been identified for Medicaid program oversight of managed care contractors: specificity of pediatric service benefits, requirements for pediatric providers contracting within networks, medical necessity standards tailored for children, quality indicators for children, appropriate payment rates for pediatric services, and promotion of high-quality care.[145] It is important (but a complex undertaking) to evaluate how contracting arrangements affect care for children. Earlier studies of Medicaid managed care focused on the difference between fee-for-service and managed care arrangements rather than on difference within managed care systems.[146] It is important to identify optimal financing and contracting arrangements within Medicaid managed care for children with special health needs and other groups of vulnerable children in particular.[147]

Despite these concerns, the transition to managed care has enabled national initiatives such as the RWJ-funded Best Clinical and Administrative Practices to facilitate innovation and improvement in delivery of care to Medicaid and SCHIP beneficiaries. Examples include efforts to identify CSHCN for purposes of coordination and quality monitoring and improving asthma care for children. Such initiatives have not been possible in fee-for-service systems. They reflect the potential value that mature managed Medicaid systems can bring to persistent gaps in quality of care among Medicaid compared to commercial plan beneficiaries.[148]

## From Social HMOs to HDOs

To overcome obstacles to comprehensive and coordinated systems of health services for high-risk children and families, new forms of managed health care must be created. This could take the form of social HMOs, or health development organizations (HDOs). The social HMO concept augments current vertically integrated medical services with additional health promotion, social services, and enhanced coordination mechanisms to produce appropriate horizontal integration.[149] Demonstration project social HMOs for the frail and elderly population have offered multifaceted risk assessment and an inclusive set of services, resources, case management, and coordination.[150] Evaluation of social HMO experience for the elderly has produced mixed outcomes.[151] Nonetheless the social HMO concept holds enormous potential for maximizing the fit between the true health needs of children and an appropriately constructed and integrated delivery system.

An extension of the social HMO concept is what has been termed a health development organization.[152] The HDO framework creates a mechanism to integrate services not only vertically and horizontally but longitudinally as well, to optimize the health development trajectory of children. HDOs would actively develop the health of the child population by using principles and practices that optimize health development trajectories. These include minimizing the influence of risk factors during a critical developmental period through targeted risk reduction and strategic use of health promotion and other protective factors. This is illustrated in Figure 15.2.

Studies of the commercial managed care sector have examined the proliferation of managed care systems that target particular populations or service needs.[153] This market-based trend toward innovation and diversification could extend to children's services and stimulate new systems of specialty care for children that previously were attempted only within public sector integration initiatives.[154]

## Conclusion

Children in the United States experience a system that can offer the latest medical advances but is also complex and often means-tested. The evolution of the U.S. health care system into distinct sectors, with fragmented services and categorical funding mechanisms, poses a significant barrier to improved organization of care. Improving the health care delivery system for children means integrating the activities of largely publicly funded community-based health services with privately delivered managed care models. A number of efforts seek to build on growing knowledge to improve the health-promoting and risk-reduction orientation of the child health system. Population-based, integrated models of service delivery systems have been developed in European nations and in localized demonstration projects in the United States. Most European countries offer universal health, developmental, and social services to children beginning at conception, including

## FIGURE 15.2. HOW RISK-REDUCTION AND HEALTH-PROMOTION STRATEGIES INFLUENCE HEALTH DEVELOPMENT.

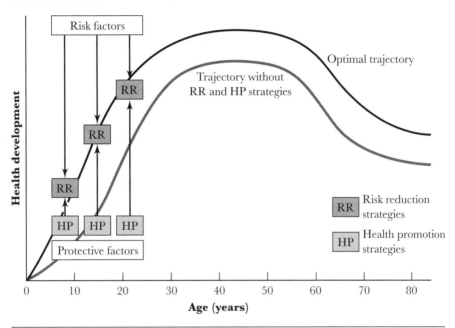

*Note:* This figure illustrates how risk-reduction strategies can mitigate the influence of risk factors on the developmental trajectory, and how health promotion strategies can simultaneously support and optimize the development trajectory. In the absence of effective risk reduction and health promotion, the developmental trajectory is suboptimal (dotted curve).

*Source:* Halfon, N., Inkelas, M., and Hochstein, M. "The Health Development Organization: An Organizational Approach to Achieving Child Health Development." *Milbank Quarterly,* 2000, *78*(3), 447–498.

nationally insured health care, maternity leave and support, and child care and development programs.[155] Because the United States has experienced a more incremental and market-based evolution of service systems, aligning incentives for health promotion among multiple public and private sectors is a more complicated challenge.

The U.S. health care system continues to produce many important innovations in addressing the special medical and developmental needs of children. Using managed care to rationalize delivery of personal medical services may substantially improve children's access to basic medical care. Recent reports from the IOM suggest that the health care system should not only be focused on diagnostic, treatment, and rehabilitation services but also improve the availability and performance of disease and disability prevention, health promotion, and developmental optimization services. This requires better measurement strategies to document service system needs and performance; service system reform strategies that can reengineer service pathways to better integrate personal health, public heath, and population health sector services; financing strategies that can facilitate and incentivize provision of these services; and efforts by states and local communities to implement these strategies.

There is opportunity during this time of great structural change to fashion more efficient delivery systems. Sufficient attention should be paid to the unique needs of children and to designing a system that meets children's needs. The move to managed care may facilitate some of the changes that are necessary to improve services delivered to children, if essential components and safeguards are included. Policy makers, health care providers, and the public at large have to consider how to ensure that children's unique needs are met under the evolving health system if health outcomes are to be improved.

## Notes

1. National Research Council and Institute of Medicine. *Children's Health, the Nation's Wealth: Assessing and Improving Child Health.* Committee on Evaluation of Children's Health. Board of Children, Youth, and Families, Division of Behavioral and Social Sciences and Education. Washington, D.C.: National Academies Press, 2004.

2. Jameson, E. J., and Wehr, E. "Drafting National Health Care Reform Legislation to Protect the Health Interests of Children." *Stanford Law and Policy Review,* 1994, *5,* 152–176; Halfon, N., Inkelas, M., and Wood, D. "Nonfinancial Barriers to Care for Children and Youth." *Annual Review of Public Health,* 1995, *16,* 447–472; Forrest, C. B., Simpson, L., and Clancy, C. "Child Health Services Research: Challenges and Opportunities." *Journal of the American Medical Association,* 1997, *277,* 1787–1793; Halfon, N., Inkelas, M., and Hochstein, M. "The Health Development Organization: An Organizational Approach to Achieving Child Health Development." *Milbank Quarterly,* 2000, *78,* 447–498.

3. Shonkoff, J. P., and Meisels, S. J. "Early Childhood Intervention: The Evolution of a Concept." In S. J. Meisels and J. P. Shonkoff (eds.), *Intervention Handbook of Early Childhood.* Cambridge, England: Cambridge University Press, 1990.

4. Hertzman, C. "The Lifelong Impact of Childhood Experiences: A Population Perspective." *Proceedings of the American Academy of Arts and Sciences, Daedalus: Health and Wealth,* 1994, *123*(4), 167–180; Sameroff, A. J., and Fiese, B. H. "Transactional Regulation and Early Intervention." In Meisels and Shonkoff (1990); Bronfenbrenner, U. "Ecology of the Family as a Context for Human Development Research Perspectives." *Developmental Psychology,* 1986, *22,* 723–742; Bronfenbrenner, U. *The Ecology of Human Development: Experiments by Nature and Design.* Cambridge, Mass.: Harvard University Press, 1979; Halfon, N., and Hochstein, M. "Life Course Health Development: An Integrated Framework for Developing Health, Policy, and Research." *Milbank Quarterly,* 2002, *80*(3), 433–479.

5. Hertzman (1994); Evans, G. "Introduction." In R. G. Evans, M. L. Barer, and T. R. Marmor (eds.), *Why Are Some People Healthy and Others Not? The Determinants of Health of Populations.*

Hawthorne, N.Y.: Aldine de Gruyter, 1994; Barker, D. J., and others. "The Relation of Small Head Circumference and Thinness at Birth to Death from Cardiovascular Disease in Adult Life." *British Medical Journal,* 1993, *306,* 422–426; Bakketeig, L. S., and others. "Pre-Pregnancy Risk Factors of Small-for-Gestational-Age Births Among Parous Women in Scandinavia." *Acta Obstetrica et Gynecologica Scandinavica,* 1993, *72,* 273–279; Werner, E. E. "High Risk Children in Young Adulthood: A Longitudinal Study from Birth to Age 32 Years." *American Journal of Orthopsychiatry,* 1989, *59,* 72–81; Freeman, J. "Prenatal and Peri-natal Factors Associated with Brain Disorders." (NIH publication no. 85–1149). Wash-ington, D.C.: U.S. Department of Health and Human Services, 1985; Kuh, D., and others. "Life Course Epidemiology." *Journal of Epidemiology and Community Health,* 2003, *57*(10), 778–783.

6. Brooks-Gunn, J., and others. "Early Intervention in Low Birthweight Premature Infants: Re-sults Through Age 5 Years from the Infant Health and Development Program." *Journal of the American Medical Association,* 1994, *272,* 1257–1262; Infant Health and Development Program. "Enhancing the Outcomes of Low-Birthweight, Premature Infants: A Multisite Randomized Trial." *Journal of the American Medical Association,* 1990, *263,* 3035–3042.

7. Shaywitz, S. E., and Shaywitz, B. A. "Dyslexia (Specific Reading Disability)." *Pediatrics in Review,* 2003, *24*(5), 147–153.

8. Karoly, L., and others. *Investing in Our Children: What We Know and Don't Know About the Costs and Benefits of Early Childhood Interventions.* Santa Monica, Calif.: RAND, 1998.

9. Brooks-Gunn and others (1994); Zigler, E. F. "Early Childhood Intervention: A Promis-ing Preventative for Juvenile Delinquency." *American Psychologist,* 1992, *47,* 997–1006.

10. Hoeckleman, R. A., and Pless, I. B. "Decline in Mortality Among Young Americans Dur-ing the 20th Century: Prospects for Reaching National Mortality Reduction Goals for 1990." *Pediatrics,* 1988, *82,* 582–595.

11. Haggerty, R. J., Roghmann, K. J., and Pless, I. B. *Child Health and the Community.* New York: Wiley, 1975; Starfield, B. "Child and Adolescent Health Measures." *Future of Children,* 1992, *2,* 25–39.

12. Halfon, N., and Berkowitz, G. "Health Care Entitlements for Children: Providing Health Services As If Children Really Mattered." In M. A. Jensen and S. G. Goffin (eds.), *Visions of Entitlement: The Care and Education of America's Children.* Albany: SUNY Press, 1993.

13. Fielding, J. E., and Halfon, N. "Where Is the Health in Health Reform?" *Journal of the Amer-ican Medical Association,* 1994, *272,* 1292–1296.

14. Jameson and Wehr (1994).

15. McGlynn, E., Halfon, N., and Leibowitz, A. "Assessing the Quality of Care for Children: Prospects Under Health Care Reform." *Archives of Pediatric and Adolescent Medicine,* 1995, *149,* 359–368.

16. Newacheck, P. W., and Halfon, N. "The Association Between Mothers' and Children's Use of Physician Services." *Medical Care,* 1986, *24,* 30–33.

17. Carnegie Task Force on Meeting the Needs of Young Children. *Starting Points: Meeting the Needs of Our Youngest Children.* New York: Carnegie Corporation of New York, 1994; Na-tional Commission on Children. *Beyond Rhetoric: A New American Agenda for Children and Fam-ilies.* Washington, D.C.: U.S. Government Printing Office, 1994.

18. National Research Council and Institute of Medicine (2004).

19. Needleman, R., and Silverstein, M. "Pediatric Interventions to Support Reading Aloud: How Good Is the Evidence?" *Journal of Developmental and Behavioral Pediatrics,* 2004, *25*(5), 352–363.

20. Daley, K. C. "Update on Sudden Infant Death Syndrome." *Current Opinion in Pediatrics,* 2004, *16*(2), 227–232.

21. Schechter, M. S. "Non-genetic Influences on Cystic Fibrosis Lung Disease: The Role of Sociodemographic Characteristics, Environmental Exposures, and Healthcare Interventions." *Seminars in Respiratory and Critical Care Medicine*, 2003, *24*(6), 639–652.

22. Halfon, Inkelas, and Hochstein (2000).

23. Select Panel for the Promotion of Child Health. *Better Health for Our Children: A National Strategy.* Washington, D.C.: U.S. Department of Health and Human Services, 1981; Harvey, B. "Why We Need a National Child Health Policy." *Pediatrics*, 1991, *87*, 1–6; Schlesinger, M., and Eisenberg, L. "Little People in a Big Policy World: Lasting Questions and New Directions in Health Policy for Children." In M. Schlesinger and L. Eisenberg (eds.), *Children in a Changing Health System: Assessments and Proposals for Reform.* Baltimore: Johns Hopkins University Press, 1990.

24. Halfon, Inkelas, and Wood (1995).

25. Lewit, E., and Monheit, A. "Expenditures on Health Care for Children and Pregnant Women." *Future of Children*, 1992, *2*, 95–114; McCormick, M. C., and others. "Annual Report of Access to and Utilization of Health Care for Children and Youth in the United States—1999." *Pediatrics*, 2000, *105*, 219–230.

26. Halfon, N., Uyeda, K., Inkelas, M., and Rice, T. *Building Bridges: A Comprehensive System for Healthy Development and School Readiness.* Los Angeles: National Center for Infant and Early Childhood Health Policy, 2004.

27. Harvey (1991).

28. Schlesinger and Eisenberg (1990).

29. National Governors Association Center for Best Practices. *A Governor's Guide to Children's Cabinets.* Washington, D.C.: NGA Center for Best Practices, 2004.

30. Grason, H., and Guyer, B. "Rethinking the Organization of Children's Programs: Lessons from the Elderly." *Milbank Quarterly*, 1995, *73*, 565–597.

31. Halfon, Inkelas, and Hochstein (2000).

32. Kahn, A. J., and Kamerman, S. B. *Integrating Services Integration: An Overview of Initiatives, Issues, and Possibilities.* (National Center for Children in Poverty.) New York: Columbia University School of Public Health, 1992.

33. Rosenblatt, A., Attkisson, C. C., and Fernandez, A. J. "Integrating Systems of Care in California for Youth with Severe Emotional Disturbance. II: Initial Group Home Expenditure and Utilization Findings from the California AB377 Evaluation Project." *Journal of Child and Family Studies*, 1992, *1*, 263–286.

34. Newacheck, P., Hughes, D., Halfon, N., and Brindis, C. "Social HMOs and Other Capitated Arrangements for Children with Special Health Care Needs." *Maternal and Child Health Journal*, 1997, *1*, 111–118.

35. Halfon and Berkowitz (1993).

36. Stoddard, J., St. Peter, R., and Newacheck, P. W. "Health Insurance Status and Ambulatory Care for Children." *New England Journal of Medicine*, 1994, *330*, 1421–1425.

37. Newacheck, P. W., and others. "The Unmet Needs of America's Children." *Pediatrics*, 2000, *105*, 989–997.

38. Stoddard, St. Peter, and Newacheck (1994).

39. Wood, D. L., and others. "Access to Medical Care for Children and Adolescents in the United States." *Pediatrics*, 1990, *86*, 666–673; Short, P. F., and Lefkowitz, D. C. "Encouraging Preventive Services for Low-Income Children: The Effect of Expanding Medicaid." *Medical Care*, 1992, *30*, 766–780.

40. Wood and others (1990); Newacheck, P. W., Hughes, D., and Stoddard, J. "Children's Access to Primary Care: Differences by Race, Income, and Insurance Status." *Pediatrics*, 1997, *97*, 26–32.

41. Lave, J. R., and others. "Impact of a Children's Health Insurance Program on Newly Enrolled Children." *Journal of the American Medical Association*, 1998, *279*, 1820–1825.

42. Olson, L. M., and others. "Children in the United States with Discontinuous Health Insurance Coverage." *New England Journal of Medicine*, 2005, *353*(4), 382–391.

43. Employee Benefit Research Institute. *Sources of Health Insurance and Characteristics of the Uninsured: Analysis of the March 1992 Current Population Survey.* (Report no. 133.) Washington, D.C.: Employee Benefit Research Institute, 1993.

44. U.S. General Accounting Office. *Medicaid: States Turn to Managed Care to Improve Access and Control Costs.* (GAO/HRD-93–46.) Washington, D.C.: U.S. Government Printing Office, 1993.

45. Newacheck, P. W., Hughes, D. C., and Cisternas, M. "Children and Health Insurance: An Overview of Recent Trends." *Health Affairs*, 1994, *14*, 244–254.

46. Kaiser Commission on Medicaid and the Uninsured. *Health Insurance Coverage in American: 2003 Data Update.* Washington, D.C.: Kaiser Family Foundation, Nov. 2004.

47. Newacheck, Hughes, and Cisternas (1994); Teitelbaum, M. *The Health Insurance Crisis for America's Children.* Washington, D.C.: Children's Defense Fund, 1994.

48. U.S. General Accounting Office (1993).

49. Kaiser Commission on Medicaid and the Uninsured (2004).

50. Kaiser Commission on Medicaid and the Uninsured (2004).

51. Kaiser Commission on Medicaid and the Uninsured (2004).

52. Kaiser Commission on Medicaid and the Uninsured (2004); Teitelbaum (1994).

53. Moyer, G. *Chartbook on Children's Insurance Status: Tabulations of the March 1998 Current Population Survey.* Washington, D.C.: Office of Health Policy, Office of the Assistant Secretary for Planning and Evaluation, 1998; Robert Wood Johnson Foundation. *Going Without: America's Uninsured Children.* Aug. 2005. Prepared for the Robert Wood Johnson Foundation by the State Health Access Data Assistance Center and the Urban Institute. Washington, D.C.: Robert Wood Johnson Foundation, Aug. 2005.

54. Robert Wood Johnson Foundation (2005).

55. Perloff, J., Kletke, P., and Neckerman, K. "Recent Trends in Pediatrician Participation in Medicaid." *Medical Care*, 1986, *24*, 749–760; Davidson, S., and others. "Full and Limited Medicaid Participation Among Pediatricians." *Pediatrics*, 1983, *72*, 552–559.

56. U.S. General Accounting Office (1993).

57. Carrasquillo, O., Himmelstein, D. U., Woolhandler, S., and Bor, D. H. "Can Medicaid Managed Care Provide Continuity of Care to New Medicaid Enrollees? An Analysis of Tenure on Medicaid." *American Journal of Public Health*, 1998, *88*, 464–466.

58. Fairbrother, G., and others. "Churning in Medicaid Managed Care and Its Effect on Accountability." *Journal of Health Care for the Poor and Underserved*, 2004, *15*, 30–41.

59. Halfon, N., and others. "Medicaid Enrollment and Health Services Access by Latino Children in Inner-City Los Angeles." *Journal of the American Medical Association*, 1997, *277*, 636–641; Flores, G., Abreu, M., Olivar, M. A., and Kastner, B. "Access Barriers to Health Care for Latino Children." *Archives of Pediatric and Adolescent Medicine*, 1998, *152*, 1119–1125.

60. Gavin, N., and others. "The Use of EPSDT and Other Health Care Services by Children Enrolled in Medicaid: The Impact of OBRA '89." *Milbank Quarterly*, 1998, *76*, 207.

61. Ellwood, M. "The Medicaid Eligibility Maze: Coverage Expands, But Enrollment Problems Persist." (Occasional paper no. 30.) Washington, D.C.: Urban Institute, 1999. [http:// newfederalism.urban.org/ pdf/occa30.pdf].

62. Avruch, Machlin, Bonin, and Ullman (1998).

63. Tang, S. S. *Children's Health Insurance Fact Sheet.* American Academy of Pediatrics. Elk Grove Village, Ill.: AAP, July 2005.

64. Davidoff, A. J., and others. *Children Eligible for Medicaid But Not Enrolled: How Great a Policy Concern?* (Series A, no. A-41.) Washington, D.C.: Urban Institute, Sept. 2000.

65. Weinick, R. M., Weigers, M. E., and Cohen, J. W. "Children's Health Insurance, Access to Care, and Health Status: New Findings." *Health Affairs*, 1998, *17*, 127–136; Thorpe, K. E., and Florence, C. S. "Covering Uninsured Children and Their Parents: Estimated Costs and Number of Newly Insured." *Medical Care, Research and Review*, 1999, *56*, 197–214.

66. Rosenbaum, S., and others. "The Children's Hour: The State Children's Health Insurance Program." *Health Affairs*, 1998, *17*, 75–89.

67. Sardell, A., and Johnson, K. "The Politics of EPSDT Policy in the 1990s: Policy Entrepreneurs, Political Streams, and Children's Health Benefits." *Milbank Quarterly*, 1998, *76*, 175–205.

68. Dubay, L., Kenney, G., and Haley, J. *Children's Participation in Medicaid and SCHIP: Early in the SCHIP Era.* (Series B, no. B-40.) Washington, D.C.: Urban Institute, Mar. 2002.

69. Kronebusch, K., and Elbel, B. "Simplifying Children's Medicaid and SCHIP." *Health Affairs*, 2004, *23*(3), 233–246.

70. Kronebusch and Elbel (2004).

71. Lieu, T. A., and others. "Risk Factors for Delayed Immunization Among Children in an HMO." *American Journal of Public Health*, 1994, *84*, 1621–1625.

72. Cooper, P. F., and Schone, B. S. "More Offers, Fewer Takers for Employment-Based Health Insurance: 1987 and 1996." *Health Affairs*, 1997, *16*, 142–149.

73. U.S. Department of Labor. "Employee Benefits in Medium and Large Establishments." Bulletin 2422. Washington, D.C.: Bureau of Labor Statistics, 1993.

74. Fox, H. B., and Newacheck, P. W. "Private Health Insurance Coverage of Chronically Ill Children." *Pediatrics*, 1990, *85*, 50–57.

75. Inkelas, M., Ahn, P., and Larson, K. *Experiences with Health Care for California's Children with Special Health Care Needs.* Los Angeles: UCLA Center for Healthier Children, Families, and Communities, 2004.

76. Valdez, R. *The Effects of Cost Sharing on the Health of Children.* (RAND publication no. R-3720-HHS.) Santa Monica, Calif.: RAND, 1986.

77. Valdez, R., and others. "Prepaid Group Practice Effects on the Utilization of Medical Services and Health Outcomes for Children: Results from a Controlled Trial." *Pediatrics*, 1989, *83*, 168–180.

78. Halfon, Inkelas, and Wood (1995).

79. Newacheck, P. W. "Characteristics of Children with High and Low Usage of Physician Services." *Medical Care*, 1992, *30*, 30–42; Wood, D. L., Corey, C., Freeman, H. E., and Shapiro, M. F. "Are Poor Families Satisfied with the Medical Care Their Children Receive?" *Pediatrics*, 1992, *90*, 66–70; Newacheck and Halfon (1986); Guendelman, S., and Schwalbe, J. "Medical Care Utilization by Hispanic Children: How Does It Differ from Black and White Peers?" *Medical Care*, 1986, *24*, 925–940; Wolfe, B. L. "Children's Utilization of Medical Care." *Medical Care*, 1980, *18*, 1196–1207; Dutton, D. B. "Explaining the Low Use of Health Services by the Poor: Costs, Attitudes, or Delivery Systems?" *American Sociological Review*, 1978, *43*, 348–368; Aday, L. A., and Andersen, R. M. "A Framework for the Study of Access to Medical Care." *Health Services Research*, 1974, *9*, 208–220.

80. Halfon, Inkelas, and Wood (1995); Newacheck (1992); Wood, Corey, Freeman, and Shapiro (1992); Dutton (1978).

81. Wood, Corey, Freeman, and Shapiro (1992); Riley, A. W., and others. "Determinants of Health Care Use: An Investigation of Psychosocial Factors." *Medical Care*, 1993, *31*, 767–783; Lieu, T. A., Newacheck, P. W., and McManus, M. A. "Race, Ethnicity, and Ac-

cess to Ambulatory Care Among U.S. Adolescents." *American Journal of Public Health*, 1994, *83*, 960–965.

82. Halfon and others (1997); Flores, Abreu, Olivar, and Kastner (1998); Holl, J. L., and others. "Profile of Uninsured Children in the United States." *Archives of Pediatric and Adolescent Medicine*, 1995, *149*, 398–406.

83. Olson, L. M., and others. "Overview of the Content of Health Supervision for Young Children: Reports from Parents and Pediatricians." *Pediatrics*, 2004, *113*(6), 1907–1916; Inkelas, Ahn, and Larson (2004).

84. Orr, S. T., Charney, E., and Straus, J. "Use of Health Services by Black Children According to Payment Mechanism." *Medical Care*, 1988, *26*, 939–947.

85. Rawlings, J. S., and Weir, M. R. "Race- and Rank-Specific Mortality in a U.S. Military Population." *American Journal of Diseases in Children*, 1992, *146*, 313–316; Margolis, P. A., and others. "The Rest of the Access-to-Care Puzzle." *Archives of Pediatric and Adolescent Medicine*, 1995, *149*, 541–545.

86. Starfield, B., and others. "Consumer Experiences and Provider Perceptions of the Quality of Primary Care: Implications for Managed Care." *Journal of Family Practice*, 1998, *46*, 216–226; Starfield, B. "Evaluating the State of Children's Health Insurance Program: Critical Considerations." *Annual Review of Public Health*, 2000, *21*, 569–585.

87. Halfon, Inkelas, and Wood (1995).

88. Kogan, M. D., and others. "The Effect of Gaps in Health Insurance on Continuity of a Regular Source of Care Among Preschool-Aged Children in the United States." *Journal of the American Medical Association*, 1995, *274*, 1429–1435; Halfon and others (1997); Rosenbach, M., Irvin, C., and Coulam, R. "Access for Low-Income Children: Is Health Insurance Enough?" *Pediatrics*, 1999, *103*, 1167–1174.

89. Starfield (2000).

90. Starfield, B., and Newacheck, P. W. "Children's Health Status, Health Risks, and Use of Health Services." In M. J. Schlesinger and L. Eisenberg (eds.), *Children in a Changing Health System*. Baltimore: Johns Hopkins University Press, 1990; Bearinger, L. H., Wildey, L., Gephart, J., and Blum, R. W. "Nursing Competence in Adolescent Health: Anticipating the Future Needs of Youth." *Journal of Professional Nursing*, 1992, *8*, 80–86; Blum, R. W., and Bearinger, L. H. "Knowledge and Attitudes of Health Professionals Toward Adolescent Health Care." *Journal of Adolescent Health Care*, 1990, *11*, 289–294.

91. Friedman, L. S., Johnson, B., and Brett, A. S. "Evaluation of Substance-Abusing Adolescents by Primary Care Physicians." *Journal of Adolescent Health Care*, 1990, *11*, 227–230; Singer, M. I., Petchers, M. K., and Anglin, J. M. "Detection of Adolescent Substance Abuse in a Pediatric Outpatient Department: A Double-Blind Study." *Journal of Pediatrics*, 1987, *111*, 938–941; Goldberg, I. D., Roghmann, K. J., McInerny, T. K., and Burke, J. D. "Mental Health Problems Among Children Seen in Pediatric Practice: Prevalence and Management." *Pediatrics*, 1984, *73*, 278–293.

92. Costello, E. J. "Primary Care Pediatrics, and Child Psychopathology: A Review of Diagnostic, Treatment, and Referral Practices." *Pediatrics*, 1986, *78*, 1044–1051.

93. Office of Technology Assessment. *Adolescent Health. Vol. III: Cross-Cutting Issues in the Delivery of Health and Health-Related Services*. (OTA-H-469.) Washington, D.C.: U.S. Government Printing Office, 1991; Singer, Petchers, and Anglin (1987); Kamerow, D., Pincus, H., and MacDonald, D. "Alcohol Abuse, Other Drug Abuse, and Mental Disorders in Medical Practice." *Journal of the American Medical Association*, 1986, *255*, 2054–2057.

94. Halfon, N., and others. "Developmental Assessments in the Pediatric Office." Pediatric Academic Societies' annual meeting, Baltimore, May 4-7, 2002.

95. Hughes, D., and Rosenbaum, S. "An Overview of Maternal and Child Health Services in Rural America." *Journal of Rural Health,* 1989, *5,* 299–319.

96. Dutton, D. "Children's Health Care 1981: The Myth of Equal Access." In *Better Health for Our Children. Vol. 4: Select Panel for the Promotion of Child Health.* (DHHS publication no. PHS 79–55071.) Washington, D.C.: Department of Health and Human Services, 1981.

97. Short and Lefkowitz (1992).

98. Halfon, N., Newacheck, P. W., Wood, D., and St. Peter, R. "Routine Emergency Room Use for Sick Care by U.S. Children." *Pediatrics,* 1995, *98,* 28–34.

99. Chang, R. K., and Halfon, N. "Geographic Distribution of Pediatricians in the United States: An Analysis of the Fifty States and Washington DC." *Pediatrics,* 1997, *100,* 172–179.

100. Kindig, D., and others. "Trends in Physician Availability in 10 Urban Areas from 1963 to 1980." *Inquiry,* 1987, *24,* 136–146.

101. Berman S, and others. "Factors That Influence the Willingness of Private Primary Care Pediatricians to Accept More Medicaid Patients." *Pediatrics,* 2002, *110*(2 Pt. 1), 239–248.

102. Orr, S. T., Charney, E., Straus, J., and Bloom, B. "Emergency Room Use by Low Income Children with a Regular Source of Health Care." *Medical Care,* 1991, *29,* 283–286; Kasper, J. D. "The Importance of Type of Usual Source of Care for Children's Physician Access and Expenditures." *Medical Care,* 1987, *25,* 386–398; and Halfon, Newacheck, Wood, and St. Peter (1995).

103. Butler, J. A., Winter, W. D., Singer, J. D., and Wenger, M. "Medical Care Use and Expenditures Among Children and Youth in the United States: An Analysis of a National Probability Sample." *Pediatrics,* 1985, *76,* 495–507.

104. Kasper (1987).

105. Schlesinger, M. "On the Limits of Expanding Health Care Reform: Chronic Care in Prepaid Settings." *Milbank Quarterly,* 1990, *64,* 189–215.

106. Halfon, N., and Hochstein, M. "Developing a System of Care for All: How the Needs of Vulnerable Children Inform the Debate." In R. K. Stein (ed.), *Health Care for Children: What's Right, What's Wrong, What's Next?* New York: United Hospital Fund of New York, 1997.

107. Rosenbaum, S., and Darnell, J. *Medicaid Section 1115 Demonstration Waivers: Approved and Proposed Activities as of November 1994.* Washington, D.C.: Center for Health Policy Research, George Washington University, 1994.

108. Perry, D. "Children's Health Insurance: Beyond Medicaid Coverage." *Health Policy and Child Health,* 1995, *2*(Supplement), 1–4.

109. Newacheck, P. W., Halfon, N., and Inkelas, M. "Monitoring Expanded Health Insurance for Children: Challenges and Opportunities." *Pediatrics,* 2000, *105,* 1004–1007.

110. Cooper and Schone (1997).

111. Halfon, Inkelas, and Hochstein (2000).

112. Halfon and Hochstein (1997); Barnett, W. S., and Escobar, C. M. "Economic Costs and Benefits of Early Intervention." In S. J. Meisels and J. P. Shonkoff (eds.), *Handbook of Early Childhood Intervention.* New York: Cambridge University Press, 1992; Olds, D. "Home Visitation for Pregnant Women and Parents of Young Children." *American Journal of the Diseases of Children,* 1992, *146,* 704–708.

113. Halfon and Hochstein (1997); Starfield (1992); Starfield and Newacheck (1990).

114. Wagner, J. L., Herdman, R. C., and Alberts, D. W. "Well-Child Care: How Much Is Enough?" *Health Affairs,* 1989, *8,* 147–157.

115. Olds, D., and others. "Effect of Prenatal and Infancy Nurse Home Visitation on Government Spending." *Medical Care,* 1993, *31,* 155–174; Olds, D., and others. "Long-Term Ef-

fects of Home Visitation on Maternal Life Course, Child Abuse and Neglect, and Children's Arrests: Fifteen Year Follow-up of a Randomized Trial." *Journal of the American Medical Association*, 1997, *278*, 637–643; Barnett and Escobar (1992); Berrueta-Clement, J. R., and others. *Changed Lives: The Effects of the Perry Preschool Program on Youths Through Age 19.* Ypsilanti, Mich.: High/Scope, 1984; and Karoly and others (1998).

116. Karoly and others (1998).

117. Halfon, Inkelas, and Hochstein (2000).

118. Starfield (1992).

119. Child Welfare League of America. *Standards for Health Care Services for Children in Out-of-Home Care.* Washington, D.C.: Child Welfare League of America, 1988.

120. Green, M. (ed.). *Bright Futures: National Guidelines for Health Supervision of Infants, Children, and Adolescents.* Arlington, Va.: National Center for Education in Maternal and Child Health, 1994.

121. Physician Payment Review Commission. *Annual Report to Congress—1995.* Washington, D.C.: Physician Payment Review Commission, 1995.

122. McGlynn, E. A., and Halfon, N. "Overview of Issues in Improving Quality of Care for Children." *Health Services Research*, 1998, *33*, 977–1000; McGlynn, Halfon, and Leibowitz (1995); Institute of Medicine. *Protecting and Improving Quality of Care for Children Under Health Care Reform: Workshop Highlights.* Washington, D.C.: Institute of Medicine, 1994.

123. U.S. General Accounting Office. *Preventive Care for Children in Selected Countries.* (GAO/HRD-93–62.) Washington, D.C.: U.S. Government Printing Office, 1993.

124. Wood, D., Saarlas, K. N., Inkelas, M., and Matyas, B. "Immunization Registries in the United States: Implications for the Practice of Public Health in a Changing Health Care System." *Annual Review of Public Health*, 1999, *20*, 231–255.

125. McGlynn and Halfon (1998).

126. Institute of Medicine (1994).

127. DuPlessis, H. M., Inkelas, M., and Halfon, N. "Assessing the Performance of Community Systems for Children." *Health Services Research*, 1998, *33*, 1111–1142.

128. DuPlessis, Inkelas, and Halfon (1998); Halfon, N., and others. *California Health Report.* (RAND publication DRU-1592-TCWF.) Santa Monica, Calif.: RAND, 2000.

129. Grason, H., and Guyer, B. *MCH Quality Systems Functions Framework.* Baltimore, Md.: Johns Hopkins School of Hygiene and Public Health, 1995.

130. Newacheck, Hughes, Brindis, and Halfon (1995).

131. Dutton (1981); Lion, J., and Altman, S. "Case-Mix Differences Between Hospital Outpatient Departments and Private Practice." *Health Care Financing Review*, 1982, *4*, 89–98; Fleming, N. S., and Jones, H. C. "Practice and Billing Patterns by Site of Care in a Medicaid Program." *Journal of Ambulatory Care Management*, 1985, *8*, 70–80; Halfon, N., and Newacheck, P. W. "Childhood Asthma and Poverty: Differential Impacts and Utilization of Health Services." *Pediatrics*, 1993, *91*, 56–61; St. Peter, R., Newacheck, P. W., and Halfon, N. "Access to Care for Poor Children: Separate and Unequal?" *Journal of the American Medical Association*, 1992, *267*, 2760–2764.

132. The Henry J. Kaiser Family Foundation. "Medicaid Managed Care Enrollees as a Percent of State Medicaid Enrollees, as of December 31, 2004." statehealthfacts.org (accessed Oct. 2, 2005).

133. Simpson, L., and Fraser, I. "Children and Managed Care: What Research Can, Can't, and Should Tell Us About Impact." *Medical Care, Research and Review*, 1999, *56*(Suppl. 2), 13–36; Claxton, G., Feder, J., Shactman, D., and Altman, S. "Public Policy Issues in Nonprofit Conversions: An Overview." *Health Affairs*, 1997, *16*, 9–28.

134. Hughes, D. C., and Luft, H. S. "Managed Care and Children: An Overview." *Future of Children*, 1998, *8*, 25–38; Szilagyi, P. G. "Managed Care for Children: Effect on Access to Care and Utilization of Health Services." *Future of Children*, 1998, *8*, 39–59.

135. Freund, D., and others. "Evaluation of the Medicaid Competition Demonstrations." *Health Care Financing Review*, 1989, *11*, 81–97.

136. Mauldon, J., and others. "Rationing or Rationalizing Children's Medical Care: Comparison of a Medicaid HMO with Fee-for-Service Care." *American Journal of Public Health*, 1994, *84*, 899–904.

137. Szilagyi, P. G., and Schor, E. L. "The Health of Children." *Health Services Research*, 1998, *33*, 1001–1039.

138. Horwitz, S. M., and Stein, R.E.K. "Health Maintenance Organizations vs. Indemnity Insurance for Children with Chronic Illness: Trading Gaps in Coverage." *American Journal of Diseases of Children*, 1990, *144*, 581–586.

139. Scholle, S. H., and others. "Changes in Medicaid Managed Care Enrollment Among Children." *Health Affairs*, 1997, *16*, 164–170; West, D. W., Stuart, M. E., Duggan, A. K., and DeAngelis, C. D. "Evidence for Selective Health Maintenance Organization Enrollment Among Children and Adolescents Covered by Medicaid." *Archives of Pediatric and Adolescent Medicine*, 1996, *150*, 503–507.

140. Cartland, J.D.C., and Yudkowsky, B. K. "Barriers to Pediatric Referral in Managed Care Systems." *Pediatrics*, 1992, *89*, 183–192.

141. Fox, H. B., Wicks, L. B., and Newacheck, P. W. "Health Maintenance Organizations and Children with Special Health Needs: A Suitable Match?" *American Journal of Diseases in Children*, 1993, *147*, 546–552.

142. Fox, H. B., and McManus, M. A. *Strategies to Enhance Preventive and Primary Care Services for High-Risk Children in Health Maintenance Organizations.* Washington, D.C.: Child and Adolescent Health Policy Center, 1995.

143. McGlynn and Halfon (1998).

144. Holahan, J., Rangarajan, S., and Schirmer. M. "Medicaid-Managed Care Payment Rates in 1998." *Health Affairs*, 1999, *18(3)*, 217–227.

145. Fox, H. B., and McManus, M. A. "Improving State Medicaid Contracts and Plan Practices for Children with Special Health Needs." *Future of Children*, 1998, *8*, 105–118.

146. Szilagyi (1998).

147. Ireys, H. "Children with Special Health Care Needs: Evaluating Their Needs and Relevant Service Structures." (Background paper for Institute of Medicine.) Baltimore: Johns Hopkins University, 1994; Simpson and Fraser (1999).

148. Thompson, J. W., and others. "Quality of Care for Children in Commercial and Medicaid Managed Care." *Journal of the American Medical Association*, 2003, *290*(11), 1486–1493.

149. Halfon and Berkowitz (1993).

150. Newacheck, Hughes, Halfon, and Brindis (1997).

151. Leutz, W. N., Greenlick, M. R., and Capitman, J. A. "Integrating Acute and Long-Term Care." *Health Affairs*, 1994, *13*, 58–74.

152. Halfon, Inkelas, and Hochstein (2000).

153. Robinson, J. C. "The Future of Managed Care Organization." *Health Affairs*, 1999, *18*, 7–24.

154. Halfon, Inkelas, and Hochstein (2000).

155. Williams, B. C., and Miller, C. A. "Preventive Health Care for Children: Findings from a 10-Country Study and Directions for United States Policy." *Pediatrics*, 1992, *89*(Suppl.), 983–998; Kahn and Kamerman (1992).

CHAPTER SIXTEEN

# MENTAL HEALTH SERVICES AND POLICY ISSUES

Susan L. Ettner
Janet C. Link

Mental disorders are both common and costly to society. In a given year, about 30.5 percent of the adult U.S. population suffer from a mental disorder, with about 6.3 percent suffering from a serious disorder.[1] The direct costs of treatment for mental disorders are substantial. In 2001, the costs associated with treating mental disorders other than dementia and mental retardation were estimated to be $85 billion, or 6.2 percent of total health care costs.[2]

Furthermore, mental illness is often accompanied by drug and alcohol abuse. In any year, 15 percent of adults with mental illness have comorbid substance disorders.[3] Among those with severe mental illness, the lifetime prevalence of co-occurring substance abuse disorders reaches 50 percent.[4] In 2001, the total cost of treating substance abuse added $18.3 million to the costs associated with treating mental health disorders.[5]

In addition to the direct treatment costs of mental health and substance abuse (MH/SA) disorders, indirect costs to individuals, employers, and society are enormous. The Global Burden of Disease Study found that neuropsychiatric conditions account for 24 percent of all disability-adjusted life-years in the Americas.[6] Although mental illness is not associated with a high mortality rate, it often has its onset in early adulthood, affecting what would normally be the most productive working years. Mental illness reduces work productivity and the employment rate[7] and increases absenteeism.[8] Other social costs associated with mental health and substance disorders are violence,[9] homelessness,[10] child abuse,[11] motor vehicle accidents,[12] teenage pregnancy,[13] incarceration,[14] and marital instability.[15]

Pharmacological advances in treating mental illness began in the 1950s and continue improving our ability to care for these disorders in an effective as well as cost-effective manner.[16] Yet despite the large costs that untreated mental illness imposes on society and the great advances in treatment made so far, use of mental health services is poorly matched to need. Although discrepancies depend on how one defines need,[17] one possibility is to examine the percentage of those who receive services in terms of the severity of their disorder (Table 16.1). Even though only 40.5 percent of adult Americans with a serious mental health or substance abuse disorder receive any treatment for these conditions, 14.5 percent of adults without a diagnosable disorder receive some form of behavioral health care.[18]

Some of the barriers to mental health care are stigma, geographic inaccessibility of providers, financial constraints because of inadequate insurance coverage, and the failure of health care providers to identify the mental health needs of their patients.[19]

In addition to the substantial access barriers facing the patients who are in greatest need of treatment, substandard quality of care and inappropriate treatment have been long-standing concerns in the mental health sector, dating from the inhumane treatment of the mentally ill in the "lunatic asylums" of the 1700s and 1800s[20] and continuing into the present, with revelations regarding excessive use of restraints and seclusion within some psychiatric facilities.[21] In outpatient settings, one study reported that only 30 percent of individuals with a depressive or anxiety disorder receive appropriate treatment.[22] Another study reported that among individuals with serious mental illness, only 15 percent receive minimally adequate treatment.[23]

## TABLE 16.1. MISMATCH BETWEEN USE AND NEED FOR MENTAL HEALTH SERVICES.

|  | Percentage of U.S. Population with Diagnosis | Percentage with Diagnosis Who Received Mental Health (MH) Treatment |
|---|---|---|
| Serious MH disorder | 6.3 | 40.5 |
| Moderate MH disorder | 13.5 | 37.2 |
| Mild MH disorder | 10.8 | 23.0 |
| None | 69.5 | 14.5 |

*Source:* Kessler, R., and others. "Prevalence and Treatment of Mental Disorders, 1990 to 2003." *New England Journal of Medicine,* 2005, *352*(24), 2515–2523.

These access and quality issues suggest the need for a fundamental rethinking of our current mental health policy. This chapter first presents an overview of the nature and treatment of mental illness in the United States. Next, it summarizes the historical development of the financing and delivery of mental health services. It then explains some of the ways in which mental health care differs from health care in general, suggesting the need for separate consideration of mental health services in the policy debate. Areas of concern for special populations are then described. The chapter concludes with a discussion of a few of the important issues facing mental health policy makers.

# Overview of Mental Illness and the Mental Health Services System

Who are the "mentally ill"?

The surgeon general's report on mental health[24] defines mental disorders as "conditions characterized by alterations in thinking, mood or behavior associated with distress and/or impaired functioning." Common manifestations of mental disorders are anxiety, which is characterized by feelings of fear and dread; psychosis, including hallucinations and delusions; mood disturbances, such as prolonged periods of extreme sadness or euphoria; and cognitive impairment, or the inability to organize, process, and recall information.[25] Table 16.2 presents the annual and lifetime prevalence of some of the most prevalent or disabling mental health disorders among adults.[26]

Distinctions are drawn among (1) mental health problems below the threshold for a standard diagnosis, (2) all diagnosable mental illnesses, (3) serious mental illness (SMI), and (4) severe and persistent mental illness (SPMI). Standard diagnoses are based on criteria outlined in the *Diagnostic and Statistical Manual of Mental Disorders* (DSM), published by the American Psychiatric Association. Serious mental illnesses are those interfering with social functioning; severe and persistent mental illnesses are chronic in addition to being serious. Examples of SPMI are schizophrenia, bipolar disorder, certain types of major depression, panic disorder, and obsessive-compulsive disorder.[27] Whereas 23.9 percent of adults suffer from a mental disorder in a given year, about 5.4 percent of adults suffer from SMI and 2.6 percent of adults suffer from SPMI (Figure 16.1).[28] People with persistent and serious mental disorders face the greatest challenges in attempting to live normal lives and are frequently the focus of mental health policy initiatives.

Because of our poor understanding of the etiology of mental disorders, interventions to prevent mental illness are less well developed than in other areas of medicine. Those prevention programs that exist in mental health have traditionally

## TABLE 16.2. PREVALENCE OF MENTAL HEALTH AND SUBSTANCE ABUSE DISORDERS.

|  | 12-Month Prevalence (Percentage) | Lifetime Prevalence (Percentage |
|---|---|---|
| Mood disorders | 11.3 | 19.3 |
|    Major depression | 10.3 | 17.1 |
|    Mania | 1.3 | 1.6 |
|    Dysthymia | 2.5 | 6.4 |
| Anxiety disorders | 19.3 | 28.7 |
|    Generalized anxiety disorder | 3.1 | 5.1 |
|    Panic disorder | 2.3 | 3.5 |
|    Social phobia | 7.9 | 13.3 |
|    Posttraumatic stress disorder | 3.9 | 7.6 |
| Nonaffective psychosis | 0.3 | 0.5 |
| Substance abuse or dependence | 11.3 | 26.6 |
| Any mental health or substance abuse disorder | 30.9 | 49.7 |

*Source:* Kessler, R., and others. "The Epidemiology of Adult Mental Disorders." In B. L. Levin, J. Petrila, and K. D. Henessy (eds.), *Mental Health Services: A Public Health Perspective.* New York: Oxford University Press, 2004.

## FIGURE 16.1. ESTIMATED TWELVE-MONTH PREVALENCE OF MENTAL HEALTH DISORDERS, SERIOUS MENTAL ILLNESS, AND SEVERE AND PERSISTENT MENTAL ILLNESS.

**Overview of mental health treatment**

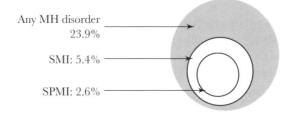

Any MH disorder 23.9%

SMI: 5.4%

SPMI: 2.6%

*Source:* Kessler, R., and others. "The 12-Month Prevalence and Correlates of Serious Mental Illness (SMI)." In R. W. Manderscheid and M. A. Sonnenschein (eds.), *Mental Health, United States, 1996.* Center for Mental Health Services. (DHHS pub. no. SMA96-3098.) Washington, D.C.: Superintendent of Documents, U.S. Government Printing Office, 1996.

focused on children. Thus, mental health services for adults consist primarily of treatment of existing disorders, both active treatment and custodial care. Active treatment of mental illness falls primarily into two categories: psychosocial interventions (employing various forms of psychotherapy) and pharmacotherapy (use of psychotropic drugs). Less frequently, electroconvulsive therapy is used. In addition, persons with SPMI often require a range of supportive services: income support, assisted housing, family intervention, vocational rehabilitation, and others.

Financing and delivery of mental health services is exceptionally fragmented. Financing sources include private, state, and federal funding streams from multiple sectors such as health, social welfare, housing, criminal justice, and education.[29] In addition to the financial complexities, mental health care is delivered in multiple settings, among them physicians' offices, general hospitals, specialty hospitals, mental health clinics, nursing homes, and other residential programs. Given the fragmentation of the delivery system and the diverse needs of people with severe and chronic mental disorders, case management services are often necessary to ensure that these patients receive the full range of services required for them to lead a relatively normal life.

## Financing and Delivery of Mental Health Services: 1800s to 1980s

To better understand many of the inadequacies and barriers to treatment in the current mental health system, it is helpful to understand its development since the 1800s. Much of the fragmentation of the current system results from financing and delivery mechanisms that developed over time without coordination. This section describes the rise and peak of state mental hospitals, the period of deinstitutionalization, the growth of insurance for mental health care, and the emergence of behavioral mental health care in the 1980s.

Mental hospitals began to appear as urbanization flourished in the early nineteenth century. Whereas prior to urbanization, individuals were predominantly cared for by their family, those with severe mental illness living in more densely populated areas were now perceived as a threat to their community and sent away to isolated asylums.[30] Throughout most of the nineteenth century, financial responsibility for mental hospitals was divided between state legislatures and local governments. State legislatures were generally responsible for financing construction and renovation of the facilities; local governments were responsible for reimbursing hospitals for the cost of care of each patient.[31] This system of divided responsibilities created perverse incentives, as hospitals faced pressure from local communities to discharge patients in a timely fashion to save money.[32]

In an effort to improve the quality of care for these patients, states began to assume all financial responsibility for mental hospitals starting in the late 1800s. This shift in funding, however, created new incentives that changed the patient case mix of the hospitals. Local communities recognized an unprecedented opportunity to shift the financial burden of senile, elderly individuals and others with long-term care needs from local almshouses to the state mental hospitals.[33] Between 1880 and 1920, the population in almshouses substantially declined, while the number of individuals in mental hospitals with long-term care needs grew dramatically. Consequently, the care provided in mental hospitals became much more custodial in nature. This shift in patient case-mix subsequently changed the link between psychiatrists and state mental hospitals, as many psychiatrists were interested in providing therapeutic treatments more than custodial care. Thus, throughout the early 1900s, more psychiatrists began seeking employment outside of mental hospitals.[34]

During the 1940s, there were two important events that further influenced the delivery and financing of mental health services: World War II and the passage of the National Mental Health Act (NMHA) in 1946. The treatment of military personnel suffering from combat-related mental illnesses led some psychiatrists to emphasize the social dimensions of mental disorders. Military psychiatrists also found that early treatment in a noninstitutional setting could produce good outcomes.[35] Additionally, passage of the NMHA gave the federal government a role in funding research, training, and development of new mental health programs.[36] The NMHA led to establishment of the National Institute of Mental Health in 1949.[37]

By the 1950s, mental health services were generally provided in two separate settings: isolated custodial asylums and outpatient settings. Those with severe mental illness who could not be safely cared for on their own or by family continued to be treated in custodial asylums, in which very few psychiatrists worked.[38] The size of public mental hospitals reached a peak in 1955, with a resident census of 558,922.[39] Outpatient care, on the other hand, was generally supplied by psychiatrists to affluent patients who were culturally attracted to therapy.[40]

During the late 1950s and 1960s, several important factors converged to give birth to the "deinstitutionalization" period. The emphasis in psychiatry on socio-environmental factors and life experience as causes of mental illness, the popular belief that early intervention in the community could prevent later hospitalization, allegations of abuse and neglect within state psychiatric hospitals, the consumer advocacy movement, and development of new antipsychotic drugs all contributed to the push to move individuals from state hospitals into the community.[41]

In 1963, the Community Mental Health Center (CMHC) Act expanded the role of the federal government in financing mental health services by furnishing grants to states to construct outpatient mental health clinics. Although CMHCs were supposed to help ease the transition of individuals from state hospitals to the community during this period of deinstitutionalization, many failed to live up to this promise.[42] Many of the new outpatient facilities were used by patients with less severe emotional and personal problems who had never previously accessed the mental health system. Moreover, little effort was made to coordinate aftercare services to individuals with SPMI who had been discharged from state hospitals.[43] Financial support from the federal government under the CMHC Act was converted to a block grant for states in 1981 and became a smaller portion of state mental health funds.[44] As of 2002, the federal mental health block grant constituted only 1.5 percent of revenue for state mental health agencies.[45]

Even though the CMHC act did not live up to its promise of facilitating deinstitutionalization, the passage of other federal programs assisted with this transition. Three of the most important programs were Medicaid, Social Security Disability Insurance (SSDI), and Supplemental Security Income (SSI). The passage of Medicaid in 1965 constituted an important source of insurance for many of those with SMI and SPMI. Because individuals discharged from state hospitals were likely to be unemployed and uninsured, Medicaid often financed their outpatient psychiatric treatment. Medicaid also enabled states to shift the care of the elderly with mental health problems from state hospitals to long-term care nursing facilities.[46] Inclusion of persons with mental disability in the SSI and SSDI programs further supported deinstitutionalization, on the assumption that these federal payments would lend enough financial support for those previously hospitalized.[47] Other programs such as public housing and food stamps offered additional resources to this population. Although the availability of resources through local, state, and federal programs enabled many individuals with mental disability to successfully transition into the community, a sizeable number fell through the cracks of the disjointed system, especially those with co-occurring mental health and substance abuse disorders. Increased homelessness and incarceration of those with SPMI are two of the most devastating consequences of an inadequate safety net for this population.[48]

In the 1980s, additional changes in the mental health services system began to emerge and define many of the important policy issues that still exist today. Private MH/SA insurance expanded, but employers and insurers controlled their liability by applying greater limitations for MH/SA services than for general medical services.[49] Managed behavioral health care emerged in the private sector in response to escalating costs, overuse of inpatient hospitalization, and a variable treatment environment characterized by poorly defined standards of care.[50] Enrollment in MBHOs continued to climb as employers and public systems were pressured to curb the growth in mental health and substance abuse treatment expenditures.[51]

## Financing and Delivery of Mental Health Services: 1990s to Present

The U.S. Congress declared the 1990s to be the "decade of the brain," because of the improved biological understanding of mental illness through advances in neuroscience, behavioral science, and genetics.[52] Following introduction of the first antidepressant in the class known as selective serotonin reuptake inhibitors (SSRIs)—fluoxetine (Prozac)—into the market in 1987, a wave of new-generation "blockbuster" psychotropic medications soon followed in the 1990s. New antidepressant and antipsychotic drugs with better tolerated side effects enabled treatment of many mental health disorders to become more feasible in an outpatient setting and more accessible to those who would have been unable to tolerate the side effects of the older-generation medications. For example, between 1987 and 1997 the number of people treated in an outpatient setting for depression increased more than 300 percent, and the percentage of individuals with depression who used antidepressants rose from 37 percent to 75 percent.[53] As a result of the greater role of psychotropic drugs and the diminishing prominence of institutionalized care, prescription drugs went from accounting for 7 percent of total expenditures in 1991 to 21 percent in 2001 (Figure 16.2), while spending on specialty hospitals decreased from 23 percent to 11 percent of total expenditures during this same time period.[54]

Inpatient care decreased from 38 percent of mental health expenditures in 1991 to 22 percent in 2001, while outpatient care grew from 38 to 52 percent over this time period (Table 16.3).[55] Mental health expenditures in residential settings, including nursing homes and other programs, remained constant at 19 percent.

### FIGURE 16.2. DISTRIBUTION OF MENTAL HEALTH PAYMENTS BY TYPE OF PROVIDER.

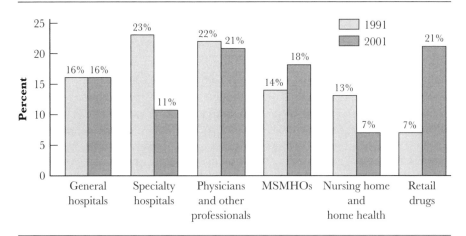

*Note:* * MSMHO = Multiservice mental health organization.

*Source:* Mark, T., and others. *National Expenditures for Mental Health and Substance Abuse Treatment, 1991-2001.* Rockville, Md.: U.S. Department of Health and Human Services, Substance Abuse and Mental Health Services Administration, 2005.

### TABLE 16.3. MENTAL HEALTH EXPENDITURES
### BY LOCATION OF SERVICE.

| | Year (Percentage) | |
|---|:---:|:---:|
| | 1991 | 2001 |
| Inpatient | 38 | 22 |
| Outpatient | 38 | 52 |
| Residential | 19 | 19 |
| Insurance administration | 5 | 6 |

*Source:* Mark, T., and others. "U.S. Spending for Mental Health and Substance Abuse Treatment, 1991–2001." *Health Affairs,* Web exclusive, Mar. 29, 2005, W5-133-W5-142. Published by Project HOPE. [http://www.projecthope.org].

The reduction in overall use of inpatient services was concomitant with shifts in the setting of inpatient care. Prior to the 1970s, most inpatient mental health care was offered within psychiatric hospitals directly owned and operated by the states. Starting in the 1970s, there was a strong move from state psychiatric hospitals into other settings—general hospitals, private psychiatric hospitals, and psychiatric units within general hospitals—which grew from 664 to 1,516 between 1970 and 1992.[56] This move was fueled in part by the closing of public facilities in many parts of the country on account of state budget deficits, deteriorating physical facilities, and the perception that direct public provision of services was less efficient than contracting with private parties to provide the services (known as the make-versus-buy debate). Between 1972 and 2000, the number of state and county psychiatric beds dropped precipitously, from 361,765 to 54,000.[57] More state psychiatric hospitals were closed in the 1990s than in the 1970s and 1980s combined, although the rate of public psychiatric hospital closures is slowing in the current decade.[58]

An important trend in the financing of mental health services since the early 1990s has been the change in distribution of mental health expenditures by payer (Table 16.4).

Between 1991 and 2001, the role of the public sector expanded, while the role of the private sector shrank. Medicaid accounted for 19 percent of all mental health expenditures in 1991, but it surpassed all other sources of funding by 2001, making up 27 percent of expenditures. In contrast, other state and local spending decreased from 27 to 23 percent of expenditures. Both Medicare and other federal spending—Veterans Affairs, Department of Defense, federal block grants—accounted for a constant percentage of expenditures between 1991 and

### TABLE 16.4. MENTAL HEALTH EXPENDITURES BY PAYER.

|  | 1991 (Percentage) | 2001 (Percentage) |
|---|---|---|
| Public sector | 57 | 63 |
| Medicare | 7 | 7 |
| Medicaid | 19 | 27 |
| Other federal spending | 5 | 5 |
| Other state and local spending | 27 | 23 |
| Private sector | 43 | 37 |
| Private insurance | 22 | 22 |
| Out-of-pocket | 15 | 13 |
| Other private funds | 6 | 3 |

*Source:* Mark and others (2005), pp. W5-133-W5-142.

2001, at 7 percent and 5 percent respectively.[59] Private insurance accounted for only 22 percent of mental health expenditures in 1991 and 2001. Thus in contrast to the medical care sector, where the main focus of policy for working-age adults and their families is the private insurance market, mental health policy is often centered on governmental actions.

It is important to note that many individuals in need of mental health services seek help outside of the formal health care sector. Regier and others[60] coined the term "the de facto mental health system" to describe delivery of mental health services in four sectors: the mental health specialty sector, the general medical sector, the human services sector, and the voluntary support sector. The human services sector comprises social welfare programs and services located within correctional institutions, schools, and religious settings. The voluntary support network sector includes self-help groups and other consumer organizations.[61] Informal caregivers also play an important role in the care of the mentally ill.[62]

## Health Care Policy: Is Mental Health Different?

Although many of the policy questions around delivering and financing mental health services mirror those for medical care, mental health is characterized by certain features that set it apart from medical care and have implications for attempting to subsume mental health into broader health care policies. This section summarizes what is different about mental health care.

## Stigma

Although stigma does not usually pose a problem of access for treating a medical condition, it is a substantial barrier to seeking care for mental health problems,[63] particularly in the specialty sector.[64] Historically, a disorder with no known etiology was treated as a mental health problem and stigmatized.[65] Despite the public's increasing understanding of the nature of mental illness, fear, avoidance, and discrimination are still common reactions to people with mental illness.[66] For this reason, the surgeon general's report and the President's New Freedom Commission on Mental Health report identified overcoming stigma as one of the most important steps to improving mental health treatment in the United States.[67] With the development of more effective psychotropic medications having fewer side effects,[68] psychiatry is becoming increasingly medicalized. The shift toward a medical model for treatment of psychiatric disorders may eventually lessen stigma, though at the possible cost of reducing support for psychosocial interventions.

## High Rate of Treatment in the General Medical Sector

Patients with psychiatric disorders often seek care for their condition in the primary care sector instead of the mental health specialty sector. A comparison of data from the National Comorbidity Survey (NCS), conducted between 1990 and 1992, and the NCS Replication Study (NCS-R), conducted between 2001 and 2003, shows an increase in the overall frequency of mental health treatment during the year prior to the interview, from 12.2 percent to 20.1 percent of adults aged eighteen to fifty-four years.[69] Yet even in 2003, only 32.9 percent of those with a diagnosable psychiatric disorder received any treatment.[70] Even among patients with the most serious disorders, very few received any mental health specialty care: only 14.4 percent received services in the psychiatric sector and 19.4 percent in the sector for other mental health services (for instance, psychologists). In contrast, 22.1 percent received some form of mental health care in the general medical sector.[71]

The degree to which primary care providers and other generalists can effectively substitute for mental health specialists in treating psychiatric disorders is controversial.[72] Mental health treatment furnished by generalists tends to focus on psychotropic drug prescriptions, with about two-thirds of such drugs prescribed by primary care providers and medical specialists other than psychiatrists.[73] Evidence is mixed on the relative efficacy of primary versus specialty care for management of psychotropic medication, with one study showing primary care to be of equivalent efficacy[74] and others of lower[75] efficacy. Episodes of mental health treatment in the general medical sector tend to be shorter and less costly than episodes involving mental health specialty care.[76] Mental health specialists may, however, offer more appropriate care.[77] For example, one study reported that among those with a probable depressive or anxiety disorder, only 19 percent of those who saw primary care providers received appropriate care. Among those who saw a mental health specialist, however, 90 percent received appropriate care.[78] A review of generalist versus specialty care of depression and a range of other disorders concluded that specialty care was superior.[79]

Even though the issue of substitution between generalists and specialists arises in other areas of medicine as well, mental health services may be particularly prone to delivery through the general medical sector, because of three factors. The first is the stigma associated with visiting a mental health specialty provider such as a psychiatrist. The second is that insurance benefits are often structured in such a way as to favor providing mental health services as part of a primary care visit.[80] The third is the geographic maldistribution[81] and inadequate supply of mental health specialists in many parts of the United States.[82] Distance and provider supply have been shown to influence mental health services utilization and the choice between specialist and generalist care.[83]

## Role of State and Local Governments in Financing and Delivery

The public sector has always played a larger role in delivering and financing mental health services than it has for medical care. Although the closing or downsizing of state mental hospitals became commonplace in the 1990s, public hospitals continue to play a critical role in delivering mental health care. Only about 26 percent of non-federal general hospitals in the United States are run by state and local government,[84] but about 36 percent of psychiatric hospitals are public.[85] Currently 217 state psychiatric hospitals remain open, accounting for about one-third of state mental health budgets.[86]

In 2001, public funding accounted for 63 percent of all mental health spending, but only 45 percent of all health care spending.[87] The differences between sources of financing are particularly pronounced for direct state and local funding, accounting for 23 percent of all mental health expenditures versus 7 percent of general health expenditures in 2001.[88] As is typical for programs implemented at the state level, there is wide variation in mental health agency expenditures per capita, ranging from $398 in the District of Columbia to $26 in West Virginia in 2001.[89] Public financing of mental health services has been argued to be partly a response to the external costs imposed on society by mental illness and addictive disorders, including unemployment, crime, violence, and homelessness.[90] The availability of publicly funded services may, however, amount to a disincentive for employers to offer behavioral health care benefits to workers.[91] Furthermore, the heavy reliance of mental health services on state and local funding makes those services vulnerable to severe budget cuts whenever the state economy is doing poorly.

## Lack of Parity: Private Insurance Coverage

Private insurance coverage for mental health and substance abuse treatment tends to be much less generous than for medical care. Most employers restrict coverage of behavioral health care to a greater degree than coverage of medical care.[92] Although the disparity may be declining over time,[93] as recently as 2002 5 percent of small firms and 1 percent of large firms did not offer any mental health benefits, despite offering medical coverage to their employees.[94] Employers routinely impose higher cost-sharing requirements and institute other restrictions that do not apply to medical care, such as limiting the number of outpatient visits (typically twenty) or inpatient days (usually thirty). One implication of differential coverage is that an employee who develops breast cancer can get most of her treatment reimbursed, while a comparable employee with onset of bipolar disorder (another chronic, costly, and partially heritable disorder) cannot.

Differential coverage may be due in part simply to stigma or discrimination, but there are economic explanations for the phenomenon as well, including the safety-net coverage offered by the public sector, "moral hazard," and adverse selection.[95] The demand response to enhanced insurance coverage, known as moral hazard, has been shown to be substantially larger for mental health services than medical care under fee-for-service systems.[96] The RAND Health Insurance Experiment, a randomized study of the effect of insurance on health care costs conducted in the premanaged care era, found that mental health care was about 50 percent more responsive to patient cost sharing than medical care spending was.[97] The greater responsiveness of mental health service utilization to subsidies may reflect greater uncertainty about the value of these services. It may also reflect the desirability of certain types of behavioral health care among populations with less acute need for such services. As one example, most people will not choose to undergo cardiac surgery in the absence of clear-cut indications for such treatment, even if it is fully covered by their insurance. In contrast, free psychotherapy might well prove highly attractive to many well-educated, psychologically minded individuals with no diagnosable psychiatric disorder. Anecdotal evidence about the popularity of Prozac and other SSRIs among people without a standard diagnosis of a depressive disorder suggests that in the absence of direct controls (utilization review, or "gatekeeping") more generous coverage of behavioral health care could lead to increased use among a wider population than was originally intended.

In addition to moral hazard, insurers may be reluctant to offer generous mental health and substance abuse benefits because of the potential for adverse selection. Individuals suffering from mental illness have been shown to have higher medical as well as behavioral health care costs.[98] Moreover, the chronic nature of many mental disorders suggests that there is greater potential for a patient to self-select into the insurance plans offering the best behavioral health care benefits. In contrast, patients and insurers cannot predict very well which patients will experience acute medical conditions during the next year, eliminating the potential both for those patients to self-select into generous insurance plans and for insurers to avoid enrolling them. Plans seeking to avoid enrolling a disproportionate number of patients with behavioral health care needs often engage in a rush to the bottom, resulting in minimal coverage of these services.

One proposed remedy is to mandate benefits, which would allow insurers to offer coverage without fear of attracting all of the costly patients. Mandated benefits cannot, however, prevent all forms of cream skimming and dumping. For example, managed care organizations (MCOs) may try to discourage patients with mental illness from enrolling by purposely trying not to develop a reputation for providing high-quality behavioral health care, by engaging in strict utilization review that effectively limits covered benefits, or by limiting provider networks so that a long waiting period for a mental health specialty visit effectively rations care.

## Lack of Parity: Medicare and Medicaid Coverage for Beneficiaries

Differential coverage of mental health and medical care can be seen not only with private insurance but with publicly funded programs as well. Medicare and Medicaid insurance are particularly important sources of insurance coverage for those with serious and persistent mental illness, since their capacity for gainful employment is impaired. Although they are less likely to be covered by employer-based insurance, they often qualify for disability-related income support and health insurance benefits through SSI or SSDI. These programs play a large role in covering those with physical disability as well. However, mental illnesses such as schizophrenia and bipolar disorder have earlier onset than many medical disorders, leading to a high proportion of disability related to mental illness. For example, about 22 percent of disabled Medicare beneficiaries qualify on the basis of psychiatric impairment.[99] Thus it is important to understand the limitations of public insurance coverage of mental health services relative to medical care.

Although the Omnibus Budget Reconciliation Act of 1989 removed the last of Medicare's payment limits for outpatient mental health care, Medicare continues to impose a 50 percent co-payment rate for outpatient mental health services other than initial diagnostic services and psychotropic drug management, in contrast to the usual 20 percent co-insurance rate for medical care. Moreover, in an effort to prevent states from shifting the cost of psychiatric hospital care onto the federal government,[100] Medicare limits lifetime coverage of psychiatric hospital care to 190 days, although no such restrictions are placed on general hospital days, including a stay in a specialty psychiatric unit within a general hospital.

Prior to the passage of the Medicare Prescription Drug, Improvement, and Modernization Act (PL 108-173) in 2003, Medicare's failure to cover outpatient prescription drugs had a serious impact on the out-of-pocket costs for those with mental illness. Beginning in January 2006, however, Medicare pays a portion of the cost of outpatient prescription drugs through private plans. This new coverage will likely be beneficial for Medicare enrollees who have mental disorders, because drug therapy is often a critical component of treatment. The new Medicare drug benefit has limitations, however, that may continue to pose financial barriers to some individuals in need of drug therapy (see Chapter Twenty, on Medicare reform, for details).

Medicaid offers more comprehensive coverage of outpatient mental health care than Medicare and pays for most prescription drugs. Its coverage of psychiatric inpatient facilities is less generous, perhaps because of the desire to avoid having federal funds replace direct state and local funding. The federal government prohibits state Medicaid programs from covering care provided to adults from age twenty-two to sixty-four within "institutions for mental disease," or IMDs (psychiatric hospitals and nursing homes specializing in psychiatric services). Although an exception to this exclusion occurs for the elderly because Medicaid is the secondary payer after Medicare, the exception is not always granted for children.

Differential coverage of mental health and medical care, or psychiatric and general hospital stays, puts beneficiaries at risk for high out-of-pocket costs and also distorts incentives. As one example, the IMD exclusion amounts to an incentive for states to treat Medicaid beneficiaries in need of inpatient mental health services in general medical wards, rather than psychiatric hospital settings. It has also been cited as one reason for the reluctance of nursing homes to diagnose and treat mental disorders among patients, for fear of meeting the IMD definition and losing Medicaid funding.[101]

## Managed Behavioral Health Care

Managed behavioral health organizations (MBHOs), also known as behavioral health care carve-outs, are essentially specialized managed care organizations that cover only mental health services (and typically substance abuse services as well). MBHOs dominate the market for private mental health coverage, with 169 million enrollees in 2000, up from 70 million in 1993.[102] Medicaid and state mental health agencies also make frequent use of MBHOs by contracting out behavioral health care. The carve-out system could also become a model for Medicare in the future. Although managed care is common in medicine, with the exception of pharmaceutical benefits management companies it is rare for a particular class of health services to be managed separately from the patient's other health care. Furthermore, it is not uncommon for employers to provide medical care coverage on a fee-for-service basis while contracting with a carve-out vendor to manage behavioral health care utilization.

Carve-out vendors are sometimes, but not always, at risk for service use of the enrollees. In risk-based carve-outs, the vendor receives a capitated payment and is at full or partial risk for the actual costs of the patient population. Almost half of individuals covered by carve-outs are enrolled in risk-based programs.[103] In administrative services only (ASO) contracts, the purchaser pays the carve-out vendor a fee to manage the care of the patient population. The vendor is not at risk for use by the patients per se; however, the amount of the administrative payment can be specified to depend on the vendor's performance, so the vendor receives a reduced fee in the event that behavioral health care costs are not sufficiently contained. In either case, the vendor has a financial incentive to reduce costs. Furthermore, given the volatility of the market for behavioral health care carve-outs, the desire to develop a reputation for effectively managing care is arguably another important incentive for vendors to contain costs.[104]

## Treatment Variability

It has been argued that there is less consensus about the effectiveness of treatment in psychiatry than in other fields of medicine.[105] As a result of this uncertainty, treatment variability may be greater in mental health than medical care.[106] Importantly, the uncertainty about treatment effectiveness and the variability in treatment implementation probably contributes to the reluctance of insurers to cover mental health services and the failure of patients to obtain appropriate care.

## Information Deficits

Poor consumer information may have even greater implications for quality of care among patients with psychiatric disorders than it does for patients with medical conditions. The classic economic theory of markets is predicated on the assumption that consumers make rational choices on the basis of perfect information. If so, market forces should prevent health care providers from offering suboptimal quality, since patients would avoid these providers and eventually drive them out of the market. Yet health care markets are more often than not characterized by imperfect information; even well-educated patients frequently know little about their condition, possible courses of treatment for it, and the quality of care being given.

The assumption of perfect consumer information is particularly difficult to justify when the patients involved have psychiatric disorders. Many people suffer from cognitive and perceptual deficits that hinder their ability to compare the quality of competing health care providers and make rational market choices. Moreover, patients with psychiatric disorders are less likely to be married or have close family ties, thus lacking support from family members who might act as their advocate in choosing a health care provider. Market failures due to imperfect information are therefore likely to be exacerbated among patients with psychiatric disorders. Furthermore, the patient in greatest need of services—one with a severely disabling disorder such as schizophrenia—is precisely the one most likely to suffer impaired judgment.

# Special Populations

Poor access to mental health care is a problem for many Americans, and to some extent the reasons for inadequate treatment cut across demographic groups. However, certain issues are of particular concern for populations such as the elderly, children, minority group members, and residents of rural areas.

## Elderly

Mental disorders generally appear to be as common among older adults as younger.[107] The loss of loved ones, which is common at an older age, frequently triggers depression. Moreover, the suicide rate is highest among older Americans.[108] Yet despite their equivalent need for services, the elderly are less likely than the nonelderly to be diagnosed and treated for mental illness.[109] Even when they do obtain care, they are less likely to receive services from the mental health specialty sector.[110] Among elderly Medicare beneficiaries receiving physician services for a psychiatric condition, only 29 percent saw a specialist at least once.[111] Suboptimal use of services among the elderly is probably due to both provider and patient factors. Providers often do not recognize the signs of mental illness among the elderly, failing to distinguish it from the normal aging process.[112] Cognitive impairment and differences in how the disorders present can make mental illness difficult to diagnose among the elderly. In turn, elderly patients tend to have greater perception of stigma than the nonelderly,[113] and traveling to obtain specialty care poses greater difficulties for the elderly because of their physical frailty.

Financial barriers contribute to their lower use of behavioral health care as well, although perhaps not more so than for younger patients.

Finally, the elderly and their caregivers suffer from the added burden of Alzheimer's disease and other dementias, which increased mental health treatment expenditures by an additional 26 percent in 1996, the most recent year available for these cost estimates.[114] The prevalence of dementia rises with age, with approximately 8–15 percent of the elderly suffering from Alzheimer's disease.[115] Importantly, dementia and other organic disorders are a frequent cause of psychiatric hospitalization among the elderly.[116] Although treatment options for dementia are currently very limited, family members and other community caregivers often experience difficulty managing the behavior of these patients. These difficulties sometimes necessitate hospitalizing agitated patients simply to get them under control, even though their illness cannot be treated as effectively as other mental disorders. As with all mental illness, caregiver burden is a major concern for the family members of patients with dementia.

## Children

Unlike with the non-elderly adult population, no large-scale study to date has estimated the prevalence of mental health disorders among children and adolescents using a nationally representative sample.[117] Therefore the mental health prevalence estimates for this population must be pieced together from a number of small-scale studies that used differing methodologies and time frames. After reviewing eighteen studies, Costello and colleagues reported the median estimate for the prevalence of any psychiatric disorder among children and adolescents to be 25 percent in a three-to-six-month period.[118] Psychiatric conditions associated with severe functional impairment among adults are referred to as serious mental illness; among children these conditions are referred to as serious emotional disturbance (SED). Looking at SED, Costello and colleagues reviewed nine studies and reported the median prevalence to be approximately 11 percent in a three-to-six-month period.[119] Suicide is also a major concern among children, being the fifth leading cause of death among those aged five to fourteen.[120]

As with adults, children experience a mismatch between the need for mental health services and receipt of services. Although 6–9 percent of children ages six to seventeen receive mental health services each year, nearly 80 percent of those who need mental health services do not receive any treatment from a physician, mental health counselor, or therapist.[121] Moreover, among children with SED, one study reported that only 40 percent receive any mental health services and only 22 percent receive any specialty mental health services.[122]

Although many children in need of mental health care may not receive any services in the medical sector, some receive services within the school. Specifically, one study reported that 14 percent of youths age nine to seventeen received mental-health-related services through schools. Among those with a mental health diagnosis, 27 percent received mental-health-related services through schools compared to only 8 percent of those without a diagnosis who received such services.[123]

Several barriers to mental health care are specific to children. As with the elderly, diagnosis of mental illness is generally more difficult in the case of children and relies heavily on proxy respondents, such as parents and teachers. Second, inadequate access to specialty care among children is exacerbated by a shortage of child psychiatrists and other mental health specialists focusing on children.[124] Another problem specific to child mental health services is the lack of studies documenting the safety and efficacy of drugs for this age group, leading to concern about potentially inappropriate off-label use of psychotropic medication among children.

## Minorities

Mental disorders are generally as common among members of racial and ethnic minority groups as for nonminorities,[125] or more common, because of their higher rate of risk factors for mental illness, such as low socioeconomic status. Suicide is a particular concern among Native Americans.[126] Yet members of minority groups tend to have fewer outpatient visits than nonminorities[127] and less frequent use of mental health specialists.[128] African Americans on Medicaid who are diagnosed with depression are less likely to receive an antidepressant prescription at the time of diagnosis, and if they do, are less likely than white beneficiaries to receive a prescription for SSRIs (instead of the older tricyclic antidepressants, which have more side effects).[129] At the same time, African Americans are admitted to inpatient psychiatric care at a much higher rate than whites.[130]

Reasons for differential treatment patterns are likely to vary with the population. For example, African Americans are thought to experience greater distrust of the system,[131] while Asian Americans may find mental health services particularly stigmatizing.[132] Recently immigrated Latinos and Asian Americans are likely to experience language barriers. Some barriers to accessing care (notably financial) cut across all racial and ethnic groups but are likely to pose greater constraints for members of minority groups, who are less wealthy on average than nonminorities. As noted by Alegria and colleagues,[133] disparities in mental health status for minorities may in part be remedied by public policy focusing on social factors such as income, education, and housing.

Finally, few providers of mental health services are members of minority groups themselves,[134] and patients are less likely to drop out of treatment if a provider shares their language and ethnicity.[135] To address the issue that inadequate cultural competence is a deterrent to receiving appropriate treatment, the surgeon general has called for mental health services to be tailored to the demographic and cultural characteristics of the patient being treated.[136]

## Rural Residents

The distance to health care providers tends to be longer in rural areas, suggesting greater time and transportation costs associated with obtaining care. Furthermore, geographic accessibility of mental health specialists is limited in rural areas,[137] leading to heavier reliance on primary care providers than in urban areas.[138] Thus lack of physical proximity to providers of mental health services is a major concern among rural populations. These problems have led to proposed solutions such as "telepsychiatry," but there is not yet sufficient information to evaluate whether these innovations can address access issues on a large scale. The geographic barrier to accessing specialty services is exacerbated by the greater stigma a rural resident experiences in obtaining mental health care, since those in a rural area have less anonymity.[139]

# Current Mental Health Policy Issues

Because our focus is on government policy, this section focuses exclusively on the actions that can be taken at the federal and state levels to improve mental health care. It should be noted, though, that many of the limitations of the U.S. mental health services delivery system are best addressed through interventions aimed at patients and providers, or they stem from decisions made by private parties, such as insurers and employers.

## Safety-Net Providers

Privatization has led to caution about declining access to care for the sickest and costliest patients. Between 1970 and 1992, all of the net growth in the number of psychiatric hospitals in the United States occurred in the private sector, increasing the proportion of psychiatric hospitals run privately from 33 percent to 64 percent.[140] Concern about the financial incentives for private hospitals to skim the relatively healthy patients and dump the sickest ones has been heightened by the concurrent trend toward for-profit psychiatric hospitals, in part because of for-profit conversions and growth in for-profit psychiatric hospital chains. In contrast to the general hospital sector, in which only 13 percent of hospitals are for-profit, 43 percent of psychiatric hospitals are for-profit.[141] Although the evidence on case mix and quality differences among public, private for-profit, and private not-for-profit providers is mixed,[142] the growing dominance of private, for-profit providers in the psychiatric sector has nonetheless been controversial.[143]

Thus it is arguably premature for states to relinquish all direct control over delivering inpatient psychiatric services before ensuring that safety-net providers exist. Certainly public hospitals continue to play a critical role for the most vulnerable patients. State hospitals are among the few willing to admit patients who are violent or disruptive, who require a long stay, or who are uninsured.[144] In the absence of arrangements to guarantee access to a private hospital for these patients, it is important for states to maintain ongoing financial and political support for public psychiatric hospitals, including initiatives to improve the quality and cost-effectiveness of care given in those institutions.

## Medicare Provider Reimbursement Methodology for Inpatient Care

Of the 645,146 Medicare hospital discharges (422,131 patients) in 2000 that were related to mental health and substance abuse disorders, 17 percent were from psychiatric hospitals and about half from "distinct part" psychiatric units within general hospitals, with the remaining 33 percent being discharges from general hospital beds.[145] Unlike general hospitals, which are paid under Medicare's prospective payment system (PPS), psychiatric specialty facilities have been exempted from PPS since its introduction in 1983, because of arguments from the psychiatric community that these facilities were unlikely to be fairly reimbursed.[146] These arguments were based primarily on three factors: the diagnostic-related groups (DRGs) did not capture patients' treatment needs, no data from psychiatric hospitals was used in developing DRGs, and DRGs accounted for much less variation in length of stay and costs for psychiatric diagnoses than for medical or surgical cases.[147]

As a result, psychiatric specialty facilities were instead reimbursed under the Tax Equity and Fiscal Responsibility Act (TEFRA) of 1982, a payment methodology that used a target amount per admission. The target amount was loosely based on the facility's historical costs, and providers could apply for an increase in their target amount (for example, if they could document an increase in the acuity of their patient case mix since the target amount was set). Thus TEFRA offered fewer incentives for cost containment than PPS; it was argued that facilities with average costs well below target amounts operated under incentives similar to cost-based reimbursement.[148] Furthermore, TEFRA rules were considered by some commentators to be inequitable[149] and to permit "gaming" by general hospitals, which could decide whether or not to apply for PPS exemption for their psychiatric units and whether to treat psychiatric patients in the units or scatterbeds.[150]

As of January 1, 2005, the Centers for Medicare and Medicaid Services began to phase in a per diem prospective payment system for inpatient psychiatric facility (IPF) hospital services provided in psychiatric hospitals and distinct part units, as required by the Medicare, Medicaid and SCHIP Balanced Budget Refinement Act of 1999 (BBRA). After the three-year phase-in period is over, facilities will be paid according to a federal per diem payment amount, which is a base rate adjusted for the patient's age, DRG assignment (one of fifteen categories based on principal diagnosis), selected comorbidities, and where the day falls within the hospital stay (earlier days are paid more). Facility-level adjustments depend on the hospital's wage index factor, rural location, teaching status, existence of an emergency department, and a cost-of-living adjustment for selected states. Further adjustments are made for outliers, stop-loss payments, receipt of electroconvulsive therapy, and interrupted stays. These payment changes will affect 494 psychiatric hospitals and 1,458 exempt psychiatric units.[151]

It is important to understand the incentives inherent in Medicare's payment methodology to psychiatric specialty facilities, because reimbursement incentives may influence a psychiatric hospital's willingness to admit certain patients, or a general hospital's decision of whether to treat Medicare beneficiaries in a psychiatric unit or a scatterbed. Two points are of interest in the new prospective payment policy. The first is the need to develop a risk adjustment system that adequately distinguishes between groups of patients expected to be more or less expensive. Without ensuring that payments are "equitable" with regard to the patient's expected costs, the same objections that were raised against the original PPS system are likely to come up again. The second issue is that, unlike the general hospital PPS, the prospective payment developed for psychiatric facilities is calculated per diem, rather than per admission. This choice has huge implications in terms of the incentives to providers to contain costs, whether through greater efficiency or by skimping on quality. Probably due to the limited number of procedures and treatment options available to psychiatric patients, much if not most of the variation in the total costs of psychiatric admissions is from the variance in length of stay, rather than heterogeneity in daily costs. Payment of a per diem rate could encourage hospitals to furnish less intensive treatment but keep patients in the hospital longer, although the adjustment in per diem rate for the day of the stay may partially or fully attenuate this incentive. In addition, the change from the TEFRA payment system (which was admission-based) may result in a shift in profits, away from general hospital psychiatric units or private hospitals, which tend to have a shorter length of stay, and toward public psychiatric hospitals, which are more likely to service long-term custodial patients.

## Managed Behavioral Health Care Under Public Programs

Following the trend in private insurance, public insurance programs are rapidly moving into managed care. As of 2004, 4.6 of the forty million elderly and disabled Medicare beneficiaries were enrolled in HMOs.[152] State Medicaid programs have moved even more rapidly to enrolling beneficiaries in managed care plans. By 2003, the proportion of Medicaid beneficiaries enrolled in MCOs was 59 percent (a dramatic increase from the 14 percent in 1993), and all but three states had some form of Medicaid managed care program.[153]

In contrast to Medicare, Medicaid managed care programs are generally mandatory and often cover the disabled. Although the initial focus of Medicaid managed care programs was women and children on public assistance, as of 2000 twenty-nine states had managed care programs for disabled SSI recipients,[154] a population with a high incidence of mental illness and substance abuse. Twenty states also had non-Medicaid managed care programs that include behavioral health care.[155]

The impact of managed care on costs, quality, and health outcomes has been a strong focus of research interest in the past decade, yet we still know relatively little about the ability of MCOs to offer high-quality care for people with severe and chronic mental illnesses, or even for those with more routine behavioral health care needs.[156] It has been argued that certain types of managed care setting present a unique opportunity for improving the care of the chronically ill,[157] but the strong financial incentives of MCOs to avoid sick patients and offer minimal benefits may override their structural advantages in caring for these populations. Reservations notwithstanding, continued enrollment of publicly insured patients in managed care plans seems certain under the inexorable pressure of cost containment. The question for mental health policy makers is therefore how to structure public managed care programs to ensure the best possible access to behavioral health care.

In this context, several decisions face the public purchaser seeking to contract with a health plan to cover its beneficiary population. The first question is whether mental health and substance abuse services should be "carved in" or "carved out." Currently, Medicare managed care plans are all carve-ins, with a single capitation payment covering both behavioral health and medical care. In contrast, Medicaid programs have made extensive use of carved-out and standalone models of managed behavioral health care for their populations, even when coverage of medical care remains fee-for-service.

Persuasive arguments can be made for or against carving out behavioral health care. Arguments in favor of carve-outs[158] are that a vendor specializing in behavioral health care is better able to manage quality and costs, because of economies of scale and scope in setting up a specialty network; having a separate budget may protect funding for behavioral health care within MCOs; and some patients might be more likely to receive a diagnosis under a carve-out system in which they can be referred elsewhere by primary care physicians who avoid diagnosing mental illness in their patients because of lack of knowledge, interest, or time. More generally, carve-outs are considered a way to address some of the market failures in the financing of mental health care, notably adverse selection and moral hazard. Carving out mental health benefits from competing health plans can reduce the probability of people sorting across these health plans on the basis of mental health care need ("adverse selection").[159] In principle, carve-outs can use direct care management grounded in clinical need instead of imposing onerous cost-sharing requirements to control moral hazard.

Potential disadvantages of carving out behavioral health care are greater administrative complexity; poor integration of medical and mental health care, which may be particularly important for the elderly and others with medical co-morbidities; possible stigmatization of the carved-out services; less control over providers, because both risk-based and ASO carve-out vendors frequently contract with independent network providers paid on a fee-for-service basis; and incentives for cost shifting between the carved-in medical and carved-out behavioral health care vendors, in which case the introduction of a carve-out might not necessarily save money overall. Disruption of care may arise in the short term as patients find that their providers do not participate in the carve-out; carve-outs often save money by reducing reimbursement, but this can lead to a high rate of non-participation by providers.[160]

Reviews of the research on the cost effects of carve-outs[161] concluded that carve-outs result in both immediate drops in costs[162] and sustained drops in costs over longer periods[163], with no evidence of cost-shifting onto other sectors.[164] Carve-outs appear to increase access to mental health care by shifting the mix of services provided and lowering patient co-payment. Implementation of carve-outs increases utilization of outpatient mental health care,[165] while the number of inpatient days falls substantially.[166] There is less evidence regarding quality of care. One study found that introducing a carve-out did not alter hospital readmission rate and increased follow-up care after discharge.[167] A review of carve-outs in fifty-two plans showed appropriateness of follow-up care improving and thirty-day readmission to the hospital declining.[168] However, an additional evaluation found that a carve-out in one state Medicaid program diverted funds away from the most severely ill patients,[169] while another suggested that persons with schizophrenia improved less under a carve-out than under fee-for-service.[170]

If behavioral health care is carved out, the purchaser must decide whether to contract with a single carve-out vendor or multiple competing vendors, and whether to use risk or ASO contracts. Competition between vendors ought to increase the incentive to contain costs and offer high-quality services. In theory, this could be achieved within a capitated system by risk-adjusting payments to avoid giving incentives for enrolling healthy, low-cost patients and avoiding sick ones. In practice, however, it is difficult to adjust payments sufficiently to avoid these incentives altogether.[171] Thus it is more common to contract with only a single carve-out vendor at a time but engage in a rebidding process every few years, to establish incentives for the vendor to do a good job. An alternative is to contract with competing vendors but use mixed payment systems, or "soft" capitation contracts, rather than full capitation mechanisms so that the purchaser retains some of the risk of the patient's costs and vendors have less cause to engage in patient selection or skimping on services. In a mixed payment system, the payment equals $\alpha + \beta \times$ costs, where $0 < \beta < 1$ and $\alpha$ is a fixed payment that is independent of actual costs. Soft capitation systems are similar, in that the purchaser bears some of the risk. A per capita target amount and "risk corridors" are set for the expenditures of the carve-out vendor. If actual costs exceed the target amount, the purchaser pays a varying portion of the extra costs; typically the purchaser assumes more risk with further expenditure increases. Conversely, if the vendor's costs fall below the target amount, the purchaser retains some but not all of the difference, with the proportion increasing the further the actual costs lie below the target amount. From the point of view of the vendor, both mixed payment systems and soft capitation contracts limit the extent of the upside and the downside to capitation payments.

Given the variability in the costs of patients with behavioral health problems, the degree of risk aversion of most MCOs, and the inadequacy of risk-adjustment methodologies, using some form of risk sharing between the purchaser and the carve-out vendor is advisable. Performance-based incentives (premised on quality indicators and not just cost-containment goals) should also be incorporated into the contract whenever possible. Measuring and adjusting outcomes for risk tends to be even more difficult for behavioral health than for medical problems. As one example, mortality is a more useful outcome measure for a medical condition such as myocardial infarction than for even severe mental illness such as schizophrenia. However, both private and public efforts to measure quality of care are under way[172] and should be strongly encouraged, because the ability of behavioral health care carve-out vendors to reduce utilization cannot be interpreted either positively or negatively without corresponding information on quality and outcomes.

## Parity in Health Insurance Benefits

In the early 1990s, proponents of parity for mental health coverage in health insurance benefits began pushing for comprehensive mental health parity legislation in Congress. In 1996, a weakened version of the original bill was passed and signed into law by President Clinton.[173] Although the passage of the Mental Health Parity Act (MHPA) of 1996 (PL 104-204) represented a small victory for proponents of parity legislation, the MHPA was actually very limited in scope.[174] The MHPA prevented group health plans from placing annual or lifetime dollar limits on mental health services that are less favorable than the limits for medical services.[175] Many other benefits, however, were not addressed by the legislation, among them co-payments, deductibles, co-insurance amounts, limits on outpatient visits, and limits on inpatient days.[176] In addition, other exemptions and loopholes in the MHPA limited its effectiveness: lack of substance abuse coverage, no requirement that health plans must offer *any* mental health coverage, an exemption for employers with fewer than fifty-one employees, and exemption from the legislation if compliance increases health plan costs by more than 1 percent.[177]

In spite of these limitations, the MHPA made two noteworthy contributions in advancing the issue of mental health parity. Importantly, passage of the MHPA helped solidify the issue of parity on the national agenda. In addition, it enabled state legislatures to experiment with more comprehensive parity legislation.[178] In 1997, thirty-four states introduced their own version of mental health parity legislation;[179] by 1998, fourteen had passed parity legislation that was more comprehensive than the MHPA.[180]

Despite the success of more comprehensive parity legislation at the state level, the Employee Retirement Income Security Act of 1974 (ERISA) greatly limits the effectiveness of any state legislation about health insurance. ERISA contains a "deemer clause" that prohibits states from regulating health plans that "self-insure" by bearing the primary risk.[181] There are no exact estimates on the number of employees who have insurance through self-insured plans, but studies suggest that it lies somewhere between 33 percent and 50 percent.[182] For this reason, it is crucial that the movement for stronger parity legislation continue to move forward at the federal level.

The reluctance of health plans to increase coverage of mental health services can be traced to the concerns about moral hazard and adverse selection discussed earlier. However, to the extent that parity legislation sets a lower bound on behavioral health care benefits for all plans, such legislation should reduce the potential for patient selection into more generous plans. Furthermore, although relatively little is known about the price elasticity of demand for mental health services under managed care,[183] the tradeoff between demand-side and supply-side cost containment suggests that patient cost-sharing requirements can be reduced as long as there is a commensurate increase in utilization management by providers. Thus it has been argued that more comprehensive coverage of mental health services need not add excessively to costs, if the moral hazard is constrained by comprehensively managing care.[184]

Since passage of the MHPA, several studies have reported that comprehensive parity legislation may be more affordable than was thought during the debate prior to passage.[185] For example, one study reported that the assumptions used in the mental health parity debate in 1996 may have overstated the true costs of full parity legislation within the context of managed care by a factor of four to eight.[186] The negative corollary to this point is that in a managed care environment parity in benefits can be achieved on paper but not translated into actual practice if gatekeeping is stricter for behavioral health care than it is for medical care.

Because studies have reported that full parity legislation can be affordable under managed behavioral health care, a difficult dilemma arises. Although passage of full parity may help reduce some of the financial barriers to mental health services, as we have described, managed behavioral health care can pose barriers to access for individuals in need of mental health treatment.[187] Interestingly, a coalition (known as the Coalition for Fairness in Mental Illness Coverage) formed by the National Alliance for the Mentally Ill and the National Mental Health Association together with the American Managed Behavioral Healthcare Association and four other organizations has been at the forefront of the push for comprehensive mental health parity legislation for more than a decade.[188]

In 2003, the Paul Wellstone Mental Health Equitable Treatment Act (MHETA) was introduced into the 108th Congress. Originally, the bill required parity for all financial arrangements (co-insurance, co-payment, deductible, dollar limits), in-patient days, and outpatient visits for mental health and other medical services. Additionally, it would have eliminated a provision from the MHPA of 1996 allowing health plans to claim an exemption if the implementation resulted in a cost increase greater than 1 percent.[189] As expected, there was enormous opposition to the MHETA from employers and insurance trade groups. The most contentious issue was the potential cost increase likely to be incurred by complying with a new parity mandate. Although the Congressional Budget Office estimated that the MHETA would have caused only a 0.9 percent increase in health care premiums, opponents argued that the increase could have been as high as 17 percent.[190] Two specific provisions fostered strong opposition: inclusion of all mental health DSM-IV-R diagnoses, and elimination of the provision from the MHPA allowing health plans to claim exemption if implementation resulted in a cost increase greater than 1 percent.[191] Because of disagreement over these provisions, the Republican leadership caused the bill to die in committee. However, the bill had strong support in both chambers of the 108th Congress and would have passed if it had been brought to a vote. The Coalition for Fairness in Mental Illness Coverage is currently working with supporters in Congress to reintroduce new mental health parity legislation into the 109th session.[192]

Importantly, because parity legislation is designed to address the disparity between medical and behavioral health care coverage, it can, at most, bring mental health benefits only up to the inadequate standard currently set by medical care insurance. As Mechanic[193] notes, many of the long-term care and rehabilitative services required by individuals with mental disorders are generally not covered by private health insurance. Furthermore, parity legislation does not address the large proportion of Americans who are uninsured or publicly insured. In particular, individuals with SPMI are less likely to have insurance coverage through their own (or a spouse's) employer, so they may benefit less from parity legislation than others with less disabling conditions. Parity legislation is therefore at best a partial solution to concerns about financial barriers to behavioral health care. Mental health policy makers should prioritize not only stronger federal parity legislation that applies to all health plans and all states, but also inclusion of comprehensive mental health and substance abuse benefits in all health policy initiatives seeking to expand insurance coverage.

## Conclusion

In April 2002, President George W. Bush announced creation of a committee, known as the President's New Freedom Commission on Mental Health, to conduct a comprehensive review of mental health care in the United States for adults with SMI and children with SED. The main goal of this commission was to "recommend improvements to enable adults with SMI and children with SED to live, work, learn, and participate fully in their communities."[194] Although the president limited the scope of the commission's task by focusing on SMI and SED, many of its goals and recommendations are also applicable to those with mental illness who do not fall under these particular categories.

The findings regarding the current mental health system can be summed up in a statement from the commission to the president that accompanied the final report, released on July 22, 2003: "After a year of study, and after reviewing research and testimony, the Commission finds that recovery from mental illness is now a real possibility. The promise of the New Freedom Initiative—a life in the community for everyone—can be realized. Yet, for too many Americans with mental illnesses, the mental health services and supports they need remain fragmented, disconnected and often inadequate, frustrating the opportunity for recovery. The time has long passed for yet another piecemeal approach to mental health reform. Instead, the Commission recommends a fundamental transformation of the nation's approach to mental health care."[195]

Within the report, the commission put forth six main goals to achieve a transformed mental health system:

1. Understanding that mental health is essential to overall health, making mental health care consumer-driven and family-driven
2. Mental health care is consumer and family driven.
3. Eliminating disparities in mental health services
4. Making early mental health screening, assessment, and referral to services common practice
5. Delivering excellent mental health care and accelerating research
6. Using IT to improve access to mental health care and information

Each goal included numerous recommendations by the commission, including support for stronger federal mental health parity legislation.[196]

In spite of the commission's blunt assessment of the mental health treatment system, it is unlikely that it will result in substantial changes to the mental health system in the near future. The report did not explicitly call for the investment of new resources to accomplish these six goals.[197] Instead, the DHHS secretary directed the administrator of the Substance Abuse and Mental Health Services Administration (SAMHSA) to take charge of coordinating government agencies in implementing these recommendations. SAMHSA, however, has a very limited budget and lacks the resources to undertake such a large task.[198]

Thus, even though there is substantial value in the commission's documentation of the problems with the current mental health system, in the absence of the political will to find financial resources with which to address them, the problems are likely to remain. Individuals with severe and chronic psychiatric disorders are among the most vulnerable patient populations, having historically been neglected or mistreated. Given the limited ability of many people with severe and chronic mental illness to advocate forcefully for themselves, policy makers need to take responsibility for ensuring that these patients have adequate access to the services they need to reenter society. Of particular concern for this population are the limitations of public insurance coverage for psychiatric care, the tenuousness of the psychiatric safety-net system, and the fractured system of delivering and financing mental health services that makes it difficult for these patients to obtain the full continuum of services they need.

Access to care is also a concern for individuals with less-severe, acute disorders, many of whom are covered by employer-based insurance. The inadequate and inequitable coverage of behavioral health care under private insurance plans, the potential for dumping or denial of needed care on the part of managed care plans, shortages of mental health specialists and certain types of mental health services in many parts of the country, and stigmatization of psychiatric treatment are among the major impediments to ensuring appropriate care for this population.

# Notes

1. Kessler, R., and others. "Prevalence and Treatment of Mental Disorders, 1990 to 2003." *New England Journal of Medicine*, 2005, 352(24), 2515–2523.

2. Mark, T., and others. *National Expenditures for Mental Health and Substance Abuse Treatment, 1991–2001.* Rockville, Md.: Substance Abuse and Mental Health Services Administration, U.S. Department of Health and Human Services, 2005.

3. Kessler, R., and others. "The Epidemiology of Co-Occurring Addictive and Mental Disorders: Implications for Prevention and Service Utilization." *American Journal of Orthopsychiatry*, 1996, *66*(1), 17–31.

4. Drake, R., and Osher, F. "Treating Substance Abuse in Patients with Severe Mental Illness." In S. Henggeler and A. Santos (eds.), *Innovative Approaches for Difficult-to-Treat Populations.* Washington, D.C.: American Psychiatric Press, 1997.

5. Mark and others (2005).

6. World Health Organization. *The World Health Report 2001—Mental Health: New Understanding, New Hope.* Geneva: World Health Organization, 2001.

7. Ettner, S., Frank, R., and Kessler, R. "The Impact of Psychiatric Disorders on Labor Market Outcomes." *Industrial and Labor Relations Review*, 1997, *51*(1), 64–81; Berndt, E., and others. "Workplace Performance Effects from Chronic Depression and Its Treatment." *Journal of Health Economics*, 1998, *17*, 511–535.

8. Kessler, R., and Frank, R. "The Impact of Psychiatric Disorders on Work Loss Days." *Psychological Medicine*, 1997, *27*, 861–873.

9. Steadman, H., and others. "Violence by People Discharged from Acute Psychiatric Inpatient Facilities and by Others in the Same Neighborhoods." *Archives of General Psychiatry*, 1998, *55*, 1–9; Swanson, J. "Mental Disorder, Substance Abuse, and Community Violence: An Epidemiological Approach." In J. Monahan and H. Steadman (eds.), *Violence and Mental Disorder: Developments in Risk Assessment.* Chicago: University of Chicago Press, 1994; Eronen, M., Angermeyer, M., and Schulze, B. "The Psychiatric Epidemiology of Violent Behavior." *Social Psychiatry and Psychiatric Epidemiology*, 1998, *33*(1), 13–23.

10. Gelberg, L. "Homeless Persons." In R. Andersen, T. Rice, and G. Kominski (eds.), *Changing the U.S. Health Care System.* San Francisco: Jossey-Bass, 1996.

11. Kelleher, K., and others. "Alcohol and Drug Disorders Among Physically Abusive and Neglectful Parents in a Community-Based Sample." *American Journal of Public Health*, 1994, *84*, 1586–1590.

12. Rice, D., and others. *The Cost of Alcohol and Drug Abuse and Mental Illness.* Washington, D.C.: U.S. Government Printing Office, 1990.

13. Kessler, R. "The Social Consequence of Psychiatric Disorders." In M. J. Cox and J. Brooks-Gunn (eds.), *Conflict and Closeness: The Formation, Functioning and Stability of Families.* Hillsdale, N.J.: Erlbaum, 1999.

14. Clark, R., Ricketts, S., and McHugo, G. "Legal System Involvement and Costs for Persons in Treatment for Severe Mental Illness and Substance Use Disorders." *Psychiatric Services*, 1999, *50*(5), 641–648.

15. Kessler, R. "The Social Consequences of Psychiatric Disorders, III: Probability of Marital Stability." *American Journal of Psychiatry*, 1998, *155*(8), 1092–1096.

16. Klerman, G. "Trends in Utilization of Mental Health Services: Perspectives for Health Services Research." *Medical Care*, 1985, *23*(3), 584–597; Nemeroff, C. "Psychopharmacology of Affective Disorders in the 21st Century." *Biological Psychiatry*, 1998, *44*, 517–525.

17. Mechanic, D. "Is the Prevalence of Mental Disorders a Good Measure of the Need for Services?" *Health Affairs,* 2003, *22*(5), 8–20.

18. Kessler and others (2005); Demyttenaere, K., and others. "Prevalence, Severity, and Unmet Need for Treatment of Mental Disorders in the World Health Organization World Mental Health Surveys." *Journal of the American Medical Association,* 2004, *291*(21), 2581–2590.

19. Surgeon General. *Mental Health: A Report of the Surgeon General.* Washington, D.C.: U.S. Government Printing Office, 1999.

20. Grob, G. *The Mad Among Us: A History of the Care of America's Mentally Ill.* Cambridge, Mass.: Harvard University Press, 1994.

21. Meier, B. "A Price Too High? Deal to Save Charter Behavioral May Have Harmed It." *New York Times,* Feb. 16, 2000.

22. Young, A., and others. "The Quality of Care for Depressive and Anxiety Disorders in the United States." *Archives of General Psychiatry,* 2001, *58*(1), 55–61.

23. Wang, P., Demler, O., and Kessler, R. "Adequacy of Treatment for Serious Mental Illness in the United States." *American Journal of Public Health,* 2002, *92*(1), 92–98.

24. Surgeon General (1999).

25. Surgeon General (1999).

26. Kessler, R., and others. "The Epidemiology of Adult Mental Disorders." In B. L. Levin, J. Petrila, and K. D. Henessy (eds.), *Mental Health Services: A Public Health Perspective.* New York: Oxford University Press, 2004.

27. Surgeon General (1999).

28. Kessler, R., and others. "The 12-Month Prevalence and Correlates of Serious Mental Illness (SMI)." In R. W. Manderscheid and M. A. Sonnenschein (eds.), *Mental Health, United States, 1996.* Center for Mental Health Services. (DHHS pub. no. SMA96-3098.) Washington, D.C.: Superintendent of Documents, U.S. Government Printing Office, 1996.

29. Surgeon General (1999).

30. Surgeon General (1999); Grob, G. *Mental Illness and American Society, 1875–1940.* Princeton, N.J.: Princeton University Press, 1983.

31. Grob, G. N. "Mental Health Policy in 21st Century America." In R. Manderscheid and M. Henderson (eds.), *Mental Health, United States, 2000.* Rockville, Md.: U.S. Department of Health and Human Services, 2001; Grob (1994).

32. Grob (2001); Grob, G. *Mental Institutions in America: Social Policy to 1875.* New York: Free Press, 1973; Grob (1983).

33. Grob (2001); Grob (1983).

34. Grob (2001).

35. Grob (1994).

36. Murphy, M., and Dorwart, R. "Mental Health Policy." In D. Calkins (ed.), *Health Care Policy.* Cambridge, Mass.: Blackwell Science, 1995; Kiesler, C., and Sibulkin, A. *Mental Hospitalization: Myths and Facts About a National Crisis.* Thousand Oaks, Calif.: Sage, 1987; Grob (1994).

37. Grob (1994).

38. Mechanic (2003); Mechanic, D. *Mental Health and Social Policy: The Emergence of Managed Care* (4th ed.). Boston: Allyn and Bacon, 1999.

39. Murphy and Dorwart (1995).

40. Mechanic (2003); Grob (1994).

41. Urff, J. "Public Mental Health Systems: Structures, Goals, and Constraints." In B. L. Levin, J. Petrila, and K. D. Henessy (eds.), *Mental Health Services: A Public Health Perspective.* New York: Oxford University Press, 2004.

42. Grob (2001).

43. Grob (2001).

44. Grob (2001).

45 Lutterman, T., Hollen, V., and Shaw, R. *Funding Sources and Expenditures of State Mental Health Agencies: Fiscal Year 2002.* National Association of State Mental Health Program Directors Research Institute, Oct. 2004. [http://www.nri-inc.org/RevExp/RE02/02Report.pdf].

46. Grob (2001).

47. Grob (2001).

48. President's New Freedom Commission on Mental Health. "Achieving the Promise: Transforming Mental Health Care in America." (Final report.) Washington, D.C.: President's New Freedom Commission on Mental Health, July 2004.; Grob (2001).

49. Mechanic (2003).

50. Surgeon General (1999); Mechanic, D. "Policy Challenges in Improving Mental Health Services: Some Lessons from the Past." *Psychiatric Services,* 2003, *54*(9), 1227–1232.

51. Surgeon General (1999).

52. Surgeon General (1999).

53. Olfson, M., and others. "National Trends in the Outpatient Treatment of Depression." *Journal of the American Medical Association,* 2002, *287*(2), 203–209.

54. Mark and others (2005).

55. Mark, T., and others. "U.S. Spending for Mental Health and Substance Abuse Treatment, 1991–2001." *Health Affairs,* Web exclusive, Mar. 29, 2005, W5-133–W5-142.

56. Mechanic, D. "Emerging Trends in Mental Health Policy and Practice." *Health Affairs,* 1998, *17*(6), 82–98.

57. National Association of State Mental Health Policy Directors (NASMHPD) Research Institute. *State Profile Highlights,* no. 04-13. Washington, D.C.: NASMHPD, March 2004.

58. "Closing and Reorganizing State Psychiatric Hospitals: 2000." In NASMHPD Research Institute, *State Profile Highlight,* no. 1, Aug. 10, 2000.

59. Mark and others, "U.S. Spending . . ." (2005).

60. Regier, D., and others. "The De Facto U.S. Mental and Addictive Disorders Service System. Epidemiologic Catchment Area Prospective 1-Year Prevalence Rates of Disorders and Services." *Archives of General Psychiatry,* 1993, *50,* 85–94.

61. Regier and others (1993).

62. Beeler, J., Rosenthal, A., and Cohler, B. "Patterns of Family Caregiving and Support Provided to Older Psychiatric Patients in Long-Term Care." *Psychiatric Services,* 1999, *50*(9), 1222–1224; Lefley, H. "Aging Parents as Caregivers of Mentally Ill Adult Children: An Emerging Social Problem." *Hospital and Community Psychiatry,* 1987, *38*(10), 1063–1070; Horwitz, A. "Siblings as Caregivers for the Seriously Mentally Ill." *Milbank Quarterly,* 1993, *71*(2), 323–339.

63. Nunnally, J. *Popular Conceptions of Mental Health: Their Development and Change.* Austin, Tex.: Holt, Rinehart, and Winston, 1961; Penn, D., and Martin, J. "The Stigma of Severe Mental Illness: Some Potential Solutions for a Recalcitrant Problem." *Psychiatric Quarterly,* 1998, *69*(3), 235–247.

64. Sussman, L., Robins, L., and Earls, F. "Treatment-Seeking for Depression by Black and White Americans." *Social Science and Medicine,* 1987, *24,* 187–196; Cooper-Patrick, L., and others. "Identification of Patient Attitudes and Preferences Regarding Treatment of Depression." *Journal of General Internal Medicine,* 1997, *12,* 431–438.

65. Grob, G. *From Asylum to Community: Mental Health Policy in Modern America.* Princeton, N.J.: Princeton University Press, 1991.

66. Surgeon General (1999); Phelan, J. B., and others. "Public Conceptions of Mental Illness in 1950, in 1996: Has Sophistication Increased? Has Stigma Declined?" Paper presented at American Sociological Association meetings, Toronto, Ont., Aug. 1997; Link, B., and others. "Public Conceptions of Mental Illness: The Labels, Causes, Dangerousness and Social Distance." *American Journal of Public Health*, 1999, *89*(9), 1328–1333.

67. Surgeon General (1999); President's New Freedom Commission on Mental Health (2003).

68. Nemeroff, C. "Psychopharmacology of Affective Disorders in the 21st Century." *Biological Psychiatry*, 1998, *44*(7), 517–525.

69. Kessler (2005).

70. Kessler (2005).

71. Kessler (2005).

72. Mechanic, D. "Treating Mental Illness: Generalist vs. Specialist." *Health Affairs*, 1990, *9*(4), 61–75.

73. Pincus, H., and others. "Prescribing Trends in Psychotropic Medications: Primary Care, Psychiatry, and Other Medical Specialties." *Journal of the American Medical Association*, 1998, *279*, 526–531.

74. Simon, G. E., and others. "Treatment Process and Outcomes for Managed Care Patients Receiving New Antidepressant Prescriptions from Psychiatrists and Primary Care Physicians." *Archive of General Psychiatry*, 2001, *4*(58), 395–401.

75. Simon, G. E., and Von Korff M. "Recognition, Management, and Outcomes of Depression in Primary Care." *Archives of Family Medicine*, 1995, *2*(4), 99–105; Callies, A. L., and Popkin, M. K. "Antidepressant Treatment of Medical-Surgical Inpatients by Nonpsychiatric Physicians." *Archives of General Psychiatry*, 1987, *2*(44), 157–160.

76. Frank, R., and Kamlet, M. "Economic Aspects of Patterns of Mental Health Care: Cost Variation by Setting." *General Hospital Psychiatry*, 1990, *12*(1), 11–18; Haas-Wilson, D., Cheadle, A., and Scheffler, R. "Demand for Mental Health Services: An Episode of Treatment Approach." *Southern Economic Journal*, 1989, *56*(1), 219–232; Wells, K. B., and others. "Cost-Sharing and the Use of General Medical Physicians for Outpatient Mental Health Care." *Health Services Research*, 1987, *22*(1), 1–17; Horgan, C. "Specialty and General Ambulatory Mental Health Services: Comparison of Utilization and Expenditures." *Archives of General Psychiatry*, 1985, *42*(6), 565–572; Knesper, D., Pagnucco, D., and Wheeler, J. "Similarities and Differences Across Mental Health Services Providers and Practice Settings in the United States." *American Psychologist*, 1985, *40*(12), 1352–1369; Ettner, S., and Hermann, R. "Differences Between the General Medical and Mental Health Specialty Sectors in the Expenditures and Utilization Patterns of Medicare Patients Treated for Psychiatric Disorders." *Health Services Research*, 1999, *34*(3), 737–760.

77. Sherbourne, C. D., and others. "Subthreshold Depression and Depressive Disorder: Clinical Characteristics of General Medical and Mental Health Specialty Outpatients." *American Journal of Psychiatry*, 1994, *151*(12), 1777–1784; Wells, K., and others. "Use of Minor Tranquilizers and Antidepressant Medications by Depressed Outpatients: Results from the Medical Outcomes Study." *American Journal of Psychiatry*, 1994, *151*(5), 694–700; Sturm, R., and Wells, K. B. "How Can Care for Depression Become More Cost-Effective?" *Journal of the American Medical Association*, 1995, *273*(1), 51–58; Katz, S., and others. "Medication Management of Depression in the United States and Ontario." *Journal of General Internal Medicine*, 1998, *13*(1), 77–85.

78. Young and others (2001).

79. Donohoe, M. T. "Comparing Generalist and Specialty Care: Discrepancies, Deficiencies, and Excesses." *Archives of Internal Medicine*, 1998, *15*(158), 1596–1608.

80. Mechanic (1998).

81. Knesper, D. J., Wheeler, J.R.C., and Pagnucco, D. L. "Mental Health Services Providers' Distribution Across Counties in the United States." *American Psychologist*, 1984, *39*(12), 1424–1434.

82. Peterson, B., and others. "Mental Health Practitioners and Trainees." In R. Manderscheid and M. Henderson (eds.), *Mental Health, United States, 1998.* Rockville, Md.: Center for Mental Health Services, 1998.

83. Ettner and Hermann (1997); Horgan (1985); Shannon, G., Bashshur, R., and Lovett, J. "Distance and the Use of Mental Health Services." *Milbank Quarterly*, 1986, *64*(2), 302–330; Horgan, C., and Salkever, D. "The Demand for Outpatient Mental Health Care from Nonspecialty Providers." In R. Scheffler and L. Rossiter (eds.), *Advances in Health Economics and Health Services Research.* Greenwich, Conn.: JAI Press, 1987.

84. American Hospital Association. *Hospital Statistics.* Chicago: American Hospital Association, 1996.

85. Manderscheid, R., and Sonnenschein, M. (eds.). *Mental Health, United States, 1996.* Department of Health and Human Services publication no. (SMA) 96-3098, ed. Center for Mental Health Services. Washington, D.C.: Superintendent of Documents, U.S. Government Printing Office, 1996.

86. NASMHPD Research Institute. *State Profile Highlights*, no. 04-13. Mar. 2004.

87. Mark and others, "U.S. Spending . . ." (2005).

88. Mark and others, "U.S. Spending . . ." (2005).

89. www.statehealthfacts.org (July 3, 2005)

90. Frank, R., and McGuire, T. "Economics and Mental Health." (Working paper 7052.) Cambridge, Mass.: National Bureau of Economic Research, 1999.

91. Frank, R., Koyanagi, C., and McGuire, T. "The Politics and Economics of Mental Health 'Parity' Laws." *Health Affairs*, 1997, *16*(4), 108–119.

92. Buck, J., and others. "Behavioral Health Benefits in Employer-Sponsored Health Plans, 1997." *Health Affairs*, 1999, *18*(2), 67–78.

93. Buck and others (1999); Barry, C. L., and others. "Design of Mental Health Benefits: Still Unequal After All These Years." *Health Affairs*, 2003, *22*(5), 127–137.

94. Barry and others (2003).

95. Frank, Koyanagi, and McGuire (1997).

96. Frank and McGuire (1999).

97. Newhouse, J. *Free for All? Lessons from the RAND Health Insurance Experiment.* Cambridge, England: Harvard University Press, 1993.

98. Frank and McGuire (1999); Croghan, T., Obenchain, R., and Crown, W. "What Does Treatment of Depression Really Cost?" *Health Affairs*, 1998, *17*(4), 198–208.

99. Lave, J., and Goldman, H. "Medicare Financing for Mental Health Care." *Health Affairs*, Spring 1990, 19–30.

100. Sherman, J. "Medicare's Mental Health Benefits: Coverage, Use, and Expenditures." *Journal of Aging and Health*, 1996, *8*(1), 54–71.

101. Taube, C., Goldman, H., and Salkever, D. "Medicaid Coverage for Mental Illness: Balancing Access and Costs." *Health Affairs*, 1990, *9*, 5–18.

102. Open Minds. *Yearbook of Managed Behavioral Health Market Share in the United States, 2000–2001.* Gettysburg, Pa.: Open Minds, 2000.

103. Oss, M., Drissel, A., and Clary, J. *Managed Behavioral Health Market Share in the United States, 1997–1998.* Gettysburg, Pa.: Open Minds, 1997.

104. Goldman, W., McCulloch, J., and Sturm, R. "Cost and Use of Mental Health Services Before and After Managed Care." *Health Affairs,* 1998, *17*(2), 40–52.

105. Tischler, G. "Utilization Management of Mental Health Services by Private Third Parties." *American Journal of Psychiatry,* 1990, *147*(8), 967–973.

106. Hermann, R. C., and others. "Variation in ECT Use in the United States." *American Journal of Psychiatry,* 1995, *152*(6), 869–875; Phelps, C. "Information Diffusion and Best Practice Adoption." In J. Newhouse and A. Culyer (eds.), *Handbook of Health Economics,* vol. 1A. Amsterdam, Neth.: North Holland Press, 2000.

107. Surgeon General (1999).

108. Hoyert, D., Kochanek, K., and Murphy, S. *Deaths: Final Data for 1997.* Hyattsville, Md.: National Center for Health Statistics, 1999.

109. German, P. S., Shapiro, S., and Skinner, E. A. "Mental Health of the Elderly: Use of Health and Mental Health Services." *Journal of American Geriatric Society,* 1985, *33*(4), 246–252; NIH Consensus Conference. "Diagnosis and Treatment of Depression in Late Life." *Journal of the American Medical Association,* 1992, *268*(8), 1018–1024; Leaf, P. J., and others. "Contact with Health Professionals for the Treatment of Psychiatric and Emotional Problems." *Medical Care,* 1985, *23*(12), 1322–1337.

110. Horgan (1985); Leaf, P. J., and others. "Factors Affecting the Utilization of Specialty and General Medical Mental Health Services." *Medical Care,* 1988, *26*(1), 9–26.

111. Ettner, S., and Hermann, R. "Provider Specialty Choice Among Medicare Patients Treated for Psychiatric Disorders." Health Care Financing *Administrative Review,* 1997, *18*(3), 1–17.

112. NIH Consensus Conference (1992); Unutzer, J., and others. "Depressive Symptoms and the Cost of Health Services in HMO Patients Aged 65 Years and Older." *Journal of the American Medical Association,* 1997, *277*(20), 1618–1623.

113. NIH Consensus Conference (1992); Butler, R., and Lewis, M. *Aging and Mental Health.* St. Louis: Mosby, 1982.

114. Mark and others (1998).

115. Ritchie, K., and Kildea, D. "Is Senile Dementia 'Age-Related' or 'Aging-Related'? Evidence from Meta-Analysis of Dementia Prevalence in the Oldest Old." *Lancet,* 1995, *346,* 931–934.

116. Ettner, S., and Hermann, R. "Inpatient Psychiatric Treatment of Elderly Medicare Beneficiaries, 1990–1991." *Psychiatric Services,* 1998, *49*(9), 1173–1179.

117. Costello, E., and others. "Prevalence of Psychiatric Disorders in Childhood and Adolescence." In B. Levin, J. Petrila, and K. Hennessey (eds.), *Mental Health Services: A Public Health Perspective* (2nd ed.). Oxford: Oxford University Press, 2004, 111–128.

118. Costello and others (2004).

119. Costello and others (2004).

120. U.S. Department of Health and Human Services. *Health, United States, 2004.* (DHHS publication no. 2004–1232, table 32.) Washington, D.C.: U.S. Department of Health and Human Services, 2004.

121. Kataoka, S. H., Zhang, L., and Wells, K. B. "Unmet Needs for Mental Health Care Among U.S. Children: Variation by Ethnicity and Insurance Status." *American Journal of Psychiatry,* Sept. 2002, *159*(9), 1548–1555.

122. Burns, B. E., and others. "Children's Mental Health Service Use Across Service Sectors." *Health Affairs,* 1995, *14,* 147–159.

123. Leaf, P. J., and others. "Mental Health Service Use in the Community and Schools: Results from the Four-Community MECA Study." *Journal of the American Academy of Child and Adolescent Psychiatry,* 1996, *35*(7), 889–897.

124. Thomas, C., and Holzer, C. "National Distribution of Child and Adolescent Psychiatrists." *Journal of the American Academy of Child and Adolescent Psychiatry*, 1999, *38*, 9–15.

125. Kessler, R. C., and others. "The Epidemiology of Major Depressive Disorder Results from the National Comorbidity Survey Replication (NCS-R)." *Journal of the American Medical Association*, 2003, *289*(23), 3095–3105; Regier, D., and others. "One-Month Prevalence of Mental Disorders in the United States and Sociodemographic Characteristics: The Epidemiological Catchment Area Study." *Acta Psychiatrica Scandinavica*, 1993, *88*, 35–47.

126. Wallace, J., and others. *Homicide and Suicide Among Native Americans, 1979–1992.* (Violence Surveillance Series, no. 2). Atlanta: National Center for Injury Prevention and Control, Centers for Disease Control and Prevention, 1996.

127. Neighbors, H., and others. "Ethnic Minority Health Service Delivery: A Review of the Literature." *Research in Community and Mental Health*, 1992, *7*, 55–71; Takeuchi, D., and Uehara, E. *Ethnic Minority Mental Health Services: A Public Health Perspective.* New York: Oxford University Press, 1996.

128. Kessler (2005); Sussman, Robins, and Earls (1987); Gallo, J., and others. "Filters on the Pathway to Mental Health Care II: Sociodemographic Factors." *Psychological Medicine*, 1995, *25*, 1149–1160; Vega, W., and others. "Lifetime Prevalence of DSM-III-R Psychiatric Disorders Among Urban and Rural Mexican-Americans in California." *Archives of General Psychiatry*, 1998, *55*, 771–778; Zhang, A., Snowden, L., and Sue, S. "Differences Between Asian and White Americans: Help Seeking Patterns in the Los Angeles Area." *Journal of Community Psychology*, 1998, *26*, 317–326.

129. Melfi, C. A., and others. "Racial Variation in Antidepressant Treatment in a Medicaid Population." *Journal of Clinical Psychiatry*, 2000, *61*, 16–21.

130. Snowden, L., and Cheung, F. "Use of Inpatient Mental Health Services by Members of Ethnic Minority Groups." *American Psychologist*, 1990, *45*, 347–355.

131. Sussman and others (1987); Lin, K., and others. "Sociocultural Determinants of the Help-Seeking Behavior of Patients with Mental Illness." *Journal of Nervous and Mental Disease*, 1982, *170*, 78–85.

132. Uba, L. *Asian-Americans: Personality Patterns, Identity and Mental Health.* New York: Guilford Press, 1994.

133. Alegria, M., and others. "The Role of Public Policies in Reducing Mental Health Status Disparities for People of Color." *Health Affairs*, 2003, *22*(5), 51–64.

134. Peterson and others (1998).

135. Takeuchi, D., Uehara, E., and Maramba, G. "Cultural Diversity and Mental Health Treatment." In A. Horwitz and T. Scheid (eds.), *The Sociology of Mental Health.* New York: Oxford University Press, 1999.

136. Surgeon General (1999).

137. Peterson and others (1998).

138. Lambert, D., and Agger, M. "Access of Rural AFDC Medicaid Beneficiaries to Mental Health Services." *Health Care Financing Review*, 1995, *17*(1), 133–145.

139. Hoyt, D., and others. "Psychological Distress and Help Seeking in Rural America." *American Journal of Community Psychology*, 1997, *25*, 449–470.

140. Manderscheid and Sonnenschein (1996).

141. Levenson, A. I. "The Growth of Investor-Owned Psychiatric Hospitals." *American Journal of Psychiatry*, 1982, *139*(7), 902–907; Ettner, S. L., and Hermann, R. C. "The Role of Profit Status Under Imperfect Information: Evidence from the Treatment Patterns of Elderly Medicare Beneficiaries Hospitalized for Psychiatric Diagnoses." *Journal of Health Economics*, 2001, *20*(1), 23–49.

142. Dorwart, R., and others. "A National Study of Psychiatric Hospital Care." *American Journal of Psychiatry*, 1991, *148*(2), 204–210; Schlesinger, M., and Dorwart, R. A. "Ownership and Mental-Health Services: A Reappraisal of the Shift Towards Privately Owned Facilities." *New England Journal of Medicine*, 1984, *311*, 959–965; Mark, T. L. "Psychiatric Hospital Ownership and Performance: Do Nonprofit Organizations Offer Advantages in Markets Characterized by Asymmetric Information?" *Journal of Human Resources*, 1996, *31*(3), 631–650.

143. Levenson (1982); Dorwart and others (1991); Schlesinger and Dorwart (1984); Eisenberg, L. "The Case Against For-Profit Hospitals." *Hospital and Community-Based Psychiatry*, 1984, *35*(10), 1009–1013; Dorwart, R. A., and Epstein, S. S. "Issues in Psychiatric Hospital Care." *Current Opinion in Psychiatry*, 1991, *4*, 789–793; Dorwart, R. A., and Schlesinger, M. "Privatization of Psychiatric Services." *American Journal of Psychiatry*, 1988, *145*(5), 543–553; Levenson, A. I. "Issues Surrounding the Ownership of Private Psychiatric Hospitals by Investor-Owned Hospital Chains." *Hospital and Community Psychiatry*, 1983, *34*(12), 1127–1131; Levenson, A. "The For-Profit System." In S. S. Sharfstein and A. Biegel (eds.), *The New Economics and Psychiatric Care*. Washington, D.C.: American Psychiatric Press, 1985.

144. Fisher, W., and others. "Case Mix in the 'Downsizing' State Hospital." *Psychiatric Services*, 1996, *47*, 255–262.

145. Thompson, T. G. "Report to Congress: Prospective Payment System for Inpatient Services in Psychiatric Hospitals and Exempt Units." Secretary of Health and Human Services, 2002. [http://www.cms.hhs.gov/providers/ipfpps/rptcongress.pdf].

146. Thompson (2002).

147. Thompson (2002).

148. Cromwell, J., and others. "A Modified TEFRA System for Psychiatric Facilities." In R. Frank and W. Manning (eds.), *Economics and Mental Health*. Baltimore: Johns Hopkins University Press, 1992.

149. Cromwell, J., and others. "Medicare Payments to Psychiatric Facilities: Unfair and Inefficient?" *Health Affairs*, Summer 1991, *10*, 124–134.

150. Lave, J., and others. "The Decision to Seek an Exemption from PPS." *Journal of Health Economics*, 1988, *7*, 163–171.

151. Thompson (2002).

152. http://www.cms.hhs.gov/media/press/release.asp?Counter=941 (July 5, 2005).

153. http://www.cms.hhs.gov/medicaid/managedcare/mcsten03.pdf (July 5, 2005).

154. Substance Abuse and Mental Health Services Administration. "Managed Care Tracking System." [http://www.samhsa.gov/mc/stateprfls] (Mar. 15, 2000).

155. Substance Abuse and Mental Health Services Administration (2000).

156. Mechanic, D., and McAlpine, D. "Mission Unfulfilled: Potholes on the Road to Mental Health Parity." *Health Affairs*, 1999, *18*(5), 7–21; Pincus, H., Zarin, D., and West, J. "Peering into the 'Black Box': Measuring Outcomes of Managed Care." *Archives of General Psychiatry*, 1996, *53*, 870–877; Lurie, N. "Studying Access to Care in Managed Care Environments." *Health Services Research*, 1997, *32*(5), 691–701.

157. Wagner, E. "Managed Care and Chronic Illness: Health Services Research Needs." *Health Services Research*, 1997, *32*(5), 702–714.

158. Frank, R., McGuire, T., and Newhouse, R. "Risk Contracts in Managed Mental Health Care." *Health Affairs*, Fall 1995, *14*, 50–64.

159. Beeuwkes-Buntin, M., and Blumenthal, D. "Carve-Outs for Medicare: Possible Benefits and Risks." In R. D. Reischauer, S. Butler, and J. R. Lave (eds.), *Medicare: Preparing for the Challenges of the 21st Century*. Washington, D.C.: National Academy of Social Insurance, 1998.

160. Drake and Osher (1997); Steadman and others (1998); Swanson (1994); Eronen, Anger-meyer, and Schulze (1998); Gelberg (1996); Kelleher and others (1994).

161. Sturm, R. "Tracking Changes in Behavioral Health Services: How Have Carve-Outs Changed Care?" *Journal of Behavioral Health Services Research*, 1999, *26*(4), 360–371; Mechanic and McAlpine (1999).

162. Goldman, W., and others. "Costs and Use of Mental Health Services Before and After Managed Care." *Health Affairs*, 1998, *17*(2), 40–52; Goldman, W., and others. "More Evidence for the Insurability of Managed Behavioral Health Care." *Health Affairs*, 1999, *18*(5), 172–181; Huskamp, H. A. "How a Managed Behavioral Health Care Carve-out Plan Affected Spending for Episodes of Treatment." *Psychiatric Services*, 1998, *49*(12), 1559–1562; Iglehart, J. K. "Managed Care and Mental Health." *New England Journal of Medicine*, 1996, *334*(2), 131–135; Ma, C. A., and McGuire, T. G. "Costs and Incentives in a Behavioral Health Carve-out." *Health Affairs*, 1998, *17*(2), 53–69; Rosenthal, M. B. "Risk Sharing in Managed Behavioral Health Care." *Health Affairs*, 1999, *18*(5), 204–213.

163. Goldman and others (1999); Grazier, K. L., and others. "Effects of a Mental Health Carve-out on Use, Costs, and Payers: A Four-Year Study." *Journal of Behavioral Health Services Research*, 1999, *26*(4), 381–389; Ma and McGuire (1998); Zuvekas, S. H., and others. "The Impacts of Mental Health Parity and Managed Care in One Large Employer Group." *Health Affairs*, 2002, *21*(3), 148–159.

164. Cuffel, B. J., and others. "Does Managing Behavioral Health Care Services Increase the Cost of Providing Medical Care?" *Journal of Behavioral Health Services Research*, 1999, *26*(4), 372–380.

165. Grazier and others (1999); Zuvekas and others (2002); Merrick, E. L. "Treatment of Major Depression Before and After Implementation of a Behavioral Health Carve-out Plan." *Psychiatric Services*, 1998, *49*(12), 1563–1567.

166. Sturm, R., and others. "Mental Health and Substance Abuse Parity: A Case Study of Ohio's State Employee Program." *Journal of Mental Health Policy Economics*, 1998, *3*(1), 129–134; Zuvekas and others (2002).

167. Merrick (1998); Stein, B., and others. "The Effect of Copayments on Drug and Alcohol Treatment Following Inpatient Detoxification Under Managed Care." *Psychiatric Services*, 2000, *51*(2), 195–198.

168. Sturm, R. "Cost and Quality Trends Under Managed Care: Is There a Learning Curve in Behavioral Health Carve-out Plans?" *Journal of Health Economics*, 1999, 18(*5*), 593–604.

169. Chang, C. F., and others. "Tennessee's Failed Managed Care Program for Mental Health and Substance Abuse Services." *Journal of the American Medical Association*, 1998, *279*(11), 864–869.

170. Manning, W., and others. "Outcomes for Medicaid Beneficiaries with Schizophrenia Under a Prepaid Mental Health Carve-out." *Journal of Behavioral Health Services and Research*, 1999, *26*(4), 442–450.

171. Ettner, S., and others. "Risk Adjustment of Mental Health and Substance Abuse Payments." *Inquiry*, 1998, *35*(2), 223–239.

172. Mechanic (1998); Mechanic and McAlpine (1999).

173. "What Is the Wellstone Act?" *Wellstone Action!* [http://www.wellstone.org/network/article_detail.aspx?itemID=3138&catID=2796] (accessed March 1, 2004).

174. "What Is the Wellstone Act?" *Wellstone Action!*

175. "The Mental Health Parity Act (of 1996)." *Centers for Medicare and Medicaid Services.* [http://www.cms.hhs.gov/hipaa/hipaa1/content/mhpa.asp#statutorytext] (accessed Feb. 15, 2005).

176. "The Mental Health Parity Act (of 1996)."

177. "The Mental Health Parity Act (of 1996)."

178. Levin, B., Hanson, A., Coe, R., and Taylor, A. *Mental Health Policy: 1998 National and State Perspectives.* Tampa, Fla.: The Loius de la Parte Florida Mental Health Institute, University of South Florida, March 25, 1998. Gitterman, D., Sturm, R., and Scheffler, R. "Toward Full Mental Health Parity and Beyond." *Health Affairs,* 2001, *20*(4), 68–76.

179. Levin, Hanson, Coe, and Taylor (1998).

180. Buck, J., Teich, J., Umland, B., and Stein, M. "Behavioral Health Benefits in Employer-Sponsored Health Plans." *Health Affairs,* 1999, *18*(2), 67–78.

181. Butler, P. "ERISA Preemption Manual for State Health Policy Makers." Washington, D.C.: National Academy for State Health Policy, 2000. [http://www.statecoverage.net/pdf/erisa2000.pdf] (accessed August 28, 2006).

182. Butler (2000).

183. Frank, R., and McGuire, T. "Economics and Mental Health." (working paper 7052.) Cambridge, Mass.: National Bureau of Economic Research, 1999.

184. Goldman, W., McCulloch, J., and Sturm, R. "Cost and Use of Mental Health Services Before and After Managed Care." *Health Affairs,* 1998, *17*(2), 40–52.

185. Sing, M., and Hill, S. "The Costs of Parity Mandates for Mental Health and Substance Abuse Insurance Benefits." *Psychiatric Services,* 2001, *52*(4), 437–440.

186. Sturm, R. "How Expensive Is Unlimited Mental Health Care Coverage under Managed Care?" *Journal of the American Medical Association,* 1997, *278*(18), 1533–1537.

187. Sturm, R., and Sherbourne, C. "Managed Care and Unmet Need for Mental Health and Substance Abuse Care in 1998." *Psychiatric Services,* 2000, *51*(2), 177; Colenda, C., Banazak, D., and Mickus, M. "Mental Health Services in Managed Care: Quality Questions Remain." *Geriatrics,* 1998, *53*, 46–63; Van Voorhees, B., Wang, N., and Ford, D. "Managed Care Organizational Complexity and Access to High Quality Mental Health Services: Perspective of U.S. Primary Care Physicians." *General Hospital Psychiatry,* 2003, *25*(3), 149–157.

188. Gitterman, D., Sturm, R., and Scheffler, R. "Toward Full Mental Health Parity and Beyond." *Health Affairs,* 2001, *20*(4), 68–76.

189. Senator Paul Wellstone Mental Health Equitable Treatment Act of 2003 (S. 486), [http://thomas.loc.gov/cgi-bin/query/z?c108:S.486]; Gonzalez, G. "Parity Advocates Aim to Close Loopholes in Mental Health Parity Law; Employers, Insurers Oppose Bill." *Business Insurance,* August 9, 2004, p. 4.

190. Gonzalez (2004).

191. Gonzalez (2004).

192. Link, J. C. "Policy Update: The Effort to Pass Stronger Federal Mental Health Parity Legislation." Unpublished manuscript, University of California, Los Angeles, 2005.

193. Mechanic, D. "Emerging Trends in Mental Health Policy and Practice." *Health Affairs,* 1998, *17*(6), 82–98.

194. Iglehart, J. "The Mental Health Maze and the Call for Transformation." *New England Journal of Medicine,* 2004, *350*(5), 507–514.

195. Executive order 13263 of Apr. 29, 2002: President's New Freedom Commission on Mental Health. *Federal Register,* 2002; *67*(86), 22337–22378.

196. Executive order 13263 (2002).

197. Inglehart (2004).

198. Inglehart (2004).

CHAPTER SEVENTEEN

# WOMEN'S HEALTH

## Key Issues in Access to Health Insurance Coverage and to Services Among Nonelderly Women

Roberta Wyn
Beatriz M. Solís

A ny debate on alternative solutions to increasing coverage and improving access needs to examine the specific implications for women. Although women and men share the same need for affordable, accessible, and quality care, there are specific health concerns and patterns of use unique to women that are often overlooked. Many health conditions are particular to women, occur with greater frequency among women, or have differing consequences for women than for men. All of this affects the amount and kind of health care services needed.

Women have a large stake in how health care services are financed and delivered. A woman is typically the coordinator of care for her family and assumes the major role for her children's health care activities.[1] Furthermore, her less advantaged and less stable economic status places her at particular financial risk for the costs of medical care.

This chapter examines some of the key policy factors related to financing and delivering health services for women who are under sixty-five years of age. First, we examine women's access to health insurance coverage, including current coverage patterns, analysis of the advantages and disadvantages of the current insuring system for women, and the economic importance of coverage. Second, we examine how health insurance coverage affects women's access to care. Last, we look beyond financial barriers to other aspects of the health care system that influence access. The population is limited to the nonelderly because much of this chapter focuses on health insurance coverage. Although women sixty-five and older also face health insurance access issues, nearly all older women have health insurance coverage through Medicare; many of their insurance coverage issues therefore differ.[2]

## Women's Access to Insurance Coverage

The mechanisms for obtaining health insurance coverage are embedded in complex social and economic situations that differ between women and men and among subgroups of women. The current health insurance structure in the United States is a voluntary system that relies primarily on health insurance obtained from one's own employment or the employment of a spouse or parent, augmented by individually purchased private insurance, and public systems for eligible low-income individuals and families (Medicaid) and for certain nonelderly disabled individuals and the elderly (Medicare). This patchwork of coverage options leaves many women dependent on coverage through a spouse, reliant on a changing public system, or uninsured. Even though women have a slightly lower rate of being uninsured than men (Table 17.1), they must often rely on complicated arrangements to obtain coverage.

The main source of coverage for women and men is through employment, obtained through one's own employment or that of a spouse or parent. Pairing

### TABLE 17.1. HEALTH INSURANCE COVERAGE BY GENDER, AGES EIGHTEEN TO SIXTY-FOUR, UNITED STATES, 2003.

| Health Insurance Coverage | Women, Percentage Covered | Men, Percentage Covered |
|---|---|---|
| Uninsured | 18 | 22 |
| Employment-based coverage, primary | 39 | 51 |
| Employment-based coverage, family | 28 | 15 |
| Privately purchased | 5 | 5 |
| Medicaid | 7 | 4 |
| Other coverage[a] | 3 | 3 |
| Total | 100 | 100 |

*Note:* [a] Medicare, CHAMPUS/VA, Indian Health Services, other types of coverage.

*Source:* Authors' analysis of the March 2004 Current Population Survey.

coverage with employment connects two distributive systems: work and insurance. Thus the factors that determine the distribution of jobs in this society also determine access to employment-based health insurance coverage.[3] This places women at a disadvantage in terms of primary coverage through their own employment because they have less attachment than men to the labor market.[4] Although nearly equal proportions of nonelderly women and men have employment-based coverage (67 percent for women and 66 percent for men; Table 17.1), women are twice as likely as men to be covered by family coverage (that is, through a spouse or parent) and less likely to have coverage directly through their own employer (39 percent of women versus 51 percent of men).[5] Women are also twice as likely as men to receive Medicaid (Table 17.1) because of income and eligibility requirements that women are more likely to meet.

Patterns of insurance coverage vary considerably by racial and ethnic background (Table 17.2). Women of color are less likely than white women to have employment-based coverage. Medicaid coverage only partly compensates for these lower employment-based coverage rates.

Yet even with Medicaid serving as a safety net, gaps in coverage persist. Black, Asian American and Pacific Islander (AAPI), American Indian and Alaskan Native (AIAN), and Latina women all have a higher uninsured rate than white women.

### TABLE 17.2. HEALTH INSURANCE COVERAGE BY RACE OR ETHNICITY, WOMEN AGES EIGHTEEN TO SIXTY-FOUR, UNITED STATES, 2003.

|  | *Percentage Covered* | | | | |
|  | AAPI[a] | AI/AN[b] | Black | Latina | White |
|---|---|---|---|---|---|
| Uninsured | 22 | 21 | 22 | 38 | 14 |
| Employment-based coverage, primary | 35 | 31 | 43 | 26 | 41 |
| Employment-based coverage, dependent | 30 | 19 | 14 | 19 | 32 |
| Privately purchased | 7 | 2 | 2 | 3 | 5 |
| Medicaid | 4 | 13 | 15 | 12 | 5 |
| Other coverage[c] | 2 | 14 | 4 | 2 | 3 |
| Total | 100 | 100 | 100 | 100 | 100 |

Notes:
[a] AAPI = Asian American and Pacific Islander;

[b] AIAN = American Indian and Alaskan Native.

[c] Medicare, CHAMPUS/VA, Indian Health Services, other types of coverage.

*Source:* Authors' analysis of the March 2004 Current Population Survey.

Several other groups of women are also at greater risk of being uninsured, low-income women particularly. Approximately four in ten poor women (family income at or below the poverty level) and one-third of near-poor women (family income 101–200 percent of poverty) are uninsured.[6] Other groups at greater risk of being uninsured include younger women; those without a high school education; women who are single parents; those who are foreign-born; and women who are not employed, work part-time, or are self-employed.[7]

## Issues with Women's Current Coverage Options

Changes in both private sector and public health coverage influence women's access to health coverage. The rapid rise in health care costs can have a disproportionate effect on women. They have lower income than men and are more likely to have a health care expenditure.[8] Medicaid and the private health insurance market have seen increasing health care costs.[9] Since 2001, employers have been experiencing double-digit increases in health care premiums,[10] from 2003 to 2004 rising 11.2 percent—lower than for 2002–03 (13.9 percent) but still double-digit growth, and at a rate higher than overall inflation and wage gains. Further, and of particular consequence to women, family coverage premiums since 2000 have gone up faster (59 percent) than inflation (9.7 percent) and wage growth (12.3 percent). Given the rise in premiums, four in ten employers reported that were "very likely" or "somewhat likely" to increase the share of the premium that employees must pay for family coverage in the next two years. These rate jumps have led some employers, especially those in small firms of 3–199 workers, to question their role in and responsibility for financing health insurance for an employee's family.[11]

During this period of high premium growth, there was a decline in the percentage of workers who received health coverage from their employers (65 percent in 2001 to 61 percent in 2004), driven mainly by a decline in the number of small firms that offer coverage.[12]

Medicaid coverage is also vulnerable to economic constraints that restrict spending and growth. Medicaid is an important program for low-income women overall, constituting an important source of financing for health care, including family planning services.[13] Women's greater use of public programs and their lower income relative to men make them disproportionately affected by changes in public policy that reduce access to health-related programs. In response to budget pressures, nearly all states have implemented, or plan to implement, cost containment measures to stem the growth of Medicaid spending, through such approaches as reduced provider rates, prescription medicine cost controls, reduction in eligibility, and limitation of benefits.[14]

A major change that has occurred in Medicaid during the past decade is the shift from fee-for-service to a managed care delivery system. In 2004, 61 percent of Medicaid recipients were enrolled in managed care, an increase from 48 percent in 1997.[15] The populations enrolled in these managed care plans are primarily adults in families (the majority of whom are women) and children.

Many features of managed care, such as its focus on coordinated care and emphasis on primary care, have the potential to improve access for the Medicaid population. Yet studies comparing Medicaid fee-for-service and Medicaid managed care show mixed results, with some measures recording improvement for women enrolled in managed care and others showing little difference or a decrease in some services under certain mandatory programs.[16]

Another major change over the past decade that has affected women's access to Medicaid is passage of the Personal Responsibility and Work Opportunity Reconciliation Act of 1996 (PRWORA), known as welfare reform. This legislation replaced Aid to Families with Dependent Children (AFDC) with Temporary Assistance to Needy Families (TANF), a time-limited assistance program. This legislation also severed the automatic link between welfare and Medicaid, tying Medicaid to income and resources instead.[17]

# Cost as a Barrier

The costs of care are cited by some women as the reason for not receiving or delaying care. One study found that approximately one-quarter of women delayed or went without care during for a year because they could not afford it.[18] Women with limited resources were the most likely to report cost concerns. Cost also affected women's use of prescription medicines, with about 20 percent reporting that in a one-year period they did not fill a prescription medicine because of costs.[19]

Having insurance coverage does not guarantee that medical or preventive services are affordable. Lack of coverage for specific health services and out-of-pocket expenses for medical care and plan deductibles raise the financial risk for insured women. Low-income adults are more likely to be underinsured than those with higher income, and underinsurance leads to access problems similar to being uninsured.[20]

Despite state coverage mandates, there are benefit gaps in private coverage. For example, although most states require private plans to cover breast cancer screening, the mandate for other screenings such as cervical cancer and osteoporosis is more limited.[21] Prescription drug coverage has become standard in employer-based plans, but prescription contraceptives are less likely to be covered. Several states have taken steps to improve access. Approximately one-half of states have implemented a contraceptive coverage mandate requiring insurers to cover prescription contraceptives to the same extent they cover other prescription medicines. Some of these states include an exemption for employers or insurers having moral or religious objections to contraception.[22]

## Health Insurance Coverage and Women's Access to Services

Several studies have documented the relationship between insurance coverage and access to care.[23] Uninsured women are much less likely than those with health insurance coverage to have had a doctor visit in the past year or a regular place where they receive care. Women who lack health insurance coverage are less likely than those with coverage to receive such screenings as a blood pressure test, blood cholesterol check, clinical breast examination, mammography, or a Pap test. Many uninsured women also have low income, a factor associated with elevated risk for some of the conditions that these screenings are intended to discover. Thus the burden of paying for preventive services often falls on those women who are least able to afford such costs. Lack of insurance coverage may well force women and medical providers to prioritize urgent health care problems, compromising access to preventive screenings. This creates an ineffective health care system, one in which advances in prevention and early diagnosis are not fully and adequately used.

A further indicator of access for women is use of prenatal services. Studies have documented that uninsured women do not receive adequate prenatal services, as measured by the point during pregnancy when care was initiated and the number of physician visits throughout the pregnancy. There are large differences in access to prenatal care between uninsured and privately insured women. Even though publicly insured women receive more care than those with no coverage, it is not as much as women with private coverage.[24]

More attention is being paid to the effect of lack of health insurance on health outcomes. For example, women without health insurance coverage have a more advanced stage of breast cancer at diagnosis and, among those with local and regional disease, poorer survival than women with private coverage.[25] Other studies have shown that lack of coverage affects birth outcomes among women,[26] the risk of in-hospital mortality (for men and women),[27] and receipt of diagnostic and therapeutic procedures for coronary disease.[28]

A 2002 report by the Institute of Medicine synthesizes the research evidence contrasting the health of the insured and uninsured (both men and women) and found that those without health insurance are more likely to receive too little medical care, be in worse health and die sooner, and receive poorer care when they are in the hospital.[29] The report cites several examples of inadequate care received by the uninsured. They include how the uninsured, more often than the insured, go without cancer screening, do not receive recommendations for chronic disease management, lack regular access to medications for chronic disease management, and receive fewer diagnostic and treatment services after traumatic injury or heart attack. The report concludes that insuring the uninsured would likely promote use of timely preventive care, foster access to a regular source of care, improve health status, and reduce the risk of dying prematurely. Further, particular benefit would accrue to racial and ethnic groups and those with low income who often lack stable coverage and have the poorest health status.

## Additional Factors Affecting Use

There are other access barriers that women report in addition to the cost of services. Studies indicate the importance of having a regular connection to the health care system. Having a usual source of care is associated with women's increased use of clinical preventive services and general medical checkups, even among insured women.[30]

Access to a regular provider of care is also an important component of women's health. Women's health care has been characterized as fragmented; many women typically see more than one provider for primary care needs in part because women's health is often split into reproductive needs and all other needs.[31] Nearly half of women with a regular provider have at least one other health provider they see routinely.[32] For many women, this other provider is an obstetrician/gynecologist (ob/gyn). To facilitate access to reproductive health care, many states have required managed care plans to allow women direct access to an ob/gyn without requiring a primary care referral.[33]

Practice and referral patterns of physicians are important determinants of using clinical preventive services for women; nearly three-quarters of women who have mammograms reported a physician recommendation as the reason for the screening.[34]

Factors such as transportation problems and lack of availability of child care also impede women's access to care, as do time constraints.[35] Multiple roles and responsibilities compete for women's time. Women often make trade-offs to allocate the time and resources available. One study found that a quarter of women who did not receive a recommended clinical preventive service reported time constraints as a factor.[36]

Language and cultural barriers also affect both access to the system and services once in the system. An Institute of Medicine study assessed the extent of disparities in health care services received by racial and ethnic groups (men and women). Through a synthesis of the literature, the study found disparities in the rate of medical procedure use between racial and ethnic groups on the one hand and nonminorities on the other, and that the former received lower-quality health care, even when access-related factors such as health insurance were taken into account.[37]

## Policy Implications and Future Research

The current insurance system leaves many women uninsured; low-income women and women of color are especially at risk of not having insurance coverage. Women without insurance coverage are at serious risk of delaying or not receiving needed care and of not being screened for early detection of disease. Costs remain a barrier even for insured women, suggesting that any coverage imposing large deductibles and co-insurance obligations would hinder use of necessary services, especially for economically disadvantaged women. Lack of coverage for specific services also reduces the use of necessary care, such as preventive screenings. These problems with benefit coverage emphasize the importance of comprehensive coverage.

Particular consideration of low-income women is required in formulating new health policy regarding financing of services. For example, they have had the lowest rate of screening for certain clinical preventive and are often most vulnerable to the effects of costs. To address this problem, the Breast and Cervical Cancer Mortality Prevention Act of 1990 was passed to pay for breast and cervical cancer screening and diagnosis for uninsured and low-income women. More recently, the Prevention and Treatment Act of 2000 enables states to provide full Medicaid benefits to eligible low-income women diagnosed with breast or cervical cancer.[38]

The states play an important in addressing benefit coverage issues in the private and public sectors.[39] State policies can mandate private insurers to cover certain benefits, although these mandates apply only to certain health plans that are not "self-funded."

As well, states administer their own Medicaid programs within federal guidelines, setting policies that establish such areas as eligibility level, optional benefits, provider payment, and program expansion.

In addition to financial access to health services, organization of health care needs to facilitate access to a regular source and provider of care to increase the continuity of care women receive. Appropriate incentives need to be in place in the health care system to encourage physician promotion of primary and preventive care.

Improvement in monitoring and reporting quality-of-care indicators for women by age, race and ethnicity, primary language, and income are needed to further discover disparities and develop incentive programs and resources to improve patient care.

Consumer assessments of health care are used by health plans, health care providers, and purchasers of care (both governmental and employer groups) as an indicator of the quality of care provided to patients. These are important tools for health care providers. However, to maximize their relevance in addressing women's experiences, they need to be fielded in languages other than English and at literacy levels that reach all patients.

In addition to the financial and structural barriers that women face, many women experience competing social roles and responsibilities that interfere with their own needs for appropriate health care. They report time constraints as a deterrent to use of services. Some of these barriers can be addressed by the health care system; extending hours, bringing services into the community where women live and work, providing culturally and linguistically appropriate services, and promoting child care access could remove some of these barriers.

Facilitating access to the health care system is only part of the process of improving the health of women. Attention to the current pace of change in the health care delivery system is needed to understand women's health. If the structure of care is fragmented; lacks mechanisms to ensure comprehensive, coordinated care; and limits quality measurement or improvement activities that are relevant to women's health, this can further limit our perspective on women's health. Women's health advocates have often focused on key areas that continue to be relevant to women's health today, such as emphasis on primary care and prevention, a patient-centered or consumer approach to health care delivery with greater emphasis on communication, and service and satisfaction.[40]

Additional research is needed on the coordination and process of care once a woman is in the health care system and receiving care. We must continue to investigate disparities in access to services, treatment approaches, and clinical outcomes between women and men, and among subgroups of women, to understand and eliminate their causes in the health care system.

# Notes

1. Salganicoff, A., Ranji, U., and Wyn, R. *Women and Health Care: A National Profile.* Menlo Park, Calif.: Henry J. Kaiser Family Foundation, 2005.
2. Henry J. Kaiser Family Foundation. *Key Facts: Women and Medicare.* Menlo Park, Calif.: Henry J. Kaiser Family Foundation, 2001.
3. Jecker, N. S. "Can an Employer-Based Health Insurance System Be Just?" *Journal of Health Politics, Policy, and Law,* 1993, *18*(3), 657–673.
4. U.S. Department of Labor, Women's Bureau. "Women in the Labor Force in 2004," 2005. [www.dol.gov/wb].

5. Based on authors' analyses of the March 2004 Current Population Survey.
6. Salganicoff, Ranji, and Wyn (2005).
7. Altman, B., and Taylor, A. *Women in the Health Care System: Health Status, Insurance, and Access to Care.* (MEPS Research Findings, no. 17. AHRQ pub. no. 02-0004.) Rockville, Md.: Agency for Healthcare Research and Quality, 2001; Henry J. Kaiser Family Foundation. *Women's Health Insurance Coverage, Women's Health Policy Facts.* Menlo Park, Calif.: Henry J. Kaiser Family Foundation, 2004; Salganicoff, Ranji, and Wyn (2005).
8. Altman and Taylor (2001); U.S. Department of Health and Human Services, Health Resources and Services Administration. *Women's Health USA 2005.* Rockville, Md.: U.S. Department of Health and Human Services, 2005.
9. Kaiser Commission on Medicaid and the Uninsured. *State Budget Constraints: The Impact on Medicaid.* Washington, D.C.: Henry J. Kaiser Family Foundation, 2003.
10. Claxton, G., and others. *Employer Health Benefits: 2004 Annual Survey.* Menlo Park, ,Calif.: Henry J. Kaiser Family Foundation, and Chicago: Health Research and Educational Trust, 2004.
11. Claxton and others (2004).
12. Claxton and others (2004).
13. Rowland, D., and Salganicoff, A. *The Key to the Door: Medicaid's Role in Improving Health Care for Women and Children.* Menlo Park, Calif.: Henry J. Kaiser Family Foundation, 1999; Gold, R., Richards C., Ranji, U., and Salganicoff, A. *Medicaid: A Critical Source of Support for Family Planning in the United States.* New York: Alan Guttmacher Institute, and Menlo Park, Calif.: Henry J. Kaiser Family Foundation, 2004.
14. Kaiser Commission on Medicaid and the Uninsured (2003); Henry J. Kaiser Family Foundation. *The Medicaid Program at a Glance.* Menlo Park, Calif.: Henry J. Kaiser Family Foundation, 2005.
15. Centers for Medicare and Medicaid Services. *Managed Care Trends* (2004 Medicaid Managed Care Enrollment Report.) Washington, D.C., 2004.
16. Salganicoff, A., Wyn, R., and Solis, B. "Medicaid Managed Care and Low-Income Women: Implications for Access and Satisfaction." *Women's Health Issues,* 1998, *8,* 339–349; Garrett, B., and Zuckerman, S. "National Estimates of the Effects of Mandatory Medicaid Managed Care Programs on Health Care Access and Use, 1997-1999." *Medical Care,* 2005, *43*(7), 649-657.
17. Levin-Epstein, J. *Welfare, Women, and Health: The Role of Temporary Assistance for Needy Families.* Menlo Park, Calif.: Henry J. Kaiser Family Foundation, 2003.
18. Salganicoff, A., Beckerman, Z., Wyn, R., and Ojeda, V. *Women's Health in the United States: Health Coverage and Access to Care.* Menlo Park, Calif.: Henry J. Kaiser Family Foundation, 2002.
19. Salganicoff, Ranji, and Wyn (2005).
20. Schoen, C., Doty, M., Collins, S., and Holmgren, A. "Insured But Not Protected: How Many Adults Are Underinsured?" *Health Affairs,* 2005, Web exclusive, w5-289-w5-302, June 14, 2005.
21. Berlin, M., and others. *Women's Access to Care: A State-Level Analysis of Key Health Policies.* Washington, D.C.: National Women's Law Center, and Menlo Park, Calif.: Henry J. Kaiser Family Foundation, 2003; Henry J. Kaiser Family Foundation (2004).
22. Alan Guttmacher Institute. *Insurance Coverage of Contraceptives: State Policies in Brief.* New York: Guttmacher Institute, 2005.
23. Altman and Taylor (2001); Breen, N., and others. "Progress in Cancer Screening over a Decade: Results of Cancer Screening from the 1987, 1992, and 1998 National Health

Interview Surveys." *Journal of the National Cancer Institute*, 2001, *93*(22), 1704-1713; Salganicoff, Ranji, and Wyn (2005).

24. Institute of Medicine (IOM). *Health Insurance is a Family Matter.* Washington, D.C.: National Academies Press, 2002.

25. Ayanian, J., Kohler, B. A., Abe, T., and Epstein, A. M. "The Relation Between Health Insurance Coverage and Clinical Outcomes Among Women with Breast Cancer." *New England Journal of Medicine*, 1993, *329*(5), 326–331.

26. Braverman, P., and others. "Adverse Outcomes and Lack of Health Insurance Among Newborns in an Eight-County Area of California, 1982–1986." *New England Journal of Medicine*, 1989, *321*(8), 508–513.

27. Hadley, J., Steinberg, E. P., and Feder, J. "Comparison of Uninsured and Privately Insured Hospital Patients: Condition on Admissions, Resource Use, and Outcome." *Journal of the American Medical Association*, 1991, *265*(3), 374–379.

28. Daumit, G., Hermann, J., and Powe, N. "Relation of Gender and Health Insurance to Cardiovascular Procedure Use in Persons with Progression of Chronic Renal Disease." *Medical Care*, 2000, *38*(4), 354–365.

29. Institute of Medicine (IOM). *Care Without Coverage: Too Little, Too Late.* Washington, D.C.: National Academies Press, 2002.

30. Brown, E. R., and others. "Women's Health-Related Behaviors and Use of Preventive Services." (Report to the Commonwealth Fund.) New York: Commonwealth Fund, Commission on Women's Health, 1995.

31. Clancy, C. M., and Massion, C. T. "American Women's Health Care: A Patchwork Quilt with Gaps." *Journal of the American Medical Association*, 1992, *268*(14), 1918–1920.

32. Salganicoff, Ranji, and Wyn (2005).

33. Berlin and others (2003).

34. Romans, M. C., and others. "Utilization of Screening Mammography 1990." *Women's Health Issues*, 1991, *1*(2), 68–73.

35. Salganicoff, Ranji, and Wyn (2005).

36. Wyn, R., Brown, E. R., and Yu, H. "Women's Use of Preventive Health Services." In M. Falik and K. Scott Collins (eds.), *Women's Health: The Commonwealth Fund Survey.* Baltimore, Md.: Johns Hopkins University Press, 1996.

37. Institute of Medicine (IOM). *Unequal Treatment: Confronting Racial and Ethnic Disparities in Health Care.* Washington, D.C.: National Academies Press, 2002.

38. Berlin and others (2003).

39. Berlin and (others 2003).

40. Zimmerman, M., and Hill, S. "Reforming Gendered Health Care: An Assessment of Change." *International Journal of Health Services*, 2000, *30*(4), 771–795.

CHAPTER EIGHTEEN

# HOMELESS PERSONS

Lisa Arangua
Lillian Gelberg

Homelessness has reached crisis proportions in the United States today. It is estimated that 3.5 million people are currently without a home.[1] However, the crisis is much worse than this; 14 percent of the U.S. population (26 million people) have been homeless at some time in their lives and 5 percent (8.5 million people) have been homeless within the past five years.[2] Although the homeless are a growing and especially needy population, they are in some ways disturbingly similar to the rest of us. The majority live in central cities, but 21 percent live in suburban areas and 9 percent in rural areas.[3] Los Angeles is known as the homeless capital, although some would argue that New York holds this infamous distinction. Most of the homeless persons of Los Angeles are long-time residents of the city and are similar to housed persons in their place of birth, citizenship status, and length of residence in Los Angeles County (with 86 percent living in Los Angeles for ten years or more).[4] This chapter profiles the homeless, examines their health status and access to health care, and proposes an integrative approach for homeless health policy.

## History of Homelessness

A discussion of how the United States has dealt with the homeless is relevant because homeless policies have come full circle. The picture of the homeless population of the United States has changed over the years. Homelessness was first encountered in colonial North America because of rapid economic changes, fluctuations in immigration and seasonal and wage labor, and sickness and disease. An increasing number of families reached a level of destitution. There was no in-kind or cash aid for the destitute. As a result, the colonies became deluged with people who had marginal means to survive.[5]

In American history, there have been three basic responses to homelessness (patterned after English poor law principles): contractual relief, outdoor relief (basic assistance given outside a public institution), and public poorhouses (also known as indoor relief). In this early period of American history, a clear distinction was made between the deserving and undeserving poor—a distinction that still endures today. The principle of the deserving and undeserving poor was based on a narrowly defined perspective of individual limitations. The undeserving poor (referred to in colonial times as paupers) were considered idle and able-bodied, and their inability to support themselves or their family was an individual and moral failure. Advocates harnessed a public fear that undeserving able-bodied malingerers would "free-ride" on other citizens. Policies for the undeserving poor never focused on systemic failures as a cause of poverty but instead placed blame on the moral degeneracy of the individual. As Cotton Mather put it, "For those who indulge themselves in idleness, the express command of God unto us is, that we should let them starve."[6]

The earliest American policies on relief to the homeless or near-homeless were contractual relief and outdoor relief. One form of contractual relief was an arrangement whereby contractors signed an annual contract to house paupers in return for work in their own home or a "work house" bought by the community. Even minimally able-bodied persons on contractual relief were required to work.[7] Similar but less regulated arrangements involved public auction of paupers. Auction winners cared for paupers in their household for a year at a fixed rate of reimbursement, and the paupers acted as indentured servants.[8]

Outdoor relief provided such things as food, clothing, firewood, or a "chit" (voucher) for medical care to nearly homeless people who remained in their own home or lived with friends or relatives in the community.[9] Those in need applied for outdoor relief to a local elected official, usually called a poormaster. Both forms of homeless relief were sustained from colonial times to around the 1820s.

By the early 1800s, critics came to believe that outdoor relief in particular helped to sustain idleness and dependency. According to Alexis de Tocqueville, the outdoor relief system bred the very condition it sought to remedy: "man had a natural passion for idleness," he wrote, and by providing the means of subsistence outdoor relief freed people from an obligation to work.[10] Critics of poor relief policies sought reduction in aid as a means of encouraging work. This period

was fueled by a strong religious revival, which harbored a belief that the undeserving poor who relied on outdoor relief could be reformed.

During the 1820s and 1830s several reports produced by separate state commissions indicated that a poorhouse system would be much more efficient than
outdoor relief or contracts for the care of paupers. The Quincy Report of 1821 in
Massachusetts, the Yates Report of 1824 in New York,[11] and the Board of
Guardians of the Poor Report of 1827 in Pennsylvania resulted in laws that required use of poorhouses as opposed to contractual or outdoor relief.[12] Other
states also followed suit with similar laws. Reformers felt that the very existence
of outdoor relief deterred the able-bodied from self-sufficiency; hence relief was
a threat to the work ethic.[13] The poorhouse would require residents to work within
their capabilities. Attitudes toward the undeserving poor were best summed up in
the Royal Poor Law Commission Report of 1834, which stated that "while relief
should not be denied the poor, life should be so miserable for them that they would
rather work than accept public aid."[14] Current block grant and entitlement policies for the poor (that is, welfare and shelter relief) continue to allude to these same
principals.[15]

However, most people on relief were not the undeserving poor described by
reformers.[16] Very few of those who received relief could work. Most were in fact
single mothers, children, the aged, or the sick. At the poorhouses, mothers and
children were mixed together with substance abusers and the mentally ill. Reformers later perceived the poorhouses as a more expensive and less effective form
of relief. The rehabilitation rate was low, and mortality high.[17]

By the early 1900s, theories regarding the destitute took on a less draconian
posture. There was less emphasis on differentiating between deserving and undeserving poor. Idle, able-bodied people were considered victims of structural forces
beyond their control (limited work opportunities, poor educational upbringing,
increasingly unaffordable housing). Jacob Riis, a reporter for the *New York Tribune,*
wrote in the 1890s about the burgeoning number of homeless in New York and
how work limitations had much to do with the increase of homelessness: "The
calculation that more than nine thousand homeless young men lodge nightly along
Chatham Street and the Bowery, is not far off the way. Nearly all are young men
fresh from good homes with honest hopes of getting a start in the city and making way for themselves. Few know anything about the city and its labor pitfalls."[18]
In the classic article on the homeless in the 1918 *Annals of American Academy of Political and Social Science,* Stuart Rice, the superintendent of New York's Municipal
Lodging House, reports, "The problem with the homeless is primarily one of labor
and housing rather than of social case work. . . . The homeless work for a much
lower rate of compensation than is paid for equivalent work elsewhere. . . . They

go hither and thither to rough uncomfortable places to do the dirty work to provide civilized comforts for us. . . . only they are willing to accept the work and hours
demanded. Meanwhile, they live in the bunkhouses."[19] Rice also gives one of the
first accounts of the culture of homelessness: "Everything in the lives of homeless
men and women drives them in the direction of dependency and parasitivism. The
living and working conditions in which the homeless perform react disastrously
upon their character and even make them subject to social case treatment."[20]

These structuralist theories of the early part of the 1900s profiled the homeless as a population that was victim to external circumstance. To mitigate the
causes and consequences of homelessness would require aggressive social policies.
This viewpoint would be pitted against the individual-limitations perspective to
fuel an entrenched debate on the causes of homelessness that still exists today.

From the structuralist arguments on the homeless emerged new forms of relief that set the foundation for the U.S. social safety net system. The rationale for
these new forms of relief was that the structural forces causing the homeless condition were mutable through income maintenance and other services. The landmark Social Security Act of 1935 established the fundamental structure of the
social safety net. The Social Security Act made available retirement benefits, unemployment compensation, and health and welfare programs. These benefits furnished health and income maintenance for many of those who would otherwise
need poorhouse placement. By 1935, the poorhouse population was reduced to
the severely ill and frail elderly as well as the permanently disabled. When poorhouses as such eventually closed, they retained their population and became our
current nursing home facilities.[21]

The American social safety net system ultimately provided mainly for the
"more deserving poor": the elderly, the severely disabled, and custodial parents.
This left mostly single men to occupy the ranks of the homeless. By the early
1940s, a combination of the safety net programs and the option of soldiering during the war effort depleted the number of homeless people.[22] In the mid-1940s
and 1950s, the homeless consisted mainly of middle-aged white men who inhab-
ited skid row areas of major urban cities.[23] Skid rows, which were once a way station for transient young seasonal laborers, became populated by a more stationary
group of homeless single men working at odd jobs in and around the city. Shelters sprang up to meet some of their housing needs.[24] The typical homeless man
in skid row in the 1950s and 1960s was thought to be a hopeless alcoholic. However, sociological studies showed that the majority of men were sober, and many
worked at least part time in day-to-day jobs.[25]

Anthropologist Kim Hopper and urban planner Jill Hamberg argue that a
"perfect storm" of deindustrialization (loss of well-paid industrial jobs to cheaper
labor markets overseas), economic downturn, sharp reduction in affordable hous-

ing, and steep cuts in public programs for the poor came together beginning in the late 1970s and accelerated rapidly in the 1980s and 1990s, causing a spike in the number of people living in poverty (up 40 percent from 1978 to 1983) and a rapid rise in homelessness.[26] Reduction in welfare benefits, relative to inflation, resulted in an increase in the number of homeless families. Gentrification, a shrinking affordable housing stock, and deindustrialization resulting in massive unemployment and larger numbers of homeless who were members of minority groups. Not since the Great Depression had we seen so many homeless and such a broad cross-section of society represented.[27] The burgeoning problem of homelessness raised public interest and gave impetus to provision of public and private funds to study the causes and consequences of the homeless condition.

At the turn of the millennium, the historical record combined with a massive body of empirical evidence on the homeless to breed a new dominant integrative structuralist/individual-limitation framework in which to influence policy. The evidence revealed that the cumulative burden of multiple individual and structural limitations leaves certain individuals vulnerable to the homeless condition. Structurally, since the 1970s the intersection of a growing pool of vulnerable poor people and an ever-shrinking stock of affordable housing inevitably left those with multiple individual limitations and diminished institutional supports (familial and safety net resources) less able to compete for limited housing. Studies tracking the homeless for a two year period or more find that the vast majority of homeless people exit homelessness within a short period of time, but recidivism (those who exit homelessness but return to it) is high. It is highest among single males (50 percent) and single females (33 percent) and lowest among adults with children in their care (22 percent).[28]

Subsidized housing and subsidized supportive housing interventions reduce recidivism. The vast majority of homeless people placed in subsidized housing stay housed. A 1998 study by Marybeth Shinn found that five years after requesting shelter, 80 percent of families who received some form of subsidized housing were stably housed (defined as being in their own place for a year without a move).[29] In a six-city study in 1995, psychologist Debra Rog reported that 86 percent of families who received both subsidized housing and services were in the same housing eighteen months later.[30] The same rates were found for single homeless adults with mental illness or a substance use disorder. Researcher Cheryl Zlotnick wrote that subsidized housing and income predicted housing stability for single homeless adults, half of whom had a mental health or substance use diagnosis, but case management did not.[31] Michael Hulburt related similar results in his 1996 study of the seriously mentally ill, where subsidized housing was highly related to stability of independent living.[32] Also in New York, psychologists Tsemberis and Asmussen concluded in 1999 that a program housing individuals with serious mental illness (SMI) in their own apartments, without any prerequisites for treatment or sobriety, and with services under their control, reduced homelessness better than programs where participation in treatment was mandatory.[33]

Current federal policy aims to end chronic homelessness among single adults with a disabling condition who have experienced homelessness continuously for a year or more, or four times during a period of three years.[34] The policy directs resources to local jurisdictions to help this subgroup with permanent affordable housing and treatment for their medical, mental health, and substance abuse problems. It focuses on the 10 percent of the homeless population who endure the cumulative burden of multiple individual and structural limitations and are vulnerable to chronic homelessness.[35] For this group of heavy service users, the aim is that homelessness should be treated appropriately as a chronic relapsing disease, using similar management plans as are used for chronic medical illnesses such as diabetes.

Despite the low rate of recidivism among homeless families, there is some concern that their exclusion from current federal policy response will reduce them to an afterthought, especially as they compete for limited affordable housing resources with their chronically homeless brethren. Policy makers should extend resources to prevent chronic homelessness among homeless families—many of whom are newly homeless—who also have disabling health problems similar to the chronically homeless. Moreover, empirical evidence has shown a striking negative health, psychological, and educational impact that the homeless condition has on the lives of children.[36] This illustrates the importance of preventing and treating encounters with homelessness among impoverished families. The homeless condition should not be treated as merely part of poverty but one of the more devastating consequences of poverty that must be actively avoided in the lives of children. Much has been learned in the decades since families first entered the ranks of the homeless. Much less has been done to mitigate the causes and consequences of family homelessness.

The words of Stuart Rice in 1918 that "the problem with the homeless is primarily one of labor and housing" remain a persistent issue with the homeless today. Through a body of empirical evidence, we have developed greater understanding of potential strategies involving provision of subsidized housing, sometimes with additional services, in ending homelessness for various groups. The empirical evidence (to be made evident in this chapter) has also shown a clear link between housing and health, as well as a gradient in health among the homeless, especially among those who have become part of the culture of homelessness. What remains is the will to translate these understandings into broad policy initiatives capable of preventing homelessness and its attending health woes and ameliorating it when it occurs.

# A Profile of the Homeless

## Demographic Characteristics

Whereas in the recent past the homeless population consisted primarily of middle-aged alcoholic white men, the distant past has become prologue to the current demographic profile of a homeless population that includes women and children as well as men. About two-thirds of the currently homeless are single men (67 percent) and 20 percent are single women.[37] Further, 34 percent of homeless women and 8 percent of homeless men are currently married.[38] Fifteen percent of homeless persons are parents with children.[39] Sixty percent of homeless women and 41 percent of homeless men have at least one minor child, but of them only 39 percent of women and 3 percent of men currently have those children with them.[40]

A majority of the currently homeless are between the ages of twenty-five and forty-four. Most homeless children (62 percent) are under the age of eight. Only 1 percent of the homeless are unaccompanied youths or teen parents under the age of eighteen, and only 2 percent are older than sixty-five.[41] However, recent research suggests that the homeless population is aging. In the 1990s, the average age of the homeless was mid-30s, whereas in 2003 the average age was in the mid-40s. Older street-dwelling homeless persons have a high mortality rate (30 percent of these sixty-plus-year-olds died within the four-year observation period), raising issues of competency and guardianship to protect them.[42] With the expected doubling of the elderly in the general population over the next few decades, we can expect a doubling of the elderly in the homeless population as well.

About 23 percent of homeless persons are veterans.[43] Male veterans are at increased risk for homelessness (male veterans have 1.25 the odds of being homeless relative to male nonveterans),[44] and post-Vietnam era male veterans are most at risk for homelessness.[45] Women veterans have a much greater risk of homelessness (two to four times the odds of women nonveterans), and it was the Vietnam-era women veterans who were most at risk for homelessness.[46] The effect on onset of homelessness among men and women who have served in the military in more recent wars remains to be determined.

Homeless persons are severely lacking in the educational and financial resources necessary to access health care. Thirty-nine percent have not graduated from high school, 34 percent have a high school diploma or GED, and 28 percent have some post–high school education.[47] Further, in 1996 the mean monthly income for homeless families was $475, 46 percent of the federal poverty line for a family of three. Single homeless persons reported a mean monthly income of $348, 51 percent of the federal poverty level for one person.[48] Despite their low income, only 28 percent of homeless persons receive income maintenance.[49] Further, 55 percent do not have medical insurance, compared to 32 percent of formerly homeless persons and 17 percent of the general population.[50]

## Course of Homelessness

From a public policy standpoint, it is important to distinguish between the incidence and the course of homelessness.[51] Half of the homeless population may be considered newly homeless (homeless one year or less), and one-fifth are long-term homeless (more than two years).[52] The distinction between homeless and non-homeless-impoverished is not a clear one, since people cycle in and out of homelessness during their lifetime.[53] However, most preventive policies have focused on the conditions of the long-term homeless (mental illness, substance abuse, and criminal activity), a population overrepresented in enumeration samples of homeless persons. The consequences of focusing on the long-term homeless are not only punitive policies that attribute social problems to individual shortcomings, as the history of homeless policies attests to, but policies that have limited impact on the incidence of homelessness. This distinction between long-term and short-term homelessness redirects policy to focus on variations in the homeless population—why people become homeless, why some cycle in and out of homelessness, and why some remain homeless for a long period of time—rather than focusing on providing housing as a first step.[54] For example, in New York City shelters, even though recurrent shelter stays for homeless women were related to (1) a history of domestic violence, (2) young women giving birth within the past year, (3) having young children, or (4) having children who are not with their mother or who join or leave their mother while she is in a shelter, it was having permanent housing of their own that constituted the strongest protection against cycling back into homelessness.[55]

The shortage of adequate affordable housing is the major precipitating factor for homelessness. The theory is that increases in income inequality working through the housing market is the root cause of homelessness, according to economists from the Public Policy Institute of California. A greater number of poor people creates more demand for low-cost and low-quality housing, which drives up the prices of such housing. "The resulting higher rents for abandonment-quality housing imply a higher cut-off income, below which homelessness is preferred to conventional housing."[56]

Unemployment, personal or family life crisis, rent going up out of proportion to inflation, and reduction in public benefits can also directly result in the loss of a home.[57] Early findings on the impact of recent federal welfare reform policies show that reduction or elimination of public assistance benefits resulted in homelessness.[58] Illness, on the other hand, tends to result from the homeless condition. Evidence has shown that persons with longer percentage of their lifetime spent homeless have worse health, compared to those with less percentage of their lifetime spent homeless.[59] Other indirect precipitants of homelessness are deinstitutionalization from a public mental hospital, substance abuse, and overcrowded prisons and jails from which prisoners who are not self-sufficient are often released.[60] Vangeest and colleagues offer empirical evidence to support this finding that substance abuse is not linked to homelessness directly but rather indirectly through greater disaffiliation from society (less support from family and friends, and lack of employment).[61] Once homeless, substance abusers' social disaffiliation may continue to hamper their ability to become housed again.[62] Reasons for homelessness among older adults (fifty or more) are remarkably stable over various locations (Boston in the United States; England; Melbourne, Australia): their homes were sold or needed repair, they fell behind in rent payments, a close relative died or a relationship was lost, there were tenant-neighbor disputes. As with other homeless populations, indirect causes of older persons' loss of their home included physical, mental, and alcohol problems, along with gambling problems (primarily in Australia). They became homeless through individual vulnerabilities as well as structural vulnerabilities such as welfare policy and gaps in service delivery.

Surprisingly, perceived reasons for homelessness do not differ for those who have mental illness compared to other homeless persons, suggesting that structural solutions, among them low-income housing and income support, might prevent homelessness for the mentally ill, as well as the rest of the homeless population.[63] However, on the basis of empirical correlates of homelessness, homeless persons with mental illness have "received a double dose of disadvantage—poverty with the addition of childhood instability [out-of-home placement] and violence [witnessed within the household or personally experienced violence]."[64]

## Comparison of Homeless to Low-Income Housed Populations

To begin to understand why a poor person becomes homeless, as well as the effect that lack of a home has on the health and medical care of poor populations, several case control studies have been conducted to compare the health of homeless and low-income housed populations.[65] Most of the case control studies found major vulnerabilities in the homeless population: more childhood problems, mental illness, and substance abuse. However, a longitudinal prospective study of never-homeless mothers with families who were seeking welfare in New York City did not find many differences in individual vulnerabilities between those who became homeless and those who stayed in the category of low-income-housed. Rather, structural factors differentiated whether a poor woman seeking welfare became homeless or housed: childhood poverty; being black; having housing instability as measured by living doubled up or having more mobility between living situations; and having family instability as manifested by pregnancy, recent childbirth, or domestic violence.[66] Another longitudinal study (six-month follow-up) did not find any difference in physical violence between homeless and low-income housed women.[67]

## Health Status

Lack of housing affects the health of all homeless people, whether they are newly homeless, long-term homeless, formerly homeless, or episodically homelessness. Even relatively short bouts of homelessness expose individuals to severe deprivation (hunger, lack of adequate hygiene) and victimization (physical assault, robbery, rape).[68] The homeless—adults and children—have a high prevalence of untreated acute and chronic medical, mental health, and substance abuse problems. They are exposed to illness because of overcrowding in shelters and exposure to heat and cold.[69] Further, sheltered homeless persons who have a substance abuse or mental health problem or a physical disability encounter difficulty in successfully exiting the sheltered environment.[70]

A dearth of prospective longitudinal epidemiologic research[71] makes it difficult to identify whether certain health conditions precede, cause, or result from the homeless condition. However, research has found that unstable housing—such as extreme overcrowding, substandard housing (lack of heat, dilapidated living conditions), or loss of housing—contributes significantly to poor health outcomes, and that stable housing plays a critical role in improving these health conditions.[72]

The significant impact housing has on health produces striking differences in the health outcomes between the homeless and their housed counterparts. A significant gradient in health emerges when we compare the homeless to their poor but stably housed peers. Homeless mothers were more likely than poor but stably housed mothers to experience spousal abuse, child abuse, drug use, and mental health problems.[73] In contrast, when we compare homeless mothers (living on the streets or in shelters) to their marginally housed peers (living temporarily in low-cost residential hotels, apartments, or private homes—doubling up with relatives or friends), a contrasting picture emerges. There is no significant difference in the mental and physical health of homeless mothers and their poor but marginally housed peers.[74]

A common theme in the literature on homeless adults' health is that homeless history—number of homeless episodes, length of time homeless, and living in unsheltered conditions—has profound effects on the health and use of health services of homeless adults. An accumulating body of research has shown that unsheltered homeless adults and homeless adults with a longer length of homelessness have poorer physical health than their sheltered or recently homeless counterparts do. Compared to those in shelter, unsheltered homeless adults are more likely to use illegal drugs or alcohol, have been victimized, and have experienced an accident or injury.[75] Similarly, unsheltered women are more likely to report fair or poor health status, be engaged in risky sex, and have higher rates of victimization, poor mental health, no injection drug use, and alcohol use—compared to sheltered women.[76] Finally, adults experiencing extended homelessness are twice as likely to die compared to those with shorter episodes.[77] This relationship between housing and health is important and suggests why we must view the entire ecology of homelessness, including the impact of lack of housing on well-being, rather than focus exclusively on the health and mental health problems of the homeless.

## Physical Health

Homeless people are subject to the same risk factors for physical illness as the general population, but they may be exposed to excessive levels of such risk and also experience risk factors unique to homelessness. Risk factors include excessive use of alcohol, illegal drugs, and cigarettes; sleeping in an upright position (resulting in venous stasis and its consequences); extensive walking in poor-fitting shoes; and inadequate nutrition.[78]

Further, homelessness itself is physically dangerous. The homeless are at risk for assault and victimization, as well as exposure to the elements. Homeless people are at great risk of being victimized for lack of personal security, whether they live in a shelter or outdoors. Moreover, they are exposed to communicable diseases such as tuberculosis and common illnesses such as asthma and flu in the shelter environment.[79]

Consequently, the homeless have a much higher rate of physical illness than the general population. About 37 percent of homeless persons report having poor health, compared to 10 percent in the general population.[80] Among homeless persons, those who are older, women, people with less education, and those who indicate a physical or mental health condition are more likely to report their health status as fair or poor. Length of time homeless is negatively associated with perceived health status by homeless persons. One-third to one-half of homeless adults have at least one chronic condition.[81] Thus illness appears to be taking its toll, preventing some of the homeless from escaping their predicament. For example, one-quarter of homeless adults report that their poor health prevented them from working or going to school.[82]

Age-adjusted mortality is very high for homeless persons.[83] In Philadelphia, homeless men and women who were living in shelters or outdoors had 3.5 times the age-adjusted mortality rate as the general population. Of any homeless subgroup, white men were most likely to die.[84] In New York City, homeless men and women living in shelters had two to three times the age-adjusted mortality rate as the general population of that city. The authors state, "The only group with a mortality rate (1713/100,000) comparable to that of our homeless sample was poor Black men in Harlem, where an earlier study documented death rates exceeding those of rural areas in the world's lowest-income countries."[85] In Boston, the average age at death for homeless persons having contact with the Boston Health Care for the Homeless Program was forty-seven years.[86] In Toronto, homeless men in shelters have higher mortality than the general male population of Toronto (8.3 times for ages eighteen to twenty-four, 3.7 times for twenty-five to forty-four, and 2.3 times for forty-five to sixty-four).[87] Some of the mortality disparities for homeless women in Toronto were even greater than for men, with the death rate five to thirty times greater than their housed counterparts in the fourteen-to-forty-four-year-old groups.[88]

The main cause of death for the younger women in Toronto shelters was HIV/AIDS and drug overdose.[89] Among homeless men, prior use of injectable drugs, incarceration, and chronic homelessness increased the likelihood of death.[90] Risk factors for death among homeless patients in another study in Boston in forty Health Care for the Homeless clinics include AIDS, renal disease, symptomatic HIV, history of cold-related injury, liver disease, arrhythmia, substance abuse, and chronic homelessness.[91] On the basis of the rate and constellation of health problems and high incidence of mortality, the homeless resemble the general population that is ten years older than the homeless population's own chronological age.[92]

Homeless children experience a higher number of acute illness symptoms, notably fever, ear infection, diarrhea, and asthma. Mothers of homeless children are more likely than their housed counterparts to report that their children are in fair or poor health.[93] For example, in New York City 40 percent of homeless children have asthma, six times the rate for the general population; for most of the homeless children, the asthma is severe and undertreated.[94]

The most common self-reported physical illnesses among homeless adults are arthritis, rheumatism, or joint problems. The next most common self-reported medical conditions are chest infection, cold, cough or bronchitis, high blood pressure and problems walking, lost limb, and other handicaps.[95] From objective clinic reports, the most common physical illnesses among homeless adults are infectious diseases; dental, vision, and skin and ear problems; gastrointestinal diseases; female genitourinary problems; and inadequate nutrition, immunization, and cancer screening.[96] Deficient immunization, though not a physical illness, reflects the lack of preventive health care in this population.[97]

## Contagious Diseases

Contagious diseases, such as tuberculosis[98] and HIV infection,[99] are much more common among the homeless than the general population. Prevention, diagnosis, and treatment of these diseases among homeless populations must be a high priority for health care, housing, and social service providers.

***Tuberculosis.*** The prevalence of positive tuberculosis skin testing (test for lifetime exposure to tuberculosis) among homeless adults ranges from 21 percent in Palo Alto[100] to 32 percent in San Francisco[101] and Los Angeles,[102] to 43 percent in New York.[103] These rates of latent TB prevalence are three to six times greater than the 5–10 percent prevalence of TB infection among the general population.[104] Active tuberculosis among the homeless aged twenty-five to forty-four may be as high as twenty times that of the general population.[105] The rate of active tuberculosis among men in a New York shelter clinic is 6 percent;[106] more than half of it is due to primary tuberculosis and not reactivation of old disease.[107]

Positive tuberculosis skin tests have been found to be related to duration of homelessness, living in crowded shelters or single-room occupancy hotels, and increasing age. Homeless persons with active tuberculosis were more likely than housed persons with this infection to be located in western and southern states; be born in the United States; be incarcerated at the time of diagnosis; have alcohol abuse, injection, or noninjection drug use; and be co-infected with HIV (34 percent). Further, they were more likely to be infectious, resulting in great risk to other homeless as well as housed persons.[108] Tuberculosis is harder to treat among the homeless because of the difficulty of screening, following, and maintaining tuberculosis treatment among this population, and because many have multidrug-resistant organisms. However, several measures have been successful in curbing the spread of tuberculosis: annual screening of all homeless people to identify and treat cases with active disease and to reduce transmission to homeless as well as other persons; screening to identify and treat cases with latent disease to prevent reactivation disease; directly observed therapy to ensure completion of therapy and prevention of multidrug-resistant tuberculosis; and use of electronic medical records across systems of care to identify outbreaks of tuberculosis, and to identify and treat those who have moved or were lost to follow-up whose tuberculosis treatment has not been completed.

***Hepatitis C and B.*** Hepatitis C (HCV) is a serious infectious disease emerging in the homeless population with a frequency much greater than in the general population. Estimated lifetime rates of hepatitis C for the homeless are 22 percent in a convenience sample of homeless and impoverished adults in Los Angeles,[109] 26 percent in a probability sample of homeless adults in the Skid Row of Los Angeles,[110]

32 percent in a mobile medical clinic in Manhattan,[111] 42 percent[112] to 44 percent[113] among homeless veterans in VA domiciliary programs, and 50 percent among homeless male clinic patients in Los Angeles.[114] This is in contrast to the 1.8 percent prevalence of HCV infection in the United States.[115]

The major risk factor for HCV among the homeless is drug use, particularly injection drug use.[116] Other correlates of HCV in homeless male patients include sharing razors and toothbrushes, and receipt of tattoos.[117] Sexual transmission has not been found to be a risk factor for hepatitis C.[118]

Hepatitis C poses a great challenge to society and the medical care profession. Most persons infected with HCV are asymptomatic for years and therefore might not come to the attention of the medical care system. Still, during that asymptomatic period, they are at risk of spreading the disease to others and engaging in health behaviors that could worsen the course of their disease (obesity, alcohol intake, tobacco smoking). Consequently, access to primary care at all stages of hepatitis C is critical to identify cases, provide counseling to prevent the spread to others, proscribe behaviors that could worsen the course of their disease, conduct hepatitis A and hepatitis B vaccination (co-infection with these viruses could lead to fulminant hepatitis and death), and monitor the course of their illness for timing of appropriate referral to specialty care with a hepatologist. However, there are long waiting lists for specialty care clinics that treat impoverished persons with hepatitis C. Most of the regimens that treat hepatitis C are tricky for homeless people given that the treatment often results in major side effects requiring a safe home environment to rest and have close monitoring. Further, since depression is exacerbated by the regimen, existing depression is a cautionary criterion for HCV treatment. Many of the homeless have depression and might not qualify for treatment. Existing drug abuse or alcohol abuse is also a cautionary criterion for HCV treatment. Given the high rate of substance abuse among homeless persons, many who are infected with HCV might not be eligible for hepatitis antiviral treatment. An explosion of costs due to hepatitis C is expected because of the high incidence of hepatitis C in the homeless population, lack of availability of treatment, the growing number of persons with long years of infection, and hepatitis C being the leading cause of liver transplantation in the United States. There are costs to individuals who become symptomatic and do not obtain hepatitis C treatment and consequently experience reduced functional ability and increased morbidity. There are also costs to society, which must pay for expensive recurrent hospitalization for chronic liver disease in these individuals.

The homeless also inordinately experience hepatitis B,[119] another serious disease affecting the liver. Rates of lifetime hepatitis B range from 23 percent in a Palo Alto[120] and 34 percent in a Los Angeles[121] VA domiciliary program to 47 percent in a mobile medical clinic in Manhatten.[122] Few homeless persons are vaccinated for hepatitis B, suggesting that immunization programs to cover adults are necessary.

*HIV.* HIV infection among the homeless is much more common than in the housed population. Studies reveal an HIV infection rate of 9–10.5 percent among San Francisco's homeless and marginally housed adults.[123] Among the homeless in that city, HIV seroprevalence was 6.3 percent among women,[124] similar to the rate of 6.2 percent among homeless persons with comorbid mental illness and substance abuse.[125] Risk factors for HIV infection include being black, injection drug use, and chronic homelessness.[126] In contrast, HIV in the general population nationally is estimated at between 0.3 percent and 0.4 percent.[127] The rate of HIV in homeless clinic populations varies greatly: 0.9 percent (1.3 percent for men and 0.1 percent for women)[128] in a treatment sample of homeless clients of a primary care clinic in Denver, 15 percent among patients of a mobile medical clinic in Manhattan,[129] and 1.8 percent among homeless veterans in a VA domiciliary program.[130]

HIV is the major cause of death among the adult homeless population. In a treatment sample of 17,292 homeless adult clients of the Boston Health Care for the Homeless Program, AIDS was the leading cause of death among those age twenty-five to forty-four.[131] Not only does homelessness increase a person's risk for HIV ninefold but HIV increases the risk for homelessness by three times. This suggests that both HIV prevention and homeless prevention programs must continue to target homeless populations with high-risk behaviors for HIV.[132] Given their high risk factors for HIV, there need to be enhanced efforts to mass-screen homeless populations for HIV. Current (past twelve months) HIV testing range from 52 percent among homeless youths[133] and 57 percent among homeless person with serious mental illness[134] to 68 percent among homeless women.[135] Homeless persons must have screening for HIV and continuity of care that maximizes sustained antiretroviral therapy, thus reducing the risk of death for homeless persons with HIV.[136]

## Women's Health

Homeless women are severely lacking in women's health services. However, pregnancy and recent births are risk factors for becoming homeless.[137] Despite their lack of a home, many homeless women have children; yet only 29 percent of women with children under eighteen years of age had their children living with them. Substance abusers and the chronic homeless were least likely to have their children living with them.[138]

Whereas many homeless women wish to have children, those interested in contraception often experienced significant barriers in their effort to prevent pregnancy. Among homeless women interviewed in Los Angeles, 41 percent had used no contraceptive method of any kind during the past year, although the average reported frequency of vaginal intercourse during that time was once per week.[139] Fewer than 10 percent use condoms regularly, despite lifestyles that place them at great risk for AIDS and other sexually transmitted diseases.[140] Many are willing to use long-term forms of birth control such as depoprovera. Fewer than 5 percent had ever used a female condom, but 38 percent of all homeless women and 73 percent of homeless youths said they were willing to try them.[141] This suggests that the female condom might be an alternative to the male condom for homeless women in STD and pregnancy prevention. The most commonly cited deterrents to contraceptive use (mentioned by 20–27 percent of women) were side effects, fear of potential health risks, and partner's dislike of contraception and cost.[142] Still, the opportunities for some kind of prevention are great. Among homeless family planning clinic users, 60 percent had a history of a sexually transmitted disease and 28 percent had a history of pelvic inflammatory disease (PID)[143]; among homeless women in the community 48 percent had a history of an STD and 22 percent had a history of PID.[144]

Homeless women undergo little cancer screening. Half of homeless women age forty or older received a clinical breast exam in the past year,[145] compared to 77 percent of the general population. Further, 32–47 percent[146] of homeless women age forty or older living in California received a mammogram in the past year, compared to 73 percent of housed women.[147] Further, 54 percent[148] to 55 percent[149] of homeless women in California received a Pap smear in the past year, compared to 77 percent of women in the U.S. general population and 67 percent in the California general population.[150] Lower use of Pap smears is alarming given that a history of abnormal Pap smears was reported by 23 percent of homeless family planning clinic users[151] and 26 percent of homeless women sampled from the community.[152]

Regarding homeless women's obstetrical history, 76 percent of them have had at least one natural child.[153] Homeless women are more likely to be pregnant (11 percent of homeless adults, 24 percent of sixteen-to-nineteen-year-old homeless youths) than their poor, but housed, peers (5 percent).[154] Ethnic disparities exist in homelessness. Twenty percent of all African American women request emergency shelter around the years of their index birth. In addition, homeless women are more likely to receive inadequate prenatal care than are poor but housed women (56 percent versus 15 percent).[155]

Homeless women in New York City are more likely than impoverished housed women to have low-birthweight newborns (16 percent versus 7 percent).[156] Similarly, in Los Angeles homeless women had higher rates of premature birth (19 percent vs. 10 percent of the general population) and low-birthweight babies

(17 percent vs. 6 percent of the general population).[157] In Toronto, homeless or underhoused women had a much higher incidence of premature, low-birthweight, and small-for-gestational-age infants, and their risk was greatly multiplied if they were substance users.[158] In New York City, infant mortality was highest among the homeless (24.9 per 1,000 live births) as compared to poor housed women (16.6 per 1,000 live births), and nonpoor housed women (12.0 per 1,000 live births).[159]

## Violence

Homeless persons suffer disproportionately from violent and abusive behavior in the United States. More than half of homeless individuals report having been criminally victimized while homeless,[160] in contrast to 37 percent of the general population who have been victimized in the past year. Homeless men experience somewhat more recent physical victimization than homeless women (20 percent vs. 18 percent respectively). However, homeless women experience considerably more recent sexual violence (9 percent vs. 1 percent respectively).[161] In a recent study, 13 percent of homeless women report being sexually assaulted or raped in the past year,[162] compared to 2.7 percent of women in the general population.[163] Having housing, even marginal housing, reduced sexual violence among impoverished women.[164]

Serious mental illness (SMI) is a significant predictor of victimization for homeless men and women. Forty-four percent of homeless persons with SMI have been criminally victimized within the past two months.[165] Among seriously mentally ill homeless people, recent victimization is a predictor of future victimization as well as increased length of time homeless.[166] Moreover, the comorbidity of SMI and substance abuse aggravate victimization among homeless persons.[167]

Victimization prior to age eighteen is also prevalent among homeless persons. Twenty-two percent of the homeless were physically abused, and 13 percent were sexually abused as a child or youth.[168] Child physical and sexual abuse history is also found to be a strong precursor to adult homelessness[169] and to homeless adult violence.[170] A homeless person with mental illness is more likely to have experienced sexual or physical abuse as a child. Mental illness and substance abuse for homeless women were associated with a history of both physical and sexual child abuse. By contrast, for homeless men only mental illness was associated with a history of physical child abuse.[171] In a sample of homeless veterans in a substance abuse rehabilitation program, childhood physical or sexual abuse among both women and men, and current physical or sexual abuse among women (but not men), was associated with suicidal ideation or suicide attempts.[172] Moreover, there is overlapping evidence that the prevalence of childhood abuse in homeless women with serious mental illness is substantially higher than among homeless women in general. Further, the intensity of exposure to that violence contributes to the severity of their psychiatric symptoms.[173] Childhood abuse as well as out-of-home placement predict homelessness among poor people[174] and substance dependence among the homeless.[175]

## Homeless Youths

Current estimates of the number of homeless youths range from one hundred thousand to half a million.[176] The 1999 Second National Incidence Studies of Missing, Abducted, Runaway, and Throwaway Children (NISMART-2), a national household and juvenile facility probability survey, found that 1,682,900 youths had a runaway or throwaway episode in that year.[177] Eight percent of adolescents in a nationally representative sample of youths reported they were homeless at least one night in the past twelve months.[178]

The federal definition of *homeless children and youth* differs somewhat from the definition of *homeless adults*. Homeless children and youth are defined by the Education for Homeless Children and Youth Program of Title VII-B of the McKinney-Vento Homeless Assistance Act (42 USC 11431 et seq.; McKinney-Vento Act). The program was originally authorized in 1987 and most recently was reauthorized by the No Child Left Behind Act of 2001. The McKinney-Vento Act defines homeless children and youth as individuals who lack a fixed, regular, and adequate nighttime residence and (in contrast to the definition of adult homelessness) includes those who are sharing the housing of other persons because of loss of housing, economic hardship, or a similar reason (sometimes referred to as being doubled-up).

Youths become homeless largely as a result of persistent family dysfunction and conflict, specifically parental neglect, physical or sexual abuse, family substance abuse, and family violence.[179] However, many homeless youths are still in contact with their families. A large proportion of their social network is made up of family and friends, and they are receiving social support from their family and friends from home. The majority (65 percent) of newly homeless youths do return home within their first year of homelessness, usually to live with a parent.[180]

Given their homelessness and other life problems, it is not surprising that homeless youths suffer from mental health problems.[181] They include poor coping skills, suicidal tendencies, substance abuse,[182] depression, and other mental health problems that result in a high rate of psychiatric hospitalization.[183] Mental disorder and victimization are especially high for LGBTU (lesbian, gay, bisexual, transgender, unsure) homeless youths.[184] The rate of LGBTU persons among homeless youths is about 20 percent or higher in larger cities.[185] Many have experienced self-mutilation (69 percent)[186] and suffer from a high level of dissociative behavior.[187] Moreover, 28 percent of street youths and 10 percent of shelter youths have participated in survival sex (sold sex for food, clothing, or shelter).[188]

Homeless youths also suffer from victimization and health problems that largely extend from their homeless condition. They experience an extremely high frequency of psychological maladjustment and victimization while homeless. Assault and robbery are reported by one-fourth to one-half of homeless youths, and rape in the past three months is reported by one in ten of these youths.[189]

Homeless youths experience physical health problems that exceed the rate among youth in the general population.[190] Hepatitis C seroprevalence was 13 percent among Montreal street youths (versus 0.8 percent in the general population)[191] and 12 percent among homeless youths in Southwest community-based settings.[192] The rate of Hepatitis B was 17 percent in Southwest community-based settings.[193] Hepatitis A was at 6 percent in two Vancouver outreach clinics[194] and 5 percent among Montreal street youths.[195] Fewer than half of homeless youths have been vaccinated against hepatitis B, but the majority are willing to receive the vaccine if offered.[196] Homeless young people also have a higher rate of HIV,[197] with seroprevalence ranging from 5 percent among homeless youths in a New York City shelter clinic[198] to 16 percent in Southwest community-based settings.[199] Homeless youths also regularly experience respiratory problems (asthma and pneumonia, scabies and trauma), other sexually transmitted diseases such as chlamydia and gonorrhea,[200] and pregnancy.[201] Homeless youths are at great risk of premature mortality—eleven times the mortality rate found in the general population of youth.[202] The deaths were most likely to occur during a period of homelessness.[203] Youths with HIV were most at risk of death, and the main causes of death were suicide and drug overdose.

Homeless youths have the highest frequency of pregnancy in the United States: for girls aged fourteen to seventeen, 48 percent of those living on the streets and 33 percent of those living in shelters reported ever having been pregnant, compared to 10 percent of those who are housed.[204] Similarly, in a Montreal study 42 percent of street youths fourteen to nineteen were pregnant at least once, and those most likely to have been pregnant had a history of severe sexual abuse and early onset of injection drug use.[205]

Homeless youths experience barriers to care specific to being adolescent; males feel that to be ill is to be weak, and females feel that being ill puts them at risk for lack of safety, not always being able to consent to their health care because they are underage and lack an adult to help them through complicated medical systems. If they are under eighteen they can apply for Medicaid, but they might not have the needed proof of parental income, and they might fear that their parents will be able to find them though the application process. Those who are eighteen or older usually do not qualify for Medicaid.

## Dental Health

A strong correlate of poverty in the United States is poor dental health. It is also one of the major health problems reported by homeless individuals. However, there are few statistics on the prevalence of dental problems specifically among homeless persons. Ninety-one percent of them who had contact with a shelter-based dental program had untreated caries. Moreover, homeless people living in the community are only one-third as likely as domiciled adults to have obtained dental care in the past year, and consequently they are twice as likely to have gross dental decay (57 percent versus 23 percent).[206] Given this high rate of dental disease, dental care should be an integral part of any health care services package developed for the homeless population. In fact, dental problems were the most important factor triggering soup kitchen users to seek out a Health Care for the Homeless Clinic.

## Mental Illness and Substance Abuse

Alcohol, drug abuse, and mental health problems among the homeless dominate the research on homeless inquiry. More than three-quarters (86 percent) of the homeless have experienced at least one alcohol, drug, or mental health problem in their lifetime, with 57 percent having mental health problems, 62 percent having alcohol problems, and 58 percent having drug problems. Psychiatric problems are also very common. Two-thirds of homeless individuals have experienced at least one alcohol (38 percent), drug (26 percent), or mental health (39 percent) problem during the past month.[207] It appears that the prevalence of lifetime mood and substance use disorders (especially cocaine abuse among women) has increased since the 1980s.[208]

One-third of homeless adults suffer from current SMI—schizophrenic disorders, affective disorders, personality or character disorders, and cognitive disorders—according to diagnostic data.[209] Further, one-third have a substance abuse disorder.[210] About 11 percent have schizophrenia, fewer than half of whom are currently receiving treatment.[211] About 17 percent have a dual diagnosis of chronic mental illness and chronic substance use.[212] These individuals pose a challenge to developing services that successfully address both aspects of their illness.[213] In addition to intrinsic illness processes, environmental stresses and homeless appearance must be considered so as to avoid inaccurate diagnosis of mental illness. These individuals may experience chronic isolation, geographical mobility, disturbed sleep, and fear of victimization; they may appear disheveled and show signs of lacking self-care, each of which could result in symptoms that might be taken for mental illness.

## Suicide

Given the high frequency of suicide within the homeless population, there is evidence suggestive of a high prevalence of inadequately treated mental illness within this population: 25 percent of homeless adults considered committing suicide, and 7 percent attempted suicide during the preceding year.[214] In a sample of veterans in an inpatient substance abuse rehabilitation program, women were more likely than homeless men to have suicidal ideation or to have made a suicide attempt.[215]

## Neuropsychological Impairment

Homeless persons commonly have neuropsychological impairment, some of which is related to a history of traumatic brain injury, mental illness, or substance abuse. The homeless suffer cognitive impairment (80 percent)[216] and mental retardation (20 percent).[217] Both conditions can have a negative impact on treatment outcomes, especially for usual treatments, which are cognitively demanding. Further, nearly one-third had reading abilities at or below the fifth grade level, suggesting that they lack sufficient basic skills to function in society.[218]

# Access to Health Care

All of this evidence shows that homelessness and the dreadful life circumstances that accompany it—inadequate housing, crowding, poor sanitation, violence, stress, exposure to drugs and violence—are salient risk factors for alarmingly poor health. This point is perhaps best represented in the finding that a homeless history—that is, a number of homeless episodes and living in unsheltered conditions—has a profound influence on the health and mortality of a homeless person.

The majority of the homeless (75 percent) have used health services in the past year,[219] which might seem to represent good access to care, but it may also underscore the poor health status of homeless people. The high level of health services use among the homeless reveals that health care may be one of several factors that could improve health outcomes for homeless persons. Ultimately, health services usage should not be considered in isolation of other powerful structural forces that affect health, such as a social and environmental context in which a person belongs.

## Use of Physical Health Services

During the past year, 63 percent of homeless persons had an ambulatory care visit, 32 percent visited an emergency room, and 23 percent were hospitalized.[220] However, 24 percent report they needed to see a doctor in the last year but were not able to,[221] and 32 percent reported being unable to obtained prescribed medication.[222] Moreover, their sources of health care use suggest inappropriate health care delivery. For example, more than half (57 percent) lack a regular source of care (a "medical home" has been acknowledged as an important indicator of access to medical care), compared to 24 percent of the poverty population in the United States and 19 percent of the general population.[223] Homeless people with a regular source of care were two-thirds less likely to have gone without needed medical care than those without,[224] and homeless women with a regular source of care had more outpatient visits and preventive health screens.[225]

The majority of the homeless seek care at places that do not offer continuous quality care. Of those who sought care in the past year, 32 percent report receiving medical care at a hospital emergency room, 27 percent at a hospital outpatient clinic, 21 percent at a community health center, 20 percent at a hospital as an inpatient, and 19 percent at a private doctor's office.[226] Some hospitalizations and emergency room visits are appropriate, but the high rate of emergency room use and hospitalization[227] in this young population suggests substitution of inpatient and emergency room care for outpatient ambulatory care services. Kushel, Vittinghoff, and Haas[228] state, in regard to their study of the homeless, that "in the United States, only persons older than 65 years had similar rates of hospitalization as those in our study, whose median age was 37 years." Making clinic visits to the Health Care for the Homeless Program reduced inappropriate ER visits by more than one-half.[229] Homeless persons' limited access to ambulatory care is due to individual factors (competing needs, substance dependence, mental illness)[230] as well as system factors (availability, cost, convenience, appropriateness of care).

Homeless adults are more likely than the general population to have had a medical hospitalization during the preceding year. For example, a Hawaiian study found that their age and sex-adjusted acute care hospitalization rate was 542 per 1,000 person-years compared to the general population rate of 96 per 1,000 person-years. In this study, homeless adults were admitted to acute care hospitals for 4,766 days compared to a predicted 640 days, resulting in costs of $2.8 million per year for excess hospitalization.[231] Further, if hospitalized, homeless adults are most likely to be admitted to a general county hospital.[232] A study in New York found that the length of a hospital stay for a homeless adult patient exceeded the mean general admission by 36 percent. About three-quarters of hospitalized homeless adults were admitted for conditions for which hospitalization is often preventable (substance abuse, mental illness, trauma, respiratory disorders, skin disorders, infectious diseases—excluding AIDS).[233] Another study found that following hospital discharge 40 percent of homeless adults were readmitted within fourteen months, usually with the same diagnosis as for the initial intake. Such hospitalization and readmission resulted in costs at a major urban hospital of more than $1.8 million during the three-month study.[234] The finding that most of the homeless inpatients were admitted for problems that could have been treated less expensively in an outpatient setting suggests difficulty in sustaining treatment intensity for homeless persons outside the hospital. These data imply an ineffective local service delivery system for the homeless population.

## Preventive Care

Homeless adults also have fewer preventive visits than the general population. For example, despite having greater risks for cancer, their screening rate was typically much lower than for the general population.[235] Regarding colon cancer screening, homeless adults fifty years and older were less likely to have ever had a lower endoscopy (23 percent vs. 47 percent for the general population), though they had a similarly low rate for fecal occult blood testing in the past year (19 percent vs. 16 percent). As for prostate cancer screening, despite the fact that the majority of homeless men are African American and thus at higher risk for prostate cancer, homeless men fifty and older were much less likely to have had screening with a prostate-specific antigen blood test in the past year (11 percent vs. 54 percent). In addition, very few homeless persons had ever been screened for skin cancer with a skin exam (24 percent ever, 15 percent past year). Homeless women have less breast and cervical cancer screening as well. This suggests that the homeless may delay seeking medical attention at a stage when severe illness could have been prevented.

## Children and Youth

Even though sheltered youths are more likely to have a regular source of care than are street youths (64 percent vs. 50 percent), the rate is much lower than for their housed counterparts (85 percent).[236] Homeless adolescents use considerable emergent services that possibly could have been avoided with early primary care; one-quarter visited an emergency room and one-fifth were hospitalized in the preceding year. Only half have ever been tested for HIV.

We need to design health service programs that facilitate health access and health promotion for homeless adolescents. All are at risk for multiple health problems, but only 28 percent used medical care services in a year.[237] Compared to their poor but housed counterparts, homeless children are more likely to use ambulatory medical services (two or more emergency department visits during the past year and more outpatient visits for well and sick care), but they are also more likely to have been hospitalized in the past year.[238] These findings highlight not only the poor health status of young homeless persons but also the need for programs for them that increase outreach efforts and improve the availability of and access to ongoing primary care services.

## Adherence to Prescribed Care

Once the homeless do get needed medical services, they may find it difficult to comply with treatment. For example, only 50 percent of homeless patients in New York City who were referred from a satellite clinic to a hospital clinic kept their appointment, and only 25 percent with cardiovascular disease remained in long-term therapy.[239] Further, in a New York City shelter only six out of fifty homeless individuals requiring isoniazid prophylaxis for tuberculosis were found to be taking their medication, and not one completed the full year of treatment.[240] Only four of thirty acutely psychotic homeless patients were taking the psychotropic medications that had been prescribed for them.[241] Lack of adherence to care, perhaps because of the unavailability of medication, is critically important for the survival of persons with HIV; in one study, risk of death was more than 250 percent higher for people receiving intermittent therapy of one to five months in comparison to people on sustained therapy for at least six months.[242]

For some conditions, most homeless adults who were screened and referred for care reported that they obtained medical care within the subsequent eight months (high blood pressure 81 percent and latent TB 78 percent ), despite the asymptomatic nature, and future rather than short-term benefit, of treatment for these conditions. However, few with dermatological or podiatric problems (44 percent) and even fewer homeless with vision impairment (33 percent) went for medical care, despite the symptomatic nature of these conditions. Barriers to seeking care for their skin or foot problems may have included a belief that medical care could not cure such problems as long as they continued living in homeless conditions. Barriers to vision care included few sources of free or low-cost glasses.[243]

Thus the success of intervention and compliance with a medical regimen is affected by the social situation of the homeless.[244] Their social conditions, competing needs, and unique lifestyles all combine to make more traditional approaches to health care delivery less effective for homeless patients even compared to poor domiciled patients. Special strategies may be needed to enhance adherence to prescribed care. For example, in one study financial incentives (five dollars, in this case) greatly increased their adherence to DOT for latent TB compared to a peer health advisor intervention or usual care (44 percent vs. 19 percent vs. 26 percent respectively completed the six months of treatment).[245] In another study, though cash incentives (five dollars) did not improve completion of preventive therapy for latent TB, those receiving the cash incentive required less staff time to follow up participants for their DOT visits.[246]

# Use of Mental Health and Substance Abuse Services

As we have noted, mental illness and substance abuse are more prevalent among homeless people than in the general population. Consequently, the majority (52 percent) of hospital admissions for homeless people were for treatment of substance abuse or mental illness, compared to 20 percent for other low-income patients.[247] A large number (15 percent to 44 percent) of homeless adults report having had a previous psychiatric hospitalization.[248] The age- and sex-adjusted rate of admission of homeless persons to state psychiatric hospitals in Hawaii was 105 per 1,000 person-years, compared to the general population rate of 0.8 per 1,000 person-years.[249]

## Ambulatory Care

Despite the high prevalence of current mental illness and prior psychiatric hospitalization, most of the homeless use existing outpatient mental health and substance abuse systems infrequently. Only 18 percent of homeless people in Baltimore's shelters had used outpatient mental health services during a six-month period,[250] and the majority of those with a previous mental hospitalization had not made an outpatient mental health visit in the past five years.[251] Although 51 percent of homeless persons with chronic mental illness had used outpatient mental health services at some time in their life, only 14 percent had used these services in the past two months.[252] Seventy-three percent of homeless clients who report inpatient treatment for mental health problems received this treatment before they became homeless.[253] These data suggest that homeless individuals who are mentally ill are in need of continuity of mental health services[254] but are not receiving these services in an outpatient setting.

The data on lack of outpatient treatment are even more striking for utilization of outpatient substance abuse services. Only 26 percent of homeless persons with recent substance abuse problems (within the past six months) used outpatient services at some time in their life, compared to 43 percent who used inpatient services.[255] Moreover, about half (52 percent) of those with recent substance abuse dependence had received treatment from the formal substance abuse treatment delivery system.[256] Recent residential treatment (past two months) for substance abuse problems was far more common than recent outpatient treatment. Only 7 percent of homeless people with substance abuse problems used outpatient substance abuse services in the past two months, compared to 16 percent who used inpatient services during this time period.[257] Even when they did use inpatient or residential services, retention was difficult for those with the greatest need for treatment. Limited use of outpatient treatment, as well as lack of any treatment use among recent substance abusers, suggests closer examination of system-level characteristics that may interfere with the homeless receiving the services they need. Outreach of mental health and substance abuse professionals to shelter settings is a start at improving access to care in dealing with mental illness and substance abuse problems among homeless persons.[258]

## Barriers to Health Care

Compounding their increased risk for disease is evidence that homeless people encounter major obstacles to obtaining needed medical and psychiatric services. About one-quarter of them stated that they needed to see a doctor in the past year but were unable to do so,[259] and more than half did not have a regular source of care.[260] Among homeless women, one-third stated they had not obtained needed medical care during the past year.[261] Some homeless people do seek care for their health problems, but certain segments of the population are less likely to obtain care even if they are sick or have a regular source of care. Those living on the streets are the least likely of all the homeless to obtain outpatient visits and preventive health screens, and even hospital inpatient care, although they are most in need.[262] Their situation is similar to the pre-Medicaid and Medicare era, when impoverished populations with acute illness had difficulty getting inpatient hospital care. Further, homeless adults with little education[263] and without health insurance are less likely to seek care even if they are sick.[264] People who are less likely to have a regular source of care are young, Hispanic, and do not have health insurance; they are long-term homeless (five or more years since last housed), have subsistence difficulties, and are socially isolated.[265] The homeless with mental health problems were less likely to seek mental health services if they had not received mental health advice or a referral from a service provider outside the mental health system, or if they had an affective disorder (such as depression).[266] Homeless persons with substance abuse problems were less likely to seek treatment for them if they did not get help accessing these services, spent more time in places that were not meant for sleeping, and lived in a service-poor environment.[267]

Delay in seeking care or lack of a regular source of care may result in health care practitioners having to manage conditions that would have been easier to treat had the individual sought help earlier or at a preventive stage. For example, homeless and poor housed women enjoyed 3.7 times the odds of having received a Pap smear in the prior year if they had a regular source of medical care.[268] Premature death might be prevented by helping homeless persons find a medical home; one-quarter of homeless persons who died in Boston had not had any medical care, inpatient or outpatient, in the year before their death.[269] However, many did have medical care prior to their death, suggesting that opportunities to prevent death might have been missed for some who did seek help.[270]

Homeless individuals face numerous problems in obtaining appropriate health care: cost, transportation, competing needs, mental illness, the homeless lifestyle, personal barriers, lack of availability of health services, medical provider bias, insufficient discharge planning from hospitals, lack of recuperative care, and so on.

## Financial Barriers

The homeless experience numerous financial barriers in accessing medical care. First, there are financial barriers and problems in satisfying eligibility requirements for health insurance. One-third[271] of homeless adults who had not obtained needed medical care stated that it was due to an inability to pay for medical services. Only one-half[272] of the homeless in the community have any form of health insurance (Medicaid, Medicare, veterans services, or private insurance), and most have no cash resources at all.[273] Although most homeless veterans are eligible for VA health benefits, almost half of them were uninsured and only one-quarter had VA insurance.[274] Lack of insurance is the major factor contributing to an inappropriate usage pattern among homeless persons. Though they are likely to have multiple barriers to obtaining needed medical care, having health insurance is often the major facilitator to receiving ambulatory care[275] and to having a regular source of care. The safety net might be able to provide care to homeless persons who are uninsured, but critical services needed to treat their condition might not be available in the safety net—and, tragically, their conditions might go untreated.

## Lack of Transportation

Accessible transportation to medical facilities is often unavailable to the homeless.[276] If they live in the inner city with concentrated homeless services, transportation might not be an issue for them. However, if they live in dispersed areas throughout the city, they must often take multiple buses to get to needed medical care. Since most homeless persons have a number of health care problems, the health care sites for all of their medical problems might not be located in the same facility or even the same part of town, further complicating their transportation problems. Long travel time to medical care was cited by one-third of homeless women as a key barrier to obtaining medical care.[277]

## Competing Needs

The homeless have competing needs. They may well place greater priority on fulfilling their basic needs for food, shelter, and income than on obtaining needed health services or following through with a prescribed treatment plan.[278] Although we typically think of homeless people as having an inordinate amount of time on their hands, they must often deal with the varied schedules and locations of several service facilities to ensure that all their needs are met.[279] For instance, it is not uncommon for a homeless person to begin the day early in the morning by lining up at a free meal program for breakfast, then walking to the next meal program to join the long line for lunch, and then walking back to the shelter to wait in line once again in hope of securing a bed for the night. Even medical care for an active disease may seem less important than other needs, and preventive health care often loses out completely. For example, many homeless children are reported not to have up-to-date immunizations[280] and are less likely to be up to date on immunizations than poor, housed children.[281] One-half to one-third of homeless individuals who said they had not obtained needed medical care stated it was because their medical problem was not sufficiently serious to warrant their attention.[282]

## Barriers Caused by Mental Illness

Those homeless individuals who experience psychological distress as well as disabling mental illness may be in the greatest need of health services and yet may be the least able to obtain them.[283] Whereas homeless veterans with substance abuse problems were more likely than other veterans to make a medical visit, they as well as homeless veterans with schizophrenia or other psychotic disorders were less likely to make multiple visits, suggesting that they were not staying connected to medical care.[284] The effect of mental illness on barriers to care is not uniform across all types of mental health problems; for example, homeless persons with schizophrenia are less likely to receive preventive care than are homeless people with depression.[285]

Why might homeless persons with mental illness encounter barriers to obtaining medical care? Reasons might include[286] individual characteristics of mental illness such as paranoia, disorientation, unconventional health beliefs, lack of social supports, lack of organizational skills to gain access to needed services, or fear of authority figures and institutions as a result of previous institutionalization. Access to care and follow-through with referrals and prescribed care might be hampered by limited education and low literacy, as well as developmental discrepancies that are due to developmental delay or cognitive impairment.[287] Further, mentally ill homeless adults often require scarce services that address multifaceted problems, among them mental illness, substance abuse, physical illness, criminality, and such social service-related problems as housing and employment.[288]

What are needed are nontraditional services that fulfill basic needs before addressing psychodynamic issues. Comprehensive case management and permanent housing are needed to address such homeless mentally ill persons' housing, social support, employment, vocational rehabilitation, mental health, and physical health needs. Such services might be best furnished by a multidisciplinary team and health service center in a supportive housing environment.

## Conditions of Homelessness

The conditions of street life themselves may affect compliance with medical care. There is usually a lack of proper sanitation;[289] no stable place to keep medications safe, intact, and refrigerated; insufficient potable water; and an inability to obtain the proper food for a medically indicated diet such as diabetes mellitus or hypertension.[290] Having fewer positive social supports,[291] homeless persons often do not have anyone who can transport them to a clinic or care for them if needed after giving birth or experiencing a major illness.[292]

Further, though most of the homeless are long-term residents of their community, many are quite mobile within a city in their search for subsistence resources. This residential mobility makes continuity of care difficult.[293] Keeping follow-up appointments—necessary for continuous, comprehensive care—is difficult for homeless people thanks to their competing needs and particular time orientation.[294]

## Survival Strategies

Homeless people sometimes present barriers to their own care. Because exhibiting toughness is necessary to survive on the streets, the homeless may deny they have health problems in an attempt to maintain a sense of their own endurance.[295] Some may actually be afraid to venture out of the immediate geographical area to which they have become accustomed, thus limiting access to medical services in other areas. They may be too embarrassed to have medical professionals see them because of their poor personal hygiene. They may fear that their meager financial resources will be taken away to pay for the medical care they receive. Fear of authority figures and need for control of situations concerning themselves are additional factors that keep homeless people from seeking medical care.[296] For example, homeless undocumented immigrants have reason to fear that medical providers will call in Immigration and Naturalization authorities; runaway teenagers and homeless women with children may fear child protective service workers; and drug abusers or criminal offenders may fear the police. Creative strategies are needed to reach out to homeless people to initiate health prevention and disease promotion as well as help manage their acute and chronic health problems, especially providing food, clothing, and advocacy to assist with negotiating the often complicated medical bureaucracy.

## Limited Availability and Accessibility of Appropriate Health Care

When identifying health care availability for the homeless, it is important to distinguish between severity of homelessness and types of available health care. The majority of homeless people fall within the category of newly homeless. They are generally housed in shelter settings, and their health status is similar to their poor but housed counterparts. The chronically homeless are often street-dwelling, and, as has been mentioned, face the greatest health challenges.

The primary care system does not entirely provide adequate services for either of these groups. The health care safety net system does not adequately respond to the needs of the poor generally. For instance, the health safety net system usually does not provide onsite comprehensive health services for the poor (mental health, substance abuse, reproductive health, ancillary services); nor does the system typically screen for these issues. Many primary care settings are not set up to treat the chronically street-dwelling homeless patient. Chronically homeless people generally seek medical care late in the course of their disease or only for traumatic or life-threatening conditions. The chronically homeless typically require advocates (case managers, or formerly homeless persons) to help them broker their initial and ongoing access to the health system. The current primary care system is not equipped with case management or intensive outreach services to connect chronically homeless people to a medical home to reduce barriers to medical care. Thus the primary care safety net system generally is not set up to adequately address the health needs of the newly homeless or the chronically homeless.

## The Health Care Profession

Homeless people may sense that the medical profession itself is a barrier to obtaining needed medical care. Medical providers may consider homeless people to be undesirable patients because of their poor hygiene or their mental illness,[297] or because of assumptions that they come to the hospital for shelter and not for a medical problem.[298] Clinic directors reported that in more than 50 percent of clinics physician recruitment was hampered by poor working conditions, inadequate salaries, physician bias against working with the homeless, and the lack of respect this work receives from the medical profession.[299] Being treated with lack of respect does not encourage follow-up care or compliance with care.

Health care practitioners may view various aspects of health care quite differently than do their homeless patients. The attitudes of homeless patients regarding establishing priorities, adhering to schedules, and keeping appointments can differ from those of their providers, setting up the possibility of conflict and failure.[300] Clinicians often automatically base a treatment plan on the assumption that the patient has a home. However, most homeless lack reliable access to a place where they can recuperate (in bed, if indicated) and properly store medication. Ordinary, uncomplicated postclinic care such as cleansing wounds with soap and hot water may be extremely difficult to implement. Prescribed dietary regimens, which may involve taking medication with meals, are impractical if patients are without a reliable place to store groceries. Because shelters, free meal programs, and garbage cans are unreliable sources of nutritious food, homeless people have little control over what they eat. Needles and medications with recreational use are highly valued on the street and can make homeless patients a target for victimization.[301]

## Lack of Adequate Discharge Planning

For homeless inpatients and those who are imprisoned, there is inadequate discharge planning. Nearly everyone who is homeless at admission remains homeless at discharge. However, one third of people housed on admission may become homeless by the time of discharge, suggesting that housing status is not static and should be reassessed during the hospital stay. Further, for most inpatients who are homeless (77 percent), the medical provider may not be aware that they were homeless and so can not adequately prepare for their housing needs.[302] As a result, homeless inpatients are discharged directly from the hospital to the streets. Even homeless mothers are often discharged to the streets with their newborn infants soon after childbirth.[303] They may be discharged with "prescriptions they can't fill." Thus, readmission of homeless patients to hospitals is not uncommon.[304] This suggests the need for routine collection of information on housing status using standardized definitions of homelessness,[305] as well as determination of ability to pay for prescribed medications with a plan to give these people free medications. Discharge planning as they reenter the community from prison or jail is also needed to prevent further homelessness. Yet many local laws make it illegal to supply housing built with public funds to anyone with a history of a felony or certain misdemeanors.

## Lack of Recuperative Services

There are insufficient recuperative services for homeless patients. If inappropriately discharged from the hospital, they are often unable to manage the necessary recuperation. Recuperation cannot be adequately managed on the streets or accommodated in shelters. Few health centers that care for the homeless offer recuperative care services because of the cost as well as restrictive licensing in many cities. Reports by hospital staff indicate that longer hospital stays among homeless patients are primarily due to lack of housing. The leading cause of a long stay cited was placement problems among homeless psychiatric patients. Public hospitals have been under a court order since 1991 to place all such patients in supportive housing at the time of discharge. However, because of a shortage of supportive housing in New York City, and the continued downsizing of state psychiatric hospitals, this housing placement process can be delayed for months. Physicians also reported delaying discharge of homeless patients who required follow-up care, knowing that their access to ambulatory care and a clean environment or their compliance with treatment might be limited.[306]

# Federal Health Programs and Housing Models for Homeless People

A variety of programs have been developed to address the health care needs of the homeless, but there is no effort to integrate these systems or ensure permanent funding. Without adequate and permanent funding, their support is in jeopardy every year. Within the federal government, most of the services fall under the umbrella of the 1987 Stewart B. McKinney Homeless Assistance Act, the first comprehensive federal legislation to address the health, education, and social welfare needs of homeless people. In this section, we focus on several programs that have addressed the health of the homeless.

## Health Care for the Homeless Program

Federal efforts to provide medical services to the homeless population are primarily conducted by the Health Care for the Homeless Program. Community health centers supported by the 1985 Robert Wood Johnson Foundation/Pew Memorial Trust Health Care for the Homeless Program (HCH programs), subsequently covered by the McKinney Act, have addressed many of the access and quality of care issues raised in this chapter.

A critical aspect of the program is outreach. Teams of health care professionals bring a range of services to the homeless in shelters, hotels, meal programs, beaches and parks, train and bus stations, religious facilities, and other places where they are found. This reduces barriers to care such as lack of transportation, insufficient information about available facilities, and psychological problems. Outreach teams are typically based in health care centers, to which clinicians can refer homeless patients who need additional medical attention. A walk-in appointment system reduces access barriers at these medical facilities. Medical care, routine laboratory tests, substance abuse counseling, and some medications are furnished free of charge.

HCH programs try to employ staff (physicians, nurses, case mangers, pharmacists, dentists, and so on) who are nonjudgmental and sympathetic to the social problems of homeless people. Physicians and nurse practitioners aim to build trusting relationships with homeless patients. This requires patience. HCH providers try to treat homeless patients with as much respect as affluent patients are customarily given in a private doctor's office. This encourages effective intervention, better compliance, and higher quality and continuity of care. Providers are expected to look beyond the presenting problem and intervene on many fronts, some of which do not lie within the traditional boundaries of medicine. At the same time, they need to realize that some homeless patients will not want to address anything other than the problem for which they are seeking care, at least at first.

Medical providers are usually in the primary care disciplines, to enable them to treat the common problems faced by homeless people. They need to recognize and treat (or refer for treatment) most common primary care problems that are medical, mental, or social in nature. This includes inadequate vaccination, routine health maintenance and prevention, developmental delay, depression and anxiety, substance abuse, physical and emotional abuse, trauma, skin infestation, peripheral vascular disease, malnutrition and failure to thrive, anemia, dental decay, podiatry problems, vision impairment, and social problems (lack of food, shelter, a place to wash up, employment, child care).

Providers often work in teams made up of case managers, nurses, nurse practitioners, social workers, and physicians. The case manager coordinates treatment and referrals for homeless patients. Referral networks of community groups and public agencies are called on for problems that the health center does not have the capability to treat, in particular basic needs for shelter, food, and clothing; subspecialty health problems, including SMI and substance abuse; social problems such as lack of income, public benefits, health insurance, and employment, as well as legal problems; emergency care; and hospital care. Transportation vouchers (for public transportation, taxis, or ambulances) are often employed to transport homeless patients to this network of referral facilities. In addition, some facilities make available showers, food, and clothing, as well as health education and preventive care programs. Since many of the homeless are uninsured and do not have the financial means to purchase medication, in house "community pharmacies" of donated medications are located in some clinics. Respite care is furnished by a few of these facilities,[307] where the average length of stay is two weeks.[308]

National evaluations of the HCH programs have been conducted. Results reveal that availability and accessibility of services was accomplished to a certain degree; the program treated 23 percent of homeless persons in smaller cities, but only 8 percent in larger ones. The HCH programs were reasonably successful at the difficult task of maintaining continuity of care for homeless patients. Half of their clients were seen on more than one occasion. Contacts with clients with a chronic medical condition average 4.5 (with two-thirds being seen more than once), whereas contacts with the remaining clients averaged 2.3. Patients with targeted chronic medical conditions including tuberculosis, hypertension, and peripheral vascular disease; diabetes; and seizure disorders were seen about every two weeks for a period of two to three months. In comparison, patients without targeted conditions stayed in the system on average about one month.

There is some evidence that the HCH program also provides comprehensive care. Although 47 percent of patient encounters were for primary care services, 25 percent were for case management and social services, and 28 percent were for substance abuse, mental health, and dental services or referrals to a hospital or specialist. Currently, there are limited data on the health status outcomes of the HCH program.

Periodic national evaluations of HCH programs have been limited. The dearth of formal evaluations results not only from limited resources and variability in population and program characteristics but also from obstacles in conducting outcome-based cost-benefit analysis. A primary goal of HCH programs is to increase access to outpatient services and decrease utilization of costly inpatient services. However, access to services may actually result in higher use and greater cost (for lab tests, medication, specialty referrals, and hospitalization) as problems going untreated are uncovered. Another goal of HCH programs is to improve health outcomes to decrease long-term costs. However, HCH projects do not have control over the availability of all necessary resources that have a direct impact on improved health outcomes for homeless persons, such as affordable housing, livable income, or other needed social services. HCH programs are currently relying on client-based evaluations (that is, patient satisfaction), instead of broad-based evaluations to inform policy, but more comprehensive cost-benefit and outcomes-based analyses are needed.

## Supported Housing Models

The "housing first model" is currently promoted for making housing available for homeless people. It emphasizes provision of immediate permanent housing and supportive services onsite, including social services, mental health care, and substance abuse treatment. In contrast, the predominant service delivery model for the homeless, the "continuum of care model" moves homeless individuals as they progress along a continuum of care from emergency shelter to transitional shelter to permanent housing. The continuum-of-care policy was passed during the Clinton administration and promoted local coordination, filling gaps in service availability, and much-needed increases in resources. Under the model, homeless individuals transition to the next stage of housing depending on how well they do in the recommended service plan or (when applicable) substance abuse or mental health treatment plan.

The housing-first model places the homeless person in stable permanent housing from the start. Sometimes this housing is located in a scatter site among the general population communities, and sometimes it is located in the communities that already have homeless services, as in integrated housing developments.[309] Services are brought to the individual and are transitioned according to the preferences, readiness, and progress of the person. Instead of being transitioned from living situation to living situation, depending on the stage on the continuum, in the housing-first model social services are transitioned over time. Other elements in some housing-first programs are provision of permanent housing at the first contact with a homeless person rather than starting with emergency shelter as the first form of housing. Further, some housing-first programs use a low-demand housing model. This does not require service utilization, participation in activities, or sobriety as a requirement of housing. It does, though, require a few simple rules, notably paying for a portion of the rent (usually with Supplemental Security Income or SSI), not destroying property, not being violent, and having a "harm reduction approach to substance use." Considering homeless persons' preferences is a keystone for the housing-first model. This fits with some of the empirical data that suggest homeless persons with comorbid mental illness and substance abuse prefer independent living, in contrast to their clinicians' recommendations for group housing.[310]

Recent research has found that in the housing-first model, in contrast to the continuum-of-care model, individuals are more likely to obtain housing earlier and stay stably housed.[311] No differences between the models were found in mental illness or substance use. An evaluation of the New York City Pathways to Housing supported housing program found that 88 percent of the experimental subjects (all of whom had psychiatric disabilities) were housed after five years, in contrast to 47 percent of subjects in the control group continuum-of-care model.[312] There is some evidence that participants in the housing-first model are most motivated and most likely to use support services just before and immediately after they achieve housing.[313] Although policy must take into account interventions that create sustained long-term housing self-sufficiency, the policy must also consider that for some subgroups of the homeless population such self-sufficiency may not be possible.

# Homeless Health and Medical Care: Future Work

The massive body of health research on the homeless, developed over the course of the past two and half decades, shows that homeless persons as a group are exposed to the highest level of virtually all social and environmental risk factors for health, and as a result they pose a serious public health concern. However, health service providers have not solved the vast constellation of homeless health issues, for reasons that go beyond the fact that their programs are underfunded and unable to meet demand. The homeless are heavy users of ambulatory and inpatient health services, reflecting their excessive need. Moreover, the homeless will almost inevitably harbor society's most devastating emerging diseases and at a high rate. A preoccupation with health services serving as a magic bullet that prevents or cures the homeless of myriad adverse health conditions is misguided. It distracts us from the more fundamental issue of why the homeless are sick in the first place. The dominant integrative policy paradigm of structural (contextual) and individual (vulnerabilities, health risk behavior) limitations presented in the early part of this chapter offers a framework in which to address these fundamental issues.

To more fully understand the structural and individual limitations that sustain adverse health conditions among the homeless, it is best to discuss each limitation in detail. We draw on the research to look at the salient factors that have created and defined the structural context and individual effects for which adverse health conditions have emerged and are sustained.

## Structural Context

The most fundamental structural cause of adverse health among the homeless is the homeless condition itself and its association with housing. There is a longstanding relationship between housing and health in public health circles. Generally speaking, the risk of poor health as it is associated with housing is not randomly distributed in the population; instead, it is inversely correlated to income.[314] Economically disadvantaged people such as the homeless live in more crowded housing situations[315] and are exposed to more environmental toxins[316] than their poor but stably housed or middle-income counterparts. Housing quality is also inversely related to income.[317] Ethnic minorities also suffer disproportionate environmental health risk owing to housing conditions,[318] although a few studies reveal no link between income and environmental quality.[319]

Recognition of the impact of poor housing on health is not recent. In his 1842 Report on the Sanitary Condition of the Labouring Population of Great Britain, Edwin Chadwick established a link between the appalling living conditions of the poor and their ill health.[320] In the middle of the nineteenth century, pathologist Rudolf Virchow advised city leaders that poorly maintained, crowded housing was associated with higher infectious disease transmission.[321] Friedrich Engels, in his study of the working class in England, noted that "there is ample proof that the dwellings of the workers who live in the slums, combined with other adverse factors, give rise to many illnesses."[322] "Slum clearance" and improving the quality of housing and sanitation were important components of nineteenth- and early-twentieth-century campaigns to control typhus, tuberculosis, and other infectious diseases.[323] In the early 1800s, the relationship between housing conditions and health was recognized among public health practitioners in the United States[324] and Europe[325] and led to the rise of the sanitary reform movement.

Researchers of the homeless have assembled a significant amount of convincing evidence to document the structural links between housing and health among the homeless. Most of these studies have been cross-sectional in nature. The cumulative impact housing has on health in these studies is typically measured by comparing chronic versus recently homeless persons. Chronic homelessness is uniquely and positively associated with a number of gynecological symptoms,[326] preterm and low-birthweight babies,[327] and forcible rape in the past twelve months among homeless women.[328] Quality of housing is measured by comparing sheltered versus unsheltered homeless. Unsheltered homeless persons are more likely to have poorer mental health, use illegal drugs, have an acute skin injury, report daily alcohol use, be victimized, and experience an accident or an injury[329] than sheltered homeless persons. Studies that are more recent prove the structural argument by relating health directly to homelessness over time. Using data from a two-year longitudinal cohort of persons with addiction, Kertesz and colleagues found that chronic homelessness was associated with especially poor mental (but not poor physical) health over time.[330] A two-year study of street-dwelling homeless with serious mental illness (SMI) in New York City found that movement to stable housing and supportive services greatly reduced psychiatric symptoms for SMI homeless. In their sixteen-month longitudinal study of homeless persons in Alameda County California, Irene Wong and her colleagues found that the level of psychological distress was responsive to change in objective housing circumstances, with attainment of domicile status being associated with fewer distress symptoms.[331]

Public health practitioners have renewed interest in housing. It parallels a growing concern in ecological approaches to the study of complex health problems and examination of the social determinants of health and the causes of persistent socioeconomic, racial, and ethnic disparities in health.[332] Several recent reports have demonstrated the value of considering multilevel (individual, family, social network, community, state) determinants of a variety of health outcomes.[333] Public health advocates have emphasized the importance of creating interventions that address these influences on health[334] and of using ecological approaches that seek change in both the physical and the social environment, at various levels of organization.

## Individual Behavioral Choices and Vulnerabilities

How does the structural context in which homeless people reside influence risky individual behavioral choices? Who is most vulnerable to adverse health outcomes because of these choices? By the very token of not having permanent housing, the homeless of course endure some level of vulnerability. Those in society who are most vulnerable to the homeless condition are the ones least likely to prevail in competing for limited affordable housing resources. This is the group most likely to endure a chronicity of homelessness. They leave their station in life and enter homelessness with an established set of vulnerabilities.

A seminal study by Caton and colleagues gives us a clearer sense of this homeless group. Caton followed a group of newly homeless single adult men and women in New York City shelters for an eighteen-month period to determine risk factors associated with long-term homelessness. Lifetime DSM-IV Axis I disorder and lifetime substance use disorder were diagnosed at baseline in about half this total sample of newly homeless.[335] The widespread prevalence of these disorders profiles the set of vulnerabilities for which people enter homelessness. Those newly homeless who were able to exit homelessness ultimately had greater social and human capital. They were younger, better psychosocially adjusted, recently or currently employed, and income earners. Those who had adequate family support, no current drug treatment, and no arrest history experienced a shorter duration of homelessness.[336] The results convey an impression of the long-term homeless as a highly vulnerable, greater-risk-taking population. The fact that no current drug treatment and no lifetime drug use history predicted shorter homeless stays implies greater risk taking on the part of the long-term homeless. Drug treatment serves as a proxy for more serious drug use, whereas lifetime drug use (tried drugs at least once at any time in their life) also captures the casual and one-time user of drugs with shorter stays in facilities for the homeless. The finding that no arrest history, a marker for deviant behavior, was associated with shorter homeless stays again suggests higher risk-taking behavior on the part of the long-term homeless.

To faithfully apply the dominant integrative approach to the adverse health outcomes of the homeless means that we cannot view individual risk-taking behavior within the framework of individual rational choice. Historically, the individual rational choice model has profoundly influenced health and social policies regarding the homeless and the poor in general. Under this model falls the notion that people bear full responsibility for their own morbidity and mortality. Hence, choice occurs in a vacuum, and the structural context in which people reside does not matter. Perhaps a more appropriate model for our purposes is that of *institutional rational choice*. This examines how the institutions and social structure in which individuals find themselves situated generate preferences.[337]

Much of what is to be explained in health services research requires the institutional or structural component because institutions constrain what is possible and structurally suggest individual interests. Institutions do this in two ways. First, by constraining what is possible—indeed, what is probable—they shape interests. Second, the interests of any individual are given by her relationship to others—that is, her position within the social structure.[338] The setting or context in which individuals find themselves helps to generate, or structurally to suggest, both their choices and their actions to realize their interests.[339] The homeless first enter their condition with a set of vulnerabilities that prevent them from affording prevailing housing rentals—an institutional structure that is no fault of theirs. They find themselves in overcrowded or substandard living situations, typically in areas of concentrated poverty. If their homeless stay becomes long-term, they develop relationships with others in their social context and are faced with an increasingly strong set of social norms that influence or reinforce their risk-taking behaviors.

Research on those homeless people most vulnerable to serious adverse health outcomes is primarily based on cross-sectional studies. Because homelessness has persistently cultivated a pocket of endemicity for communicable disease, we focus here on major current communicable diseases in society. Homeless people most vulnerable to HCV positivity were those with greater homelessness severity, a history of substance use (IDU and non-IDU), recent IDU-related behaviors including equipment sharing, other forms of sharing (toothbrushes, razors), tattoos, sexually transmitted diseases, a jail or prison history, and greater age.[340] Homeless persons most vulnerable to HIV seroprevalence included those with lower education, those with a prison history, white sex traders, racial minorities, those who engaged in recent receptive anal sex, syringe sharing, transfusion, those who had five or more recent sexual partners, and female crack users who gave sex for drugs.[341] Homeless people who were more vulnerable to TB included black males, those aged thirty to fifty-nine, and those who had a history of incarceration or drug abuse.[342] This evidence makes it apparent that the primary risk factors for communicable disease are either measures of persistent homelessness (such as homeless severity) or overlap with many of the risk factors associated with persistent homelessness (being male, having a history of incarceration or substance abuse, and so on). The structural effects such as persistent lack of housing and substandard housing therefore seem to have some influence on the health of homeless people. Other structural effects that are associated with persistent homelessness, such as the social norms within a community of long-term homeless, may further shape risky behaviors to invoke these disease consequences.

The striking impact that homelessness confers on the health of children also makes them a group vulnerable to structural impacts. Structural resources that target families (income maintenance, affordable housing benefits) typically enable homeless families to have short homeless stays. Female-headed adults in homeless families are similar to poor housed families on many health measures.[343] However, compared to poor housed children, homeless children consistently experience more health problems. Homeless children are sick four times as often as other poor children and experience more acute and chronic illness.[344] About 26 percent of all children and 33 percent of children under age five become ill more often during episodes of homelessness.[345] More than 20 percent of homeless preschoolers have emotional problems serious enough to require professional care, and 47 percent of homeless school age children have problems such as anxiety, depression, and withdrawal, compared to 18 percent of other poor children.[346] The evidence on the health of homeless children shows a strong relationship between environment and health. Young children, given their lower immunity compared to adults, may be more susceptible to the impact of their housing environment on health, even with short bouts of homelessness.

Recent federal, state, and metropolitan initiatives to end homelessness target the persistently homeless.[347] The U.S. Congress appropriated $35 million to assist chronically homeless adults in fiscal year 2003 and proposed double that amount for FY2005.[348] Additionally, funding from the Department of Housing and Urban Development now prioritizes housing the chronically homeless. However, the striking impact that the homeless condition has on the lives of children illustrates the importance of preventing and treating encounters with homelessness among impoverished families. As a result, homeless children should not be left out of the federal response to ending homelessness. Moreover, the policy response to ending homelessness should consider structural factors that could continue to impede health, even once formerly homeless individuals are permanently housed. For instance, the HUD's Moving to Opportunities Fair Housing Demonstration Project, which relocated public housing residents in high-poverty neighborhoods to less-poor neighborhoods, found that moving significantly lowered psychological distress among adults and anxiety and depressive disorders among children.[349] Thus certain structural factors, such as neighborhood effects on health, should not be excluded from the national and local policy response on ending homelessness.

## The Integrative Approach as a Policy Paradigm

Any policy response to the health of the homeless must consider an approach that combines structural factors (situational context in which health is influenced and occurs) and individual factors (risk factors and vulnerabilities, such as risky behavior, that influence health). The persistent and widening gap in health disparities among the homeless is largely the result of health policies that have been traditionally based on altering individual behavior as a means of improving the health circumstances of the homeless. However, this approach ignores the environmental and economic structures, social and cultural norms, and institutions that shape decision-making processes to facilitate and perpetuate patterns of behavior. An integrative approach combines individual and structural factors to probe beyond myopic models to broader motivational assumptions. This approach would examine such factors as refinement of housing codes to reflect current knowledge of healthful housing, adding measures of housing quality and satisfaction in local health department reports, the collaboration of public health representatives in local urban planning processes, and encouraging neighborhood collective efficacy and organizational participation to mobilize communities around issues of neighborhood and health conditions. In this sense, the integrative model can take a leading role in setting priorities for social, economic, and health policy to better promote health among society's most vulnerable members.

## Future Research

The current direction for health research in the United States accommodates the new integrative approach (structural and individual) for homeless research and policy. The National Institutes of Health have been the largest funder of research on the homeless. For more than two decades, the NIH has invested millions of dollars in research that has amassed information on the composition, health needs, and health service use of the homeless population. The ultimate intent of this research has been to improve the health of the homeless. However, available research has not been translated into practice. Issues such as the large volume of conflicting research results, constraints on physicians' time, and lack of policies to foster implementation have served as barriers to translating research results into practical and sustaining practice.

The NIH Roadmap outlines translation of research advances using expanded research partnerships and integrated research networks in the context of a patient-centered approach, consistent with recent recommendations from the Institute of Medicine. The NIH Roadmap marks a paradigm shift in health research, from one that traditionally focused on homogeneous clinical and biological questions about the human organism to population-based interventions that deal with human behaviors, health priorities, economic and social structures, laws, and cultures that are heterogeneous across settings. The paradigm shifts largely resulted from research results that lacked relevance in the community setting and remain unaccepted by the communities that might benefit from them. Traditional terms of funding supports forced researchers to focus on generalizable research questions and results and then move onto the next project. Community engagement has become a strategic imperative within the new dominant paradigm of health research. The new paradigm requires community stakeholder involvement in the entire research process, which enables research priorities and research results to become more relevant and actionable in local situations for those that would apply them.

The integrative approach (structural and individual) to addressing issues of the health of the homeless effectively accommodates the new NIH paradigm for health research. The integrative approach offers a framework in which to focus research questions on the health of homeless persons, while the new NIH research paradigm imparts the structure for which answers to these research questions will be translated into practice within the community. Both the integrative model on homeless health issues and the new NIH research paradigm focus on a population health approach. These complementary models allow individuals from the community (clinical practitioners, policy makers, urban planners, homeless people themselves ) to (1) come together around a common purpose; (2) examine research questions about the homeless that involve individual behaviors and the political, environmental, economic, and social context; and (3) make decisions and develop confidence in their ability to solve their own problems. Ultimately, these complementary models will help develop much-needed information on which services work, for which homeless groups, in which communities, and at what costs, all critical elements for effective and economically efficient public policies regarding the homeless.

## Conclusion

Columbia University public health professor Ilan Meyer states it well: "The study of social and economic factors in public health may have unintended consequences that, paradoxically, serve to preserve disparities rather than eliminate them. This can occur because public health research transports social issues into the health domain, where they are examined through the narrow prism of health relevance instead of within their political, social, and economic contexts. We refer to this as the 'public healthification' of social problems, akin to the 'medicalization' and 'healthism' that have occurred with the advance of biomedicine in the last century."[350]

Perhaps of greatest concern is that our nation seems to have come to accept homelessness as just another negative aspect of modern life, similar in this way to violent crime. It is difficult for health policy makers to address the problems of the homeless population when public support for homeless people is weak at best. Perhaps advocates for the homeless have done a disservice by focusing on homeless people's medical, mental health, and substance abuse problems and needs rather than on the core issues of lack of low-income housing as well as the breakdown of social cohesiveness and community relations in this country. Gary Blasi suggests that

> Mass homelessness is now seen as an acceptable feature of American life. Institutional forces have been aggravated by conservative political forces, aimed at demonstrating either that homelessness is not much of a problem after all, or that such problems as there are, flow from the personal and moral failures of those who are homeless. Advocates for homeless people, as some of them now recognize, bear considerable responsibility for reinforcing some distortions and introducing others. Indeed it is possible (although by no means uncertain) that by redefining extreme poverty in terms of homelessness, by advocating for "the homeless" rather than for the extremely poor (including those with disabilities), and by paying inadequate attention to questions of race, advocates unwittingly harmed the ultimate cause they believed they were serving: alleviating the human suffering that attends extreme deprivation.[351]

# Notes

1. Burt, M., and others. *Homelessness: Programs and the People They Serve: Summary Report.* Washington, D.C.: Interagency Council on Homelessness, 1999.
2. Link, B., and others. "Lifetime and Five Year Prevalence of Homelessness in the United States." *American Journal of Public Health,* 1994, *84,* 1907–1912.
3. Burt and others (1999).
4. Cousineau, M. "Comparing Adults in Los Angeles County Who Have and Have Not Been Homeless." *Journal of Community Psychology,* 2001, *29,* 693–701.
5. Katz, M. *In the Shadow of the Poorhouse.* New York: Basic Books, 1986.
6. Trattner, W. *From Poor Law to Welfare State* (4th ed.). New York: Free Press, 1989.
7. "The Poorhouse Story." 2005. [http://www.poorhousestory.com/history.htm] (accessed Mar. 22, 2006).

8. "Poorhouse Story" (2005).

9. Katz (1986).

10. Trattner (1989).

11. Rothman, D. J. (ed.). *The Almshouse Experience: Collected Reports:* includes *Quincy Report of 1821 and Yates Report of 1824*. New York: Arno Press and *New York Times*, 1971.

12. Katz, M. *In the Shadow of the Poorhouse: A Social History of Welfare in America* (rev. ed.). New York: Basic Books, 1996.

13. Katz (1986).

14. Trattner (1989).

15. Katz, M. (ed.). *The Undeserving Poor: From the War on Poverty to the War on Welfare*. New York: Pantheon Books, 1990.

16. Katz (1986).

17. Katz (1986).

18. Riis, J. *How the Other Half Lives*. New York: Scribner, 1890.

19. Rice, S. A. "The Homeless." *Annals of the American Academy of Political and Social Science*, 1918, *77*, 140–153.

20. Rice (1918).

21. Katz, M. B. "Poorhouses and the Origins of the Public Old Age Home." *Milbank Memorial Fund Quarterly/Health and Society*, 1984, *62*, 110–140.

22. Kusmer, K. L. *Down and Out, on the Road: The Homeless in American History*. New York: Oxford University Press, 2002.

23. Bahr, H. M. *Skid Row: An Introduction to Disaffiliation*. New York: Oxford University Press, 1973.

24. Bahr (1973).

25. Blumberg, L. U., Shipley, T. E., and Borsky, S. *Liquor and Poverty: Skid Row as a Human Condition*. New Brunswick, N.J.: Rutgers Center for Alcoholic Studies, 1978; Bogue, D. *Skid Row in American Cities*. Chicago: University of Chicago Press, 1963.

26. Hopper, K., and Hamberg, J. "The Making of America's Homeless: From Skid Row to New Poor, 1945–1985." In R. G. Bratt, C. Hartman, and A. Meyerson (eds.), *Critical Perspectives on Housing*. Philadelphia: Temple University Press, 1986.

27. Baxter, E., and Hopper, K. *Private Lives/Public Spaces: Homeless Adults on the Streets of New York*. New York: Institute for Social Welfare Research, 1981.

28. Culhane, D., and Kuhn, R. "Patterns and Determinants of Public Shelter Utilization Among Homeless Adults in New York City and Philadelphia." *Journal of Policy Analysis and Management*, 1998, *17*, 23–43; Wong, Y. I., and Piliavin, I. "A Dynamic Analysis of Homeless-Domicile Transitions." *Social Problems*, 1997, *44*, 408–423.

29. Shinn, M., and others. "Predictors of Homelessness Among Families in New York City: From Shelter Request to Housing Stability." *American Journal of Public Health*, 1998, *88*, 1651–1657.

30. Rog, D., Holupka, C., and McCombs-Thornton, K. "Implementation of the Homeless Families Program: 1. Service Models and Preliminary Outcomes." *American Journal of Orthopsychiatry*, 1995, *65*, 502–513.

31. Zlotnick, C., Robertson, M., and Lahiff, M. "Getting off the Streets: Economic Resources and Residential Exits from Homelessness." *Journal of Community Psychology*, 1999, *27*, 209–224.

32. Hurlburt, M., Wood, P., and Hough, R. "Providing Independent Housing for the Homeless Mentally Ill: A Novel Approach to Evaluating Long-Term Longitudinal Housing Patterns." *Journal of Community Psychology*, 1996, *24*, 291–310.

33. Tsemberis, S., and Asmussen, S. "From Streets to Homes: The Pathways to Housing Consumer Preference Supported Housing Model." *Alcoholism Treatment Quarterly*, 1999, *17*, 113–132.

34. U.S. Department of Housing and Urban Development (HUD). "Notice of Funding Availability (NOFA) for the Collaborative Initiative to Help End Chronic Homelessness." 2002. [http://www.hud.gov/offices/cpd/homeless/apply/2002nofa/index.cfm].

35. Kertesz, S. G., and others. "Homeless Chronicity and Health-Related Quality of Life Trajectories Among Adults with Addictions." *Medical Care*, 2005, *43*, 574–585.

36. Homes for the Homeless. *Homeless in America: A Children's Story.* New York: Institute for Children and Poverty, 1999; National Center on Family Homelessness. "Homeless Children: America's New Outcasts." 1999. [www.familyhomelessness.org/fact_children.pdf].

37. Burt and others (1999).

38. Koegel, P., and Burnam, A. *The Course of Homelessness Study: Aims and Designs.* Rockville, Md.: National Institute of Mental Health, 1991.

39. Burt and others (1999).

40. Burt and others (1999); Cowal, K., and others. "Mother-Child Separations Among Homeless and Housed Families Receiving Public Assistance in New York City." *American Journal of Community Psychology*, 2002, *30*, 711–730.

41. Burt and others (1999).

42. O'Connell, J. J., and others. "Old and Sleeping Rough: Homeless Persons on the Streets of Boston." *Care Management Journals*, 2004, *5*, 101–106.

43. Burt and others (1999).

44. Gamache, G., Rosenheck, R., and Tessler, R. "The Proportion of Veterans Among Homeless Men: A Decade Later." *Social Psychiatry and Psychiatric Epidemiology*, 2001, *36*, 481–485.

45. Rosenheck, R., Frisman, L., and Chung, A. "The Proportion of Veterans Among Homeless Men." *American Journal of Public Health*, 1994, *84*, 466–469.

46. Gamache, G., Rosenheck, R., and Tessler, R. "Overrepresentation of Women Veterans Among Homeless Women." *American Journal of Public Health*, 2003, *93*, 1132–1135.

47. Burt and others (1999); Link and others (1994).

48. Burt and others (1999).

49. Burt and others (1999).

50. Burt and others (1999).

51. Phelan, J., and Link, B. "Who Are 'the Homeless'? Reconsidering the Stability and Composition of the Homeless Population." *American Journal of Public Health*, 1999, *89*, 1334–1338.

52. Burt and others (1999).

53. Koegel, P. "Through a Different Lens: An Anthropological Perspective on the Homeless Mentally Ill." *Culture, Medicine and Psychiatry*, 1992, *16*, 1–22.

54. Phelan and Link (1999).

55. Metraux, S., and Culhane, D. "Family Dynamics, Housing and Recurring Homelessness Among Women in New York City Homeless Shelters." *Journal of Family Issues*, 1999, *20*, 371–396.

56. Quigley, J., Raphael, S., and Smolensky, E. *Homelessness in California.* San Francisco: Public Policy Institute of California, 2001.

57. Mojtabai, R. "Perceived Reasons for Loss of Housing and Continued Homelessness Among Homeless Persons with Mental Illness." *Psychiatric Services*, 2005, *56*, 172–178.

58. Nunez, R., and Cox, C. "A Snapshot of Family Homelessness Across America." *Political Science Quarterly*, 1999, *114*, 289–299.

59. Arangua, L., Andersen R., and Gelberg, L. "The Health Circumstances of Homeless Women in the United States." *International Journal of Mental Health*, 2005, xx.

60. Brickner, P. W., and others (eds.). *Health Care of Homeless People*. New York: Springer, 1985.

61. Vangeest, J., and Johnson, T. "Substance Abuse and Homelessness: Direct or Indirect Effects?" *Annals of Epidemiology*, 2002, *12*, 455–461.

62. Zlotnick, C., Tam, T., and Robertson, M. J. "Disaffiliation, Substance Use, and Exiting Homelessness." *Substance Use and Misuse*, 2003, *389*, 577–599.

63. Mojtabai (2005).

64. Mojtabai (2005).

65. Weinreb, L., Goldberg, R., and Lessard, D. "Pap Smear Testing Among Homeless and Very Low-Income Housed Mothers." *Journal of Health Care for the Poor and Underserved*, 2002, *13*, 141–150; Wenzel, S. L., and others. "Physical Violence Against Impoverished Women: A Longitudinal Analysis of Risk and Protective Factors." *Women's Health Issues*, 2004, *14*, 144–154.

66. Shinn and others (1998).

67. Zlotnick, Tam, and Robertson (2003).

68. Link and others (1994).

69. Fischer, P., and Breakey, W. "Homelessness and Mental Health: An Overview." *International Journal of Mental Health*, 1986, *14*, 6–41.

70. Culhane and Kuhn (1998).

71. Shinn and others (1998); Roy, E., and others. "Mortality in a Cohort of Street Youth in Montreal." *Journal of the American Medical Association*, 2004, *292*, 569–574; Caton, C. L., and others. "Risk Factors for Long-Term Homelessness: Findings from a Longitudinal Study of First-Time Homeless Single Adults." *American Journal of Public Health*, 2005, *95*, 1753–1759.

72. Bauman, K. "Shifting Family Definitions: The Effect of Cohabitation and Other Non-family Household Relationships on Measures of Poverty." *Demography*, 1999, *36*, 315–325.

73. Wood, D., Valdez, R. B., Hayashi, T., and Shen, A. "Homeless and Housed Families in Los Angeles: A Study Comparing Demographic, Economic, and Family Function Characteristics." *American Journal of Public Health*, 1990, *80*(9), 1049–1052.

74. Burt and others (1999).

75. Gelberg, L., and Linn, L. "Assessing the Physical Health of Homeless Adults." *Journal of the American Medical Association*, *1989*, 262, 1973–1979; Gelberg, L., Andersen, R., and Leake, B. "The Behavioral Model for Vulnerable Populations: Application to Medical Care Use and Outcomes." *Health Services Research*, 2000, *34*, 1273–1302; Robertson, M., Zlotnick, C., and Westerfelt, A. "Drug Use Disorders and Treatment Contact Among Homeless Adults in Alameda County, California." *American Journal of Public Health*, 1997, *87*, 221–228.

76. Lim, Y., and others. "How Accessible Is Medical Care for Homeless Women?" *Medical Care*, 2002, *40*, 510–520; Wenzel, S., Andersen, R., Gifford, D., and Gelberg, L. "Homeless Women's Gynecological Symptoms and Use of Medical Care." *Journal of Health Care for the Poor and Underserved*, 2001, *12*, 323–341; Wenzel, S., Leake, B., and Gelberg, L. "Health of Homeless Women with Recent Experience of Rape." *Journal of General Internal Medicine*, 2000, *15*, 265–268; Stein, J., Lu, M., and Gelberg, L. "Severity of Homelessness and Adverse Birth Outcomes." *Health Psychology*, 2000, *19*, 524–534.

77. Barrow, S., Herman, D., Cordova, P., and Struening, E. "Mortality Among Homeless Shelter Residents in New York City." *American Journal of Public Health*, 1999, *89*, 529–534.

78. Brickner and others (1985).

79. Fischer, P. J., and others. "Mental Health and Social Characteristics of the Homeless: A Survey of Mission Users." *American Journal of Public Health*, 1986, *76*(5), 519–524.

80. Gallagher, T., Andersen, R., Koegel, P., and Gelberg, L. "Determinants of Regular Source of Care Among Homeless Adults in Los Angeles." *Medical Care*, 1997, *35*, 814–830.

81. Burt and others (1999).

82. Robertson, M., and Cousineau, M. "Health Status and Access to Health Services Among the Urban Homeless." *American Journal of Public Health*, 1986, *76*, 561–563.

83. Hwang, S. "Mortality Among Men Using Homeless Shelters in Toronto, Ontario." *Journal of the American Medical Association*, 2000, *283*, 2152–2157; Hwang, S. "Is Homelessness Hazardous to Your Health? Obstacles to the Demonstration of a Causal Relationship." *Canadian Journal of Public Health*, 2002, *93*, 407–410.

84. Hibbs, J., and others. "Mortality in a Cohort of Homeless Adults in Philadelphia." *New England Journal of Medicine*, 1994, *331*, 304–309.

85. Barrow, Herman, Cordova, and Struening (1999).

86. Hwang, S., O'Connell, J., and Brennan, T. "Causes of Death in Homeless Adults in Boston." *Annals of Internal Medicine*, 1997, *126*, 625–628.

87. Hwang (2000).

88. Cheung, A., and Hwang, S. "Risk of Death Among Homeless Women: A Cohort Study and Review of the Literature." *Canadian Medical Association Journal*, 2004, *170*, 1243–1247.

89. Cheung and Hwang (2004).

90. Barrow, Herman, Cordova, and Struening (1999).

91. Hwang, S., and others. "Risk Factors for Death in Homeless Adults in Boston." *Archives of Internal Medicine*, 1998, *158*, 1454–1460.

92. Gelberg, L., Linn, L. S., and Mayer-Oakes, S. A. "Differences in Health Status Between Older and Younger Homeless Adults." *Journal of the American Geriatrics Society*, 1990, *38*, 1220–1229.

93. Almeida, R. A., Dubay, L. C., and Ko, G. "Access to Care and Use of Health Services by Low-Income Women." *Health Care Financing Review*, 2001, *22*, 27–47.

94. McLean, D. "Asthma Among Homeless Children: Undercounting and Undertreating the Underserved." *Archives of Pediatric and Adolescent Medicine*, 2004, *158*, 244–249.

95. Burt and others (1999).

96. Burt and others (1999); Wenzel, Andersen, Gifford, and Gelberg (2001); Long, H., and others. "Cancer Screening in Homeless Women: Attitudes and Behaviors." *Journal of Health Care for the Poor and Underserved*, 1998, *9*, 276–292.

97. Wood, D., Valdez, R., Hayashi, T., and Shen, A. "Health of Homeless Children and Housed, Poor Children." *Pediatrics*, 1990, *86*, 858–866.

98. Brickner and others (1985); Zolopa, A., and others. "HIV and Tuberculosis Infection in San Francisco's Homeless Adults: Prevalence and Risk Factors in a Representative Sample." *Journal of the American Medical Association*, 1994, *272*, 455–461.

99. Zolopa and others (1994); Robertson, M. J., and others. "HIV Seroprevalence Among Homeless and Marginally Housed Adults in San Francisco." *American Journal of Public Health*, 2004, *94*, 1207–1217.

100. Cheung, R., and others. "Viral Hepatitis and Other Infectious Diseases in a Homeless Population." *Journal of Clinical Gastroenterology*, 2002, *34*, 476–480.

101. Zolopa and others (1994).

102. Gelberg, L., and others. "Tuberculosis Skin Testing Among Homeless Adults." *Journal of General Internal Medicine*, 1997, *12*, 25–33.

103. McAdam, J., and others. "The Spectrum of Tuberculosis in a New York City Men's Shelter Clinic (1982–1988)." *Chest*, 1990, *97*, 798–805.

104. Des Prez, R., and Heim, C. "Mycobacterium Tuberculosis." In G. Mandell, G. Douglas, and J. Bennett (eds.), *Principles and Practices of Infectious Diseases*. New York: Churchill Livingstone, 1990.

105. Brewer, T., and others. "Strategies to Decrease Tuberculosis in U.S. Homeless Populations: A Computer Simulation Model." *Journal of the American Medical Association*, 2001, *286*, 834–842.

106. McAdam, J., Brickner, P., and Glicksman, R. "Tuberculosis in the SRO/Homeless Population." In P. Brickner and others (eds.), *Health Care for Homeless People*. New York: Springer, 1985.

107. Barnes, P. F., and others. "Transmission of Tuberculosis Among the Urban Homeless." *Journal of the American Medical Association*, 1996, *275*, 305–307.

108. Haddad, M. B., and others. "Tuberculosis and Homelessness in the United States, 1994–2003." *Journal of the American Medical Association*, 2005, *293*, 2762–2766.

109. Nyamathi, A. M., and others. "Risk Factors for Hepatitis C Virus Infection Among Homeless Adults." *Journal of General Internal Medicine*, 2002, *17*, 134–144.

110. Gelberg, L., Robertson, M., and Andersen, R. *Hepatitis B and C Among Homeless Adults*. Rockville, Md.: National Institute on Drug Abuse (1-RO1-DA14294–01), 2001–2004.

111. Rosenblum, A., and others. "Hepatitis C and Substance Use in a Sample of Homeless People in New York City." *Journal of Addictive Diseases*, 2001, *20*, 15–23.

112. Cheung and others (2002).

113. Desai, R. A., Rosenheck, R. A., and Agnello, V. "Prevalence of Hepatitis C Virus Infection in a Sample of Homeless Veterans." *Social Psychiatry and Psychiatric Epidemiology*, 2003, *38*, 396–401.

114. Stein, J. A., and Nyamathi, A. "Correlates of Hepatitis C Virus Infection in Homeless Men: A Latent Variable Approach." *Drug and Alcohol Dependence*, 2004, *75*, 89–95.

115. Alter, M., and others. "The Prevalence of Hepatitis C Virus Infection in the United States, 1988 Through 1994." *New England Journal of Medicine*, 1999, *341*, 556–562.

116. Cheung and others (2002); Nyamathi and others (2002); Rosenblum and others (2001); Stein and Nyamathi (2004).

117. Stein and Nyamathi (2004).

118. Nyamathi, A., and others. "Presence and Predictors of Hepatitis C Virus RNA in the Semen of Homeless Men." *Biological Research for Nursing*, 2002, *4*, 22–30.

119. Klinkenberg, W. D., and others. "Prevalence of Human Immunodeficiency Virus, Hepatitis B, and Hepatitis C Among Homeless Persons with Co-Occurring Severe Mental Illness and Substance Use Disorders." *Comprehensive Psychiatry*, 2003, *44*, 293–302.

120. Cheung and others (2002).

121. Gelberg, L., and others. "Hepatitis B Among Homeless and Other Impoverished U.S. Military Veterans in Residential Care in Los Angeles." *Public Health*, 2001, *115*, 286–291.

122. Rosenblum and others (2001).

123. Zolopa and others (1994); Robertson and others (2004).

124. Robertson, M. J. "HIV Seroprevalence Among Homeless and Marginally Housed Adults in San Francisco." *American Journal of Public Health*, 2004, *94*(7), 1207–1217.

125. Klinkenberg and others (2003).

126. Robertson and others (1999).

127. McQuillan, G., and others. "Update on the Seroepidemiology of Human Immunodeficiency Virus in the United States Household Population: NHANES III, 1988–1994." *Journal of Acquired Immune Deficiency Syndrome and Human Retrovirology*, 1997, *14*, 355–360.

128. Shlay, J., and others. "Human Immunodeficiency Virus Seroprevalence and Risk Assessment of a Homeless Population in Denver." *Sexually Transmitted Diseases,* 1996, *23,* 304–311.

129. Rosenblum and others (2001).

130. Cheung and others (2002).

131. Hwang, O'Connell, and Brennan (1997).

132. Culhane, D. P., Gollub, E., Kuhn, R., and Shpaner, M. "The Co-Occurrence of AIDS and Homelessness: Results from the Integration of Administrative Databases for AIDS Surveillance and Public Shelter Utilization in Philadelphia." *Journal of Epidemiology and Community Health,* 2001, *55,* 515–520.

133. DeRosa, C. J., and others. "HIV Risk Behavior and HIV Testing: A Comparison of Rates and Associated Factors Among Homeless and Runaway Adolescents in Two Cities." *AIDS Education and Prevention,* 2001, *13,* 131–148.

134. Desai, M. M., and Rosenheck, R. A. "HIV Testing and Receipt of Test Results Among Homeless Persons with Serious Mental Illness." *American Journal of Psychiatry,* 2004, *161*(12), 2287–2294.

135. Herndon, B., and others. "Prevalence and Predictors of HIV Testing Among a Probability Sample of Homeless Women in Los Angeles County." *Public Health Reports,* 2003, *118,* 261–269.

136. Riley, E. D., and others. "Antiretroviral Therapy, Hepatitis C Virus, and AIDS Mortality Among San Francisco's Homeless and Marginally Housed." *Journal of Acquired Immune Deficiency Syndrome,* 2005, *38,* 191–195.

137. Weitzman, B. C. "Pregnancy and Childbirth: Risk Factors for Homelessness?" *Family Planning Perspectives,* 1989, *21*(4), 175–178.

138. Zlotnick, C., Robertson, M. J., and Tam, T. "Substance Use and Separation of Homeless Mothers from Their Children." *Addictive Behavior,* 2003, *28,* 1373–1383.

139. Gelberg, L., and others. "Use of Contraceptive Methods Among Homeless Women for Protection Against Unwanted Pregnancies and STD's: Prior Use and Willingness to Use in the Future." *Contraception,* 2001, *63,* 277–281.

140. Shuler, P. A., Gelberg, L., and Davis, J. E. "Characteristics Associated with the Risk of Unintended Pregnancy Among Urban Homeless Women." *Journal of the American Academy of Nurse Practitioners,* 1995, *7,* 13–22; Brickner, P., and others (eds.). *Under the Safety Net: The Health and Social Welfare of the Homeless in the United States.* New York: Norton, 1990.

141. Gelberg and others (2001).

142. Gelberg, L., and others. "Chronically Homeless Women's Deterrents to Contraception." *Perspectives on Sexual and Reproductive Health,* 2002, *34,* 278–285.

143. Brickner and others (1990).

144. Gelberg, L., Andersen, R., and Browner, C. *Access to Care for Homeless Women of Reproductive Age.* Rockville, Md.: Agency for Health Care Policy and Research (R01 HS08323), 1995–2000.

145. Long and others (1998); Chau, S., and others. "Cancer Risk Behaviors and Screening Rates Among Homeless Adults in Los Angeles County." *Cancer Epidemiology, Biomarkers and Prevention,* 2002, *11,* 431–438.

146. Long and others (1998); Chau and others (2002).

147. Chau and others (2002).

148. Long and others (1998).

149. Chau and others (2002).

150. Chau and others (2002).

151. Shuler, P. A. *Homeless Women's Holistic and Family Planning Needs: An Exposition and Test of the Nurse Practitioner Model.* (dissertation.) University of California, Los Angeles, 1991.

152. Lim and others (2002).

153. Burt and others (1999).

154. Chavkin, W., Kristal, A., Seabron, C., and Guigli, P. "The Reproductive Experience of Women Living in Hotels for the Homeless in New York City." *New York State Journal of Medicine*, 1987, *87*, 10–13.

155. Paterson, C. M., and Roderick, P. "Obstetric Outcome in Homeless Women." *British Medical Journal*, 1990, *301*, 263–266.

156. Chavkin, Kristal, Seabron, and Guigli (1987).

157. Stein, Lu, and Gelberg (2000).

158. Little, M., and others. "Adverse Perinatal Outcomes Associated with Homelessness and Substance Use in Pregnancy." *Canadian Medical Association Journal*, 2005, *173*, 615–618.

159. Chavkin, Kristal, Seabron, and Guigli (1987).

160. Burt and others (1999).

161. Burt and others (1999); Wenzel, S., Koegel, P., and Gelberg, L. "Antecedents of Physical and Sexual Victimization Among Homeless Women: A Comparison to Homeless Men." *American Journal of Community Psychology*, 2000, *28*, 367–390.

162. Wenzel, Leake, and Gelberg (2000).

163. Wenzel, Leake, and Gelberg (2000).

164. Kushel, M. B., and others. "No Door to Lock: Victimization Among Homeless and Marginally Housed Persons." *Archives of Internal Medicine*, 2003, *163*, 2492–2499.

165. Lam, J., and Rosenheck, R. "The Effect of Victimization on Clinical Outcomes of Homeless Persons with Serious Mental Illness." *Psychiatric Services*, 1998, *49*, 678–683.

166. Lam and Rosenheck (1998).

167. Wenzel, Koegel, and Gelberg (2000); Lam and Rosenheck (1998).

168. Burt and others (1999).

169. Wenzel, Koegel, and Gelberg (2000); Herman, D., Susser, E., Struening, E., and Link, B. "Adverse Childhood Experiences: Are They Risk Factors for Adult Homelessness?" *American Journal of Public Health*, 1997, *87*, 249–255.

170. Nyamathi, A., and others. "Comparison of Psychosocial and Behavioral Profiles of Victimized and Nonvictimized Homeless Women and Their Intimate Partners." *Research in Nursing and Health*, 2001, *24*, 324–335.

171. North, C., Smith, E., Pollio, D., and Spitznagel, E. "Are the Mentally Ill Homeless a Distinct Homeless Subgroup?" *Annals of Clinical Psychiatry*, 1996, *8*, 117–128.

172. Benda, B. B. "Gender Differences in Predictors of Suicidal Thoughts and Attempts Among Homeless Veterans That Abuse Substances." *Suicide and Life Threatening Behavior*, 2005, *35*, 106–116.

173. Davies-Netzley, S., Hurlburt, M., and Hough, R. "Childhood Abuse as a Precursor to Homelessness for Homeless Women with Severe Mental Illness." *Violence and Victims*, 1996, *11*, 129–142.

174. Koegel, P., Melamid, E., and Burnam, M. "Childhood Risk Factors for Homelessness Among Homeless Adults." *American Journal of Public Health*, 1995, *85*, 1642–1649.

175. Booth, B., Sullivan, G., Koegel, P., and Burnam, A. "Vulnerability Factors for Homelessness Associated with Substance Dependence in a Community Sample of Homeless Adults." *American Journal of Drug and Alcohol Abuse*, 2002, *28*, 429–452.

176. Dietz, P., and Coburn, J. *To Whom Do They Belong? Runaway, Homeless and Other Youth in High-Risk Situations in the 1990s.* Washington, D.C.: National Network for Runaway and Youth Services, 1991.

177. Molina, B. S. "High Risk Adolescent and Young Adult Populations: Consumption and Consequences." *Recent Developments in Alcoholism*, 2005, *17*, 49–65.

178. Ringwalt, C., Greene, J., Robertson, M., and McPheeters, M. "The Prevalence of Homelessness Among Adolescents in the United States." *American Journal of Public Health*, 1998, *88*, 1325–1329.

179. MacLean, M., Embry, L., and Cauce, A. "Homeless Adolescents' Paths to Separation from Family: Comparison of Family Characteristics, Psychological Adjustment, and Victimization." *Journal of Community Psychology*, 1999, *27*, 179–187.

180. Milburn, N.-G., and others. "Predictors of Close Family Relationships over One Year Among Homeless Young People." *Journal of Adolescence*, 2005, *28*, 263–275.

181. Whitbeck, L. B., and others. "Mental Disorder, Subsistence Strategies, and Victimization Among Gay, Lesbian, and Bisexual Homeless and Runaway Adolescents." *Journal of Sex Research*, 2004, *41*, 329–342.

182. Van Leeuwen, J. M., Hopfer, C, and Hooks, S. "A Snapshot of Substance Abuse Among Homeless and Runaway Youth in Denver, Colorado." *Journal of Community Health*, 2004, *29*, 217–229.

183. Roy, E., and others. "Risk Factors for Hepatitis C Virus Infection Among Street Youths." *Canadian Medical Association Journal*, 2001, *165*, 557–560; Ensign, J., and Santelli, J. "Health Status and Service Use: Comparison of Adolescents at a School-Based Health Clinic with Homeless Adolescents." *Archives of Pediatrics and Adolescent Medicine*, 1998, *152*, 20–24; Greene, J., Ennett, S., and Ringwalt, C. "Substance Use Among Runaway and Homeless Youth in Three National Samples." *American Journal of Public Health*, 1997, *87*, 229–235; Greene, J., and Ringwalt, C. "Youth and Familial Substance Use's Association with Suicide Attempts Among Runaway and Homeless Youth." *Substance Use and Misuse*, 1996, *31*, 1041–1058.

184. Whitbeck and others (2004).

185. Whitbeck and others (2004).

186. Tyler, K., Whitbeck, L., Hoyt, D., and Johnson, K. "Self-Mutilation and Homeless Youth: The Role of Family Abuse, Street Experiences, and Mental Disorders." *Journal of Research on Adolescence*, 2003, *13*, 457–474.

187. Tyler, K., Cauce, A., and Whitbeck, L. "Family Risk Factors and Prevalence of Dissociative Symptoms Among Homeless and Runaway Youth." *Child Abuse and Neglect*, 2004, *28*, 355–366.

188. Greene, J., Ennett, S., and Ringwalt, C. "Prevalence and Correlates of Survival Sex Among Runaway and Homeless Youth." *American Journal of Public Health*, 1999, *89*, 1406–1409.

189. MacLean, Embry, and Cauce (1999).

190. Green, L. W. "Ethics and Community-Based Participatory Research: Commentary on Minkler." *Health Education and Behavior*, 2004, *31*, 698–701.

191. Roy and others (2001).

192. Beech, B. M., Myers, L., Beech, D. J., and Kernick, N. S. "Human Immunodeficiency Syndrome and Hepatitis B and C Infections Among Homeless Adolescents." *Seminars in Pediatric Infectious Diseases*, 2003, *14*, 12–19.

193. Beech, Myers, Beech, and Kernick (2003).

194. Ochino, J. J., and others. "Past Infection with Hepatitis A Virus Among Vancouver Street Youth, Injection Drug Users and Men Who Have Sex with Men: Implications for Vaccination Programs." *Canadian Medical Association Journal*, 2001, *165*, 293–297.

195. Roy, E., and others. "Seroprevalence and Risk Factors for Hepatitis A Among Montreal Street Youth." *Canadian Journal of Public Health*, 2002, *93*, 52–53.

196. Lifson, A., and Halcon, L. "Substance Abuse and High-Risk Needle-Related Behaviors Among Homeless Youth in Minneapolis: Implications for Prevention." *Journal of Urban Health: Bulletin of the New York Academy of Medicine*, 2001, *78*, 690–698.

197. Walters, A. "HIV Prevention in Street Youth." *Journal of Adolescent Health*, 1999, *25*, 187–198.

198. Stricof, R., Kennedy, J., Nattell, T., and Weisfuse, I.N.L. "HIV Seroprevalence in a Facility for Runaway and Homeless Adolescents." *American Journal of Public Health*, 1991, *81*, 50–53.

199. Beech, Myers, Beech, and Kernick (2003).

200. Van Leeuwen, J., and others. "Reaching Homeless Youths for Chlamydia Trachomatis and Neisseria Gonorrhoeae Screening in Denver, Colorado." *Sexually Transmitted Infections*, 2002, *78*, 357–359.

201. Ensign and Santelli (1998); Greene, J., and Ringwalt, C. "Pregnancy Among Three National Samples of Runaway and Homeless Youth." *Journal of Adolescent Health*, 1998, *23*, 370–377.

202. Roy and others (2004).

203. Abdalian, S. E. "Street Youth Mortality: Leaning with Intent to Fall." *Journal of the American Medical Association*, 2004, *292*, 624–626.

204. Greene and Ringwalt (1998).

205. Haley, N., and others. "Characteristics of Adolescent Street Youth with a History of Pregnancy." *Journal of Pediatric and Adolescent Gynecology*, 2004, *17*, 313–320.

206. Gelberg, L., Linn, L. S., and Rosenberg, D. J. "Dental Health of Homeless Adults." *Special Care in Dentistry*, 1988, *8*, 167–172.

207. Burt and others (1999).

208. North, C. S., Eyrich, K. M., Pollio, D. E., and Spitznagel, E. L. "Are Rates of Psychiatric Disorders in the Homeless Population Changing?" *American Journal of Public Health*, 2004, *94*, 103–108.

209. Fischer and others (1986); Koegel, P., Burnam, A., and Farr, R. "The Prevalence of Specific Psychiatric Disorders Among Homeless Individuals in the Inner-City of Los Angeles." *Archives of General Psychiatry*, 1988, *45*, 1085–1092; Smith, E., North, C., and Spitznagel, E. "Alcohol, Drugs, and Psychiatric Comorbidity Among Homeless Women: An Epidemiologic Study." *Journal of Clinical Psychiatry*, 1993, *54*, 82–87.

210. Fischer and others (1986); Koegel, Burnam, and Farr (1988); Smith, North, and Spitznagel (1993); Bassuk, E., Rubin, L., and Lauriat, A. "Is Homelessness a Mental Health Problem?" *American Journal of Psychiatry*, 1984, *141*, 1546–1550; Arce, A. A, Tadlock, M. T., Vergare, M. J., and Shapiro, S. H. "A Psychiatric Profile of Street People Admitted to an Emergency Shelter." *Hospital and Community Psychiatry*, 1983, *34*, 812–817; Koegel, P., and Burnam, M. "Alcoholism Among Homeless Adults in the Inner City of Los Angeles." *Archives of General Psychiatry*, 1988, *45*, 1011–1018; Struening, E., and others. "A Typology Based on Measures of Substance Abuse and Mental Disorder." *Journal of Addiction and Disease*, 1991, *11*, 99–117.

211. Folsom, D., and Jeste, D. "Schizophrenia in Homeless Persons: A Systematic Review of the Literature." *Acta Psychiatrica Scandinavica*, 2002, *105*, 404–413.

212. Koegel, P., and others. "Utilization of Mental Health and Substance Abuse Services Among Homeless Adults in Los Angeles." *Medical Care*, 1999, *37*, 306–317.

213. Koegel, Burnam, and Farr (1988).
214. Robertson, M., Ropers, R., and Boyer, R. *The Homeless of Los Angeles County: An Empirical Evaluation.* Los Angeles: UCLA School of Public Health, 1985.
215. Benda (2005).
216. Solliday-McRoy, C., and others. "Neuropsychological Functioning of Homeless Men. *Journal of Nervous and Mental Disease,* 2004, *192,* 471–478.
217. Solliday-McRoy and others (2004).
218. Solliday-McRoy and others (2004).
219. Burt and others (1999).
220. Kushel, M. B., Vittinghoff, E., and Haas, J. S. "Factors Associated with the Health Care Utilization of Homeless Persons." *Journal of the American Medical Association,* 2001, *285,* 200–206.
221. Burt and others (1999).
222. Kushel, Vittinghoff, and Haas (2001).
223. Gallagher, Andersen, Koegel, and Gelberg (1997).
224. Lewis, J., Andersen, R., and Gelberg, L. "Health Care for Homeless Women." *Journal of General Internal Medicine,* 2003, *18,* 921–928.
225. Lim and others (2002).
226. Burt and others (1999).
227. Kushel, Vittinghoff, and Haas (2001).
228. Kushel, Vittinghoff, and Haas (2001).
229. Han, B., and Wells, B. L. "Inappropriate Emergency Department Visits and Use of the Health Care for the Homeless Program Services by Homeless Adults in the Northeastern United States." *Journal of Public Health Management and Practice,* 2003, *9,* 530–537.
230. Stein, J., Andersen, R., Koegel, P., and Gelberg, L. "Predicting Health Services Utilization in Homeless Adults: A Prospective Analysis." *Journal of Health Care for the Poor and Underserved,* 2000, *11,* 212–230.
231. Martell, J., and others. "Hospitalization in an Urban Homeless Population: The Honolulu Urban Homeless Project." *Annals of Internal Medicine,* 1992, *116,* 299–303.
232. Robertson and Cousineau (1986).
233. Salit, S., and others. "Hospitalization Costs Associated with Homelessness in New York City." (Special article.) *New England Journal of Medicine,* 1998, *338,* 1734–1740.
234. Kelly, J. T., and Goldfinger, S. M. *Homeless Inpatients: Medical, Surgical, and Psychiatric Problems.* San Francisco: University of San Francisco, 1985.
235. Chau and others (2002).
236. Klein, J. D., and others. "Homeless and Runaway Youths' Access to Health Care." *Journal of Adolescent Health,* 2000, *27,* 331–339.
237. McGuire, J. "Hoptel Equalizes Length of Stay for Homeless and Domiciled Inpatients." *Medical Care,* 2000, *38,* 1003–1010.
238. Almeida, Dubay, and Ko (2001).
239. Brickner, P. W., and Kaufman, A. "Case Finding of Heart Disease in Homeless Men." *Bulletin of the New York Academy of Medicine,* 1973, *49,* 475–484.
240. McAdam, Brickner, and Glicksman (1985).
241. Bassuk, Rubin, and Lauriat (1984).
242. Riley and others (2005).
243. Gelberg, Andersen, and Leake (2000).
244. Gallagher, Andersen, Koegel, and Gelberg (1997).

245. Tulsky, J. P., and others. "Adherence to Isoniazid Prophylaxis in the Homeless: A Randomized Controlled Trial." *Archives of Internal Medicine,* 2000, *160,* 697–702.

246. Tulsky, J. P., and others. "Can the Poor Adhere? Incentives for Adherence to TB Prevention in Homeless Adults." *International Journal of Tuberculosis and Lung Disease,* 2004, *8,* 83–91.

247. Salit and others (1998).

248. Koegel, Burnam, and Farr (1988); Gelberg, L., Linn, L., and Leake, B. "Mental Health, Alcohol and Drug Use, and Criminal History Among Homeless Adults." *American Journal of Psychiatry,* 1988, *145,* 191–196.

249. Martell and others (1992).

250. Fischer and others (1986).

251. Gelberg, Linn, and Leake (1988).

252. Koegel and others (1999).

253. Burt and others (1999).

254. Lamb, H. R., and Bachrach, L. L. "Some Perspectives of Deinstitutionalization." *Psychiatric Services,* 2001, *52,* 1039–1045.

255. Koegel and others (1999).

256. Koegel and others (1999).

257. Koegel and others (1999).

258. Bradford, D. W., and others. "Can Shelter-Based Interventions Improve Treatment Engagement in Homeless Individuals with Psychiatric and/or Substance Misuse Disorders?" *Medical Care,* 2005, *43,* 763–768.

259. Burt and others (1999).

260. Gallagher, Andersen, Koegel, and Gelberg (1997).

261. Lewis, Andersen, and Gelberg (2003).

262. Lim and others (2002).

263. Stein, Andersen, Koegel, and Gelberg (2000).

264. Lim and others (2002).

265. Gallagher, Andersen, Koegel, and Gelberg (1997).

266. Koegel and others (1999).

267. Koegel and others (1999).

268. Weinreb, Goldberg, and Lessard (2002).

269. Hwang, S., and others. "Health Care Utilization Among Homeless Adults Prior to Death." *Journal of Health Care for the Poor and Underserved,* 2001, *12,* 50–58.

270. Hwang and others (2001).

271. Lewis, Andersen, and Gelberg (2003).

272. Burt and others (1999).

273. Koegel, P., and Gelberg, L. "Patient-Oriented Approach to Providing Care to Homeless Persons." In D. Wood (ed.), *Delivering Health Care to Homeless Persons: The Diagnosis and Management of Medical and Mental Health Conditions.* New York: Springer, 1992, 16–29.

274. Kushel, Vittinghoff, and Haas (2001).

275. Kushel, Vittinghoff, and Haas (2001).

276. Robertson and Cousineau (1986).

277. Lewis, Andersen, and Gelberg (2003).

278. Gallagher, Andersen, Koegel, and Gelberg (1997); Lewis, Andersen, and Gelberg (2003); Gelberg, L., and Linn, L. "Social and Physical Health of Homeless Adults Previously Treated for Mental Health Problems." *Hospital and Community Psychiatry,* 1988, *39,* 510–516; Gelberg, L., Gallagher, T. C., Andersen, R. M., and Koegel, P. "Competing Priorities as

a Barrier to Medical Care Among Homeless Adults in Los Angeles." *American Journal of Public Health*, 1997, *87*, 217–220.

279. Koegel and Gelberg (1992).

280. Almeida, Dubay, and Ko (2001).

281. Almeida, Dubay, and Ko (2001).

282. Robertson and Cousineau (1986).

283. Gelberg and Linn (1988); Folsom, D.,and others. "Medical Comorbidity and Receipt of Medical Care by Older Homeless People with Schizophrenia or Depression." *Psychiatric Services*, 2002, *53*, 1456–1460.

284. Desai, M., Rosenheck, R., and Kasprow, W. "Determinants of Receipt of Ambulatory Medical Care in a National Sample of Mentally Ill Homeless Veterans." *Medical Care*, 2003, *41*, 275–287.

285. Folsom and others (2002).

286. Gelberg, L., and Linn, L. "Psychological Distress Among Homeless Adults." *Journal of Nervous and Mental Disease*, 1989, *177*, 291–295.

287. Health Care for the Homeless Clinicians' Network. *Adapting Your Practice: General Recommendations for the Care of Homeless Patients*. Nashville, Tenn.: National Health Care for the Homeless Council, 2004.

288. Gelberg and Linn (1988).

289. Baxter and Hopper (1981).

290. Hwang, S., and Bugeja, A. "Barriers to Appropriate Diabetes Management Among Homeless People in Toronto." *Canadian Medical Association Journal*, 2000, *163*, 161–165.

291. Health Care for the Homeless Clinicians' Network (2004).

292. Koegel and Gelberg (1992); Health Care for the Homeless Clinicians' Network (2004).

293. Koegel and Gelberg (1992).

294. Koegel and Gelberg (1992).

295. Koegel and Gelberg (1992).

296. Stark, L. "Barriers to Health Care for Homeless People." In R. Jahiel (ed.), *Homelessness: A Prevention Oriented Approach*. Baltimore: Johns Hopkins University Press, 1992.

297. Folsom and others (2002).

298. Baxter and Hopper (1981).

299. Doblin, B., Gelberg, L., and Freeman, H. "Patient Care and Professional Staffing Patterns in McKinney Act Clinics Providing Primary Care to the Homeless." *Journal of the American Medical Association*, 1992, *267*, 698–701.

300. Koegel and Gelberg (1992).

301. Koegel and Gelberg (1992).

302. Tsai, M., Weintraub, R., Gee, L., and Kushel, M. "Identifying Homelessness at an Urban Public Hospital: A Moving Target?" *Journal of Health Care for the Poor and Underserved*, 2005, *16*, 297–307.

303. Stark (1992).

304. Stark (1992).

305. Tsai, Weintraub, Gee, and Kushel (2005).

306. Salit and others (1998).

307. Brickner and others (1985); Gundlapalli, A., and others. "It Takes a Village: A Multidisciplinary Model for the Acute Illness Aftercare of Individuals Experiencing Homelessness." *Journal of Health Care for the Poor and Underserved*, 2005, *16*, 257–272.

308. O'Connell, J., and Lebow, J. "AIDS and the Homeless of Boston." *New England Journal of Public Policy*, 1992, *8*, 541–556.

309. Hopper, K., and Barrow, S. "Two Genealogies of Supported Housing and Their Implications for Outcomes Assessment." *Psychiatric Services*, 2003, *54*, 50–54.

310. Schutt, R. K., Weinstein, B., and Penk, W. E. "Housing Preferences of Homeless Veterans with Dual Diagnoses." *Psychiatric Services*, 2005, *56*, 350–352.

311. Metraux, S., Marcus, S., and Culhane, D. "The New York-New York Housing Initiative and Use of Public Shelters by Persons with Severe Mental Illness." *Psychiatric Services*, 2003, *54*, 67–71.

312. Tsemberis, S., and Eisenberg, R. "Pathways to Housing: Supported Housing for Street-Dwelling Homeless Individuals with Psychiatric Disabilities." *Psychiatric Services,* 2000, *51*, 487–493.

313. Pollio, D. E., and others. "Service Use over Time and Achievement of Stable Housing in a Mentally Ill Homeless Population." *Psychiatric Services*, 2000, *51*, 1536–1543.

314. Thiele, B. "The Human Right to Adequate Housing: A Tool for Promoting and Protecting Individual and Community Health." *American Journal of Public Health*, 2002, *92*, 712–715.

315. Myers, D., Baer, W., and Choi, S. "The Changing Problems of Overcrowded Housing." *Journal of the American Planning Association*, 1996, *62*, 66–84.

316. Evans, G. W., and Kantrowitz, E. "Socioeconomic Status and Health: The Potential Role of Environmental Risk Exposure." *Annual Review of Public Health, 2002, 23*, 303–331.

317. Mayer, S. E. "Trends in Economic Well-Being and the Life Chances of America's Children." In G. Duncan and J. Brooks-Gunn (eds.), *Consequences of Growing up Poor.* New York: Russell Sage Foundation, 1997.

318. Frumkin, H. "Minority Workers and Communities." In R. Wallace (ed.), *Maxcy-Rosenau-Last Public Health and Preventive Medicine.* Stamford, Conn.: Appleton and Lange, 1998.

319. Elliott, M. R., Wang, Y., Lowe, R., and Kleindorfer, P. "Environmental Justice: Frequency and Severity of U.S. Chemical Industry Accidents and the Socioeconomic Status of Surrounding Communities." *Journal of Epidemiology and Community Health*, 2004, *58*, 24–30.

320. Chadwick, E. "Report on the Sanitary Condition of the Labouring Population of Great Britain by Edwin Chadwick, 1842." M. Flinn (ed.). Edinburgh, Scotland: University Press, 1965.

321. Rosen, G. *A History of Public Health.* New York: MD Publications, 1965.

322. Engels, F. *The Condition of the Working Class in England.* New York: Panther Books, 1969.

323. Byrne, D., and Keithly, J. "Housing and the Health of the Community." In R. Burridge and D. Ormandy (eds.), *Unhealthy Housing: Research, Remedies and Reform.* New York: Spoon Press, 1993.

324. Melosi, M. V. *The Sanitary City: Urban Infrastructure in America from Colonial Times to the Present.* Baltimore: Johns Hopkins University Press, 2000.

325. Wohl, A. S. *Endangered Lives: Public Health in Victorian Britain.* Cambridge, Mass.: Harvard University Press, 1983.

326. Wenzel, Andersen, Gifford, and Gelberg (2001).

327. Stein, Lu, and Gelberg (2000).

328. Wenzel, Leake, and Gelberg (2000).

329. Gelberg and Linn (1989); Gelberg, Andersen, and Leake (2000).

330. Kertesz (2005).

331. Wong, Y.-L.P.I. "Stressors, Resources, and Distress Among Homeless Persons: A Longitudinal Analysis." *Social Science and Medicine*, 2001, *52*, 1029–1042.

332. Berkman, L., and Kawachi, I. (eds.). *Social Epidemiology.* New York: Oxford University Press, 2000.

333. Sampson, R., Raudenbush, S., and Earls, F. "Neighborhoods and Violent Crime: A Multi-level Study of Collective Efficacy." *Science,* 1997, *277,* 918–924.

334. Gordis, L. "From Association to Causation: Deriving Inferences from Epidemiologic Studies." In L. Gordis (ed.). *Epidemiology* (2nd ed.). Philadelphia: Saunders, 2000.

335. Caton and others (2005).

336. Caton and others (2005).

337. Marlis, E., and Kannan, M. (eds.). *Preferences, Institutions and Rational Choice.* Oxford, England: Oxford University Press, 1995.

338. Marlis and Kannan (1995).

339. Marlis and Kannan (1995).

340. Stern and Nyamathi (2004).

341. Robertson and others (2004).

342. Haddad and others (2005).

343. Browne, A., and Bassuk, S. "Intimate Violence in the Lives of Homeless and Poor Housed Women: Prevalence and Patterns in an Ethnically Diverse Sample." *American Journal of Orthopsychiatry,* 1997, *67,* 261–278.

344. Homes for the Homeless (1999).

345. Homes for the Homeless (1999).

346. National Center on Family Homelessness (1999).

347. Commission on Homelessness (Atlanta). "Blueprint to End Homelessness in Atlanta in Ten Years." [http://www.hud.gov/offices/cpd/homeless/apply/2002nofa/index.cfm] (accessed Mar. 27, 2006).

348. U.S. HUD (2002).

349. Leventhal. T., and Brooks-Gunn, J. "Moving to Opportunity: An Experimental Study of Neighborhood Effects on Mental Health." *American Journal of Public Health,* 2003, *93,* 1576–1582.

350. Meyer, I. H., and Schwartz, S. "Social Issues as Public Health: Promise and Peril." (Editorial.) *American Journal of Public Health,* 2000, *90,* 1189–1191.

351. Blasi, G. "And We Are Not Seen: Ideological and Political Barriers to Understanding Homelessness." *American Behavioral Scientist,* 1994, *37,* 563–586.

PART FIVE

# DIRECTIONS FOR CHANGE

CHAPTER NINETEEN

# MANAGED CARE AND THE GROWTH OF COMPETITION

Gerald F. Kominski
Glenn A. Melnick

As we enter the twenty-first century, managed care has become an integral part of the U.S. health care system. In the early 1990s, President Clinton presented a plan for national health care reform that was based on a modified version of managed competition first proposed by Alain Enthoven.[1] Through a combination of newly formed health alliances and competitive bidding by health plans, the incentives of the health care market would have been restructured to encourage price competition in the health care market at both the health plan and provider levels.

Although Congress enacted several significant incremental reforms during the 1990s, the failure to pass comprehensive national health care reform legislation meant that responsibility for restructuring the health care system fell primarily on the private sector and individual states. However, as the first decade of the new century unfolds, managed care appears to have been displaced as the main paradigm for market-oriented reform by consumer-directed (or -driven) health plans (CDHPs), which build on price competition but rely on the patient, not the health plan, as the key decision maker in most health care purchasing decisions.

This chapter offers a review and synthesis of the empirical literature on the effects of managed care and competition and discusses the implications of current trends.

# Models of Managed Care

Managed care has existed in the United States for more than seventy years. As early as 1932, the Committee on the Costs of Medical Care called for the practice of medicine in the United States to be reorganized into prepaid group practice.[2] This recommendation acknowledged that the incentives of fee-for-service, solo-practitioner medical practice were inefficient compared to a system where physicians coordinated their care and received a fixed payment in advance for their services. Despite these conceptual advantages, the only prominent prepaid group practice for many years was the nonprofit Kaiser Permanente health plan. During the past two decades, managed care has evolved into a broad concept encompassing a variety of managed care organizations (MCOs) or managed care plans (MCPs), some of which barely resemble prepaid group practice.

## Health Maintenance Organizations

Health maintenance organizations (HMOs) are the traditional form of managed care. Group-model HMOs contract with a single medical group to provide care to plan members, while staff-model HMOs employ physicians directly. In group-model HMOs, the medical group usually contracts exclusively with the HMO, which is known as a closed panel; that is, providers do not treat patients outside the HMO. Staff-model HMOs are by definition closed panels.

Group- and staff-model HMOs represent a traditional model of managed care that many physicians view as excessively intrusive and many consumers see as too restrictive because of their closed panels. Therefore, alternative models have evolved that allow physicians greater autonomy in how their practices are organized and permit greater choice for plan members. Network-model HMOs contract with multiple medical groups, rather than a single group, while HMOs on the independent practice association (IPA) model contract with individual physicians in solo practice. Network- and IPA-model HMOs are typically open-panel; physicians do not contract exclusively with a single HMO and may continue to treat non-HMO patients.

All forms of HMOs employ some form of gatekeeper, a primary care physician who serves as the initial point of contact for receiving care and who must authorize referrals for specialty care. However, in response to competitive pressures during the 1990s, HMOs have begun offering multiple managed care products, including other forms of managed care (described later).[3] For example, some HMOs offer an open-access product that allows self-referral within the network but imposes increased cost sharing on members who choose this option. These hybrid arrangements are likely to continue growing in response to changing perceptions of what best serves the interests of the health plans, providers, and members.

## Preferred Provider Organizations

Preferred provider organizations (PPOs) represent a less restrictive form of managed care than the HMO, mainly because they do not require primary care physicians to serve as gatekeepers and thus permit self-referral to specialists. They are generally formed by employers or insurers who contract with physicians and other providers to create a network of participating or preferred providers. These preferred providers generally agree to follow utilization management guidelines and to accept discounted fee-for-service payments as conditions for participating in the PPO. Health plan members are encouraged to use the preferred provider network through reduced cost sharing, although they are generally covered for care provided by nonparticipating physicians.

## Point-of-Service Plans

Point-of-service (POS) plans are essentially the same as the open-access HMOs we have already described, but they also offer limited coverage for self-referral outside the network. Members may choose the level of managed care they desire at the point of service, with the degree of cost sharing increasing along with freedom of choice. Members in these three-tier plans who use a gatekeeper (HMO tier) have the lowest co-payments, while those self-referring to network providers (PPO tier) have higher co-payments, and those seeking care outside the network (POS tier) have the highest co-payments.

# Growth of Managed Care

Without question, managed care has grown substantially since the early 1970s, when Paul Ellwood's advocacy of health maintenance organizations[4] was translated into national policy as the HMO Act of 1973. This legislation gave federal grants and loans to federally qualified HMOs to promote their expansion. More importantly, it required employers with twenty-five or more employees already offering health insurance coverage to offer at least two HMO options, thus promoting the growth of managed care. By the time Harold Luft published his seminal book on HMO performance in 1981, slightly more than seven million U.S. residents were enrolled in HMOs,[5] and almost half of all HMO members were concentrated in California in a single network, the Kaiser Foundation Health Plans.[6]

By 1990, enrollment in HMOs increased fivefold to about thirty-five million in almost seven hundred HMOs across the United States. As the 1990s came to an end, HMO enrollment (including enrollment in POS plans) had more than doubled again, to an estimated eighty-one million, or about 25 percent of the U.S. population.[7] Since then, HMO and POS enrollment has declined to an estimated sixty-six million as of 2004.[8] This decline is largely due to the growth of PPOs and has been attributed by many analysts to a managed care backlash (to be discussed).

Among individuals who obtained health insurance through their place of employment, 97 percent were enrolled in some form of managed care as of 2005. But enrollment in PPOs among individuals with employment-based coverage has increased from 28 percent in 1996 to 61 percent in 2004, while enrollment in HMOs has declined from 31 percent to 21 percent during the same period.[9]

A number of factors explain the rapid proliferation of managed care during the past two decades. A primary driving force clearly has been employers seeking lower-cost alternatives to indemnity insurance for their employee health benefit plans. At the start of this period of growth, the cost advantages of HMOs were most thoroughly documented by Luft, who found that the long-term cost savings of HMOs were primarily attributable to a lower rate of hospitalization, rather than improved productivity or lower input costs.[10] Thus, although the empirical evidence did not suggest that HMOs would produce substantial savings, they nevertheless gave employers an alternative to the inflationary incentives of indemnity-based, fee-for-service health benefits.

In the early years of managed care, employees faced a complex decision in choosing whether to enroll in an HMO. One major advantage was a reduction in out-of-pocket expenditures associated with most HMOs. Prior to the mid-1980s, however, this financial advantage was offset by having a limited choice of providers and by having to obtain gatekeeper approval before seeking specialty care. These disadvantages of the traditional HMO spurred development of less-restrictive forms of managed care, such as PPOs and POS plans. Advocates of managed care cite this ability of the industry to innovate and create new products that vary across markets in response to consumer demand as a major advantage of market-driven reform.

In addition to these cost considerations on the part of employers and employees, managed care also has the potential to improve quality of care, at least in part because of the financial incentives facing providers. In theory, managed care has the potential to improve coordination of care through clinical management of entire episodes of care, develop information systems to assist in care coordination, identify and eliminate wasteful or ineffective practices, and identify and manage care for the costliest conditions (such as those involving chronic illness).

In summary, HMOs as the primary form of managed care grew rapidly until the end of the 1990s and are now experiencing declining enrollment nationally in favor of less restrictive forms of managed care.

## The Managed Care Backlash

At the beginning of the 1990s, HMOs were the centerpiece of President Clinton's proposal for health care reform in the United States. By the end of the decade, HMOs enrollment had peaked and analysts were discussing the emergence of a managed care backlash.[11] Although the causes of this backlash were complex, a major factor was dissatisfaction on the part of HMO members with the increasing sense of restriction regarding their choice of providers and treatments, fueled by several highly visible law suits filed against HMOs alleging unlawful denial of care.[12]

The policy response to this popular backlash resulted in various proposals for legislation that would have created a "patients' bill of rights" during the period from 1998–2001. Although none of these bills were enacted at the national level, the threat of such legislation during this period led to voluntary changes in HMO products that resulted in "open access" HMOs permitting self-referral to specialty care with prior approval from the patient's primary care provider.

These changes in the fundamental functions of HMOs, combined with the decline in HMO enrollment that began in 2000, led one health economist (Jamie Robinson) who has written extensively on managed care to conclude in 2001 that the United States was witnessing the end of managed care.[13] According to Robinson, despite the economic success of managed care it has become a cultural and political failure and is being abandoned in favor of an emerging model of consumer-centered or patient-directed health care system, in which individuals are empowered with both information and sufficient competing choices to make cost-effective decisions about health care. Of course, not all health economists agree that managed care has been an economic success.[14] In contrast to declining managed care enrollment, high-deductible health plans, either alone or combined with Health Reimbursement Accounts or Health Savings Accounts, are expected to grow rapidly during the remainder of this decade. Whether this trend represents the end of managed care or simply a reformulation of the role of managed care in the U.S. health care system remains to be seen. In any event, since the last edition of this book managed care is no longer being viewed as the central component of market-based health care reform. But what does the evidence show about how managed care and competition have actually changed the health care system?

## California and the Development of Competitive Markets

An essential element of the development of the managed care market is competition among health plans and the interaction between health plans and consumers. These interrelationships can have important implications for ongoing product innovation and the overall development of the managed care market. To better understand this process, it is instructive to examine the evolution of the managed care market in California and its impact on restructuring the state's health care system.

In June 1982, the California legislature adopted what was to become model legislation for the nation, designed to encourage price competition in the health care sector. The law explicitly permitted formation of health plans that contracted with selected, or "preferred," providers. This legislation allowed the state's Medicaid program, known as MediCal, as well as private insurance companies to contract with a subset of licensed hospitals to which it would channel its enrollees in return for signing participating contracts. The contracts often required price concessions and increased utilization review oversight in order to control both price and use of health services. The law allowed the growth of HMOs and created the conditions necessary for the formation of PPOs.

In the early 1980s, fewer than 20 percent of the state's insured population were enrolled in managed care plans (most of them being in the Kaiser Permanente HMO). In the years following introduction of the law, the number of plans in California peaked at more than one hundred. Through increased competition and ongoing consolidation as the market matures, the number of plans has been substantially reduced; as of the end of 2005, forty-two full-service plans were licensed to operate in the state.[15]

With the passage of California's selective contracting law, health insurance plans had greater flexibility to develop alternative health insurance patterns and to test design features in order to attract subscribers. This increased competition in the health insurance market led to a burst of innovation and a proliferation of choices available to consumers. For example, PPOs grew rapidly by offering a wide choice of providers in their networks. In addition, they combined this feature with lower monthly premiums (compared to prevailing standard fee-for-service indemnity plans) and financial incentives to use network providers, while still affording some financial coverage for out-of-network utilization. The number of people voluntarily selecting these plans that include some reduction in their choice of provider grew dramatically. At the same time, innovations in the HMO market were being tested. The number of HMOs competing with Kaiser and with PPOs grew rapidly.

The new HMOs differed dramatically from Kaiser in ways that made them attractive to both providers and consumers. Physicians could join an HMO either as individuals or as part of an IPA or group practice. Hospitals, likewise, could contract with the plans selectively. Consumers had a choice of private providers in these plans, and the monthly premium was generally less than with conventional indemnity plans.

During this same period, employers began changing their fringe benefit contribution rates for health insurance, requiring employees to pay more from their monthly paycheck if they selected a plan with higher premiums. The response of consumers to these changes has been remarkable. Voluntary enrollment in managed care plans grew so rapidly that within ten years a majority of the privately insured population had joined some type of managed care plan offering lower monthly premiums in return for some restrictions on choice of provider. This shift from general indemnity health insurance to managed care plans requiring consumers to accept some restrictions on providers and hospitals was largely caused by market forces, but it was also assisted by government action encouraging those forces. The basis for this dramatic restructuring of the health care system is the increased role of price competition in the health care sector among providers and health insurance plans, and more efficient pricing in the health insurance market.

As might be expected, the supply side of the health market also underwent dramatic changes. As the number of people joining managed care health plans grew, health plans had to add capacity to their provider networks to handle the increased volume. Consequently, the percentage of physicians and hospitals contracting with managed care plans has increased substantially. The growth in enrollment in health plans gives the plans greater bargaining power when negotiating with providers for participation in their networks. To counter this growing power on the part of health plans, providers began consolidating to form their own networks. These networks allowed expanded primary care capacity within local areas as well as wider geographic coverage. California continues to have the largest HMO penetration rate in the United States, with an estimated 47.8 percent in 2004.[16]

## Impact of Managed Care and Competition

In the traditional setting, hospitals compete on the basis of services, technology, and amenities to attract physicians and their patients.[17] Physicians' ability to deliver quality care and compete for patients depends in part on the range of services they can provide. Hospitals partially control the range of available services by deciding in which specialized equipment, staff, and services to invest. In negotiating with hospitals, physicians can increase their bargaining leverage by credibly threatening to shift their patients to another hospital. Hospitals, in turn, can remove admitting privileges from physicians who do not bring in many patients. Lack of admitting privileges to a highly regarded local hospital could put a physician at a competitive disadvantage.

# Price Competition Among Insurers

Introducing selective contracting and managed care risk contracts changes the economic incentives faced by both insurers and providers. The ability to assemble preferred provider networks endows insurers with the potential power to channel patients away from more expensive providers. Insurers, competing with one another for subscribers, have both a financial incentive and the benefit of economies of scale to search the market for an optimal mix of high-quality and low-price providers. Under such conditions, insurers can leverage excess capacity and competitive hospital market conditions to negotiate lower prices with health care providers.

In theory, effective use of the selective contracting mechanism can generate savings for insurers, thereby leading to price advantages over other insurers who pay "too much." Such price advantages could be important in building or maintaining a subscriber base in a competitive insurance market. However, selective contracting plans operate under constraints that in all likelihood prevent them from choosing providers solely by price. If payers use only a price criterion in choosing providers, they may assemble too limited a network, thereby putting themselves at risk of diminishing their subscriber base because of unacceptable quality or access. Thus payers must assess the relative consumer attractiveness of individual hospitals before choosing which hospitals to exclude for reasons of high price.

Faced with the pressure to reduce prices or risk being excluded from an insurer's network, providers must also balance tradeoffs in negotiating with selective contracting plans. They must assess their importance to the insurer's network, which determines the likelihood of being excluded should they refuse to grant requested price concessions. Their ability to retain patients should the contract not be offered influences their bargaining position.

Insurers may also face competitive pressure on their premiums, depending on how price-sensitive purchasers are in selecting health insurance. Managed competition and other market-oriented reforms are founded on the assumption that in markets with a sufficient amount of choice among competing health insurers competition on the basis of price (that is, premiums) will constrain growth in health expenditures. Of course, this assumption itself presumes that purchasers are sufficiently price-sensitive to seek lower-cost insurers, all things being equal.

Previous research on the early effects of selective contracting in California indicates that restructuring the health care market can lead to increased price competition and lower cost growth in the hospital industry. Melnick, Zwanziger, Bamezai, and Pattison found that increasing price sensitivity on the part of buyers has resulted in improved price competition among hospitals, leading them to offer price discounts to secure contracts with managed care plans.[18] Hospitals lowered their costs when faced with competitive pressure on their prices exerted by managed care plans.[19]

Previous published studies showing that competition can lead to smaller increases in hospital costs and prices have been limited in several ways. Because they were done soon after the introduction of price competition, they do not address the question of whether cost-containment effects can be sustained over a long period of time, or if they are simply a one-time reduction followed by increases at previous rates.

Zwanziger, Melnick, and Bamezai addressed the question of whether price competition in California resulted in a long-term and sustained reduction in hospital expenditures in two related studies.[20] These analyses were designed to isolate and compare the effects of competition on hospital revenues prior to and following the growth of managed care plans and selective contracting. They found that in the period from 1983 to 1997, hospital expenses in the most competitive markets were 18.4 percent lower than in the least competitive markets, while revenue in the least competitive markets was 19.4 percent lower than in the most competitive ones. They conclude that competition resulting from selective contracting has had a sustained effect, although the potential impact of reduced expenses and revenue on hospital quality is unclear.

The RAND Health Insurance Experiment (HIE) yielded the first scientifically valid estimates of individual price sensitivity to level of copayment and deductible for individual health services. But the HIE did not specifically look at price sensitivity to premiums, since individuals in that study were randomly assigned to a number of insurance plans. Of course, determining the price elasticity of demand for health insurance is a difficult task. Most studies cannot adequately control for unobserved differences among insurance plans and unobserved characteristics among those selecting the plans, and thus they are subject to selection bias. Nevertheless, several recent studies have been able to examine price sensitivity to premiums.

Dowd, Feldman, and Coulam examined the impact of level of out-of-pocket premiums on Medicare beneficiaries under the Medicare+Choice program.[21] Using county-level data, they found that a $10 change in out-of-pocket premiums, relative to the lowest premium plan in the market, produced a four percentage point decline in market share for health plans. The same $10 change in out-of-pocket premiums increased the probability of switching plans by 16 percent. The authors point out that although price sensitivity of Medicare beneficiaries is lower than for nonretirees, their findings suggest sufficient price sensitivity to impose competitive restraints on premium increases.

Atherly, Dowd, and Feldman used individual-level data to examine the impact of out-of-pocket premiums on Medicare beneficiaries and found less price sensitivity than in the previous study.[22] In this case, they found that a $10 increase in out-of-pocket premiums was associated with only a 0.62 percent decline in market share. They also found that low-income beneficiaries were more price-sensitive than those with high incomes, a not unexpected finding. Commenting on the discrepancy between their two studies, they concluded that the lack of price sensitivity based on individual-level data might not be sufficient to drive high-cost insurance plans from the market.

Buchmueller found a similar price elasticity of demand for health insurance using data on retirees from a single large employer.[23] He found that a $5 increase in out-of-pocket premiums was associated with a 0.4 percentage point decline, on average, in market share. The price sensitivity of single retirees was greater than for married retirees, with a $5 increase in out-of-pocket premiums resulting in a 1.5 percentage point decline in market share. Strombom, Buchmueller, and Feldstein found greater price sensitivity among employees in the University of California system, with a $5 increase in out-of-pocket premiums associated with a 3.2 percentage point decline among all health insurers, and a 7.6 percentage point decline among managed care plans.[24]

## Hospital Prices

Despite rapid growth in health plans that feature selective contracting, there is very little empirical evidence in the literature concerning its effects on hospital prices. The desired outcome is lower prices, but some researchers caution that endowing insurers with substantial market power could have a negative impact. For instance, Pauly suggests that in areas where an insurer commands a large share of the health insurance market, it may exploit its position to gain greater discounts.[25] Hospitals in these areas may be so hampered by revenue constraints that serious reduction in quality of care could occur, or financial losses could eventually threaten their viability.

Several studies have addressed these issues both theoretically and empirically.[26] One of the best empirical tests of these issues was conducted by Staten, Dunkelberg, and Umbeck.[27] They evaluated the effects of hospital market structure and insurer market share on the discount rate that hospitals offered to gain acceptance into the newly formed Blue Cross of Indiana PPO. They compared historical charges with the initial proposed bid for each hospital to calculate the discount rate. These discount rates were regressed on two alternative measures of hospital market structure (sole hospital in the county, or number of hospitals in the county) and two alternative measures of Blue Cross market share (Blue Cross share of the individual hospital's volume, and Blue Cross share of the private market). The ratio of inpatient days per bed for a one-month period was included as a measure of capacity use. The study found that hospitals located in counties with more competitors offered greater discounts and that higher Blue Cross share at either the hospital or the market level did not significantly lower the proposed discounts offered by hospitals.[28]

Melnick, Zwanziger, Bamezai, and Pattison conducted a study of hospital prices that was designed to produce an improved empirical test of these issues.[29] The results indicated that prices paid to hospitals in the Blue Cross of California PPO network, after controlling for hospital product differences, were strongly influenced by the competitive structure of the hospital market. Hospitals located in less competitive markets were able to secure higher prices. The estimated value of the coefficient for the Herfindahl-Hirschman index (HHI), a measure of market competition, was 0.11–0.13. To illustrate the effect of the HHI on prices, consider a market where a merger leads to three competitors becoming two. Assuming that the competitors have equal market shares, the HHI would change from 0.33 to 0.50, an increase of 50 percent. Such a reduction in the level of competition would lead, on average, to an estimated price increase of approximately 9 percent.

These findings on the relative bargaining position of the hospital and the PPO offer some insight into payer strategies for network design and network pruning. They suggest that consolidating a payer's business in fewer hospitals produces offsetting price effects. The consolidation increases the importance of the PPO to the hospital, enabling the PPO to extract bigger price discounts. At the same time, however, the payer becomes more dependent on those hospitals and must eventually pay them higher rates. Hospital mergers and consolidations in a competitive market also contribute to higher prices, even among nonprofits.[30]

High-occupancy hospitals in markets with little excess capacity receive much higher prices than expected. These results are particularly striking since neither hospital occupancy nor the average occupancy of the other hospitals in the market individually affects prices. Only a relatively small number of hospitals have a high occupancy rate, defined as 75 percent or greater. Still, the results show how important the availability of excess capacity is to the PPO in maintaining a credible threat to move patients elsewhere. If this spare capacity becomes too small, the negotiated price paid by the PPO increases dramatically.

The results illustrate some of the subtleties involved in developing hospital networks. In general, it pays for plans to contract with midsized hospitals where they can gain greater leverage with the same patient volume than in larger hospitals, which can absorb a greater number of Blue Cross patient-days without becoming too dependent on a single payer. In addition, these findings suggest that increased consolidation among plans leads to greater hospital cost savings because the importance of a single hospital diminishes with increasing plan size. Factors other than minimum price are important for the PPO to consider in determining the configuration of its networks.

Kralewski and others identified factors that affect the ability of HMOs to secure hospital discounts.[31] By analyzing hospital-HMO contracts, hospital operating characteristics, and market conditions, they determined that the level of risk sharing, the number of hospitals within a five-mile radius, the proportion of the population enrolled in HMOs, and the number of HMOs operating in the metropolitan statistical area (MSA) were directly related to the ability of HMOs to offer discounts. Further analysis showed that higher cost sharing by enrollees, a larger number of hospitals within a five-mile radius, and more HMOs operating within an MSA results in greater discounts. This suggests that competitive HMO markets do lead to price concessions for hospital services. Hospitals are using discounts as one way to attract HMO business and garner market share.

In addition, Feldman, Kralewski, Shapiro, and Chan found that in competitive health care markets hospitals have to compete with each other for managed care patients by offering discounts for inpatient services.[32] Specifically, staff- and network-model HMOs can extract larger discounts from hospitals compared to an IPA or a group-model HMO because they usually have higher patient enrollment.

HMOs, however, do not always seek the services of hospitals offering the lowest prices. Another study by Feldman and colleagues found that HMOs use different criteria in contracting with hospitals.[33] Low prices, an important element, nonetheless are only one aspect taken into consideration. Of six HMOs reviewed in this study, four network- and group-model HMOs placed price as the most important factor and sought discounts intensely, while two IPA-model HMOs focused more on access and quality rather than seeking the lowest prices. Consequently, these two HMOs contracted with more hospitals within the community.

## Health Care Expenditures

Since the time of rapid growth in managed care in the early 1980s, several studies have further confirmed the original findings summarized in Luft's work on HMO performance.[34] The best overall summaries of the empirical literature regarding the impact of managed care since 1980 have been conducted by Miller and Luft.[35] Their latest summary of the literature supports earlier findings that

HMOs use fewer resources, but most of the effect now is attributable to shorter length of hospital stay rather than to lower admission rate, as was found in Luft's earlier work. The most significant finding was from the Medical Outcomes Studies, which found admission rates 26–37 percent lower in HMOs.[36]

Discussion of the savings of managed care relative to indemnity insurance is quickly diminishing as a relevant issue in the United States. Given the substantial portion of the population already enrolled in managed care, a more relevant question for the future is, Can competition between health plans control the rate of growth in health care expenditures?[37] As we have discussed, there is empirical evidence that competitive markets have had a lower rate of growth in hospital expenditures. Other evidence supports the conclusion that total health care expenditures grew more slowly in California relative to the rest of the nation in the mid-1990s owing to the increasingly competitive market.[38] However, a number of markets continue to have little competition, and 37 percent of employees nationwide are offered only a single health plan by their employers.[39] Therefore the conditions for managed competition still do not exist in many areas of the United States.[40] Consequently, despite the proliferation of managed care, its potential for containment of national health expenditures has not been fully realized. In fact, Luft and Miller conclude that HMOs have not achieved what their proponents promised, namely, improved quality at a lower cost.[41]

## Quality of Care

During the 1990s, California was in the forefront in developing a health care market based not only on price competition but also on value-based purchasing.[42] The efforts of several large purchasing groups, notably the California Public Employees Retirement System (CalPERS, representing state, county, and municipal employees), the University of California (UC), the Pacific Business Group on Health (PBGH, representing fifty large private and public purchasers), and PacAdvantage (formerly the Health Insurance Plan of California, a purchasing cooperative representing small employers and administered by PBGH), were central to transforming the market. PBGH (which includes CalPERS and UC) played a central role in collecting enrollee satisfaction data, requiring that Health Plan Data and Information Set (HEDIS) data made available by participating health plans be audited independently, and conducting several independent surveys assessing health plan performance (including provider satisfaction with health plans).[43] The California Office of Statewide Health Planning and Development (OSHPD), and more recently PBGH, sponsored several major studies to develop risk-adjusted measures of hospital outcomes for individual clinical conditions, such as acute myocardial infarction and coronary artery bypass graft surgery, that are then published as public report cards.[44]

The capacity for meaningful quality reporting is now well established and the extensive efforts to measure and report quality indicators are documented and discussed elsewhere in this volume (Chapters Six, Seven, and Eight). Nevertheless, a fundamental question still remains: Is the overall quality of managed care plans better than that of indemnity plans? Again, Miller and Luft have conducted the most thorough review of the existing literature.[45] The findings from their 2002 review of the literature are consistent with their previous reviews, indicating that the evidence regarding HMOs and quality is rather mixed. Access to care and member satisfaction are generally lower, use of preventive services is generally higher, but measures of clinical quality are equally favorable and unfavorable. With regard to frail Medicare beneficiaries and those with chronic conditions, the pattern toward worse quality reported in their previous literature review continues to be supported by more recent studies.[46] Regarding the impact of competition, at least one recent study found that market-based reforms intended to increase price competition among hospitals in New Jersey produced a higher mortality rate among heart attack patients.[47]

Miller and Luft conclude that two decades of mixed findings regarding quality of care in HMOs may be impossible to overcome without fundamental changes in clinical processes and health information systems.[48] Their assessment of the less-than-stellar performance of HMOs after two decades of evidence and their gloomy forecast for the future of managed care may in fact be a major reason for the managed care backlash discussed earlier.

## Conclusions

Managed care clearly produced a revolution in the U.S. health care delivery system.[49] The elements of managed competition, outlined by Enthoven more than two decades ago, have slowly evolved in various markets throughout the country, most notably in California. Managed care has become entrenched in the health care market, and the predominant form of health care delivery, albeit in continuously evolving organizational forms. Along with its rapid growth during the 1990s, managed care has also experienced an increasing level of popular dissatisfaction and bad publicity since the late 1990s and throughout the early 2000s, as newspapers and other media constitute regular outlets for some of the most common complaints against managed care.

National health expenditures and health insurance premiums have continue to grow rapidly since 1997,[50] after a period of unprecedented slow growth during the mid-1990s that was viewed by many advocates of managed care as evidence that competition was finally working to contain overall health care costs. As a result, dissatisfaction with managed care as a cost-containment strategy has shifted national interest toward other market-based reforms, specifically, consumer-directed health plans. Whether the managed care industry will be able to realize its potential for high-quality care at lower cost after two decades of mixed performance now seems in doubt.

The potential for selection bias continues to be an important issue, particularly given the inadequate status of risk-adjustment mechanisms. The promise of managed care and managed competition is difficult to realize fully unless health plans have incentives to enroll all levels of risk. Although adequate risk-adjusted payment systems have been developed for hospital inpatient and outpatient services under the Medicare program, risk-adjusting capitation rates has proven more difficult,[51] primarily because of the difficulty in identifying a priori who in the population is likely to experience high-cost acute events. This continues to be an area of important research, particularly under the Medicare program, which risk-adjusts payments to health plans for beneficiaries enrolled in HMOs.

The empirical literature indicates that competition in the hospital sector can lead to lower hospital costs and lower prices for major purchasers. Third-party plans that use selective contracting (PPOs and HMOs) can leverage competitive market conditions to negotiate lower prices with hospitals. But how these insurance plans design and manage their hospital networks is important in determining the benefits ultimately derived by the consumers of health care services. The effectiveness of selective contracting as a cost and price control method is highly dependent on the existence of a sufficient level of competition in the market. This suggests that both third-party payers through their contracting activities and government agencies through regulatory oversight must ensure that market conditions remain competitive.

Given recent declines in HMO enrollment and the shift in national attention toward consumer-directed health plans, perhaps the time has come for a new paradigm of managed care that focuses on improved health promotion, disease prevention, quality, and outcomes, without the expectation of lower costs. In other words, it may be time for HMOs to truly focus on health maintenance. In the current health care market, that could bestow a significant competitive advantage, particularly in contrast to self-managed, consumer-directed care.

# Notes

1. The elements of managed competition were first described in Enthoven, A. C. "Consumer Choice Health Plan: A National Health Insurance Proposal Based on Regulated Competition in the Private Sector." *New England Journal of Medicine*, 1978, *298*, 709–720; and

later refined in Enthoven, A. C., and Kronick, R. "A Consumer-Choice Health Plan for the 1990s." *New England Journal of Medicine,* 1989, *320,* 29–37, 94–101.

2. Committee on the Costs of Medical Care. *Medical Care for the American People: The Final Report.* Chicago: University of Chicago Press, 1932.

3. Gold, M., and Hurley, R. "The Role of Managed Care 'Products' in Managed Care 'Plans.'" *Inquiry,* 1997, *34,* 29–37; and Gabel, J., Whitmore, H., Bergsten, C., and Grimm, L. "Growing Diversification in HMOs, 1988–1994." *Medical Care Research and Review,* 1997, *54,* 101–117.

4. Ellwood, P. and others. "Health Maintenance Strategy." *Medical Care,* 1971, *9,* 291–298.

5. Luft, H. S. *Health Maintenance Organizations: Dimensions of Performance.* New York: Wiley, 1981. See also Luft, H. S. "How Do Health-Maintenance Organizations Achieve Their 'Savings'?" *New England Journal of Medicine,* 1978, *298,* 1336–1343.

6. Gruber, L., Shadle, M., and Polich, C. "From Movement to Industry: The Growth of HMOs." *Health Affairs,* 1988, *7,* 197–208.

7. InterStudy Publications. [http://www.hmodata.com].

8. InterStudy. *Competitive Edge Report.* Spring 2005, reported on Kaiser Family Foundation State Health Facts Website. [http://www.statehealthfacts.kff.org].

9. Claxton, G., and others. *Employer Health Benefits: 2005 Annual Survey.* Menlo Park, Calif.: Kaiser Family Foundation, and Chicago: Health Research and Education Trust, 2005. [http://www.kff.org/insurance/7315/upload/7315.pdf].

10. Luft (1981).

11. Blendon, R. J., and others. "Understanding the Managed Care Backlash." *Health Affairs,* July–Aug. 1998, *17,* 80–94; Enthoven, A. C., and Singer, S. J. "The Managed Care Backlash and the Task Force in California." *Health Affairs,* July–Aug. 1998, *17,* 95–110. An entire special issue of the *Journal of Health Care Politics, Policy, and Law* was dedicated to the topic in October 1999.

12. Peterson, M. A. "Introduction: Politics, Misperception, or Apropos?" *Journal of Health Politics, Policy, and Law,* 1999, *25,* 873–886.

13. Robinson, J. C. "The End of Managed Care." *Journal of the American Medical Association,* 2001, *285,* 2622–2628.

14. Miller, R. H., and Luft, H. S. "HMO Plan Performance Update: An Analysis of the Literature, 1997–2001." *Health Affairs,* 2002, *21,* 63–86.

15. California Department of Managed Health Care. [http://www.dmhc.ca.gov].

16. InterStudy (2005).

17. Newhouse, J. P. "Toward a Theory of Non-Profit Institutions: An Economic Model of a Hospital." *American Economic Review,* 1970, *60,* 4–74; Pauly, M. V., and Redisch, M. "The Not-for-Profit Hospital as a Physicians' Cooperative." *American Economic Review,* 1973, *63,* 87–99; Harris, J. "The Internal Organization of Hospitals: Some Economic Implications." *Bell Journal of Economics and Management Science,* 1977, *8,* 467–482; and Ellis, R. P., and McGuire, T. G. "Provider Behavior Under Prospective Reimbursement: Cost Sharing and Supply." *Journal of Health Economics,* 1986, *5,* 129–151.

18. Melnick, G. A., Zwanziger, J., Bamezai, A., and Pattison, R. "The Effects of Market Structure and Hospital Bargaining Position on Hospital Prices." *Journal of Health Economics,* 1992, *11,* 217–233.

19. Robinson, J. C. "Decline in Hospital Utilization and Cost Inflation Under Managed Care in California." *Journal of the American Medical Association,* 1996, *276,* 1060–1064; Robinson, J. C. "HMO Market Penetration and Hospital Cost Inflation in California." *Journal of the*

*American Medical Association*, 1991, *266*, 2719–2723; and Melnick, G. A., and Zwanziger, J. "Hospital Behavior Under Competition and Cost Containment Policies: The California Experience." *Journal of the American Medical Association*, 1988, *260*, 2669–2675.

20. Zwanziger, J., Melnick, G. A., and Bamezai, A. "Cost and Price Competition in California Hospitals, 1980–1990." *Health Affairs*, 1994, *13*, 118–126; and Zwanziger, J., Melnick, G. A., and Bamezai, A. "The Effect of Selective Contracting on Hospital Costs and Revenues." *Health Services Research*, 2000, *35*, 849–867.

21. Dowd, B. E., Feldman, R., and Coulam, R. "The Effect of Health Plan Characteristics on Medicare+Choice Enrollment." *Health Services Research*, 2003, *38*, 113–135.

22. Atherly, A., Dowd, B. E., and Feldman, R. "The Effect of Benefits, Premiums, and Health Risk on Health Plan Choice in the Medicare Program." *Health Services Research*, 2004, *39*, 847–864.

23. Buchmueller, T. "Price and the Health Plan Choices of Retirees." *Journal of Health Economics*, 2006, *25*, 81–100.

24. Strombom, B. A., Buchmueller, T. C., and Feldstein, P. J. "Switching Costs, Price Sensitivity, and Health Plan Choice." *Journal of Health Economics*, 2002, *21*, 89–116.

25. Pauly, M. V. "Monopsony Power in Health Insurance: Thinking Straight While Standing on Your Head." *Journal of Health Economics*, 1987, *6*, 73–81.

26. Pauly (1987); Pauly, M. V. "Reply: A Response to Market Share/Market Power Revisited." *Journal of Health Economics*, 1988, *7*, 85–87; Pauly, M. V. "Market Power Monopsony, and Health Insurance Markets." *Journal of Health Economics*, 1988, *7*, 111–128; Staten, M., Dunkelberg, W., and Umbeck, J. "Market Share and the Illusion of Power: Can Blue Cross Force Hospitals to Discount?" *Journal of Health Economics*, 1987, *6*, 43–58; and Staten, M., Umbeck, J., and Dunkelberg, W. "Market Share/Market Power Revisited: A New Test for an Old Theory." *Journal of Health Economics*, 1988, *7*, 73–83.

27. Staten, Umbeck, and Dunkelberg (1988).

28. Although the paper by Staten and colleagues (1988) offered the first analysis of hospital prices under PPO arrangements, it has several important limitations. The dependent variable, the discount rate, was calculated using the initial bid proposed by the hospital and not the final price agreed between the PPO and the hospital. Thus their measure is likely to overestimate the final price agreed on by hospitals in the PPO contract.

29. Melnick, Zwanziger, Bamezai, and Pattison (1992).

30. Keeler, E., Melnick, G. A., and Zwanziger, J. "The Changing Effects of Competition on Non-Profit and For-Profit Hospital Pricing Behavior." *Journal of Health Economics*, 1999, *18*, 9–86; and Melnick, G. A., Keeler, E., and Zwanziger, J. "Market Power and Hospital Pricing: Are Nonprofits Different?" *Health Affairs*, May–June 1999, *18*, 167–173.

31. Kralewski, E., and others. "Factors Related to the Provision of Hospital Discounts for HMO Inpatients." *Health Services Research*, 1992, *27*, 133–153.

32. Feldman, R., and others. "Effects of HMOs on the Creation of Competitive Markets for Hospital Services." *Journal of Health Economics*, 1990, *9*, 207–222.

33. Feldman, R., Kralewski, J., Shapiro, J., and Chan, H. C. "Contracts Between Hospitals and Health Maintenance Organizations." *Health Care Management Review*, 1990, *15*, 47–60.

34. Luft (1981).

35. Miller, R. H., and Luft, H. S. "Managed Care Plan Performance Since 1980: A Literature Analysis." *Journal of the American Medical Association*, 1994, *271*, 1512–1519; Miller, R. H., and Luft, H. S., "Does Managed Care Lead to Better or Worse Quality of Care?" *Health Affairs*, 1997, *16*, 7–25; and Miller and Luft (2002).

36. Greenfield, S., and others. "Variations in Resource Utilization Among Medical Specialties and Systems of Care: Results from the Medical Outcomes Study." *Journal of the American Medical Association*, 1992, *267*, 1624–1630.

37. Enthoven, A. C. "Why Managed Care Has Failed to Contain Health Costs." *Health Affairs*, 1993, *12*, 28–43.

38. Melnick, G. A., and Zwanziger, J. "State Health Care Expenditures Under Competition and Regulation, 1980 through 1991." *American Journal of Public Health*, Oct. 1995, *85*, 1391–1396; Robinson, J. C. "Health Care Purchasing and Market Changes in California." *Health Affairs*, 1995, *14*, 118–130; and Enthoven, A. C., and Singer, S. J. "Managed Competition and California's Health Care Economy." *Health Affairs*, 1996, *15*, 40–57.

39. Claxton and others (2005).

40. Marquis and Long (1999).

41. Miller and Luft (2002).

42. Luft, H. S. "Modifying Managed Competition to Address Cost and Quality." *Health Affairs*, 1996, *15*, 24–38.

43. Pacific Business Group on Health. "PBGH's Commitment to Quality Improvement." [http://www.pbgh.org/PBGH_folder/quality.html].

44. See, for example, Parker, J. P., and others. *The California Report on Coronary Artery Bypass Graft Surgery 2003 Hospital Data*. Sacramento: California Office of Statewide Planning and Development, Feb. 2006. Other reports available [http://www.oshpd.state.ca.us/HQAD/Outcomes/index.htm].

45. Miller and Luft (2002).

46. See, for example, Wholey, D. R., Burns, L. R., and Lavizzo-Mourey, R. "Managed Care and the Delivery of Primary Care to the Elderly and the Chronically Ill." *Health Services Research*, 1998, *33*(2), Part II, 322–353; Escarce, J. and others, "Health Maintenance Organizations and Hospital Quality for Coronary Artery Bypass Graft Surgery." *Medical Care Research and Review*, 1999, *56*, 340–362; and Pourat, N., Kagawa-Singer, M., and Wallace, S. "Are Managed Care Medicare Beneficiaries with Chronic Conditions Satisfied with Their Care?" *Journal of Aging and Health*, 2006, *18*, 70–90.

47. Volpp, K.G.M., and others. "Market Reform in New Jersey and the Effect on Mortality from Acute Myocardial Infarction." *Health Services Research*, 2003, *38*, 515–533.

48. Miller and Luft (2002).

49. Marquis and Long (1999); Bodenheimer, T., and Sullivan, K. "How Large Employers Are Shaping the Health Care Marketplace." *New England Journal of Medicine*, 1998, *338*, 1003–1007, 1084–1087; and Kuttner, R. "The American Health Care System: Employer-Sponsored Health Insurance." *New England Journal of Medicine*, 1999, *340*, 248–252.

50. National health expenditures as a percentage of GDP grew from 13.6 percent in 1997 to 16.0 percent in 2004. See Smith, C., Cowman, C., Heffler, S., Catlin, A., and the National Health Accounts Team. "National Health Spending in 2004: Recent Slowdown Led by Prescription Drug Spending." *Health Affairs*, 2006, *25*, 186–196. Employment-based health insurance premiums doubled between 1998 and 2005. See Claxton and others (2005).

51. Newhouse, J. P. "Risk Adjustment: Where Are We Now?" *Inquiry*, 1998, *35*, 122–131; and Dudley, R. A., Rennie, D. J., and Luft, H. S. "Population Choice and Variable Selection in the Estimation and Application of Risk Models." *Inquiry*, 1999, *36*, 200–211.

CHAPTER TWENTY

# MEDICARE REFORM

Gerald F. Kominski
Jeanne T. Black
Thomas H. Rice

Medicare was enacted in 1965 as a compromise on the road toward a comprehensive system of national health insurance. Like most great compromises, its original design reflected prevailing concepts about health benefits and health care delivery that have changed substantially in the last forty years. As the second largest social insurance program in the United States after Social Security, Medicare continues to bestow tremendous benefit to beneficiaries and their families, who might otherwise individually bear the entire health care costs associated with aging. More than a safety net, Medicare gives seniors and the disabled access to the highest-quality health care. But in the first decade of the twenty-first century, forty years after its enactment, Medicare is facing several significant challenges that threaten the very principles on which the program was originally based.

This chapter begins with a review of the origins of Medicare as an alternative, incremental strategy developed after decades of failed attempts to enact comprehensive national health insurance.[1] We then discuss how Medicare has evolved, including its benefit structure and payment mechanisms, to meet various challenges since its enactment in 1965. Next we review the current challenges facing Medicare, including the demographic threat to its long-term solvency. Finally, we discuss recent changes to Medicare enacted as part of the Medicare Prescription Drug, Improvement, and Modernization Act of 2003, including the new prescription drug benefit and efforts to transform Medicare from a defined benefits program to one based on defined contributions.

# Origin and Philosophy of Medicare

The United States stands alone among developed nations in not providing universal health coverage to its population. Proposals for national health insurance in the United States were first made before World War I. Following the Great Depression, every decade of the twentieth century saw major proposals put forward that failed to win approval in the U.S. Congress. At the root of these failures are fundamental ideological differences between liberal and conservative policy makers. Historically, liberals have advocated a system of social insurance, while conservatives have favored a welfare approach that extends assistance only to those who cannot fend for themselves in the private market.

The theory of social insurance recognizes that the benefits and costs of capitalism are not equally distributed within society, and that in a democracy government has a role in tempering the impact of a competitive market economy on individuals.[2] Thus the United States has social insurance programs to cushion the financial impact of occupational injuries, unemployment, and poverty in old age. In general, social insurance programs share three principles:

1. Pooled risk, because serious illness, injury, or job loss is unpredictable
2. Redistribution of income through the tax system, to achieve affordable coverage for all
3. National administration, to ensure universal access

Although the United States has failed to adopt a system of universal coverage for all residents, it does have a program of social health insurance for its elderly population. The Medicare program, enacted on July 30, 1965, as Title XVIII of the Social Security Act, is the most important piece of health insurance legislation in U.S. history. Its passage raises a fundamental question: Why was Medicare enacted rather than universal health insurance? To answer this question, and to understand how Medicare evolved as well as current proposals for its reform, requires a brief review of the history of national health insurance initiatives in the United States.

The first efforts to promote national health insurance in the United States grew out of the Progressive movement that emerged during the first decade of the twentieth century. Those efforts were based on European models of compulsory social insurance, first enacted into law by Chancellor Otto von Bismarck of Germany in 1883. The leaders of the American Medical Association (AMA), having positive views of the German and British systems, initially were supportive of the Progressives' efforts.[3] However, the AMA soon found that local medical societies were vehemently opposed. By 1920, the medical profession solidified its opposition to comprehensive health reform, a position that it maintained throughout the remainder of the twentieth century. Conversely, organized labor, which initially feared that government programs such as compulsory social insurance would lessen workers' need to join labor unions, later became an outspoken advocate of national health insurance.

Calls for health reform to address rising medical costs are not a recent phenomenon. In 1927, eight private foundations established the Committee on the Costs of Medical Care. The committee's final report, published in 1932, called for reorganizing health care delivery into prepaid medical group practice, and for promoting experiments in voluntary health insurance. Voicing its opposition, the *Journal of the American Medical Association* editorialized against "the forces representing the great foundations, public health officialdom, social theory—even socialism and communism" that were threatening the "sound practice of medicine."[4]

Following the Great Depression, President Franklin Delano Roosevelt established the Committee on Economic Security. Its recommendations formed the basis for the package of social legislation known as the New Deal, which included the Social Security Act of 1935. However, the committee's consideration of health insurance brought an immediate storm of criticism from the AMA. As a result, Roosevelt did not publicly support national health insurance, fearing that passage of his entire program—and his reelection—could be jeopardized by its inclusion. At the same time, the AMA, suspicious of future government involvement in health care, began to support the private, voluntary hospital insurance programs begun by Blue Cross and commercial insurance companies, and state Blue Shield programs for surgical and medical expenses.[5]

Despite the failure to enact a national health insurance program as part of the New Deal, support for such a program remained strong in Congress. Every year between 1939 and 1951, a comprehensive health insurance bill sponsored by Sen. Robert Wagner (D-N.Y.), Sen. James Murray (D-Mont.), and Rep. John Dingell, Sr. (D-Mich.) was introduced into Congress. Over this thirteen-year period, the Murray-Wagner-Dingell bills never received enough support to be reported out of committee, and thus these bills never reached a vote on the floor of the House or Senate. In 1948, Harry Truman campaigned for president on a Fair Deal platform that included national health insurance. Once elected, however, he was unable to overcome the opposition of a coalition of Republicans and Southern Democrats. The AMA mounted a nationwide campaign promoting the horrors of "socialized medicine," and several supporters of national health insurance failed to win reelection in 1950.[6]

By the early 1950s, Truman's advisors in the Federal Security Agency (now the Department of Health and Human Services) were convinced that a new strategy was necessary. They concluded that progress toward national health insurance required a more limited, incremental approach. Popular support for the Social Security program meant that a health insurance program for the elderly stood the greatest chance of approval. Linking a program of Medicare to Social Security had the added benefit of avoiding the stigma associated with a welfare program and portraying Medicare as analogous to private insurance for which the beneficiary has paid.

A program to address the needs of the elderly was also more difficult for the AMA to oppose. In the words of Robert M. Ball, who worked on the initial Medicare proposals and later became a Social Security Commissioner:

> The elderly were an appealing group to cover first in part because they were so ill suited for coverage under voluntary private insurance. They used on average more than twice as many hospital days as younger people but had only about half as much income. Private insurers, who set premiums to cover current costs, had to charge them much more, and the elderly could not afford the charges. Group health insurance, then as today, was mostly for the employed and was just not available to the retired elderly. The result of all this was that somewhat less than half of the elderly had any kind of health insurance, and what they had was almost always inadequate. . . . So the need was not hard to prove, nor was it difficult to prove that voluntary individual insurance was not only not meeting the need, but that it really could not meet the need.[7]

In order to win political support, it also was crucial for Medicare not to be viewed as a threat to the existing health care delivery or financing system. The program was positioned as a solution to the financial difficulties of the elderly that resulted from use of medical services, particularly costly hospitalization, rather than one that would comprehensively address their health needs. As a strategy to temper the AMA's opposition, physician services were not included in the initial Medicare proposals.

Between 1958 and 1963, numerous Congressional hearings and intense lobbying took place on the subject of Medicare. Although it was now generally accepted that there was strong public support for a program of health insurance for the elderly, there was vociferous debate between social insurance and welfare advocates regarding the benefits and structure of the program and whether it should be administered by the federal government or by the states. President John F. Kennedy strongly supported providing hospital insurance for the elderly through the Social Security program. However, he was unable to obtain the support of the majority on the House Ways and Means Committee, which had authority for proposed legislation requiring new federal expenditures and whose members included a conservative coalition of Republicans and Southern Democrats opposed to expansion of federal programs. Finally, the landslide Democratic victories in the 1964 elections led President Lyndon Johnson to make hospital insurance for the elderly the first piece of legislation introduced into both houses of Congress as part of his Great Society program.

Competing bills were submitted and considered by the Ways and Means Committee. Under the chairmanship of Rep. Wilbur Mills (D-Ark.), a surprising compromise was reached. The Medicare program would provide hospital insurance to all Social Security beneficiaries on the basis of the Blue Cross model and voluntary insurance for physician services along the lines of the health plan for federal employees offered by Aetna Life Insurance. Conservatives had hoped to limit Medicare to state programs serving the very poor elderly. However, in the final bill benefits for the poor were expanded to cover all ages, to be administered as a joint federal-state program known as Medicaid.

In summary, Medicare emerged out of frustrated efforts to pass national health insurance that began in the early part of the twentieth century. Its proponents conceived it as a social insurance program, and they hoped and expected that it would be the foundation for incremental expansion to other populations and additional benefits. But the compromises that led to its passage masked these philosophical underpinnings and sowed the seeds for many of the conflicts over Medicare's design and financing that continue into the present.

## Evolution of Medicare

The original Medicare program included two parts, Hospital Insurance (Part A) and Supplementary Medical Insurance (Part B). The major benefits covered under Part A were 90 days of hospital care per episode[8] of care plus 60 lifetime reserve[9] days, 100 days of posthospital care per episode in a skilled-nursing facility (SNF) if preceded by an inpatient admission, 100 posthospital home health visits per year, and 190 lifetime days of inpatient psychiatric care. Hospice benefits were added later, and home health care was shifted to Part B. Part B covered most physician services, outpatient hospital services, and durable medical equipment. There was no coverage for outpatient prescription drugs, nor any limit on a beneficiary's out-of-pocket expenses. The original Medicare benefits package remains essentially unchanged, with the exception of a new outpatient prescription drug benefit that began in 2006 (to be discussed).

Medicare is financed by a combination of payroll taxes, general revenues, and beneficiary contributions. Part A is a true social insurance program, with eligibility based on payment of payroll taxes that are mandatory for all workers.

All beneficiaries eligible for Part A are also eligible for Part B, but participation is voluntary and requires monthly premium payments, which are deducted directly from Social Security checks. These premiums are set to be approximately 25 percent of Part B costs, with the remainder contributed by federal general revenues. Both Part A and Part B require beneficiary cost sharing. For Part A, this includes a deductible for the first day of hospital care plus coinsurance for hospital care beyond sixty days, and coinsurance for SNF care beyond twenty days as well as for durable medical equipment provided by a home health agency. Part B has an annual deductible and requires 20 percent coinsurance for most services.[10]

Part B intentionally diverges from the social insurance model; it is voluntary and is financed in part by current beneficiary premiums. The political opponents of social insurance for physician services accepted their inclusion in a separate voluntary insurance plan to preempt future efforts to expand the social insurance component of Part A.

Medicare's framers also knew that political support for the program required that it be modeled on the existing system of health care delivery and financing. As a result, hospital reimbursement followed the existing form of cost-based agreements with the Blue Cross system, and insurance companies served as payment intermediaries. Similarly, fearing physician refusal to participate in the program, Part B did not establish a fee schedule. Instead, it established payments based on a modified version of the physician's "usual, customary, and reasonable (UCR)" fees charged to privately insured patients; Medicare's version was known as "customary, prevailing, and reasonable (CPR)" charges. To reassure physicians that the physician-patient relationship would remain intact, Part B allowed physicians to bill patients directly, with the patient to seek payment from the government. In addition, physicians could bill patients for the difference between Medicare's allowed charge for a service and the physician's usual charge, a practice known as balance billing.

Once Medicare had been enacted, implementing it was an enormous task. To ensure passage and smooth implementation, Medicare's developers made accommodations to a wide range of interest groups. One result of these compromises was rapid growth in Medicare expenditures. The cost-based hospital reimbursement system and CPR physician payment system were predictably inflationary, and both hospital charges and physician fees increased sharply in the program's early years. However, the program's initial emphasis was on removing financial barriers to care, not on changing the delivery or financing of the health care system. In 1972, Medicare was expanded to cover individuals with end-stage renal disease and disabled people under age sixty-five who had been receiving Social Security disability benefits for two years.

During the 1970s, the rising cost of health care was a growing national concern, and it shaped concerns about the future of Medicare for the next two decades. National health expenditures as a percent of Gross Domestic Product (GDP) rose from 7.1 percent in 1970 to 8.9 percent in 1980.[11] Medicare's share of national health care costs grew from 10.5 percent to 15.2 percent over the same period.[12] Following the failure of various national health insurance proposals in the 1970s and of legislative and voluntary efforts to control hospital costs, the Medicare program began to adopt a new stance toward provider payment beginning in the mid-1970s. Medicare sponsored several demonstration projects during this period to develop incentive reimbursement programs for hospitals that would encourage greater efficiency and cost containment. Beginning in the 1980s, Medicare received increased Congressional scrutiny because of the growing federal budget deficit. The stage was thus set for Medicare to adopt new policies aimed at restraining costs.

In 1983, the Health Care Financing Administration (the federal agency responsible for Medicare and Medicaid, now the Centers for Medicare and Medicaid Services) implemented a prospective payment system (PPS) for hospitals. Rather than paying hospitals according to their retrospective costs, PPS paid them a fixed amount related to the patient's reason for admission, categorized according to a classification system known as diagnosis-related groups (DRGs). PPS had an immediate effect on hospital utilization; length of stay decreased more than 10 percent between 1983 and 1985, and admissions declined as hospitals shifted procedures to the outpatient setting.[13]

Medicare also implemented price controls and global expenditure targets for payment of physician services beginning in 1992. The Medicare Fee Schedule (MFS), based on the resource-based relative value scale (RBRVS) developed at Harvard University, had as explicit goals redistribution of payments from surgical to primary care services as well as from urban to rural practitioners. Both the DRG and RBRVS approaches have been adopted by commercial insurance plans as successful cost-containment measures.[14]

Despite successful implementation of hospital and physician price controls, Medicare continued to face challenges in the 1990s, since expenditures continued to grow at a faster rate than revenues. This led to concerns about the long-term solvency of the program, which according to projections in the mid-1990s would be in a deficit position by the year 2001. To address this impending financing crisis, the Balanced Budget Act (BBA) of 1997 was enacted with strong bipartisan support. The BBA included a number of measures aimed at controlling Medicare spending as well as creation of Medicare Part C (called Medicare+Choice) to offer more options for Medicare beneficiaries to join health plans. In 1998, the growth rate in

Medicare expenditures fell to an unprecedented 1.5 percent,[15] and Medicare costs actually decreased in the six months ending in March 1999.[16] However, by 2000, lawmakers were facing political pressure to return some of these savings from providers seeking higher payments, from health plans seeking higher capitation rates, and from beneficiaries seeking expanded benefits. The Medicare Prescription Drug, Improvement, and Modernization Act (MMA) of 2003 addressed many of these stakeholder demands. In addition to adding a long-overdue prescription drug benefit to Medicare, the MMA increased payments to hospitals and health plans and introduced an improved risk-adjustment system for payments to health plans to further encourage them to enroll high-risk beneficiaries.

# Is Medicare Facing a Crisis?

There is no question that the Medicare program faces formidable challenges in the coming decades. As with U.S. health care costs overall, Medicare expenditures have risen steadily as a proportion of GDP. The aging of the baby boom generation is expected to create enormous additional demands. The Medicare benefit package, envisioned initially as just a first step toward comprehensive coverage, has become increasingly inadequate to meet beneficiaries' health needs. The policy question is whether these challenges represent a crisis that requires a radical solution, or whether continued incremental changes will maintain and improve the program as they have in the forty years since its inception. This section discusses the demographic and utilization factors that contribute to rising Medicare costs, forecasts of Medicare insolvency, and the rising financial burden on beneficiaries.

## Demographics

The most significant threat to the future of the Medicare program is the aging of the U.S. population. As the baby boom generation (those born between 1946 and 1964) reaches retirement age between 2011 and 2029, this demographic bulge will create an enormous financial burden on Medicare. The number of beneficiaries is estimated to rise from approximately forty million in 2000 to seventy-eight million in 2030.[17] Though the population age sixty-five to seventy-nine may nearly double between 2000 and 2050, those eighty and older will be the fastest-growing segment of the elderly, increasing as much as 244 percent.[18]

Demographic changes have political and social implications for the Medicare program in addition to their economic impact.[19] Demographic projections depend on assumptions regarding mortality, fertility, and immigration. Average life expectancy increased throughout the twentieth century as a result of improved standards of living as well as advances in medical care. The key question here is whether historical improvement in mortality will continue, or whether there is a genetically determined limit to the human life span. Whatever the answer to this question, further improvement in average life expectancy will increase the number of years individuals are dependent on the Medicare program.

Assumptions regarding the number of children born to women of child-bearing age affect population growth, the proportion represented by the elderly, and the ratio of tax-paying workers to the number of Medicare beneficiaries. Current forecasts use a fertility rate of slightly below replacement level, consistent with the experience of most European countries. In the long run, however, it is difficult to predict the impact of economic conditions on fertility as well the impact of increased immigration.

In a country with a below-replacement fertility rate, population growth results from both increased longevity and immigration. In 2002, foreign-born residents represented 11.5 percent of the U.S. population, and 22.0 percent of the population were either foreign-born or had one or both parents who were.[20] Most immigrants to the United States in the twenty-first century will belong to ethnic groups currently identified as minorities. Immigrants generally have a higher fertility rate than the native-born population, 83.7 per 1,000 in 2004 versus 56.7 per 1,000.[21] Therefore immigration may increase the proportion of younger workers in the population. The U.S. fertility rate has declined overall, so that the combined number of children and the elderly relative to the size of the working age population (that is, the dependency ratio) is forecast to be lower in 2050 than it was in 1960.[22]

Because Medicare is a public program for a targeted population group, it is subject to unique political pressures not experienced by universal health care programs. In countries with national health insurance, the risk pool includes the entire population, of which the elderly are a relatively small proportion. Expenditures for individuals under age sixty-five are already counted in the system, so the effect of a growing number of individuals reaching age sixty-five is simply the incremental cost of health care for sixty-five-year-olds versus sixty-four-year-olds. In contrast, the baby boom generation will create a huge budgetary impact in the United States, because most beneficiaries transition from private insurance (or no coverage) to public insurance when they become eligible for Medicare. The European countries and Japan have already absorbed the health costs of a population that aged more rapidly than that of the United States. Though there have been signs of strain and incremental reforms in their health systems, these countries continue to furnish universal coverage, and cost pressures have not resulted in radical restructuring.[23]

## Costs

A generally accepted means of assessing trends in health care expenditures is to examine their relationship to national GDP. Between 1975 and 1995, Medicare expenditures exceeded GDP growth by 3.5 to 4.0 percent per year.[24] Consequently, the Medicare program became an ever larger proportion of the national economy. The trustees of the Part A and Part B trust funds are required by law to make an annual report to Congress that forecasts future expenditures and revenue. The addition of the Part D drug benefit and increased payments to Medicare Advantage plans under the MMA of 2003 have increased forecasts of Medicare spending relative to the economy. The latest trustees' report forecasts that Medicare expenditures will increase from 2.6 percent of GDP in 2004 to 7.5 percent in 2030.[25]

Price, volume, and intensity of service all play a role in medical expenditures. Both the PPS and MFS were mechanisms to limit provider payment and reduce utilization. These approaches to price controls have been effective, but they do not address other underlying determinants of continuing expenditure growth— that is, the diffusion of medical technology and the increasing intensity of services. The growth in health care costs of the elderly has been primarily due to technology driving increasing intensity of services consumed per capita.[26] Analysts differ in their assumptions about how individuals will use services in the future, and the evidence is contradictory. Factors that would increase costs include the oldest old being far more likely to be institutionalized or to require assistance with activities of daily living.

In addition, utilization rates for procedures such as angioplasty and hip replacement among Medicare beneficiaries have increased dramatically over the past ten years, with some of the largest increases in the population age eighty-five and older. Will the average eighty-five-year-old consume fewer resources because she will be healthier? Or, will she consume the same or more because she will have bypass surgery and a hip replacement in order to continue playing tennis?

Finally, many chronic conditions are not strongly associated with mortality, so that increased longevity will mean more people living with chronic conditions such as dementia.[27] On the other hand, several factors support the notion that per capita use of services may decline as the population ages. For example, a large proportion of Medicare costs is incurred in the last year of a beneficiary's life; thus increased longevity means that the cost of dying will be spread over a longer period of time. In addition, the cost of dying is lower for the oldest old.[28] The costs for a ninety-three-year-old who dies of pneumonia in a nursing home are less than those for a sixty-eight-year-old who dies in the intensive care unit of complications from open heart surgery. In addition, advances in treatment and improved understanding of risk factors can delay the onset of some chronic conditions.[29]

Efforts to reduce growth in the price and volume of services, whether through regulation or competition, were the focus of Medicare reform efforts in the 1980s and 1990s. With the addition of a prescription drug benefit as part of the MMA of 2003, controlling program expenditures will continue to be a challenge facing the Medicare program during the next decade.

## Forecasts of Insolvency

The Medicare Part A Trust Fund has been forecast to become insolvent many times during its history. The frequent declarations of a crisis in Medicare can be explained in part by the nature of economic forecasts. Forecasting requires assumptions about demographics, economic growth, worker productivity, health care costs, and other important variables. Small differences in assumptions compound over time, with the result that analysts' forecasts can vary significantly and change dramatically from year to year. Nevertheless, the Medicare trustees are required by law to project the funds' status seventy-five years into the future. Considering the changes that have occurred since the 1930s in medicine, in technology generally, in society, and in the world economy, it is obviously absurd to expect long-term forecasts to be reliable.

Reliable short-term estimates are also difficult to produce. In 1996, the Part A Trust Fund was projected to be bankrupt in 2001.[30] However, the reimbursement changes mandated by the BBA of 1997 were more successful than anticipated in restraining Medicare costs, and by the time of the 1999 trustees' report bankruptcy of the trust fund had been put off until 2015.[31] The 2005 annual report concludes that the trust fund will remain solvent until 2020, even with the addition of the prescription drug benefit.[32] These vastly different forecasts illustrate just how sensitive these projections are to changes in the economy as well as expenditure patterns among Medicare beneficiaries.

## Benefit Gaps and Rising Out-of-Pocket Expenditures

The Medicare benefit package was modeled after the private health plans of the 1960s, with Part A analogous to Blue Cross hospital coverage and Part B to Blue Shield coverage of physicians' services. The private "Medigap" market developed to offer supplementary insurance, similar to major medical policies sold by many private insurers. Medicare as originally designed was not intended to cover all the medical expenditures of the elderly. Early estimates were that it would pay about 40 percent.[33] In 2002, it was estimated to cover 45 percent of medical and long-term care costs.[34] The program has always required beneficiaries to contribute a significant amount toward their covered medical benefits in the form of the part

B premium as well as deductibles and coinsurance. However, noncovered services account for the majority of beneficiary out-of-pocket spending. In 2002, the largest component was the cost of long-term care (36 percent), followed by prescription drugs (22 percent).[35]

In 1965, the medical profession, which fought so strenuously against the passage of Medicare, also considered prepaid group practice to be socialized medicine and ostracized physicians who practiced in what are now called group-model HMOs. However, rising health care costs stimulated many changes in the structure of private health plans. As discussed in Chapter Nineteen, by the 1990s HMOs and other forms of managed care had replaced indemnity fee-for-service (FFS) as the predominant type of health plan design. Managed care plans eliminated the distinctions between hospital and physician benefits, which had become unwieldy as health care delivery moved increasingly into ambulatory care. They also included benefits for preventive services. Many employers also added prescription drug coverage to managed care plans as an inducement for their employees to switch from costly indemnity plans. Meanwhile, the basic structure of Medicare remained unchanged. What began as a program that mirrored private health insurance in 1965 became one with a distinctly different benefit structure by the end of the twentieth century.

As of 2000, the traditional Medicare program lacked two important benefits found in most employer-sponsored health plans: prescription drugs and catastrophic coverage. Although prescription drugs are increasingly important in treating the chronic illnesses suffered by the elderly, their cost has been rising more rapidly than that of health care overall. National health spending on prescription drugs almost tripled between 1995 and 2003. In contrast, total national health expenditures increased by only 70 percent.[36] Although 89 percent of beneficiaries in 2001 had supplemental coverage (through privately purchased Medigap policies, Medicare HMOs, employer-sponsored plans, or Medicaid),[37] 27 percent had no coverage for prescription drugs.[38] The burden of prescription drug expenses for the elderly has been exacerbated by the fact that the retail pharmacy prices paid by the elderly and others without prescription drug coverage are substantially higher than the prices negotiated by managed care plans. This gap in Medicare coverage led to enactment of a new prescription drug benefit (Medicare Part D) effective in 2006.

Medicare has no limitation on beneficiaries' out-of-pocket costs, whereas the typical private insurance plan covers all expenses after the enrollee has incurred a specified amount of co-insurance payment, up to the policy's lifetime maximum. Nor does Medicare cover long-term nursing home care, which also is not generally covered by private employer-sponsored health insurance. Although there is a small private market for long-term care insurance, most nursing home costs are paid by the Medicaid program (for those who are poor or who spend down their assets), or out of pocket by the elderly or their families. Although the need is great, there are currently no viable reform proposals to include nursing home care as part of the basic Medicare benefit package.

The poverty rate among the elderly has dropped from 28.5 percent in 1966 to 10.2 percent in 2003, equivalent to the rate in the population age eighteen to sixty-four.[39] However, health care costs have risen much faster than the incomes of the elderly. Therefore out-of-pocket costs represent an increasing proportion of income—the very condition Medicare was enacted to ameliorate. In 1998, average out-of-pocket costs for Medicare beneficiaries represented 19 percent of median income, with this proportion projected to rise to 30 percent by 2025,[40] not including expenditures for long-term care.

## Reforming Medicare

During the 1990s, the Clinton administration consistently supported use of the private market to achieve cost savings and promote innovation in delivering health services. The Medicare+Choice program was established as part of the BBA of 1997 to expand private sector health plan options for Medicare beneficiaries. Managed care plans participating in Medicare+Choice (renamed Medicare Advantage as part of the MMA of 2003) must cover the basic package of Medicare benefits. They compete within a given market on the basis of supplemental benefits such as prescription drugs, provider networks, and customer service. However, they do not compete on price. Beneficiaries continue to pay the same basic Part B premium, and their total cost sharing cannot be greater than that of traditional Medicare. All plans within a county are paid the same rate per beneficiary, with adjustment for health status and other risk factors. As the name implied, Medicare+Choice gave many beneficiaries the choice between traditional Medicare and a managed care plan similar to that offered by employers in the private sector, while preserving the basic entitlements of the original Medicare program. As of 2005, almost 4.8 million beneficiaries were enrolled in managed care plans, down from a peak enrollment of 6.3 million in 2000.[41]

Since the passage of Medicare in 1965, the political values of the United States have shifted fundamentally. Whereas government was once viewed as a positive force for social change, the prevailing climate holds that government is inefficient and that markets can better meet the desires of individual consumers. This orientation, coupled with cyclic forecasts of trust fund insolvency, has led some policy makers to assert that the Medicare program requires radical restructuring if it is to survive in the new century. Supporters of the role of government, on the other hand, argue that continued innovation in payment systems, improvement in chronic disease management, taking advantage of the federal government's purchasing power, and other incremental steps can both reform Medicare and preserve its function as a social insurance program.

## Expanding Benefits

By the turn of the century, there was bipartisan agreement that the Medicare benefits package should be updated to reflect changes in the needs of the elderly and in the practice of medicine. Yet past experience shows how difficult it is to devise a benefit that is not prohibitively expensive and is perceived by beneficiaries as meeting their needs. In June 1988, Congress passed the Medicare Catastrophic Coverage Act (MCCA); by November 1989 it was repealed. The MCCA expanded Part A benefits (reducing the beneficiary liability for hospital co-payments, increasing the SNF benefit, and expanding home health and hospice benefits), capped out-of-pocket expenses for Part B, and provided drug benefits (subject to a deductible and coinsurance).[42] Unlike existing Medicare benefits, however, it was designed to be budget-neutral for the federal government. Rather than increase the Social Security payroll tax, the MCCA was to be financed entirely by beneficiary premiums. Further departing from prior Medicare policies, the premium schedule was progressive, based on adjusted gross income. Following the principles of social insurance, the catastrophic coverage was compulsory, designed to afford the most protection for those with the greatest medical expenses and the lowest income.

The lobbying efforts to repeal this legislation stemmed from a number of factors, including its complexity and the resulting difficulty in communicating its benefits, pharmaceutical industry opposition, and lack of consumer understanding of the purpose and value of catastrophic coverage. Opposition was strong among the affluent elderly; they were satisfied with existing private Medigap policies and were least likely to need the protections of the new legislation.[43] At its founding in 1965, Medicare was established as a universal program. With the repeal of the MCCA, the public rejected a means-tested approach to expanding Medicare in which well-off beneficiaries would finance benefits for the vulnerable. This experience contained lessons for policy makers that applied to further expansion of Medicare benefits, including prescription drug coverage.

Beginning in 1999, rising awareness of the financial burden of drug costs on the elderly led to bipartisan support for a Medicare prescription drug benefit. The availability of prescription drug coverage was the reason many beneficiaries initially had enrolled in Medicare+Choice plans.[44] However, this coverage was not available to all enrollees, and its comprehensiveness eroded in the late 1990s as managed care plans experienced difficulty sustaining profitability in this line of business.

In 2003, 69 percent of enrollees in Medicare+Choice plans had prescription drug coverage.[45] That same year, 21 percent of Medicare+Choice plans limited drug coverage to $500 or less and 64 percent to $1,000 or less. In addition, co-payments for generic drugs typically were $10 or less, but for brand-name drugs about three-quarters of enrollees paid $20 or more per prescription.[46] The proportion of employers furnishing retiree coverage for Medigap or Medicare+Choice premiums also has declined. Large employers (those with more than one thousand employees) are the most likely to offer retiree benefits, but the proportion doing so dropped from 66 percent in 1988 to 38 percent in 2003.[47] Individual Medigap plans that include prescription drug coverage are beyond the financial reach of most beneficiaries. As a result, in 2000 almost half of Medicare beneficiaries lacked drug coverage for some or all of the year.[48]

## Medicare Part D—Prescription Drug Benefit

The Medicare Prescription Drug, Improvement, and Modernization Act (MMA) was signed into law in 2003. Although it included a number of provisions, the key component was an outpatient prescription drug benefit, beginning in January 2006. Along with lack of long-term care coverage, most observers viewed this as the program's major coverage gap—one that had become especially conspicuous with the recent surge in drug spending among seniors. As we have noted, a previous Medicare prescription drug benefit was enacted in 1988 but repealed the next year before being implemented.[49]

The prescription drug benefit, although ultimately approved by Congress, followed a most contentious debate. In general, Republican supporters favored a benefit that would be administered through the private insurance system on the basis of market forces, whereas Democratic detractors called for a government-administered benefit based on the federal government negotiating drug prices. Under the legislation that was approved, those beneficiaries wishing drug coverage obtain it either through a Medicare managed care plan (previously Medicare+Choice, now renamed Medicare Advantage) or through a stand-alone prescription drug plan. Interestingly, the latter had not been marketed previously, largely because insurers were concerned about adverse selection into such a product. The drug benefit is voluntary, like Part B coverage, but it differs in that one must explicitly choose to purchase the benefit rather than the benefit being the default. Dual-eligible beneficiaries who received drug coverage from state Medicaid programs are automatically eligible for, and enrolled in, a prescription drug plan.

The legislation is perhaps most noted for its unusual benefit structure including what has been dubbed the "doughnut hole." After paying a monthly premium estimated to be about $32 per month, the benefit looks like this (with the doughnut analogy in parentheses):

- A $250 annual deductible before the benefit kicks in (the person has not begun to eat the doughnut)
- 75 percent insurance coverage for the next $2,000 per year in covered prescription drug benefits (the part of the doughnut before the hole is consumed)
- A $2,850 gap in coverage; that is, no coverage for annual prescription drug spending between $2,250 and $5,100 per year (the doughnut hole)
- 95 percent coverage for annual spending in excess of $5,100 (the part of the doughnut after the hole is consumed)

This benefit may be unlike any other in the annals of insurance, so an explanation is order. Because drug costs are so high, and because Congress did not want to spend more than $400 billion over the first ten years of the benefit (although current cost estimates turn out to be much higher), it needed a way to contain costs but at the same time ensure that most enrollees would enjoy some of the benefits. The solution was to have a low deductible so that most would see some of the benefits in the second bullet point above. However, it was too expensive to provide that level of coverage for all spending over the deductible; hence the doughnut hole. Near-full coverage then recommences once annual expenses reach the truly catastrophic level of $5,100 annually; this will benefit an estimated 10 percent of enrollees.[50]

Health plans and insurers selling the benefit must conform to certain rules, including provision of a minimum of two or more drugs in a particular therapeutic class. They are allowed to establish formularies of covered drugs and use their purchasing power to negotiate lower prices with drug manufacturers. Government is not allowed to negotiate prices, in sharp contrast to other programs such as the Veterans Administration and Medicaid. In addition, in order to try to ensure that a cross-section of seniors (rather than a group of predominantly sicker ones) sign up for the benefit, those who do not enroll during an open enrollment period will face a 1 percent increase in premiums every month they wait.

A final key provision concerns subsidies for low-income beneficiaries. Individuals who have income below 150 percent of the federal poverty level and who meet certain asset restrictions will receive substantial discounts with respect to both premiums and cost-sharing requirements. For example, a person dually eligible for Medicare and Medicaid with income below 100 percent of the poverty level would pay no premiums, and just $1 per prescription for generic drugs and $3 per prescription for brand-name drugs.

At the time of writing, the drug benefit has been in effect only two months, so many questions remain:

- How popular will the benefit be with program beneficiaries? Will they enroll in droves, as with Part B, or will many think that the benefit is too skimpy to justify the premiums? (In fact, the average beneficiary would benefit in the long run, as the benefit is subsidized by about 75 percent.) So far, enrollment is much lower than projected by the government.
- Will the large number of plans offering coverage be confusing overall to Medicare beneficiaries, and if so, will that keep enrollment down? In Los Angeles County, in 2006 there were eighty-five choices of drug plans available: thirty-eight Medicare Advantage plan choices offered by eighteen companies and forty-seven stand-alone prescription drug plans offered by another eighteen companies. This is not just an urban phenomenon. In Arkansas, beneficiaries had to choose among forty prescription drug plans offered by fifteen companies.
- Will there be adverse selection into the program? How will the late-enrollment penalty (should it not be extended or repealed) affect who signs up?
- Will market forces be successful in keeping drug prices down? How will these prices compare to those secured by large government buyers, such as the Veterans Administration?
- Will employers continue to provide retiree drug benefits in the wake of the Medicare benefit? (The legislation includes subsidies that are intended to induce them to retain previous coverage.)
- Will there be any political fallout when many beneficiaries find themselves in the doughnut hole and receive no reimbursements for their drug purchases? It has been estimated that 6.9 million beneficiaries will have drug expenses that fall into the doughnut hole in the first year of the program's operation.[51]

## Privatizing Medicare Premium Support

Under the MMA of 2003, Congress took several significant steps to further privatize the Medicare program, both by relying on the private market for the prescription drug benefit and by enhancing payment rates to health plans under Medicare Advantage to encourage beneficiaries to enroll in Medicare managed health plans. In addition, the MMA also includes provisions for a demonstration project beginning in 2010 to establish payments to health plans based on competitive bidding. This competitive bidding approach is built on the "premium support" proposal for Medicare reform proposed in 1995.[52]

Traditional fee-for-service Medicare is a defined benefits program, in which all beneficiaries are guaranteed a defined set of benefits regardless of ability to pay or health status. As health care costs rise and the beneficiary population increases, this system creates an open-ended financial obligation for the federal government. Policy makers who seek to limit this obligation have proposed replacing the current program with a defined contribution or voucher approach. In its purest form, defined contribution would limit the obligation of the federal government by giving beneficiaries a fixed dollar amount with which they would purchase their own health insurance in the private market. The amount of the government contribution would be adjusted for inflation using a standard economic indicator such as the Consumer Price Index (CPI) or the GDP. Thus federal Medicare expenditures would be fixed at a targeted level, equal to the government's contribution multiplied by the number of eligible beneficiaries, and beneficiaries would pay any difference between the cost of the plan they chose and the federal contribution. If health care costs continue their historical pattern of rising faster than GDP, the financial risk for these increased costs would be shifted to beneficiaries.

Noting that a strict voucher approach would not be viable either politically or programmatically, economists Henry Aaron and Robert Reischauer proposed a version of the defined contribution approach termed premium support.[53] There are two crucial assumptions underlying this approach: private sector competition is the best means to restrain the rate of cost increases in the Medicare program; and the federal government's financial obligation should be limited in order to impose fiscal discipline on the program and avoid the need for future tax increases to support Medicare.

Under the premium support system, the federal government and beneficiaries would share the risk of rising health care costs. The federal contribution would not be tied to an external economic indicator but would instead be based on bids submitted by private sector health plans seeking to participate in the Medicare program. The traditional Medicare program would be retained, but it would be required to compete with private health plans.

In theory, premium support would offer beneficiaries greater choice, enabling them to select the health plan that best met their needs. Because they would pay the difference between the premium support contribution and the cost of their chosen plan, beneficiaries would have a financial incentive to choose a plan that offered the best value in terms of cost and quality. The beneficiary's required contribution would replace the current Part B premium as well as eliminate the need for Medigap coverage under the traditional program.

As was mentioned, Congress has authorized a demonstration project of premium support in up to six metropolitan areas (to be determined) starting in 2010. This demonstration is certainly a major step toward ultimate privatization of

Medicare, but the potential savings that might accrue through true competition among plans could be more than offset by the increased costs of furnishing incentives (that is, sufficiently high payment rates) to ensure adequate participation by health plans in the six market areas. There also is ongoing, strong opposition to this provision of the MMA among Congressional Democrats.

## Conclusion

Medicare was implemented in 1965 as an incremental step toward national health insurance in the United States. Forty years later, it survives as the country's second largest social insurance program and is likely to continue well into the twenty-first century as a separate program. The fundamental challenges facing the future of Medicare are how to finance the projected growth in enrollment and the increased costs of technology, and whether ongoing efforts to privatize the program will stabilize it financially.

When Medicare was enacted, a founding principle was that it was supposed to reflect mainstream medicine and health insurance, including mainstream delivery and payment methodologies. One obvious question regarding the future of Medicare is whether various reform proposals are consistent with this original principle. Despite the substantial movement during the past two decades toward defined contributions for pension benefits in the private sector, defined contribution plans for health benefits are still not common, although recent developments to encourage Health Savings Accounts may fundamentally change the nature of employment-based coverage during the next decade. Before beginning a grand experiment with the future of Medicare, however, perhaps policy makers should wait until the private market fully embraces consumer-directed health plans.

In the meantime, incremental efforts to expand benefits and offer additional subsidies to low-income beneficiaries are likely to reduce existing disparities within the program and improve the health and financial stability of those who are most vulnerable. Congress may also need to revisit the MMA of 2003 to address its costs, which are already projected to far exceed the original estimates of about $400 billion over its first ten years, as well as other aspects of the legislation, which shortly after implementation appeared to be both poorly understood and problematic.

## Notes

1. This section draws heavily on Marmor, T. R. *The Politics of Medicare* (2nd ed.). New York: Aldine De Gruyter, 2000; and to a lesser extent on Hirshfield, D. S. *The Lost Reform: The*

*Campaign for Compulsory Health Insurance in the United States from 1932 to 1943*. Cambridge, Mass.: Harvard University Press, and Commonwealth Fund, 1970.

 2. Dionne, E. J. "Medicare's Social Contract: Social Insurance Commentary." In R. D. Reischauer, S. Butler, and J. R. Lave (eds.), *Medicare: Preparing for the Challenges of the 21st Century*. Washington, D.C.: National Academy of Social Insurance, 1998.

 3. Ball, R. M. "Medicare's Social Contract: Reflections on How Medicare Came About." In Reischauer, Butler, and Lave (1998).

 4. Fishbein, M. "The Committee on the Costs of Medical Care." *Journal of the American Medical Association*, 1932, *99*, 1950–1952.

 5. Marmor (2000).

 6. Marmor (2000).

 7. Ball (1998), p. 31.

 8. An episode of care starts with an inpatient admission and ends sixty days after discharge from a hospital or skilled-nursing facility. Thus beneficiaries can have multiple episodes per year.

 9. Lifetime reserve days are a pool that can be used if a beneficiary has an inpatient episode exceeding ninety days. Lifetime reserve days cannot be replaced once used.

10. For 2006, the Part A deductible for inpatient hospital care was $952 per episode and coinsurance was $238 per day for the sixty-first through ninetieth days. Skilled-nursing facility coinsurance was $119 per day for the twenty-first through the hundredth days. The Part B premium was $88.50 per month, and the deductible was $123 per year. See Centers for Medicare and Medicaid Services, "Medicare Premiums and Deductibles for 2006." Sept. 16, 2005 [http://www.cms.hhs.gov/apps/media/press/release.asp?Counter=1557].

11. Health Care Financing Administration, Office of the Actuary. "National Health Expenditures, Aggregate, Per Capita, Percent Distribution, and Annual Percent Change by Source of Funds: Calendar Years 1960–98." n.d. [http://www.hcfa.gov/stats/nhe-oact].

12. Health Care Financing Administration.

13. Moon, M. *Medicare Now and in the Future*. Washington, D.C.: Urban Institute Press, 1996.

14. Carter, G. M., Jacobson, P. D., Kominski, G. F., and Perry, M. J. "Use of Diagnosis-Related Groups by Non-Medicare Payers." *Health Care Financing Review*, 1994, *16*, 127–158.

15. Pear, R. "'98 Medicare Growth Slowest Since Program Began in '65." *New York Times*, Jan. 12, 1999, p. A1.

16. Pear, R. "With Budget Cutting, Medicare Spending Fell Unexpectedly." *New York Times*, May 4, 1999, pp. A20, A24.

17. Kaiser Family Foundation. "Medicare Chartbook 2005" (3rd ed.). [http://www.kff.org/medicare/upload/Medicare-Chart-Book-3rd-Edition-Summer-2005-Report.pdf].

18. U.S. Census Bureau, Population Division. "National Population Projections." [http://www.census.gov/population/www/projections/natsum.html].

19. For further discussion of this topic, see Friedland, R. B., and Summer, L. *Demography Is Not Destiny, Revisited*. Washington, D.C.: Georgetown University Center on an Aging Society, Mar. 2004.

20. Schmidley, A. D., and Robinson, J.G.*U.S. Census Bureau, Measuring the Foreign-Born Population in the United States with the Current Population Survey: 1994–2002*. (Working Paper no. 73.) Washington, D.C.: U.S. Census Bureau Population Division, Oct. 2003. [http://www.census.gov/population/documentation/twps0073/twps0073.pdf].

21. U.S. Census Bureau. *Fertility of American Women, June 2004*. Washington, D.C.: Current Population Reports, P20–555, Dec. 2005. [http://www.census.gov/prod/2005pubs/p20–555.pdf].

22. "2005 Annual Report of the Board of Trustees of the Federal Old-Age and Survivors Insurance and Disability Insurance Trust Funds." Table V.A.2. Washington, D.C.: U.S. Government Printing Office, Apr. 5, 2005 [http://www.ssa.gov/OACT/TR/TR05/tr05.pdf].

23. See Ikegami, N., and Campbell, J. C. "Japan's Health Care System: Containing Costs and Attempting Reform." *Health Affairs*, May–June 2004, *23*, 26–36; Reinhardt, U., Hussey, P., and Anderson, G. "U.S. Health Care Spending in an International Context." *Health Affairs*, May-June 2004, *23*, 10–25.

24. Fuchs, V. "Health Care for the Elderly: How Much? Who Will Pay for It?" *Health Affairs*, Jan.–Feb. 1999, *18*, 11–21.

25. "2005 Annual Report of the Board of Trustees of the Federal Hospital Insurance and Federal Supplementary Health Insurance Trust Funds." [http://www.cms.hhs.gov/Reports TrustFunds/downloads/tr2005.pdf].

26. See Fuchs (1999); and Moon (1996).

27. Wolfe, J. R. *The Coming Health Crisis: Who Will Pay for Care for the Aged in the Twenty-First Century?* Chicago: University of Chicago Press, 1993.

28. White (1999).

29. Wolfe (1993).

30. Moon (1996).

31. "1999 Annual Report of the Board of Trustees of the Federal Hospital Insurance and Supplementary Medical Insurance Trust Funds." Mar. 30, 1999. [http://www.hcfa.gov/ pubforms/ tr/hi1999/HI2.htm].

32. "2005 Annual Report of the Boards of Trustees of the Federal Hospital Insurance and Federal Supplementary Medical Insurance Trust Funds" (2005).

33. Marmor (2000).

34. Kaiser Family Foundation. *Medicare Chart Book, 2005*. Washington, D.C.: Kaiser Family Foundation, 2005.

35. Kaiser Family Foundation (2005).

36. National Center for Health Statistics. *Health, U.S., 2005*. Table 122. Hyattsville, Md.: National Center for Health Statistics.

37. Laschober, M. "Trends in Medicare Supplemental Insurance and Prescription Drug Benefits, 1996–2001." Washington, D.C.: Kaiser Family Foundation, June 2004.

38. Safran, D. G., Neuman, P., Schoen, C., and others. "Prescription Drug Coverage and Seniors: Findings from a 2003 National Survey." *Health Affairs*, Web exclusive, 2005, W5-152-W5-166.

39. Dalaker, J. *Current Population Reports. Poverty in the United States: 1998*. Table B-2. (U.S. Census Bureau, Series P60-207.) Washington, D.C.: U.S. Government Printing Office, 1999. [http:// www.census.gov/prod/99pubs/p60-207.pdf]; U.S. Census Bureau. *Statistical Abstract of the United States, 2006*. Table 696. Washington, D.C.: U.S. Census Bureau, 2006.

40. Maxwell, S., Moon, M., and Segal, M. *Growth in Medicare and Out-of-Pocket Spending: Impact on Vulnerable Beneficiaries*. (no. 430.) New York: Commonwealth Fund, 2001.

41. Kaiser Family Foundation. *Medicare Advantage Fact Sheet*. Menlo Park, Calif.: Kaiser Family Foundation, Apr. 2005.

42. Moon (1996).

43. Moon (1996).

44. Schoen, C., and others. *Medicare Beneficiaries: A Population at Risk*. New York: Commonwealth Fund, 1998 [http://www.cmwf.org/programs/medfutur/medicare_survey97_308.asp].

45. Gold, M., Achman, L., Mittler, J., and Stevens, B. *Monitoring Medicare+Choice: What Have We Learned? Findings and Operational Lessons for Medicare Advantage.* Washington, D.C.: Mathematica Policy Research, Aug. 2004.

46. Gold, Achman, Mittler, and Stevens (2004).

47. McArdle F. N., and others. "Large Firms' Retiree Health Benefits Before Medicare Reform: 2003 Survey Results." *Health Affairs,* Web exclusive, January 14, 2004, W4-7–W4-19 [http://content.healthaffairs.org/cgi/content/full/hlthaff.w4.7v1/DC1].

48. Families USA. *Cost Overdose: Growth in Drug Spending for the Elderly, 1992-2010.* Washington, D.C.: Families USA, Publication 00-107, July 2000.

49. The passage and then almost immediate repeal of the Medicare Catastrophic Coverage Act of 1988 represented a major shock to supporters of program reform. It is therefore not surprising that a full fifteen years passed before another major reform bill, the MMA, was able to attain sufficient support. Perhaps the major reason for repeal was that the bill's entire cost was borne by Medicare beneficiaries, much of it through a supplemental income tax payment on seniors with higher income. Because many of these beneficiaries already had subsidized prescription drug coverage through a former employer, they tended to view the legislation as providing little in the way of new benefits but at a substantial cost. See Rice, T., Desmond, K., and Gabel, J. "The Medicare Catastrophic Coverage Act: A Postmortem." *Health Affairs,* 1990, *9,* 75–87.

50. Mays, J., and others. *Estimates of Medicare Beneficiaries' Out-of-Pocket Drug Spending in 2006: Modeling the Impact of the MMA.* Washington, D.C.: Kaiser Family Foundation, Nov. 2004.

51. Kaiser Family Foundation. *Estimates of Medicare Beneficiaries' Drug Spending in 2006: Modeling the Impact of the MMA.* (Executive summary.) Nov. 2004 [http://www.kff.org/medicare/upload/Executive-Summary-Estimates-of-Medicare-Beneficiaries-Out-Of-Pocket-Drug-Spending-in-2006-Modeling-the-Impact-of-the-MMA.pdf].

52. Aaron, H. J., and Reischauer, R. D. "The Medicare Reform Debate: What Is the Next Step?" *Health Affairs,* 1995, *14,* 8–30.

53. Aaron and Reischauer (1995).

CHAPTER TWENTY-ONE

# PUBLIC HEALTH AND PERSONAL HEALTH SERVICES

Lester Breslow
Jonathan E. Fielding

In our current effort to reform the organization, delivery, and financing of personal health services (that is, medical care), the broad question of how these services contribute to the public health goals for our country receives little consideration. Much discussion about personal health services has focused on how to control the enormous and escalating costs of medical, physician, pharmaceutical, hospital, and other services; and how to overcome the access barriers that arise from lack of health insurance and other challenges to obtaining needed care, including ethnic discrimination, poor distribution of providers, and other problems. More recently, considerable discussion has also focused on issues of patient safety and quality of care. In deciding how these medical care system problems should be addressed, the appropriate role of public health agencies is the subject of this chapter.

Neglect of this issue probably derives from the common view that public health is concerned only with disease control by such measures as epidemiological investigation, immunization, health education, and attention to health hazards in the physical environment. Another common public misperception is that if public health agencies have any role in delivery of medical care delivery, it should be providing or financing care for the economically disadvantaged segment of the population, as the safety net.

## Public Health's Mission and Scope

A perspective on appropriate roles for public health derives from public health's mission. According to the Institute of Medicine, National Academy of Sciences, the mission is "fulfilling society's interest in assuring conditions in which people can be healthy."[1] Public health thus concerns itself with the health of the entire population and how it may be enhanced by improving the health-related conditions in which people live. It includes all the ways in which a society organizes to protect and advance the health of its members: through governmental agencies, voluntary associations, professional societies, and community groups devoted to health.

Public health efforts aim at improving three conditions that can contribute to population health: the physical environment; the social environment, including its effect on behavior; and the system of delivery of personal health care services. The physical environment, all those physical aspects of people's surroundings, profoundly affects their health. The well-known impact of working conditions, water safety, and food handling—among myriad other living circumstances—illustrates the point. Therefore modern public health has directed substantial effort toward ensuring a healthful physical environment, at first mainly focusing on ways to reduce microbial threats to health but increasingly aiming more broadly at the whole physical milieu. Historically, physical environmental control measures have been public health's most fundamental way of carrying out its mission because, once in place and maintained, they do not require specific behaviors on the part of individuals to protect their health from that source. A good example is ensuring a safe water supply.

With the twentieth-century transition from communicable to noncommunicable diseases as the predominant group of health problems, evidence has grown that people's behavior (for example, with respect to tobacco and alcohol) has a strong and often definitive influence on the disease mechanisms that cause death, disability, and the timing of disease development. In analyzing the underlying causes of death rather than the disease mechanisms involved, McGinnis and Foege found that almost two-fifths are attributable to tobacco, diet or activity patterns, and alcohol (Table 21.1).[2]

The behavior of both individuals and groups is shaped by the broader social environment, including such factors as the media, strength of family and other social relationships, sense of shared responsibility for the quality of life in the community, and beliefs. Thus the social environment strongly influences patterns of health and ill health in the population overall and in subgroups defined by gender, age, race, ethnicity, and other factors.[3]

## TABLE 21.1. ACTUAL CAUSES OF
## DEATH IN THE UNITED STATES, 1990.

| Cause | Estimates of Total Deaths | |
|---|---|---|
| | Number | Percentage |
| Tobacco | 400,000 | 19 |
| Diet and activity patterns | 300,000 | 14 |
| Alcohol | 100,000 | 5 |
| Toxic agents | 60,000 | 3 |
| Firearms | 35,000 | 2 |
| Sexual behavior | 30,000 | 1 |
| Motor vehicles | 25,000 | 1 |
| Illicit use of drugs | 20,000 | 1 |
| Total | 970,000 | 46 |

*Source:* McGinnis, J. M., and Foege, W. H. "Actual Causes of Death in the United States." *Journal of the American Medical Association,* 1993, *270,* 2207–2212.

The third major influence on the health of the population is the availability and quality of personal health services (medical care). Extensive achievements in this field during recent decades—in biochemistry, pharmacology, noninvasive testing procedures, surgical techniques, and other areas—have increased the possibility of longer and healthier lives. The often dramatized impact of these innovations on the health of an individual or small group of individuals, however, creates a tendency for society to overestimate their overall health significance. Bunker attributes only five years of the thirty-year increase in life expectancy of Americans during the twentieth century to the work of the medical care system.[4]

Public health has generally operated inconspicuously, identifying and implementing means to improve all three conditions that can advance health. Credit is rarely given for what has been accomplished through public health initiatives, in part because their success is often measured by health problems that do not occur, or whose impact is mitigated but not eliminated. Hence we take for granted that pasteurized milk is safe to drink, and that individuals with tuberculosis are identified quickly and appropriately treated so they are not a threat to the public.

There are, then, a number of reasons for public health involvement in personal health services:

1. Personal health services are increasingly effective as a means of improving a population's health, and thereby a legitimate concern of public health.

2. A substantial proportion of the population in the United States either does not have financial access to a minimum set of health care services or may lose access with change in government programs or in living circumstances such as a job move or job loss.

3. A considerable portion of the personal health services currently delivered suffer from deficiency in quality, often adversely affecting health outcomes.

4. The recent spiral in medical care costs has absorbed a disproportionate share of social resources, limiting investment to improve access to health care services as a whole, and preventing investment in other sectors (transportation, social services, housing, environmental protection, and so forth) that could potentially yield higher dividends in health at the population level.

Examination of public health's role in personal health services is therefore timely and important. Public health represents society's interest, but how should society's interests be advanced? What are the leverage points to effect change?

## Prevention in Personal Health Services

Because public health's hallmark is prevention, it has traditionally emphasized this aspect of personal health services. Historically, the medical care system has operated mainly in a complaint-response mode; people with a complaint of being sick seek a physician (or other health care provider), who responds with diagnosis and therapy. The public health pattern is different; it focuses on the entire population, with or without symptoms of being sick, and aims at maintaining health and preventing disease.

Prevention in personal health service is often divided into three categories: primary, secondary, and tertiary.

Primary prevention consists of preventing disease onset through efforts to maximize positive and minimize negative health effects of the physical and social environments, as well as to advance the application of specific preventive medical measures of proven effectiveness. Public health seeks to control air pollution as an environmental source of disease and to diminish excessive consumption of fatty foods, a behavior that can lead to cardiovascular and other diseases.

Medical care can, and increasingly does, incorporate substantial primary prevention services. Perhaps the most obvious is immunization. Vaccination against the communicable diseases of childhood, and especially recently those of adults as well such as against influenza and pneumonia, has vastly curtailed the burden for these diseases. Public health works with the medical care system, including provision of some direct public health services, to ensure protection of people against communicable diseases that can be avoided by immunization.

Because certain behavioral practices have been clearly identified as causing disease (lack of exercise, excessive alcohol consumption, and so on), public health seeks to minimize these behavior patterns. One way has been to seek incorporation of advice on such matters into a medical practice. Two problems, however, have deterred physicians from using their opportunity to help patients adopt healthful behaviors. One is the common belief among physicians that their efforts in this regard do not yield much benefit; the second is the failure of the physician payment system to compensate physicians adequately for the time involved in providing the service. Further, the benefit of physician advice on behavioral issues has not been shown for some key behaviors. However, there is good evidence indicating that physician advice for smoking cessation can have a useful effect.[5]

Secondary prevention consists of detecting and treating disease or its clear precursors at a time when an intervention to reduce the risk level can be most effective. Cervix cancer in situ is almost universally curable. Hypertension, although asymptomatic, greatly increases the risk for stroke and other cardiovascular disease if not effectively treated. Public health has therefore advocated screening to find health risk factors and disease itself as promptly after onset as possible, before adverse health effects have advanced. The number of tests to detect important risk factors or early stages of treatable conditions has expanded in the recent past. The *Guide to Clinical Preventive Services* has codified the evidence for them and makes evidence-based recommendations for clinical practice, and many medical groups and health care payers subscribe to these recommendations, in whole or in part.[6]

Managing disease that has already occurred so as to minimize the likelihood of its progressing to further damage, disability, and other possible adverse consequences, or to mortality, is sometimes called tertiary prevention. Many companies that now sell health insurance, so-called health plans, offer encouragement and assistance by specialized personnel (deemed coaches or care coordinators) to patients with chronic diseases, because they have discovered that such coaching lowers the cost of providing services to their beneficiaries and improves health outcomes.[7] This is a fast-growing aspect of the medical service system in the United States.

Probably the most rapidly increasing feature of prevention in personal health service has been inaugurated by the many major companies in the United States who have established work-site health promotion and disease prevention programs.[8] External vendors often provide these services, but some companies use their own staff. The rationale for broad adoption of these company-sponsored programs is to reduce the cost of medical services and the cost of absenteeism.

Prevention in personal health services may be considered in individual clinical situations and in community endeavors. The former involve physicians and other health care professionals in their practice with their particular patients. Increasingly, however, various disease prevention services are being offered to groups outside of the main medical care setting. For example, campaigns are undertaken to screen those at high risk for HIV with the intent of finding people with early stages of the condition and, with follow-up treatment to them, reducing the progression to AIDS. Other population-oriented programs may target schools, worksites, religious organizations, or entire communities.

Preventive personal health services have been effective in reducing some disease burdens. Probably the most obvious is seen in advances against immunizable diseases, of which smallpox eradication is the most notable example. Table 21.2, however, reveals the great success in recent decades against the acute communicable diseases that were formerly so prominent—in large part accomplished through immunization programs. Progress has occurred with respect to diphtheria, influenza, and other conditions, but much remains to be done with immunization. In addition to notable achievements in children's health, the former major chronic communicable diseases of adult life, syphilis and tuberculosis, have also declined substantially as a result of active case finding by public health agencies and medical treatment. The resurgence of tuberculosis during the late 1980s and early 1990s, however, underscores the importance of maintaining surveillance of diseases that have declined in frequency.

Less widely recognized, chronic noncommunicable disease death rates have likewise been yielding to control efforts. Table 21.3 indicates that heart disease mortality dropped by more than 40 percent during the last half of the twentieth century, and cerebrovascular disease even more sharply. Cancer mortality, though increasing until about 1990, has now declined to approximately the rate prevailing in 1970. These advances probably reflect the combined influence of both more effective personal health services and the broader public health activities.

### TABLE 21.2. DECLINE OF SELECTED ACUTE COMMUNICABLE DISEASE CASES, UNITED STATES, 1920–2000.

| Year | Smallpox | Diphtheria | Poliomyelitis | Measles |
|------|----------|------------|---------------|---------|
| 1920 | 102,128 | 147,991 | 2,338 | 469,924 |
| 1940 | 2,795 | 15,536 | 9,804 | 291,102 |
| 1960 | 0 | 918 | 3,190 | 442,000 |
| 1980 | 0 | 3 | 9 | 13,506 |
| 2000 | 0 | 1 | 0 | 176 |

*Source:* U.S. Department of Health Education and Welfare. For 1920 registration area only. Cited in D. Mechanic (ed.), *Handbook of Health, Health Care, and the Health Professions.* New York: Macmillan, 1983. National Center for Health Statistics, *Health, United States, 2003.* Hyattsville, Md.

### TABLE 21.3. DEATH RATES FROM MAJOR NONCOMMUNICABLE DISEASES, UNITED STATES, 1950–2000, SELECTED YEARS.

| Disease | Years | | | |
|---|---|---|---|---|
| | 1950 | 1970 | 1990 | 2000 |
| Heart disease | 587 | 493 | 322 | 258 |
| Cancer | 194 | 199 | 216 | 200 |
| Cardiovascular disease | 181 | 148 | 65 | 61 |

*Source:* U.S. Department of Health and Human Services. National Center for Health Statistics. Hyattsville, Md., 2003.

The latter include, first, epidemiological investigations that have disclosed the role of tobacco, obesity, increased fat consumption, excessive alcohol consumption, and increased sedentary lifestyles; and then initiation of educational and other efforts to control these factors.

Public health agencies have also been extensively involved with personal health services in seeking secondary prevention for cervix and breast cancer, and hypertensive heart disease among other conditions, through promotion and sometimes actual provision of screening for these and other noncommunicable diseases. Health departments, voluntary health agencies, and concerned physician groups have often collaborated in such endeavors.

Disease control accomplishments during the twentieth century have yielded substantively longer lives, from an average of forty-seven years in 1900 to seventy-seven years in 2000.[9] Not only are people surviving into their eighties and nineties; they are doing so with reasonably good health. In 2002, more than 90 percent of the American people assessed their health as excellent or good, not fair or poor; 78 percent of persons sixty-five to seventy-four years of age rated their health as excellent or good, as did 69 percent of those over seventy-five.[10] Thus, it is no longer appropriate to identify aging with infirmity, although the frequency of the latter does increase with age.

We are now entering what some have called a third era of health in the modern world, as distinguished from a first era when communicable diseases dominated the health scene, and a second era when chronic noncommunicable diseases prevailed.[11] We have by no means completely overcome these two sets of diseases (and never will!), but thinking about health must no longer be restricted to its opposite, that is, disease occurrence and how to deal with it. Now we can move onto considering health in the sense of the WHO Ottawa Charter definition: "a resource for everyday life."[12] People increasingly regard health as the capacity to do what they want to do in life: the fitness to climb a mountain, the cognition and memory to play bridge, the vision and hearing to enjoy an opera, or whatever. They seek health to permit them to live life as they want to, not merely to overcome diseases. Public health, including the assurance of personal health services, must now turn attention to this third era of health, to advance and maintain health in a positive sense.

## Public Health and Provision of Personal Health Services

As the principal governmental agencies for public health, local and sometimes state health departments have long administered certain personal health services directed toward health promotion and disease prevention. They have often provided prenatal care and childhood immunization services directly, particularly for those segments of the population that the private health care system seldom reaches effectively. In many locales the health department has served as planner, convener, and facilitator, helping to mobilize community resources to extend services to the economically disadvantaged. Also, in many states and communities public health departments have assumed responsibility for a broader array of personal health services for people with low income. For example, some local public health agencies carry responsibility for Medicaid and local indigent care programs.

These responsibilities are exercised in several forms. Some jurisdictions operate health plans for Medicaid eligibles and other low-income individuals, contracting with physicians, hospitals, and other providers and performing the other required functions of a managed care organization. Other jurisdictions have comprehensive personal health care delivery systems, including both inpatient and outpatient activities. In some jurisdictions the local health agency has been given statutory responsibility for health care for the indigent. The responsibility to furnish personal health care services to a substantial population without other access to medical care has become so burdensome in some jurisdictions, however, that it jeopardizes the conduct of other public-health-sponsored activities with a potentially greater impact on population health. This trend has therefore favored the tendency to separate public health departments from agencies concerned primarily with indigent medical care.

Historically, actual involvement in personal health services emerged initially as a critical aspect of public health's original task: communicable disease control. During the early part of the century, when the struggle against infectious diseases extended beyond environmental action to include developing personal immunity in individuals, health departments undertook mass smallpox vaccinations (and subsequently other immunizations). More substantial engagement in personal health services by public health agencies expanded into maternal and child health during the 1920s, as a result of the growing conviction that such services could reduce the excessively high maternal and infant death rates prevailing at that time. Then came certain diagnostic procedures, especially as technology for communicable disease control advanced. For example, tuberculin testing of tuberculosis patients' contacts and then x-raying positive reactors became an accepted public health practice. Further, health department laboratories offered communicable disease diagnostic services to physicians in their communities. Subsequently, these services expanded into other realms such as screening for diseases having congenital and environmental causes.

Advances in clinical science and corresponding improvements in medical care necessitate greater public health attention to them as means of improving health. Widespread recognition of their potential in protecting and enhancing health has led to establishing large-scale public programs of medical care for people identified as having unmet personal health service needs, thus filling substantial gaps in the mainstream delivery system. In other cases, this lack of availability of health care in a defined population has been met by making payment in the public welfare mode for personal health services that are provided to individuals meeting specific eligibility requirements for Medicaid and other targeted programs. In addition, the government may create financial incentives for private organizations to finance or provide care to populations unable to afford it. The awarding of tax-exempt status for nonprofit health care organizations, including voluntary private hospitals, was in part based on the assumption that these institutions would help meet the health needs of the poor through uncompensated care.

# Direct Medical Service Delivery by Government

Direct delivery of personal health services by government in the United States started with the U.S. Marine Hospital Service, which was established to offer care for merchant seamen in support of the nation's entry into international commerce, and to the country's early military medical services. These two agencies, for merchant seamen and military forces, have evolved into the current U.S. Public Health Service and the Armed Forces Medical System.

Over the years the federal government has assumed responsibility for directly supplying medical services to other substantial segments of the population. The Department of Veterans Affairs operates an array of medical centers, nursing units, domiciliary care units, and outpatient clinics for its beneficiaries, many of which are affiliated with academic medical centers, both to enhance the quality of care and to give training opportunities to young physicians.[13] The Indian Health Service operates (or funds the operation by Indian tribal government of) hospitals, health centers, and other types of ambulatory care unit on tribal lands throughout the country.[14]

State governments historically have provided hospital services, not for such specific segments of the population but rather for people suffering from particular conditions, such as mental illness and tuberculosis. Beds for these purposes have declined substantially over the last quarter century as tuberculosis cases fell and were also treated increasingly on an ambulatory basis, and as state hospitalization for mentally ill patients was curtailed with the notion that they would be better served in community centers. Unfortunately, the latter have not materialized to the extent needed.

Many county and city governments have offered both inpatient and outpatient general hospital services for the indigent, and emergency and some other medical services, often with financial support from state and federal sources. However, funding for these operations in recent years has usually been precarious, with financial crises common. Overall, indigent care, regardless of who provides it, tends to be uneven in extent and quality, reflecting the lack of nationally ensured services in the United States.

From 1975 to 2002, the total number of hospitals in the United States dropped 19 percent and the number of beds more than one-third; beds under federal governmental auspices fell by more than one-half, reducing the proportion from 10 to 5 percent of the total (Table 21.4). The proportion of beds operated by state and local governments remained quite steady, about one-seventh of the total. Meanwhile community nonprofit hospitals expanded their proportion of beds, now over one-half of the total; and community for-profit hospitals had doubled their share, from 5 to 11 percent. The former increase largely reflects services of community hospitals that were previously undertaken by specialized rather than general hospitals.

# Core Public Health Responsibilities

The public health care system delivers substantial amounts of medical care, particularly for the economically disadvantaged, the severely mentally ill, and the developmentally impaired. But this role is only one expression of the public health mission. Unfortunately, local fiscal authorities have often diverted what resources are appropriated for the traditional public health core functions focused on protecting and improving the health of all residents of their jurisdiction into personal health services for the poor. This reflects the strain of forty-four million Americans being without health insurance, a number that has every likelihood of con-

### TABLE 21.4. HOSPITALS, BEDS, AND
### OCCUPANCY RATES, ACCORDING TO TYPE OF
### HOSPITAL, UNITED STATES, SELECTED YEARS, 1975–2002.

|  | 1975 | 1990 | 2002 |
| --- | --- | --- | --- |
| Hospitals |  |  |  |
| Total | 6,257 | 5,721 | 5,167 |
| Federal | 382 | 337 | 240 |
| State and local government | 1,761 | 1,444 | 1,136 |
| Community, nonprofit | 3,339 | 3,191 | 3,025 |
| For-profit | 775 | 749 | 766 |
| Beds (000s) |  |  |  |
| Total | 1,073 | 1,025 | 870 |
| Federal | 132 | 98 | 50 |
| State and local government | 210 | 169 | 130 |
| Community, nonprofit | 658 | 657 | 582 |
| For-profit | 73 | 101 | 108 |
| Occupancy rate (percentage) |  |  |  |
| Total | 76.7 | 69.5 | 67.8 |
| Federal | 80.7 | 72.9 | 66.0 |
| State and local government | 70.4 | 65.3 | 64.9 |
| Community, nonprofit | 77.5 | 69.3 | 67.2 |
| For-profit | 65.9 | 52.8 | 59.0 |

*Note:* Excluded are long-term hospitals and hospital units in institutions such as prisons and college dormitories, facilities for the mentally retarded, and alcoholism and chemical dependency hospitals.

*Source:* National Center for Health Statistics. *Health, United States, 2004.* Hyattsville, Md.: National Center for Health Statistics, 2004.

tinued growth in the absence of a national policy that health care should be the right of every citizen, and in the wake of the failure of national health reform. However, the other consequence of reallocating money to what appears to be the most pressing priority (sick people without other access to urgently needed medical services) is that these funds are not available for community-oriented prevention activities. Consequently, public health can suffer a diminished ability to respond to serious public health threats such as the resurgence of tuberculosis, or the emergence of HIV/AIDS and new forms of influenza.

The growing perception that our nation had lost sight of its public health goals, allowing the public health infrastructure to fall into disarray, led to the previously cited Institute of Medicine recommendation that the public health mission be defined as "fulfilling society's interest in assuring conditions in which people can be healthy." On the basis of this mission, the report identified three principal core functions for public health: assessment, assurance, and policy development.

## Assessment

An indispensable role for a governmental public health agency is to assess the opportunities to improve the health of the population it serves. In so doing, the public health agency needs sophistication in assessing the contributions of the various determinants of health to the burden imposed on the population by ill health. An essential initial step is to collect (directly or through access to external databases) a health-and-disease profile of the population. Traditionally, assessments have targeted the major causes of morbidity, mortality, and more recently disability. In addition, health can be measured as a set of positive attributes based on the more recent definitions of health adopted by public health bodies nationally and internationally.

At the state and local levels, an ideal assessment would be to array the major causes of morbidity, disability, mortality, and lack of well-being for major segments of the population defined by age, gender, and geography, and also by race or ethnic identity. Traditionally, ill health has been arrayed according to disease (cancer, heart disease, arthritis, and so on). However, as McGinnis and Foege have proposed, a better way to consider health improvement opportunities might be to focus on the common factors that underlie many of the most burdensome health conditions (Table 21.1). These factors have in common that they can be considerably ameliorated through behavior change.

In analogous fashion, how might we judge the potential contribution of personal health services to health improvement in the overall population of a defined area and in population subgroups? The point of departure for such an exercise is to determine the proportion of the population variance in key health measures that is associated with health services. To take as a hypothetical example acquired heart disease, health services might be found to account for 10 percent of the variance in mortality and disability rates. The next step would be to determine, on the basis of the best evidence, the characteristics of health service systems and specific diagnostic and therapeutic modalities that are reproducibly associated with the best and worst outcomes.

To the degree possible, differences between the best and worst outcomes would be partitioned into problems of access to services, overuse and underuse of appropriate services, poor coordination of care, and poor technical quality of services. Developing databases that would permit this degree of problem definition remains at an early stage for most health conditions. However, a substantial investment in quality indicators, practice guidelines, and outcomes measurement should in time produce sufficient tools for public health departments to assume leadership in helping solve the problems in organizing and delivering personal health services on the part of both private and public providers.

A related role is to identify the characteristics of populations that are not receiving adequate care by virtue of diminished access, poor quality, or lack of financial resources. Traditionally, public health organizations have taken the lead in pointing out that there is a substantial segment of our population, including 8.3 million children, who do not have access to any organized source of continuing medical care or payment for such care.[15] They are largely dependent on so-called emergency services that state or local governments may provide or require other local institutions to provide. In addition, many millions work in precarious job situations where they are at risk of both job loss and loss of health insurance benefits offered by or through their employer.

Most striking, during the 1990s—a period of unprecedented economic growth in the United States—the number of uninsured continued to grow and the proportion of Americans covered by employer-related health benefits declined. Public health agencies should become the most trusted source for information on unmet service needs, the quality assurance practices used by providers, health outcomes, and the health status of subpopulations within their territory. They should also systematically assess the degree of integration of health services with other governmental and private sector services, such as education, social services, and welfare.

Tools have been developed to help public health agencies in the overall assessment and planning process. APEX (Assessment Protocol for Excellence in Public Health) and PATCH (Planned Approach to Community Health) are among these guides for assessing community health needs.[16] Many health departments are using *Healthy Communities 2000: Model Standards,* a guidebook to marrying the national objectives in Healthy People 2000 with local needs and priorities.[17]

## Assurance

The Institute of Medicine report stressed "assurance" that services necessary to achieve agreed-on goals are made available, whether by encouraging action on the part of other entities (private or public sector), or by requiring such action through regulation, or by supplying services directly. Public health agencies should involve key policy makers and the general public in determining a set of high-priority personal and communitywide health services that governments will guarantee to every member of the community. This guarantee should include subsidization or direct provision of necessary personal health services for those unable to afford them.[18]

Assurance of appropriate services for health is a central function of public health. In proposing plans to improve the health of its population, a department of public health should ensure that all groups have access to a minimum set of high-quality personal health care services. The plans should also set expectations for the performance of health care systems and health care providers.

Developing large managed care organizations with broad responsibility for the health care of defined, enrolled populations is a natural point of leverage in assuring the nation of adequate performance of the health care system. Large managed care organizations are developing clinical data systems that generate databases amenable to analysis of care outcomes and of the types of service furnished to individuals and groups defined by disease (for example, adult onset diabetes mellitus), age group (such as infants from zero to one year), income level, or geography. In addition, quality has become a basis for competition in the market for personal health services. Therefore health department leadership should include helping to define the kinds of outcome an organization should be able to show, according to best practices as recorded in the literature and ensuring dissemination of this information to consumers as well as health professionals in understandable form.

Health departments should have special expertise in setting expectations for outcomes in clinical preventive services (such as age-specific immunization rates and mammography rates by age) and in monitoring them. However, monitoring the results of services administered when a disease state is present is of equal importance. For this reason, public health agencies should also participate in setting expectations for disease and procedure outcomes, such as the mortality rate for cardiovascular disease, or frequency of complications for endoscopy or angioplasty. They may also suggest the specifications and dissemination plans for report cards that are increasingly required of health care providers, because these reports can identify problems with access and quality and yield helpful relevant information to those deciding among health plan or provider groups.

Currently, most health departments have no jurisdiction over the organizations delivering comprehensive care, except for licensing institutions and sometimes provider groups. In some areas, particularly large cities, the health department may also deliver clinical services; this presents a potential conflict of interest in setting standards or expectations for results. Nonetheless, there are existing levers that can be used to help ensure good outcomes in delivering personal health care services. The health department can help to establish a local coalition of private and public medical service purchasers that sets requirements for both the services to be provided and the service data that plans and providers must make available in a standard format. The health department can also champion the important quality assurance work of JCAHO (Joint Commission on Accreditation of Health Care Organizations) and of voluntary national and statewide groups focused on improving quality care. Additionally, the health department can take the lead in disseminating information on a required core of preventive services, such as those developed by the U.S. Preventive Services Task Force.[19] Further, the department can publicize the practice guidelines that are being developed through public and private processes, and it can urge consumers to ask questions about treatment outcomes, both in general and for specific conditions about which they are especially concerned, before selecting choices under an employer-sponsored health benefit plan.

Public health agencies should make it a central function to receive, analyze, and report on the results of quality assurance efforts in personal health services delivery. They can use their role as guardian of the public's health to publicize problems and progress alike to the public, as well as to inform providers and professional organizations about opportunities for improvement in both access and quality. Ensuring that the public has objective information on the performance of alternative health care purchasing organizations and physician groups is increasingly important as more employers adopt a passive purchaser role vis-à-vis health plans, giving employees a fixed amount of money and letting them choose among a number of locally available plans.

## Public Policy

A number of assurance functions are accomplished through participating in development of public policy. Some access data and quality-assessment requirements are being incorporated into laws or administrative regulations. Public health, as an agent of the public with the responsibility of "fulfilling society's interest in assuring conditions in which people can be healthy," should be proactive in suggesting where and what regulation is appropriate, and in commenting on proposals advanced by others.

An important public policy role is to underscore the large number of people uninsured for medical and hospital services and the continuing growth of this population. In addition to preventable deaths, lack of health insurance can lead to reduced productivity of workers, impacting both individual employers and our national competitiveness. Policy makers need to be shown that the uninsured population is much less likely to receive preventive care, seek care for serious symptoms, and have continuing sources of care. This results in failure to have problems diagnosed at an early and more treatable stage. They need to understand that making public medical services available directly to the uninsured is even more challenging as public systems are buffeted by competition from the private sector that is able to secure payment for services to specific subgroups under Medicaid and Medicare.

Identifying the opportunity to improve health outcomes through broader benefit coverage is part of a larger need to educate the public and policy makers on the key determinants of health, and on how policy options can affect these factors. In this context, almost all careful studies of determinants of health have found that personal health care services make a difference in health, but this difference accounts for a small fraction of the variance in health among populations and for most specific health conditions. Determinants with a generally larger total contribution to variance include income distribution, social factors, environmental exposure, and health behavior.

Among these items, health habits have received the most attention in recent years, but the other contributors to common diseases often display strong effects. For example, in cardiovascular disease the degree of social isolation presents risk gradients about equal in magnitude to behavioral risk factors. For most disease categories, and certainly for quality of well-being, poverty is a quantitatively more important risk factor than access to health care services or the quality of those services. In addition, economic, community, social, and political factors are the primary contributors to such major societal problems of ill health as child abuse, spousal abuse, other violence, and poor birth outcomes.

As part of this educational effort, public health departments can generate data showing that the current level of investment in medical services is disproportionate to the ability of those services to diminish the population burden of ill health. Whether the argument is for additional resources or for reallocation of existing resources to address other causal factors, the rhetoric is not likely to strike a responsive chord unless the health department can make a convincing case for what type of investment is likely to achieve greater societal returns. For example, would after-school programs for youth in areas of high risk of school dropout and gang membership be a better investment than a higher density of MRI machines, or increasing the Medicare payment for erythropoietin? Would a prenatal and postnatal home visiting program for lower-income pregnant women yield a better health return than routinely offering amniocentesis as a covered medical service benefit? Would a social marketing campaign to encourage youths to drink nonalcoholic beverages have more impact on alcoholism than more or better rehabilitation facilities?

Although there are not unequivocal answers to most of these questions, showing the effects of well-evaluated model programs is a useful initial step in this educational process.

## Expertise and Capacity

What is the interest and capacity of public health agencies at the state and local levels to assume the set of responsibilities we have outlined? The Institute of Medicine report and strong efforts by the CDC, the American Public Health Association, and national and local health officer associations to define core public health functions have raised consciousness of the role public health should play in health promotion at the community level. Barriers to assuming these important roles include restricted flexibility in use of funds (which are often channeled from categorical programs), mismatch of skills and interests between existing personnel and new priorities, and some outsiders' perception that a more limited role for public health agencies is advisable. For example, a survey of thirty-two health departments and districts in Washington State found that the self-assessed strengths of most were program management and direct provision of service. They felt that the major deficiencies were assessment functions and use of data to guide community and program planning and policy.

If public health is to ensure the health of populations, then establishing its expertise and credibility as the pathfinding organizer and lead planner in achieving this area of goals must be accorded a high priority.

## Notes

1. Institute of Medicine. *The Future of Public Health*. Washington, D.C.: National Academy Press, 1988.
2. McGinnis, J. M., and Foege, W. H. "Actual Cases of Death in the United States." *Journal of the American Medical Association*, 1993, *270*, 2207–2212.
3. Evans, R. G., Barer, M. L., and Marmor, T. R. *Why Are Some People Healthy and Others Not?* New York: Aldine de Gruyter, 1994.
4. Bunker, J. P., Frazier, H. S., and Mosteller, F. "Improving Health: Measuring Effects of Medical Care." *Milbank Quarterly*, 1994, *72*, 225–258.
5. Glynn, T. J., and Manley, M. W. *How to Help Your Patients Stop Smoking: A National Cancer Institute Manual for Physicians.* (45 DHHS PHS NIH NCI NIH Publication 93–3064.) Bethesda, Md.: National Cancer Institute, 1993.
6. U.S. Preventive Services Task Force. *Guide to Clinical Preventive Services: An Assessment of the Effectiveness of 169 Interventions.* Baltimore, Md.: Williams and Wilkins, 1989.
7. Wennberg, J. E. Personal communication, 2004.
8. Pelletier, K. "A Review and Analysis of the Clinical and Cost-Effectiveness Studies of Comprehensive Health Promotion and Disease Management Programs at the Worksite. 1995–1998. Update (IV)." *American Journal of Health Promotion*, 1999, *13*, 333–345.
9. National Center for Health Statistics. *Health, United States, 2003*. Hyattsville, Md.: NCHS, 2003.

10. National Center for Health Statistics. *Health, United States, 2004.* Hyattsville, Md.: NCHS, 2004.

11. Breslow, L. *Perspectives: The Third Revolution in Health.* In J. F. Fielding, R. C. Brownson, and N. M. Clark (eds.), *Annual Review of Public Health.* Palo Alto, Calif.: Annual Reviews, 2004.

12. "Ottawa Charter for Health Promotion." *Canadian Journal of Public Health,* 1986, *77,* 425–436.

13. U.S. Department of Veterans Affairs. *Annual Report of the Secretary of Veterans Affairs/Department of Veterans.* Washington, D.C.: U.S. Government Printing Office, 1994.

14. U.S. Department of Health and Human Services, Public Health Service. *Trends in Indian Health.* Washington, D.C.: U.S. Government Printing Office, 1994.

15. Trevino, F. M., and Jacobs, J. P. "Public Health and Health Care Reform: The American Public Health Association's Perspective." *Journal of Health Policy,* 1994, *15,* 397–406; U.S. Bureau of the Census. *Current Population Survey: Annual Social and Economic Supplement, 2006.* [http://pubdb3.census.gov/macro/032006/health/h01_001.htm] (accessed Sept. 12, 2006).

16. National Association of County Health Officials. *Assessment Protocol for Excellence in Public Health (APEX/PH).* Washington D.C.: National Association of County Health Officials, 1991; U.S. Department of Health and Human Services, Centers for Disease Control and Prevention. *Planned Approach to Community Health (PATCH).* Atlanta: Public Health Service, 1992.

17. American Public Health Association. *Healthy Communities 2000: Model Standard* (3rd ed.). Washington, D.C.: American Public Health Association, 1991.

18. Institute of Medicine (1988).

19. U.S. Preventive Services Task Force (1989).

CHAPTER TWENTY-TWO

# THE CONTINUING ISSUE OF MEDICAL MALPRACTICE LIABILITY

## Ruth Roemer

The medical insurance crises of the 1970s and 1980s were followed by a third medical insurance liability crisis in 2001–2003.[1] According to the landmark report of the Institute of Medicine *To Err Is Human*, medical malpractice results in approximately ninety-eight thousand deaths per year and countless injuries.[2] It is no surprise, therefore, that despite various efforts at health care reform the issue of medical malpractice liability continues to provoke debate and alternative proposals for modifying the tort system for handling it. They include alternative dispute resolution, enterprise liability, caps on damages, no-fault compensation, an administrative system for medical injury compensation, and apologies by physicians and hospitals for their mistakes.

Several things make this issue an aspect of any major change in the health system, whether brought about by legislation, judicial decision, or voluntary action. First is the charge that high medical malpractice insurance premiums and defensive medicine are major contributors to escalating health care costs. Second is concern about patients' rights, specifically their inability to sue managed care organizations (MCOs) for medical malpractice. Third is the long-standing dissatisfaction with the tort system's handling of medical malpractice, for its failure to compensate many victims of malpractice and deter negligent practice.

## Does Medical Malpractice Litigation Increase Costs?

With respect to the first allegation, the evidence does not support the charge that medical malpractice litigation is a major cause of the rising costs of health care. On average, physicians pay less than 4 percent of annual practice receipts for malpractice insurance. This represents less than 1 percent of total U.S. health expenditures and therefore cannot be a primary cause of the growth in expenditures.[3] With respect to the impact of defensive medicine, although some procedures may be unnecessary others are beneficial and part of cautious, conservative medical practice.[4] Moreover, some precautions may prevent mistakes, making the net economic impact of defensive medicine unclear.[5] The Office of Technology Assessment (OTA) concludes that "overall only a small percentage of diagnostic procedures—certainly less than 8 percent—is likely to be caused primarily by conscious concern about malpractice liability."[6] Much of the increased spending on health care can more reasonably be explained as expanding and proliferating medical technology and rising costs of pharmaceuticals rather than the practice of defensive medicine.[7]

## May MCOs Be Sued for Denial of Care?

With respect to the second concern, a central issue in the growth of managed care is the question of the liability of MCOs for malpractice.

MCO liability for denial or delay of care concerns those MCOs and health plans that are subject to the Employee Retirement Income Security Act of 1974 (ERISA), under which the employer furnishes or funds health benefits. ERISA applies to all employee pension, health, and other benefit plans established by private sector employers or by state-licensed insurers.[8] More than 160 million Americans are covered by ERISA plans in their workplace.[9]

On June 21, 2004, in a long-awaited decision (*Aetna* v. *Davila*), the U.S. Supreme Court held that state legislation giving patients the right to sue managed care organizations for denying coverage for treatment that a physician deemed medically necessary is completely preempted by ERISA.[10] A unanimous decision written by Justice Clarence Thomas held unconstitutional a Texas patients'-rights statute that allowed a patient to sue his MCO in a state court for denying care. The Supreme Court declared that "any state-law cause of action that duplicates, supplements, or supplants the ERISA civil enforcement remedy conflicts with the clear congressional intent to make the ERISA remedy exclusive and is therefore preempted."[11]

In a concurring opinion, Justice Ruth Bader Ginsburg, joined by Justice Stephen Breyer, called on Congress and the Supreme Court to "revisit what is an unjust and increasingly tangled ERISA regime."[12] Justice Ginsburg noted that a "regulatory vacuum" exists because state law remedies are preempted and very limited federal remedies exist under ERISA. Under ERISA, plaintiffs denied care are limited to relief in federal courts only of payment for the cost of medical care denied (which may be only the cost of an X-ray or a medication) but cannot receive damages available in state courts for injuries suffered as a result of the denial (such as lost wages or compensation for pain and suffering).[13] Thus the challenge to Congress is to pass a federal patients' rights bill, furnishing a right to sue managed care organizations in state courts.

Although the Supreme Court has now closed the door on malpractice suits against ERISA plans in state courts under current law, a trend had been also shaping up toward restricting or softening the scope of the ERISA preemption. In recent years, interpretation of the ERISA preemption had been narrowed somewhat to bar only suits for denial of care (benefits decisions) but to allow suits relating to quality of care (medical decisions)—a difficult distinction to draw.[14] Many decisions mix benefits and medical or treatment decisions, and in one such case, *Pegram* v. *Herdrich*, the U.S. Supreme Court held in a unanimous decision in June 2000 that MCOs cannot be held liable as fiduciaries under ERISA for wrongful conduct in making such mixed decisions.[15]

Further restriction of the ERISA preemption occurred in 1995 in the *Travelers* case, a unanimous decision of the U.S. Supreme Court holding that a New York statute imposing surcharges on hospitals and some health care payers, including ERISA plans, in order to create a pool of funding to cover the uninsured was not preempted by ERISA because the statute had only an indirect economic effect.[16] Some legal authorities on ERISA thought that this case might "signal a change both in methods of statutory interpretation and in the Court's willingness to allow state regulation of some aspects of health care delivery that affect ERISA plans."[17] But the 2004 decision by the Supreme Court in *Aetna* v. *Davila* dashed this hope.

Those seeking to retain the immunity from suit that ERISA has provided to self-insured plans contend that allowing such suits increases the costs of health care. Advocates for increased legal accountability of MCOs deny this contention but say that some increased cost would be acceptable to protect patients from substandard care. Earlier cases indicated a propensity of the Supreme Court to soften the ERISA preemption, but this possibility has now been foreclosed unless Congress acts to allow malpractice suits against managed care organizations for medical injuries just as they are allowed against hospitals.[18]

## Is the Tort System of Compensation Fair and Equitable?

The third concern is dissatisfaction with the tort system on the grounds that it costs too much; is an erratic, unpredictable, and inefficient method of compensating persons injured by substandard care; and fails to deter negligent practice.[19] Despite extensive state legislation designed to curb malpractice suits, the question is still unresolved as to whether the present tort system of handling medical malpractice liability meets the twin objectives of fairly and adequately compensating persons injured by substandard care and deterring negligent practice.

To examine the options available for addressing the issues concerning the medical malpractice liability system, it may be helpful first to review the medical malpractice insurance crises of the 1970s and 1980s and their sequelae—the causes, the state legislative responses that ensued, and evaluations of these legislative actions. Then we may turn to the crisis of 2001–2003 and to alternative proposals that have been advanced. Finally, some comments are offered on how best to compensate victims of substandard medical care and how best to deter negligent medical practice—a question that may become urgent with legislative or voluntary reform of the health system.

## The Malpractice Insurance Crises of the 1970s, 1980s, and 2001–2003

In the 1960s and early 1970s, the frequency and severity of medical malpractice claims increased dramatically. Claim frequency rose nationally at an average annual rate of 12.1 percent, and paid claim severity (cost per claim, including awards and out-of-court settlements) increased by 10.2 percent. In some states, the increases were even greater. In California, both the frequency and the severity increased between 1969 and 1974 at an average annual rate of nearly 20 percent.[20] Throughout the 1970s, awards rose at a rate in excess of the general rate of inflation and the cost of medical care. Between 1970 and 1975, the average malpractice award increased from $11,518 to $26,565—an average annual rate increase of 18 percent. By 1978 the average award had increased to $45,187, representing a cumulative increase of 70 percent for the three years 1976–1978.[21]

Because of this escalation in the number of malpractice claims filed and in the size of awards, the premiums for malpractice liability insurance rose astronomically—by as much as 500 percent in some states.[22] In 1974, several important insurers withdrew from the market.[23] Thus the crisis of the 1970s was not because a large number of patients were injured but instead because of a breakdown in the malpractice insurance market.[24]

As a result, many physicians without adequate insurance coverage avoided high-risk cases, limited their practice in other ways (as with obstetrician-gynecologists restricting practice to office gynecology), withdrew from emergency service or from practice altogether, or practiced without insurance coverage or with lowered coverage.[25]

The problems with availability and affordability of malpractice insurance led to formation of compulsory pooling arrangements—joint underwriting associations—to compel insurers to provide insurance for malpractice as a condition of writing other insurance.[26] These joint underwriting associations were formed to ensure insurance coverage for physicians who could not obtain insurance, by requiring insurance companies offering property and casualty insurance to underwrite insurance for a physician who could not obtain liability insurance. Patient compensation funds, funded by a surcharge on all insurers, were established in nine states to settle catastrophic claims up to a certain limit. Some physicians formed their own insurance companies. These physician-owned firms insure about 60 percent of U.S. physicians and are represented by the Physicians Insurers Association of America.[27]

In response to this crisis, many states formed commissions to investigate and report on the medical malpractice insurance crisis in their states. In nearly every state, new statutes were enacted to restrain medical malpractice suits by restricting the scope of liability, limiting the size of awards, reducing the statute of limitations, limiting contingent fees of attorneys, and introducing pretrial screening panels or arbitration to discourage "frivolous" suits.[28] These measures are discussed later in this chapter.

After 1976, the frequency of claims leveled off, but the severity of awards continued to increase.[29] By 1985, however, when the second malpractice insurance crisis occurred, malpractice insurance premiums were again rising. From 1981 to 1986, they rose 75 percent, according to the 1983 Physicians' Practice Costs and Income Survey and the 1986 Physicians' Practice Follow-up Survey.[30] Claim frequency was rising by more than 12 percent after the increase in the 1970s that led to the 1975 crisis. Between 1975 and 1984, average medical malpractice verdicts increased at nearly twice the rate of the Consumer Price Index. These events prompted a leading authority on medical malpractice to say, "The fact that claim frequency and severity have continued to rise tends to confirm the fact that the response to the last crisis did not radically change the malpractice system."[31]

This statement is confirmed by a third medical malpractice insurance crisis in 2001–2003. In these two years, according to the American Medical Association, physicians in eighteen states had great difficulty in obtaining affordable professional liability insurance, and in twenty-six additional states the situation worsened.[32] Many insurance carriers have left the field of malpractice insurance, forcing physicians to turn to joint underwriting associations for coverage.[33] In an incisive article on the new medical malpractice crisis, the authors point out that "although the statutory mission of these organizations is to assure that all physicians can obtain coverage, the rates charged by these carriers can be prohibitively high, particularly for physicians who have previously been sued."[34]

The medical malpractice insurance crises have been ascribed to medical factors, legal factors, and insurance practices. The medical factors include greater use of health services because of enactment of Medicare and Medicaid and the growth of voluntary insurance; increased use of advanced medical technology entailing greater risk; and the fact that the practice of medicine is inherently a high-risk undertaking with a certain number of adverse outcomes, regardless of negligence. Also contributing to malpractice claims are heightened expectations on the part of consumers (the "every couple expects a perfect baby" syndrome) and changes in the doctor-patient relationship as medicine becomes more highly specialized and technical, with resulting depersonalization of health services.[35]

Legal factors have also contributed to the increase in claims. Abolition or modification of the locality rule, making the acceptable standard of practice a state or national standard, tends to increase claims and make expert witnesses more available. Abolishing the charitable immunity rule that formerly insulated voluntary hospitals from suits was a factor that favored plaintiffs' suits. Another contributing factor was expanding the scope of informed consent, requiring a subjective scope of disclosure of the risks of a procedure as needed by a particular patient rather than the objective scope of disclosure afforded by what a reasonably prudent physician practicing in the same or similar circumstances would disclose. Similarly, expansion of the doctrine of respondeat superior, which imposes responsibility on an employer for an employee's wrongdoing, contributed to claim increases. States that abolished or expanded the locality rule, abolished charitable immunity, and adopted broadened informed consent and respondeat superior doctrines were found to have claim costs twice as high as states that made none of these changes.[36]

Insurance experience and practice also contributed to the crisis. In the mid-1970s a decline in the stock market reduced capital and earnings on the investments of the insurance companies. Since most companies wrote "occurrence" policies in which the insurance company would be responsible for future claims as long as the incident on which the claim was based occurred in a year for which the insurance was purchased, insurance companies had to maintain large reserves to cover the "long tail" of future claims (the period from the occurrence of the incident to the eventual claim and its disposition).

After the 1975 crisis, insurance companies generally wrote "claims made" policies, in which the physician was covered for the year for which the policy was written, leaving a long tail of uninsured liability for the physician.[37] To cover a claim made after a claims-made policy has expired, the health care provider can purchase insurance known as "tail" coverage.[38] As a result of these experiences and practices, even though insurance was available in the 1980s it was more expensive and less coverage was provided, largely because of increasing loss payments, declining interest rates, tightening of the reinsurance market, and growing awards and uncertainty about the tort system.[39]

The medical malpractice insurance crises created problems in the medical, legal, and insurance sectors of society, but the main losers were consumers. The major part of the cost of these premium increases was not paid by physicians or hospitals but instead passed on to third-party payers as part of the cost of medical and hospital service.[40]

# State Legislative Reforms

Following the medical malpractice insurance crisis of the 1970s, most states enacted various laws to restrain malpractice suits. These changed laws have been grouped as relating to (1) filing claims, (2) defining standards of medical care or burden of proof, (3) determining the amount recoverable, and (4) alternatives to court resolution of claims.[41]

## Filing Claims

In this category are a number of types of statute.

***Ad Damnum Clause Reform.*** This legislation prohibits the plaintiff from stating the amount sought to be recovered, as is traditional in pleadings, although some statutes permit the plaintiff's attorney to request a specific sum at the trial. The justification for this reform is the belief that publication of large claims is prejudicial to defendants and inappropriately influences juries.

***Limitation on Attorneys' Fees.*** Most commonly, attorneys in medical liability cases are paid a fee contingent on the outcome of the case (35–50 percent of any award made to the plaintiff plus the expenses of litigation) rather than an hourly rate. Legislative reforms establish a sliding scale (the percentage declining with the size of the award) or set a reasonable amount as approved by the court.[42]

Contingent fees are supported on the ground that they constitute an incentive for lawyers to take cases that have a reasonable likelihood of success and to refuse those in which the plaintiff is unlikely to prove that the doctor was negligent. Theoretically, contingent fees allow recourse to the courts for low-income persons, but in reality lawyers will not take a case unless a substantial award is likely.[43] Thus, the contingent-fee system tends to screen out frivolous cases, but it also denies recourse for minor injuries or for injuries to the elderly, two types that do not promise large awards. The exclusion of small cases from the court system, however, may be due to high fixed costs of suit (including the costs of expert witnesses), not to contingent fees.[44]

Contingent fees are prohibited in England and Canada, which historically have had a lower rate of malpractice litigation than the United States, although the frequency of litigation has been increasing in these countries recently.

In the United States, the Federal Tort Claims Act limits contingent fees to 25 percent, and state workers' compensation laws also regulate contingent fees. Opposition to contingent fees is urged on the ground that they stimulate excessive litigation, create a conflict of interest between attorney and client, and impede settlement of claims.[45] About half the states specify a limit on attorneys' fees or authorize the courts to set fees.[46] From a public policy point of view, limitation of the plaintiff's attorney's fee is prejudicial to claimants when defendants (physicians, hospitals, and insurers) may spend unlimited amounts for the most skilled defense. In a dissenting opinion in a case holding constitutional the California Medical Injury Compensation Reform Act (MICRA), which prescribes a sliding scale of contingency fees, Chief Justice Rose Bird of the California Supreme Court stated that the act "prohibits severely injured victims of medical negligence from paying the general market rate for legal services, while permitting defendants to pay whatever is necessary to obtain high quality representation."[47]

**Preventing Frivolous Suits.**  Legislation to discourage claims without legal merit requires the losing party in a malpractice case to reimburse the opposing party for costs if the suit is fraudulent or in bad faith. About fifteen states have such laws. Or a state may require a certificate of merit by way of an affidavit of an expert before a suit is filed.

**Pretrial Screening Panels.**  Legislation to offer mandatory or voluntary screening of malpractice cases as a prerequisite to trial is intended to discourage nonmeritorious claims. The panel's decision is not binding and does not prevent the plaintiff from filing a lawsuit. The argument in favor of pretrial screening panels is that the number of claims going to trial is reduced. In opposition is the contention that these panels add an extra step in resolving claims and do not reduce the number of suits.[48] The OTA identified twenty-two states with some form of pretrial screening.[49]

The constitutionality of pretrial screening panels has been challenged as a violation of due process and equal protection, denial of a jury trial in violation of the Seventh Amendment to the Constitution, and improper delegation of judicial authority. Generally, the legislation has been upheld as a valid exercise of the police power of the state, but in six states such statutes have been declared unconstitutional.[50]

***Statutes of Limitations.*** Many states have shortened the time within which a medical malpractice claim must be filed after an injury occurs or should have been discovered. States have also limited the latest age at which a child may bring an action, or they have specified that a statute would be suspended only until a child reached a certain age. California sets a limit of three years from the time of the injury or one year from discovery, whichever is earlier. For minors, the rule is three years or the eighth birthday, whichever is later. Longer deferred statutes of limitations are designed to protect victims of latent injuries, but some late claims may be suits to recover by retroactive application of new standards, adding to the costs of the tort system. Instead, an authority in this field recommends a short statute of limitations with additional time for discovery, as in California; to offset the incentive to conceal injuries, physicians should be required to pay an uninsurable fine for fraud or concealment of a negligent injury.[51]

## Defining Standards of Care and Burden of Proof

In this category are five types of statute.

***Standards of Care.*** Statutes specifying the applicable standard of care in a malpractice suit, whether community, state, or national, were passed as the old locality rule was replaced by state or national standards. One reason for changing the strict locality rule was the difficulty in finding physicians willing to testify against their local colleagues; expanding the locality rule enabled plaintiffs to engage national experts.[52]

***Qualifications of Expert Witnesses.*** Some statutes specify the qualifications for an expert witness. For example, Ohio requires that an expert witness spend 75 percent of professional time in the active practice of his or her specialty.[53]

*Clinical Practice Guidelines.* Many specialty boards have developed clinical practice guidelines, and the federal government has supported development of guidelines. Since such guidelines represent professional consensus on appropriate procedures, they may be applicable in medical malpractice cases, despite the possibility of courts excluding them as evidence because of the rule against hearsay evidence or admitting them only as part of expert testimony.

At least three states—Maine,[54] Minnesota, and Vermont—have passed legislation that permits guidelines to be used as a defense in malpractice litigation, under certain circumstances. Both Maine and Minnesota bar the plaintiff from introducing the guidelines as evidence that the physician failed to meet the standard of care. Vermont permits guidelines to be admitted in evidence by either the plaintiff or defendant in mandatory malpractice arbitration. Concern is expressed that guidelines may not reflect changes in medical practice promptly; that there is a potential for conflict among national, state, and institutional guidelines; and that these conflicts may hinder rather than help solve issues in medical liability.[55]

*Informed Consent.* The expansion in the 1970s of the doctrine of informed consent to a more patient-oriented standard has led some states to enact legislation specifying what information must be given to the patient or specifying professional or customary standards of disclosure as a defense.[56]

*Res Ipsa Loquitur.* The legal doctrine of res ipsa loquitur ("the thing speaks for itself") was expanded in the 1970s from an inference of negligence to a presumption of negligence, which shifts the burden of proof from the plaintiff to the defendant and requires the defendant to show that the injury did not result from the defendant's negligence. This expanded application was found to place defendants at a disadvantage, with the result that some states have prohibited or limited use of the doctrine.[57]

## Determining Amounts Recoverable

This category comprises six types of statute.

*Joint and Several Liability.* About two-thirds of the states have modified the rule on joint and several liability, which allows the plaintiff to sue all defendants responsible and recover from each in proportion to fault (joint liability) or to sue any one defendant and recover the total amount, with that defendant able to recover from the other defendants for their shares (several liability). In some states, several liability was abolished. More commonly, the statutes limit several liability depending on the degree of the defendant's or plaintiff's fault or the ability of other defendants to pay the claim. For example, in Iowa, if the defendant is less than 50 percent responsible for all damages, he or she is liable only for his or her proportion of the damages; but if the responsibility is more than 50 percent, the defendant can be held severally liable for the entire amount of the damages.[58]

*Collateral Source Offsets.* The collateral source rule is a rule of evidence that prevents introducing evidence that the plaintiff has health or disability insurance covering the same injury. This rule originated at a time when individuals privately provided such coverage; the view was that the prudent person should not be penalized and the wrongdoer should not be relieved of liability because this would negate the deterrent effect of the penalty. The rule is opposed on the ground that recovery from multiple sources produces a windfall for the plaintiff (although in reality most health and disability policies require the plaintiff to reimburse the insurer for any payments received from the tort system).

At least thirty states have modified the collateral source rule, either to require juries to be informed about payment from other sources or to mandate an offset from the award for all or some of the collateral benefits. Also, a statute may be an exception to modification of the collateral source rule, allowing exclusion of collateral source benefits where the health care insurer has the right of subrogation, that is, the right to recover payment from an award in a tort action.[59]

*Itemized Jury Verdicts.* Requiring juries to itemize the various components of an award for damages instead of issuing a lump-sum figure is designed to promote objective and realistic awards by juries and permit subsequent analysis of verdicts.[60] Thus, with itemized jury verdicts, the economic components of an award (past and future medical expenses, past and future income loss) and noneconomic components (pain and suffering, bereavement, loss of consortium, loss of parental or filial support, and punitive damages) are clearly set forth.

*Caps on Damages.* Caps on damages may set a limit on noneconomic damages only (such as pain and suffering), or put a total cap on both economic and noneconomic damages.

More than half the states place some limit on noneconomic damage awards. These limits range from $250,000 to $750,000.[61] Some states specify exceptions; the Michigan cap does not apply to cases in which the patient has an injury to the reproductive system or has lost a bodily function.[62] Since no clear guidelines exist for assessing compensation for pain and suffering, proposals have been made to establish specific guidelines based on the age of the victim and the severity of the injury.

Only eight states have a cap on total damages, both economic and noneconomic. Permitted damages in these states range from $500,000 to $1 million. Four of these states have patient compensation funds.[63]

Statutory limits on damage awards are the subject of controversy and constitutional challenge. As of 1993, supreme courts in fifteen states had held caps on damages unconstitutional as a denial of due process or equal protection.[64]

A recent wave of decisions has invalidated caps on damages as a violation of provisions of the state constitution, most commonly as a violation of the right to a jury trial.[65] For example, in holding unconstitutional the $500,000 cap on noneconomic damages in the Oregon Tort Claims Act, the supreme court of Oregon stated that the cap "violates the injured party's right to receive an award that reflects the jury's factual determination of the amount of the damages as will fully compensate (plaintiffs) for all loss and injury to them."[66]

The supreme courts of Illinois, Kentucky, and New Hampshire have made similar decisions, and on Aug. 16, 1999, the Ohio Supreme Court, in a four-to-three decision, held unconstitutional a broad 1996 law designed to limit damage suits by capping damages, shortening the statute of limitations in certain suits, and otherwise curtailing damage suits.[67] In many states, these decisions have fomented a struggle between the legislature and the courts on change in the civil justice system, with business groups calling for limitation on liability lawsuits and the courts invalidating them on state constitutional grounds.

Other states, however, have upheld limits on noneconomic damages.[68] In 1985 the California Supreme Court, as mentioned, upheld the $250,000 limit on noneconomic damages in MICRA, the prototype of statutory caps on damages, on the ground that the limit is rationally related to the state's interest in reducing malpractice costs. Chief Justice Bird issued a stinging dissent, stating that victims of severe medical injury have been singled out to bear the bulk of relief in the medical malpractice insurance crisis, and the $250,000 limit on noneconomic damages cannot withstand any meaningful level of judicial scrutiny.[69]

Caps on damages have been popular because it is claimed that they reduce liability insurance premiums for providers by limiting insurers' liability for large claims.[70] Premiums in states with caps on awards were found to be an astonishing 17.1 per cent lower than in states without caps.[71] Still, even states with caps experienced a rise in premiums.[72] But arguing against caps is that they weaken the purpose of malpractice litigation: compensation for injury. As one legal authority states, "Malpractice premiums unaccompanied by lower rates of injury are not savings to society but, rather, transfer payments from injured patients to health care providers. . . . MICRA-style flat caps selectively penalize the neediest cases. . . ."[73]

Therefore caps on damages are not the panacea for reform of the medical malpractice problem, as some have urged.

***Punitive Damages.*** Punitive damages may be imposed in a case of intentional, gross, or egregious negligence. Those who favor punitive damages in a malpractice action emphasize their deterrent effect; those who oppose punitive damages state that allegations of gross negligence are used for bargaining in settlement negotiations and that such conduct is more appropriately regulated by licensing bodies, institutional review committees, or the criminal justice system.[74] Some reformed statutes abolish punitive damages in any suit for compensation for negligence; others limit punitive damages in various ways (limiting the amount, paying the punitive damage award to the state instead of permitting a windfall to the plaintiff, restricting the contingency fee on a punitive damage award to reduce the incentive for pursuing such claims).[75]

***Periodic Payments.*** By 1987, twenty-one states had enacted provisions requiring or allowing periodic payments of an award.[76] Periodic payments benefit the defendant and the insurer by reducing the cost of a large award and permitting modification of the award in the event the injured person dies, thus eliminating a windfall to the beneficiaries. Periodic payments benefit the injured person by ensuring availability of funds and avoiding the risk of mismanagement of a large lump sum.

## Evaluations of State Legislative Reforms

A number of studies have examined the effects of the various reforms described in the previous section. Of them, the OTA selected six principal empirical studies that examined the impact of tort reform in two or more states to ascertain whether these reforms reduced the frequency of medical malpractice claims, the size of awards or payments, or the level of medical malpractice insurance premiums, all of these collectively called "malpractice cost indicators."[77]

The OTA concluded that only two reforms significantly reduced one or more of the malpractice cost indicators: caps on damage awards, and mandatory collateral source offsets. No significant impact was found in three reforms: limits on attorneys' fees, mandatory or discretionary periodic payments, and restricting the use of res ipsa loquitur. Other reforms that were found to have mixed (some positive findings and some negative) or isolated effects (only one significant result) are restricting statutes of limitation, establishing pretrial screening panels, limiting the doctrine of informed consent, and allowing costs awardable in frivolous suits.

Regarding use of practice guidelines as the standard of care, OTA predicts that practice guidelines may not be appropriate as a means of tort reform but that their development may be important in determining the standard of care under the existing tort system.

In its 1994 report on defensive medicine, the OTA offers further evaluation of various strategies in malpractice reform, particularly with respect to their impact on practicing defensive medicine. OTA concludes that tort reforms that tinker with the current system retaining personal liability of the physician are likely to be more successful in limiting the direct costs of malpractice—claim frequency, payment per paid claim, and insurance premiums—than in altering physician behavior. Use of practice guidelines is not a panacea, OTA states, but the guidelines may reduce defensive medicine because they offer guidance for the courts on standard of care.

## Criticisms of the Tort System

An important criticism of the tort system of handling medical malpractice is the small fraction of the premium dollar that reaches the injured person. In 1976, a landmark report of the Special Advisory Panel on Medical Malpractice in New York state found that of total medical malpractice premiums only 25–40 percent goes to the claimant, and most of this payout goes to claimants with large claims.[78] In 1986, a RAND study found that only 50 percent of total malpractice costs reach the injured person—much less than is received by the victims of other tort-based systems.[79]

Another criticism is the small proportion of injured patients who are compensated. In 1985, Danzon reported that the incidence of malpractice is much greater than the frequency of claims.[80] In 1991, the Harvard Medical Practice Study found that not more than 6.25 percent, and possibly fewer than 1 percent, of those injured receive compensation for medical injuries. Most victims of relatively minor injuries, and most victims of even severe injuries who are over sixty-five, receive no compensation.[81] The universe of injuries includes those due to adverse outcomes of the disease or medical procedures and those due to negligence. For those due to negligence, only a small proportion of patients injured sue; of those who sue, a smaller proportion receives any compensation. Figure 22.1, adapted by the OTA from J. R. Posner's work, depicts this experience.[82]

A recent analysis of data from the National Practitioners' Data Bank (NPDB) by the Public Citizen Health Research Group for the period 2002–2004 found that very few doctors were responsible for the vast majority of malpractice payouts.[83] Only 5.5 percent of doctors are responsible for 57.3 percent of medical malpractice payouts to patients. Nearly 83 percent of doctors have never had a malpractice payout since the NPDB was created in 1990. Moreover, doctors with repeated malpractice payouts suffer infrequent disciplinary action. Only 8.3 percent of doctors who made two or more malpractice payouts were disciplined by

## FIGURE 22.1. MEDICAL INJURIES, NEGLIGENT CONDUCT, AND MALPRACTICE CLAIMS.

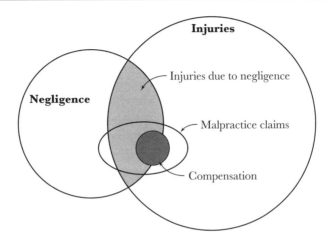

*Source:* Office of Technology Assessment. *Impact of Legal Reforms on Medical Malpractice Costs.* (OTA-BP-H-19.) Washington, D.C.: U.S. Government Printing Office, Oct. 1993, p. 9. Adapted from Posner, J. R. "Trends in Medical Malpractice Insurance, 1970–1985." *Law and Contemporary Problems,* 1986, *49*(2), 37.

their state licensing boards, and only 11.4 percent of doctors who made three or more malpractice payouts were disciplined by their state licensing boards. On the basis of this information, Public Citizen Health Research Group concludes that the real medical malpractice crisis today is inadequate patient safety, not lawsuits or the legal system.

Halley points out that the piecemeal measures adopted after each crisis make recovery by an injured person more difficult and restrict the awards obtained. Halley writes: "In this view, tort reform compounds the other undesirable features of the tort approach: the lottery effect, yielding overcompensation to a few injured patients, and under compensation or no compensation to a larger number; long delays for those finally obtaining compensation; great system expense, since attorneys for the plaintiffs and the defense and insurers receive the major share of the premium dollar; and the increasing hardships of adversarial tort litigation. As a consequence, there has been considerable interest in new approaches, although none of these has obtained widespread support, and the level of such interest has always been crisis-driven."[84]

Despite the inequities and even injustices of the tort system for handling medical malpractice, it has persisted, with only the piecemeal changes we have described, because, as consumer advocates point out, it is "often the only practical means available to patients for exposing, punishing, and deterring substandard medical practice."[85]

# Alternatives to the Tort System

Various alternatives have been proposed. The five main types can be summarized as (1) alternative dispute resolution (ADR), which includes conciliation, mediation, and arbitration; (2) enterprise liability; (3) no-fault insurance, which includes medical adversity insurance and "neo-no-fault" insurance; (4) apologizing and an early offer system; and (5) the Model Medical Accident Compensation System, patterned after the workers' compensation system.

## Alternative Dispute Resolution

ADR is a nonjudicial process that includes conciliation (bringing the parties together), mediation (bringing the parties together and suggesting possible solutions),[86] and arbitration (holding a hearing at which the parties present their cases and an award is made). The most important of these is arbitration, which may be voluntary or mandatory, binding or nonbinding, an independent proceeding, or related to a court case.

Arguments in favor of arbitration are that it resolves claims quickly, reduces costs, permits greater access for small claims, and reduces the burden on the courts.

Arguments against arbitration are that it may favor providers if a provider is a member of the arbitration panel, it may not compensate the injured person adequately, it may reduce the provider's incentive to lower the incidence of malpractice because the private arbitration process avoids the stigma of a court suit, agreements to arbitrate may not be fully understood by the patient and thus may give an unfair advantage to the provider, and the informality of arbitration hearings may violate the due process rights of the parties.[87]

Experience with alternative dispute resolution is still limited. The courts have encouraged its use. Some state statutes allow binding, irrevocable arbitration agreements in medical malpractice cases, or, as in California, private agreements may lead to arbitration. In 1981, authorities in the field pointed out that arbitration has the advantages of accommodating all case types; offering various arbitration arrangements; and being expeditious, economical, and generally acceptable, so that it should be considered "not alone as a procedural alternative to litigation but as a substantive contribution to resolution of medical issues."[88]

Despite these alleged advantages of arbitration, concern has arisen that delay in the arbitration process and the ability of providers to select favorable arbitrators may prejudice injured patients. For example, in *Engalla* v. *Kaiser Permanente Medical Group*,[89] a mandatory arbitration case involving excessive delays in appointing an arbitrator, the California Supreme Court held that Kaiser Permanente's failure to comply with the time requirements of the arbitration agreement would allow this case to be heard in court, but the California Supreme Court did not invalidate the mandatory arbitration system generally. In accordance with recommendations of a blue ribbon advisory panel appointed by Kaiser Permanente following this decision, Kaiser Permanente has reformed its arbitration process to include an independent administrator, use of a single neutral arbitrator, early mediation, explicit deadlines, and a broad advisory panel.[90] The increasing popularity of new strategies for conflict resolution may impel a resurgence of alternative dispute resolution of medical liability.

## Enterprise Liability

Related to alternative dispute resolution is the concept of enterprise liability, which allows patients, providers, and health care institutions to enter into a contract placing all liability for the physician's action on the health care institution.

Those favoring contracting for enterprise liability argue that it encourages health care institutions to strengthen their quality control measures, reduces the cost of liability insurance and improves the physician-patient relationship by eliminating the threat of suit, reduces the need for defensive medicine, promotes early and more certain awards, and cuts insurers' administrative costs by reducing the number of individual policies and claims.

Against contracting for enterprise liability are the arguments that it does not cover all patients, the courts may look unfavorably on the contracts as an unfair limitation on the tort rights of patients, and consumers are not sufficiently informed or sufficiently powerful to protect their interests in contract negotiations.[91]

There are several arguments advanced for enterprise liability.[92] First, the current system suffers from the well-known deficiencies of failing to compensate many injured patients and failing to deter negligence. Moreover, certain practices of malpractice insurers, such as not basing premiums on individual experience but rather on location and specialty, minimize incentives for quality improvement.[93] Second, the organizational unit that is ultimately responsible for efficient health care should also bear financial liability for malpractice so that it can include the cost of patient harm in its calculations. Third, placing liability for malpractice in the high policy-making level of the organizational unit tends to decrease defensive medicine, which has been estimated to cost about 8 percent of diagnostic procedures.[94]

Fourth, imposing liability at the high level of the organizational unit may also promote equity by encouraging policies that benefit the many with cost-effective procedures, rather than the few with expensive procedures.[95] Fifth, imposing liability on health plans follows from a capitated payment system, since health plans must bear the cost of future medical care from the present payment, and enterprise liability would require plans to incorporate the cost of malpractice awards in their calculations.[96] Sixth, health plans are in a position to reduce the incidence of malpractice through organizational and managerial strategies. Finally, an integrated delivery system may have the capacity to arrange for sharing liability among numerous units in a health plan network.

Proponents of enterprise liability contend that such a system promotes quality by improving relations between health plans and health care professionals, promoting teamwork, and relieving physicians to some extent of the extremely negative experience of malpractice suits.

Despite the apparent cogency of these arguments, many questions are unanswered. Is enterprise liability feasible in the absence of comprehensive health care reform? Which enterprise should be responsible: the health plan, or the hospital or other enterprise directly involved in delivering health care?[97] What inequities result from the operation of different health plans? In a mixed health care system—part managed care and part traditional practice—how is malpractice liability handled fairly? Notwithstanding the theoretical appeal of many of the arguments for enterprise medical liability, can such a system realistically be implemented? Can it withstand legal challenge? Does it prejudice the injured patient by shifting liability to a powerful and invisible defendant? Moreover, now that the Supreme Court has denied patients the right to sue their managed care organizations in state courts,[98] enterprise liability as a means of reforming the tort system seems doomed.

## No-Fault Compensation

The essence of the no-fault approach is that it is a compensation system that eliminates proof of negligence as a basis for collecting damages. As Grad points out, a no-fault system would recognize the fact that the risk of medical injury is inherent in modern medicine and would permit compensation for all such injuries, irrespective of negligence.[99]

In 1976–77, the California Medical Association and the California Hospital Association sponsored the Medical Insurance Feasibility Study in California to determine the economic feasibility of a pure no-fault system. This study is important for showing that adverse outcomes of medical care, although numerous, are finite and can be identified. The study found that 82 percent of adverse outcomes were class I adverse outcomes, involving complications of treatment (including giving drugs to patients). Class II adverse outcomes—the effects of incomplete or delayed diagnosis or treatment—accounted for only 15 percent of adverse outcomes.[100] Most no-fault systems now in use around the world cover only class I adverse outcomes and not class II outcomes. It is therefore suggested that since class I injuries account for 82 percent of total adverse outcomes, a no-fault system applicable to that 82 percent might be worthwhile, leaving class II outcomes in a residual fault-based liability system.[101]

In support of a no-fault insurance system, it would extend compensation to more injured persons, deliver compensation more promptly, avoid the substantial cost of proving negligence, make similar compensation available to patients with similar injuries, and create incentives for improving the quality of care by defining the causes of untoward outcomes and means of avoiding them and by basing insurance premiums on each provider's experience rating.

Those against a no-fault insurance system urge consideration that it may cost more than the current system because more people will be compensated; although the question of negligence is eliminated, the question of causation remains; it requires work to define the compensable events and the compensation schedule; the system covers only economic damages, not pain and suffering, although the compensation schedule might reflect some elements of pain and suffering; it removes a deterrent to substandard care; it may cause some providers to refuse to accept high-risk patients; and it may be complex in resolving claims involving multiple providers.[102]

Next we turn to two forms of limited no-fault insurance: medical adversity insurance and neo-no-fault insurance.

***Medical Adversity Insurance.*** In 1973, Havighurst and Tancredi proposed a no-fault approach that they called "medical adversity insurance."[103] The proposal would identify those injuries that deserve compensation, calling them "designated compensable events." The proposal aimed to improve the quality of care by defining categories of untoward outcomes and the means for avoiding them. Although this system has not been implemented, benefits claimed for it are the impact on the quality of medical care (it generates a listing, specialty by specialty, of potential adverse effects of various procedures), administrative savings derived by avoiding court suits, and reduction of emotional stress and stigma for all parties.[104]

***Neo-No-Fault Insurance.*** Another variation on the no-fault system is neo-no-fault.[105] The essence of this proposal is to encourage early out-of-court settlement for the actual economic losses and use the money that would have been spent on litigation and pain and suffering to pay for adequate injury compensation. This proposal differs from pure no-fault because the tort system is retained as an alternative.[106]

Under this proposal, a provider facing a malpractice claim has the option of offering the claimant, within 180 days after the claim is filed, periodic payment or a lump sum approved by the court as compensation for economic losses, including medical expenses, rehabilitation, and lost wages not covered by other insurance. Certain disincentives to sue would prevail: recovery is allowed only for wanton conduct, the standard of proof required is higher (not the usual standard in civil cases of preponderance of the evidence, but rather proof by clear and convincing evidence), limitation of noneconomic damages, and a penalty on the plaintiff of having to pay the defendant's costs if the claimant is awarded less than the noneconomic loss offered by the defendant.

The advantage of this proposal is that it produces prompt payment for economic loss in return for giving up the right to sue. But in egregious cases with great pain and suffering, the claimant would be permitted to bring a tort action.

***Examples of U.S. No-Fault Systems.*** Three examples of limited no-fault systems exist in the United States.

In 1986, Congress enacted the National Childhood Vaccine Injury Act of 1986, with its no-fault compensation system for children injured as a result of side effects of immunization against childhood diseases. The legislation was designed to encourage vaccine manufacturers to increase their production of vaccines, which had declined dangerously because of the industry's fear of malpractice suits. Compensation is payable by the federal government on the basis of strict liability, that is, without regard to fault or negligence by the manufacturer or the administering physician.[107]

Two states, Virginia and Florida, have enacted no-fault compensation systems for birth-related neurological injuries. The Virginia Birth-Related Neurological Injury Compensation Act of 1987 was designed to make liability insurance for obstetrician-gynecologists affordable and available by taking claims for certain catastrophically injured newborns out of the tort system, thus permitting quicker compensation and increasing access to obstetrical care.[108]

Compensation is awarded only for those infants who meet a narrow statutory definition of injury to the spinal cord or brain—caused by deprivation of oxygen or mechanical injury in the course of labor, delivery, or resuscitation in the immediate postdelivery period in a hospital—that rendered the infant permanently "motorically disabled" and developmentally or cognitively disabled such that assistance in all activities of daily living is required, and that was not caused by congenital or genetic factors, degenerative neurological disease, or maternal substance abuse. The injury must have been caused by a physician who was participating in the program or at a participating hospital.

The program is funded by an annual assessment of $250 per licensed physician, voluntary assessments of $5,000 per participating physician, and $50 per delivery for participating hospitals, not to exceed $150,000 in any twelve-month period.[109]

The procedure is as follows. The claimant files a claim with the Workers' Compensation Commission and serves a petition on the fund that administers the program and determines whether the claim falls within the definition of the statute. If the fund finds that the injury is compensable, the commission issues an order without a hearing and sends the case to a medical review panel of three qualified and impartial physicians, which makes a recommendation to the commission as to whether the case is covered by the act. If the fund determines that the case does not fall within the definition, then the commission holds a hearing at which the panel's recommendation is given considerable but not determinative weight.[110] Awards are made according to statutory provisions.

The plaintiff has no option of an alternative remedy if the delivery was performed by a participating hospital, but final appeal may be made to the Virginia Court of Appeals. By the end of 1992, only four claims had been filed under this program.

The Florida Birth-Related Neurological Injury Compensation Act was passed in 1988; though similar to that of Virginia, it differs in several respects. The claim must be filed within five years, instead of ten; and it is not required that the infant need assistance in all activities. A hospital is protected from liability only if the delivery is done by a participating physician, so hospitals either require their physicians to participate or pay the physician's assessment. Thus, about 90 percent of obstetricians in Florida participate.[111]

A thorough study of the experience under these no-fault, birth-injury statutes found that the number of cases is small, perhaps because of lack of outreach and the option remaining of choosing to sue in tort. The study also found that no-fault cases are resolved more quickly than tort suits, and that no-fault's low administrative costs are related to using only a few expert hearing officers and medical consultants.[112] The study concluded that no-fault programs are feasible and produce major gains in efficiency. In the opinion of the authors of the study, a broader no-fault injury program covering more eligible cases would improve both compensation and deterrence, though this outcome depends on the details of implementation of the statutes.[113]

### Experience with No-Fault Insurance in Other Countries.

Three countries have adopted systems of no-fault compensation for personal injury: New Zealand, Sweden, and Finland.

Since 1974, New Zealand has had a comprehensive system of compensation for all personal injuries, whether they occur at work, on the highway, in the home, in the hospital, or anywhere else. The scheme was introduced because of varying results for people with equal problems and equal needs, because many people received no compensation for injuries, and because extravagant and drawn-out adversary techniques reduced compensation to claimants.[114]

The intent of the scheme is to compensate all instances of physical or mental harm caused by accident but excluding those arising from illness or old age. The scope of the scheme is broad, but excluded are (1) the effects of a cardiovascular or cerebrovascular episode unless it is work-related and the result of undue strain, or unless the episode results from an injury by accident; and (2) physical or mental damage caused exclusively by disease, infection, or the aging process.[115]

Administered by a nonprofit, autonomous governmental organization (the Accident Compensation Corporation), the New Zealand program, as of 1989, compensated for total disability, in periodic payments, at a level of 80 percent of earnings up to a ceiling of $976 per week. Proportionate adjustments are made for partial disability. The benefit level is fixed at 80 percent to create an incentive for rehabilitation. Payments are made for disability, adjusted for inflation, until age sixty-five, when pensions take over.

In addition to payment for loss of earnings, reasonable costs of medical and dental treatment are covered, as well as reasonable costs of transport to the doctor or hospital for initial treatment and for further rehabilitative treatment, rehabilitation, and retraining assistance; payment for reasonable cost of necessary constant personal attention of the injured person following the accident; lump sum for permanent physical disability; lump sum for pain and suffering; lump sum to dependent spouse and dependent children; and other benefits.[116]

The program is financed by contributions from employers and employees and the self-employed, together with payments from owners of motor vehicles, and a small supplement from general taxation.

The New Zealand system has enjoyed wide public support. New Zealand has not experienced the growth in defensive medicine or the harm to the doctor-patient relationship associated with malpractice suits. As for the effect on the quality of medical practice, the Right Honorable Sir Owen Woodhouse, who is largely responsible for introducing and promoting the New Zealand compensation system, said that "it is a strange argument that physicians need to be made fearful of court actions in order to maintain those professional standards upon which their whole livelihood will depend. Certainly there are no signs in New Zealand that medical standards have deteriorated in the years during which the comprehensive scheme has been operating."[117]

On January 1, 1975, Sweden introduced a voluntary patient insurance scheme administered by a consortium of insurers headed by Scandia Life. The scheme is funded and paid by the county councils on a per capita basis. Injured patients may elect to bring an action in tort or may receive compensation under the patient compensation program without having to prove fault.[118] The program was not enacted by the Swedish government but is the result of an agreement between the Federation of County Councils and a consortium of Swedish insurers. Although the program is generally described as no-fault, it is not strictly so because error underlies most payments: "Such an error, however, does not have to be proved negligent; error may be assumed where the outcome is unusual."[119]

In January 1978, Sweden introduced a pharmaceutical scheme, which is also a voluntary, nonstatutory system covering injuries from vaccination and blood products. Impelled by the threat of legislation, the program is paid for by the drug industry, and premiums are based on each company's market share.

Five types of injury are covered under the Swedish compensation system: (1) treatments, (2) timing and accuracy of diagnosis, (3) accidents, (4) infections, and (5) injuries caused by diagnostic procedures. To be compensated, an individual must have reported sick for a minimum of fourteen days or been hospitalized for at least ten days, or have suffered permanent injury, or died. Compensation is paid for loss of income and for medical care, with indemnities for pain and suffering and permanent disfigurement.

The philosophy of the Swedish system is based on the principles of tort law in that injuries, complications, or undesired results as an unavoidable consequence of the illness or necessary treatment are not covered. Compensation is paid whether or not the error of judgment or clinical practice was negligent; therefore doctors and nurses are willing to admit errors and encourage patients to file claims.[120]

The claims process is simple, inexpensive, and easy to administer. The patient has the right to take an appeal to a claims panel, which meets for a day about twelve times a year. If the claims panel rejects the appeal, the patient's final resort is to submit the claim to arbitration.

Finland has introduced comprehensive pharmaceutical and treatment injury insurance modeled after the Swedish system. The Patient Injury Act of 1986 permits payments for loss of earnings, loss of amenities, and pain and suffering. Ninety-three percent of all medical care is provided by the state. Compensation is payable for any injury that has arisen from examination, treatment, or any similar action, or neglect of the same; that has been caused by an infection connected with examination or treatment; or that has been caused by accident connected with examination or treatment, occurring during ambulance transport, or resulting from a defect in medical equipment.

The scheme is financed through insurance, which doctors and other health providers must obtain. The Patient Insurance Association issues policies and handles claims and settlements. Failure to carry insurance makes the uninsured provider liable for ten times the normal premium. If a provider is uninsured, the Patient Insurance Association pays the patient and then collects the increased premium.[121]

In Finland, the Patient Injury Act of 1986 has eliminated the need to prove negligence entirely. In Sweden, negligence need be proved only if the injured person elects to sue in tort instead of seeking compensation through the patient insurance program. But because the damages paid under the insurance program are the same as those recoverable in tort, there is little incentive to sue.[122]

***Apologizing and an Early Offer System.*** In the United States, experience has shown that openness and apologizing by the doctor for a mishap, without admitting fault, can sometimes mitigate the harsh feelings that lead to a lawsuit. Or such communication can sometimes decrease the damages awarded.[123]

Increased emphasis on patient safety has also led to more transparency about an untoward outcome. This, in turn, has led to early offer programs in which patients and the health care organization have incentives to negotiate a private settlement immediately after an adverse event.

## The Model Medical Accident Compensation Act

Finally, we turn to the proposal for a system of medical accident compensation that applies the principles of workers' compensation to medical injury compensation.[124] In the belief that administrative or agency compensation is theoretically and realistically the solution for the medical professional liability dilemma, Halley and colleagues have advanced a model statute authored by Bryce B. Moore, former director of the Kansas workers' compensation program, and supported by extensive research by the Midwest Institute for Health Care and Law.

Like workers' compensation, the Model Medical Accident Compensation System involves a trade-off: it extends benefits to a larger number of injured individuals than are compensated currently in exchange for restricting the tort system. The administrative process is designed for prompt, limited, and certain compensation for an increased number of injured individuals, avoiding the delay, costs, and uncertainties of court procedures. A greater proportion of the premium dollar would go to the injured person than occurs under the adversarial process. Attorneys may represent claimants and providers in the administrative process.

Definition of the medical injury or compensable event is not through a schedule of compensable events but rather through review of individual cases, applying the standard of reasonable care. Proof of negligence is not required, but the concept of medical error or "fault" (responsibility for an outcome) is retained to distinguish compensable events from progression of the disease or unavoidable consequences of treatment. Administrative determination by the Medical Accident Compensation Board replaces adversarial tort litigation and the jury. The determination of compensable events is made by the Medical Accident Compensation Board, assisted by an expert review panel.

Payment of all compensation claims is guaranteed through requirements that health care providers carry insurance and through a Recovery Guarantee Fund. There are three methods of funding: (1) purchase of an insurance policy by an individual provider, (2) provider self-insurance (usually for an institution), and (3) membership in a group-funded self-insurance pool (a less-expensive method than individual purchase of insurance).

The Recovery Guarantee Fund is established in the state treasury to ensure payment of compensation in the event a provider is uninsured or unable to pay the benefits under the act. Payments from the fund are not expected to be large, because health care providers generally carry the required insurance, just as most employers carry the appropriate workers' compensation insurance.

Benefits are based on economic loss with equivalent compensation for claimants without ascertainable earnings, such as housewives, homemakers, retired persons, and children. Benefits include those for medical care and rehabilitation, temporary and permanent personal disability, death benefits, and burial expenses. Calculation of permanent personal injury benefits is based on the highest of three percentages: loss of the claimant's earning ability, overall reduction in the claimant's health level, and functional disability to the body as a whole.

The cost of an administrative system is an important concern because of the anticipated increase in the number of compensated injuries. These increased payments may be offset by the greater efficiency of the system and by cost controls built into the system: maximum limits on liability, a two-year statute of limitations on filing a claim, credit for duplicate payments (no windfall to the claimant from collateral sources), limitation on attorneys' fees, and so on.

The act allows appeal to the courts from a decision of the board. As in workers' compensation, appeals are based on the record of proceedings before the board. The courts have jurisdiction to determine whether the board has made a correct finding under the act.

Most important are provisions built into the model act to promote acceptable quality of health care. Separate from the compensation provisions are others for strengthened state agencies that conduct surveillance of medical practice, institutional review procedures, and other peer review mechanisms. Quality assurance is linked to the data-collection functions of the board, which are connected to state and national data banks.

## Medical Malpractice Reform in the U.S. Context

The many proposals for change in the tort system of handling medical malpractice liability break down into three main types: (1) piecemeal reforms, or tinkering with the tort system; (2) no-fault compensation systems; and (3) an administrative program of compensation modeled on the workers' compensation system.

Twenty years' experience with piecemeal reforms has made only minor improvements in the tort system, which fails to compensate many injured persons; pays only 25–40 percent of total premium cost to injured persons; and is fraught with delays, high costs, and inequities among injured persons suffering from the same or similar injuries. Careful evaluation of the effects of piecemeal reform has confirmed their minimal benefits. The repeated recurrence in the 1980s, the 1990s, and in 2001–2003 of the medical malpractice insurance crisis of the 1970s attests to the need for an alternative approach.

No-fault compensation systems are currently operating in the federal vaccine compensation program and in two states for compensation for birth-related neurological injuries. Examples of the no-fault approach exist in automobile insurance. Although the compensable event is clearly defined in automobile accidents, definition of potentially compensable medical events requires more work. The Medical Insurance Feasibility Study, sponsored by the California Medical Association and the California Hospital Association in the late 1970s, showed that it is possible to define potentially compensable events and that a no-fault system of medical injury compensation is feasible.[125] From a policy point of view, the well-documented report of New York's Special Advisory Panel on Medical Malpractice in 1976 strongly recommended a compensation system that does not pay damages for injuries caused by malpractice but rather compensates for bad medical results.[126]

The experience of New Zealand, Sweden, and Finland with their differing no-fault systems of medical injury compensation shows the rationality, equity, and public acceptance of no-fault systems. The systems of health insurance and social security benefits in these countries, however, are much more all-encompassing than those in the United States.

Despite the soundness of the no-fault approach and the appeal of neo-no-fault in retaining the option of a suit in tort, political realities seem to militate against adoption of this alternative. Objections to the no-fault approach were detailed earlier in this chapter, but the principal countervailing force lies in the power of the special interests that would be affected by adopting this approach (mainly insurance companies and trial lawyers).

In view of these realities, a feasible and rational alternative is the Model Medical Accident Compensation Act, patterned after the workers' compensation program and designed to be an administrative system for reasonable and rapid compensation for medical injuries. Even though workers' compensation may be in need of some modernization itself (such as increased benefits and strengthened rehabilitation provisions), few people would dream of ever returning to the tort system for redress of occupational injuries and diseases. Administrative law is increasingly the means in the United States for handling technical problems requiring expertise and prompt resolution. It is an appropriate vehicle for solving the problem of medical injury compensation. Extensive research and investigation have explored the economic, constitutional, and medical features of such a system, and precedents exist in other administrative law programs.

Regardless of when and how medical malpractice liability reform should be undertaken, the fundamental issue is quality of care.[127] No system of medical care can eliminate all adverse outcomes, a certain number of which are inevitable in high-technology medicine, and no system can eliminate all bad actors and all substandard performance; but strategies can be adopted to monitor and continually improve the quality of care. The Model Medical Accident Compensation Act contains provisions on data collection and surveillance of care that can strengthen current protections of the quality of care.

Enacting national health insurance that ensures universal coverage of the total population may reduce the propensity to sue because all medical care, including that needed because of adverse outcomes of earlier care, will be covered. Patient anger with the health care system—a necessary ingredient for a lawsuit—may be reduced by universal coverage.[128] Malpractice suits may also be restrained as health maintenance organizations and third-party administrators introduce quality control measures such as Kaiser Permanente's Report Card on Quality of Care to strengthen the existing quality system of state licensure, disciplinary actions, and peer review processes.

In 1986, an authority on medical malpractice called the current system not a compensation system but a liability system, pointing out that (1) our current system fails as a compensation system, (2) evidence is lacking that it has any deterrent effects, and (3) the costs of liability coverage and administration are too high.[129] Nearly twenty years later, with health care reform still on the national agenda, the climate of opinion may indeed be favorable for rationalizing our handling of medical injury compensation by adopting an administrative system that is more equitable and less costly than the tort system.

# Notes

1. Liang, B. A., and Ren, L. "Medical Liability Insurance and Damage Caps: Getting Beyond Band Aids to Substantive Systems Treatment to Improve Quality and Safety in Healthcare." *American Journal of Law and Medicine*, 2004, 30(4), 501–541.

2. Kohn, L. T., and others. *To Err Is Human: Building a Safer Human System.* Washington, D.C.: Institute of Medicine, 2001.

3. U.S. Congress, Office of Technology Assessment (OTA). *Impact of Legal Reforms on Medical Malpractice Cost.* (OTA-BP-H-19.) Washington, D.C.: U.S. Government Printing Office, 1993.

4. Aaron, H. J. *Serious and Unstable Condition: Financing America's Health Care.* Washington, D.C.: Brookings Institution, 1991. The OTA states that "most defensive medicine is not of zero benefit." U.S. Congress, OTA. *Defensive Medicine and Medical Malpractice.* (OTA-H-602.) Washington, D.C.: U.S. Government Printing Office, 1994.

5. Aaron (1991). For uncertainty about the effects of defensive medicine, see Studdert, D. M., Mello, M. M., and Brennan, T. M. "Medical Malpractice." *New England Journal of Medicine,* 2004, *350*(3), 283–292.

6. OTA (1994), p. l.

7. Aaron (1991); Strunk, B. C., and Ginsburg, P. B. "Tracking Health Care Costs: Trends Turn Downward in 2003." *Health Affairs,* 9 June 2004, W4-354–W4-362.

8. Butler, P. A. *ERISA Preemption: Manual for State Health Policymakers.* Washington, D.C.: Alpha Center, National Academy for State Health Policy, 2000.

9. Armitage, J. L. "Pegram v. Herdrich: HMO Physicians as Fiduciaries." *De Paul Journal of Health Care Law,* 2002, *5*(2), 341–363.

10. *Aetna* v. *Davila* and *Cigna* v. *Calad,* 124 S. Ct. 2498 (2004). See Mariner, W. F. "The Supreme Court Limitation of Managed Care Liability." *New England Journal of Medicine,* 2004, *351*(13) 1347–1352.

11. 124 Ct. 2488, and Westlaw, p. 8 of 17.

12. 124 Ct. 2488 at Westlaw p. 15 of 17.

13. See Rosenblatt, R. E., Law, S. A., and Rosenbaum, S. *Law and the American Health Care System.* Westbury, N.Y.: Foundation Press, 1997.

14. See, for example, *Dukes* v. *U.S. Healthcare, Inc.,* 57 F. 3rd 350 (3rd Cir. 1995), cert. denied 116 S. Ct. 564 (1995); Pear, R. "Series of Rulings Eases Constraints on Suing HMOs." *New York Times,* Aug. 15, 1999, pp. 1, 19; Jacobson, P. D., and Pomfret, S. D. "ERISA Litigation and Physician Autonomy." *Journal of the American Medical Association,* 2000, *283*(7), 921–926.

15. 530 U.S. 211, 120 S.Ct. 2143 (June 12, 2000). See Mariner, W. K. "What Recourse?— Liability for Managed-Care Decisions and the Employee Retirement Income Security Act." *New England Journal of Medicine,* 2000, *343*(8), 592–596.

16. *New York State Conference of Blue Cross and Blue Shield Plans* v. *Travelers Ins. Co.,* 115 S. Ct. 1671 (1995).

17. Rosenblatt, Law, and Rosenbaum (1997), p. 195; Geyelin, M. "Courts Pierce HMO's Shield Against Lawsuits." *Wall Street Journal,* Apr. 30, 1999, pp. B1, B4; Rosenbaum, S., Frankford, D. M., and Moore, B., "Who Should Determine When Health Care Is Medically Necessary?" *New England Journal of Medicine,* 1999, 340(3), 299–232.

18. *Darling* v. *Charleston Community Memorial Hospital,* 33 Ill. 2d 326, 211 N.E. 2d 253 (1965).

19. U.S. General Accounting Office (GAO). "Medical Malpractice: No Agreement on the Problems or Solutions." (Report to Congressional Requesters; GAO/HRD 86-50.) Washington, D.C.: U.S. General Accounting Office, 1986; Harvard Medical Practice Study. *Patients, Doctors and Lawyers: Medical Injury Malpractice Litigation and Patient Compensation in New York: The Report of the Harvard Medical Practice Study to the State of New York.* New York: New York Health Department, 1990; Sage (1997).

20. Danzon, P. M. *The Frequency and Severity of Medical Malpractice Claims*. (RAND publication R-2870-ICJ/HCFA.) Santa Monica, Calif.: Institute for Civil Justice, RAND, 1982.
21. Danzon, P. M. *Medical Malpractice: Theory, Evidence, and Public Policy*. Cambridge, Mass.: Harvard University Press, 1985; Jacobson, P. D. "Medical Malpractice and the Tort System." *Journal of the American Medical Association*, Dec. 15, 1989, *262*(23), 3320–3327.
22. Danzon (1985).
23. Grad, F. P. "Medical Malpractice and Its Implications for Public Health." in R. Roemer and G. McKay (eds.), *Legal Aspects of Health Policy: Issues and Trends*. Westport, Conn.: Greenwood Press, 1980.
24. Danzon (1985).
25. Halley, M. M. "Tort Law Impact on Health Care." In M. M. Halley, R. J. Fowks, B. C. Bigler, and D. C. Ryan (eds.), *Medical Malpractice Solutions and Proposals for Injury Compensation*. Springfield, Ill.: Thomas, 1989.
26. Danzon (1985).
27. Bigler, E. C. "Medical Professional Liability in the United States." In Halley, Fowks, Bigler, and Ryan (1989).
28. Danzon (1985).
29. Danzon (1982).
30. Rosenbach, M. L., and Stone, A. G. "Malpractice Insurance Costs and Physician Practice, 1981–1986." *Health Affairs*, Winter 1990, *9*, 176–185.
31. Danzon (1985), Preface.
32. Melio, M. M., Studdert, D., and Brennan, T. A. "The New Medical Malpractice Crisis." New England Journal of Medicine, 2003, *348*(23), 2281–2284.
33. Melio, Studdert, and Brennan (2003).
34. Melio, Studdert, and Brennan (2003).
35. Grad (1980); Danzon (1982).
36. Danzon (1982); Jacobson (1989).
37. Bigler (1989).
38. U.S. GAO (1986).
39. Halley, M. M. "Tort Law Impact on Healthcare." In Halley, Fowks, Bigler, and Ryan (1989).
40. Grad (1980).
41. Halley, M. M. "Tort Reform: The Response to Crisis." In Halley, Fowks, Bigler, and Ryan (1989).
42. U.S. GAO (1986).
43. Law, S., and Polan, S. *Pain and Profit: The Politics of Malpractice*. New York: HarperCollins, 1978.
44. Danzon, P. M. *Contingent Fees for Personal Injury Litigation*. (Prepared for Health Care Financing Administration.) Santa Monica, Calif.: U.S. Department of Health, Education, and Welfare, and RAND, 1980.
45. Danzon (1985).
46. OTA (1993).
47. *Roa v. Lodi Medical Group*, 37 Cal. 3d 920, 211 Cal. Rptr. 77, 695 P. 2d 164 (1985).
48. Halley, "Tort Reform . . ." (1989).
49. OTA (1993).
50. Danzon (1985); OTA (1993).
51. Danzon (1985).

52. OTA (1993).

53. U.S. GAO (1986).

54. In incorporating into state law twenty practice guidelines for four specialties (anesthesiology, emergency medicine, obstetrics and gynecology, and radiology), the Maine legislature sought to resolve malpractice claims by eliminating the need to establish the standard of practice and hoped to control health care costs by reducing the incentive to perform unnecessary tests and procedures. See U.S. GAO. *Medical Malpractice: Maine's Use of Practice Guidelines to Reduce Costs.* (GAO/HRD-94-80.) Washington, D.C.: U.S. General Accounting Office, 1993.

55. OTA (1993).

56. OTA (1993).

57. Halley, "Tort Reform . . ." (1989).

58. OTA (1993); Halley, "Tort Reform . . ." (1989).

59. OTA (1993); Halley, "Tort Reform . . ." (1989).

60. Halley, "Tort Reform . . ." (1989).

61. Studdert, Mello, and Brennan (2003).

62. OTA (1993).

63. OTA (1993).

64. OTA (1993).

65. Glaberson, W. "State Courts Sweeping away Laws Curbing Suits for Injury." *New York Times,* July 16, 1999, pp. 1, 13; Glaberson, W. "Looking for Attention with a Billion-Dollar Message." *New York Times,* July 18, 1999, Week in Review, p. 3. See, for example, *Sofie* v. *Fiberboard Corp.,* 112 Wash. 2d 636, 771 P. 2d 711 (Wash. 1989); *Moore* v. *Mobile Infirmary Assign,* 592 So. 2d 156 (Ala. 1991); *Bolton* v. *Deveau,* 1999 N.H. Lexis 338 (New Hampshire Apr. 21, 1999).

66. *Lakin* v. *Senco Products,* 1999 WL 498088, *10,29 (Or., July 15, 1999).

67. Glaberson, W. "Ohio Supreme Court Voids Legal Limits on Damage Suits." *New York Times,* Aug. 17, 1999, p. A9.

68. OTA (1993). See, for example, *Pulliam* v. *Coastal Emergency Services of Richmond,* 357 Va. 1, 509 S.E.2d 307 (1999).

69. *Fein* v. *Permanente Medical Group,* 38 Cal. 3d 137, 695 P. 2d 665, 687 (1985).

70. Sage, W. M. "Medical Liability and Patient Safety." *Health Affairs,* 2003, *23*(4), 27–36; Liang, B. A., and Ren, L. "Medical Liability Insurance and Damage Caps: Getting Beyond Band Aids to Substantive Systems Treatment to Improve Quality and Safety in Healthcare." *American Journal of Law and Medicine,* 2004, *30*(4), 501–541.

71. Thorpe, K. E. "The Medical Malpractice 'Crisis': Recent Trends and the Impact of State Tort Reforms." *Health Affairs,* Jan. 21, 2004, W4-20–W4-30.

72. Poisson, E. S. "Addressing the Impropriety of Statutory Caps on Pain and Suffering: Awards in the Medical Liability System." *N. Carolina Law Review,* 2004, *82*(2) 759–796.

73. Sage (2003), p. 32.

74. Halley, "Tort Reform Law Impact on Health Care" (1989).

75. Halley, "Tort Reform . . ." (1989); Law, S. A. "A Consumer Perspective on Medical Malpractice." *Law and Contemporary Problems,* 1986, *49*(2), 306–320.

76. Halley, "Tort . . ." (1989); OTA (1993).

77. OTA (1993). The six studies analyzed are Adams, E. K., and Zuckerman, S. "Variation in the Growth and Incidence of Medical Malpractice Claims." *Journal of Health Politics, Policy, and Law,* 1984, *9*(3), 475–488; Barker, D. K. "The Effects of Tort Reform on Medical Malpractice Insurance Markets: An Empirical Analysis." *Journal of Health Politics, Pol-*

*icy, and Law,* 1992, *17*(1), 143–161; Blackmon, G., and Zeckhauser, R. "State Tort Reform Legislation: Assessing Our Control of Risks." In P. H. Schuck (ed.), *Tort Law and the Public Interest.* New York: Norton, 1991; Danzon, P. M. "The Frequency and Severity of Medical Malpractice Claims: New Evidence." *Law and Contemporary Problems,* 1986, *49*(2), 57–84; Sloan, F. A., Mergenhagen, P. M., and Bovbjerg, R. R. "Effects of Tort Reforms on the Value of Closed Medical Malpractice Claims: A Microanalysis." *Journal of Health Politics, Policy, and Law,* 1989, *14*(4), 663–689; Zuckerman, S., Bovbjerg, R. R., and Sloan, F. "Effects of Tort Reforms and Other Factors on Medical Malpractice Insurance Premiums." *Inquiry,* 1990, *27*(2), 167–182.

78. Report of the Special Advisory Panel on Medical Malpractice (Jan. 1976), discussed at length in Grad (1980).

79. Thorpe, K. E. "The Medical Malpractice 'Crisis': Recent Travels and the Impact of State Tort Reforms." *Health Affairs,* Jan. 21, 2004, W-20–W4-3.

80. Danzon (1985).

81. Harvard Medical Practice Study (1990).

82. OTA (1993), figure adapted from Posner, J. R. "Trends in Medical Malpractice Insurance, 1970–1985." *Law and Contemporary Problems,* 1986, *49*(2), 37.

83. Public Citizen Health Research Group. *Health Letter,* 2005, 21(6), 12.

84. Halley, "Tort Reform . . ." (1989).

85. Law and Polan (1978).

86. See Metzloff, T. B., Peeples, R. A., and Harris, C. T. "Empirical Perspectives on Mediation and Malpractice." *Law and Contemporary Problems,* 1997, *60*(1), 107; Dauger, E. A., and Marcus, L. J. "Adapting Mediation to Link Resolution of Medical Malpractice Disputes with Health Care Quality Improvement." *Law and Contemporary Problems,* 1997, *60*(1), 185.

87. U.S. GAO (1986); Fowks, R. J. "Arbitration." In Halley, Fowks, Bigler, and Ryan (1989).

88. Ladimer, I., Solomon, J. C., and Mulvihill, M. "Experience in Medical Malpractice Arbitration." *Journal of Legal Medicine,* 1981, *2*(4), 433–470; quote on p. 452.

89. *Engalla* v. *Kaiser Permanente Medical Group,* 938 P. 2d 903 (Cal. 1997).

90. Sage (1997).

91. Sage, W. M., Hastings, K. E., and Berenson, R. A. "Enterprise Liability for Medical Malpractice and Health Care Quality Improvement." *American Journal of Law and Medicine,* 1994, *20*(1 and 2), 1–28; Abraham, K. S., and Weiler, P. S. "Enterprise Medical Liability and the Choice of the Responsible Enterprise." *American Journal of Law and Medicine,* 1994, *20*(1 and 2), 29–36.

92. These arguments are drawn from Sage, Hastings, and Berenson (1994).

93. Sage, Hastings, and Berenson (1994), citing Danzon (1985) and Darling, L. L. "The Applicability of Experience Rating to Medical Malpractice Insurance." (Note.) *Case Western Reserve Law Review,* 1987–88, *38*, 255, 261–265.

94. U.S. Congress, OTA. *Defensive Medicine and Medical Malpractice.* (OTA-H-602.) Washington, D.C.: U.S. Government Printing Office, 1994. See also Sage, Hastings, and Berenson (1994), citing a 1992 study by Lewin-VHI, estimating that malpractice reform might save $25–76 billion in unnecessary tests and procedures over a five-year period. Rubin, R., and Mendelsohn, D. "Estimating the Costs of Defensive Medicine." In Lewin-VHI, Oct. 21, 1992.

95. Sage, Hastings, and Berenson (1994).

96. Sage, W. M. "Enterprise Liability and the Emerging Managed Health Care System." *Law and Contemporary Problems,* 1997, *60*(2), 159–210.

97. Abraham and Weiler (1994).

98. *Aetna* v. *Davila* and *Cogna* v. *Calad*, 124 S. Ct. 2496 (2004).

99. Grad (1980).

100. Mills, D. H. "The Case for and Against Pure No-Fault." In Halley, Fowks, Bigler, and Ryan (1989). The original study is *Report on the Medical Insurance Feasibility Study,* sponsored by California Medical Association and California Hospital Association (D. H. Mills, administrator, editor, and contractor). San Francisco: Sutter, 1977.

101. Mills (1989).

102. OTA (1993); Danzon (1985).

103. Havighurst, C. C., and Tancredi, L. E. "'Medical Adversity Insurance'—a No-Fault Approach to Medical Malpractice and Quality Assurance." *Insurance Law Journal*, Feb. 1974, *613*, 69–97.

104. Tancredi, L. R. "Designated Compensable Events." In Halley, Fowks, Bigler, and Ryan (1989).

105. O'Connell, J. "Neo No-Fault Remedies for Medical Injuries: Coordinated Statutory and Contractual Alternatives." *Law and Contemporary Problems*, 1986, *49*(2), 125–141.

106. O'Connell, J. "Neo No-Fault: Settling for Economic Losses." In Halley, Fowks, Bigler, and Ryan (1989).

107. National Childhood Vaccine Injury Act, P.L. no. 99–660, sec. 311, 100 Stat. 3755, 1986; Grad, F. P. *The Public Health Law Manual* (2nd ed.). Washington, D.C.: American Public Health Association, 1990.

108. Virginia Birth-Related Neurological Injury Compensation Act of 1987, Va. Code Ann., Sec. 38.2-5000-5021 (1993); Institute of Medicine. *Medical Professional Liability and the Delivery of Obstetrical Care. Vol. I and Vol. II: An Interdisciplinary Review.* V. P. Rostow and R. J. Bulger (eds.). (Division of Health Promotion and Disease Prevention, Committee to Study Medical Professional Liability and the Delivery of Obstetrical Care.) Washington, D.C.: National Academy Press, 1989).

109. Institute of Medicine (1989).

110. OTA (1993).

111. Florida Birth-Related Neurological Injury Compensation Act of 1988, Fla. Stat., sec. 766. 303–315 (1994); OTA (1993). For an informative description of the experience with the Virginia and Florida statutes, see "No-Fault Malpractice Reform, An Unproven Rx for Medical Liability." *State Health Notes*, Apr. 4, 1994, pp. 4–5.

112. Bovbjerg, R. R., Sloan, F. A., and Rankin, P. J. "Administrative Performance of 'No-Fault' Compensation for Medical Injury." *Law and Contemporary Problems*, 1997, *60*(2), 71.

113. Bovbjerg, R. R., and Sloan, F. A. "No-Fault for Medical Injury: Theory and Evidence." *University of Cincinnati Law Review,* 1998, *67*(1), 55, 123.

114. Woodhouse, Sir O. "The New Zealand Experience." In Halley, Fowks, Bigler, and Ryan (1989).

115. Woodhouse (1989).

116. U.S. GAO (1986).

117. Woodhouse (1989), p. 179.

118. Brahams, D. "The Swedish and Finnish Patient Insurance Schemes." In Halley, Fowks, Bigler, and Ryan (1989); GAO (1986).

119. Brahams (1989), p. 186.

120. Brahams (1989).

121. Brahams (1989). See also Kokkonen, P. "No-Fault Liability and Patient Insurance: The Finnish Patient Injury Law of 1986." *International Digest of Health Legislation*, 1986, *40*(1), 241–246.

122. Brahams (1989).

123. Kiger, P. J. "The Art of Apology." *Workforce Management*, Oct. 2004, 57–62 [www.workforce.com]; Zimmerman, R., "Doctors' New Tool to Fight Lawsuits: Saying I'm Sorry." *Wall Street Journal*, May 18, 2004, pp. 1, 14.

124. This section is based on four chapters in Halley (1989).

125. Mills (1989), in Halley, Fowks, Bigler, and Ryan (1989).

126. Grad (1980).

127. Liang, B. A., and Ren, L. "Medical Liability Insurance and Damage Caps: Getting Beyond Band-Aids to Substantive Systems Treatment to Improve Quality and Safety in Healthcare." *American Journal of Law and Medicine*, 30(4), 501–541.

128. Lander, L. *Defective Medicine: Risk, Anger, and the Malpractice Crisis.* New York: Farrar, Straus & Giroux, 1978.

129. Bovbjerg, R. R. "Medical Malpractice on Trial: Quality of Care Is the Important Standard." *Law and Contemporary Problems*, 1986, *49*, 321–347.

CHAPTER TWENTY-THREE

# ETHICAL ISSUES IN PUBLIC HEALTH AND HEALTH SERVICES

Pauline Vaillancourt Rosenau
Ruth Roemer

The cardinal principles of medical ethics[1]—autonomy, beneficence, and justice—apply in public health ethics but in somewhat altered form. Personal autonomy and respect for autonomy are guiding principles of public health practice as well as of medical practice. In medical ethics, the concern is with the privacy, individual liberty, freedom of choice, and self-control of the individual. From this principle flows the doctrine of informed consent. In public health ethics, autonomy, the right of privacy, and freedom of action are recognized insofar as they do not result in harm to others. Thus from a public health perspective autonomy may be subordinated to the welfare of others or of society as a whole.[2]

Beneficence, which includes doing no harm, promoting the welfare of others, and doing good, is a principle of medical ethics. In the public health context, beneficence is the overall goal of public health policy and practice. It must be interpreted broadly, in light of societal needs, rather than narrowly, in terms of individual rights.

Justice—whether defined as equality of opportunity, equity of access, or equity in benefits—is the core of public health. Serving the total population, public health is concerned with equity among various social groups, with protecting vulnerable populations, with compensating persons for suffering disadvantage in health and health care, and with surveillance of the total health care system. As expressed in the now-classic phrase of Dr. William H. Foege, "Public health is social justice."[3]

This chapter concerns public health ethics as distinguished from medical ethics. Of course, some overlap exists between public health ethics and medical ethics, but public health ethics, like public health itself, applies generally to issues affecting populations, whereas medical ethics, like medicine itself, applies to individuals. Public health involves a perspective that is population-based, a view of conditions and problems that gives preeminence to the needs of the whole society rather than exclusively to the interests of single individuals.[4]

Public health ethics evokes a number of dilemmas, many of which may be resolved in several ways, depending on one's standards and values. The authors' normative choices are indicated. Data and evidence are relevant to the normative choices involved in public health ethics. We refer the reader to health services research wherever appropriate.

To illustrate the concept of public health ethics, we raise several general questions to be considered in different contexts in this chapter:[5]

- What tensions exist between protection of the public health and protection of individual rights?
- How should scarce resources be allocated and used?
- What should the balance be between expenditures and quality of life in the case of chronic and terminal illness?
- What are appropriate limits on using expensive medical technology?
- What obligations do health care insurers and health care providers have in meeting the right-to-know of patients as consumers?
- What responsibility exists for the young to finance health care for older persons?
- What obligation exists for government to protect the most vulnerable sectors of society?

We cannot give a clear, definitive answer that is universally applicable to any of these questions. Context and circumstance sometimes require qualifying even the most straightforward response. In some cases, differences among groups and individuals may be so great and conditions in society so diverse and complex that no single answer to a question is possible. In other instances, a balance grounded in a public health point of view is viable. Sometimes there is no ethical conflict at all because one solution is optimal for all concerned—for the individual, the practitioner, the payer, and society. For example, few practitioners would want to perform an expensive, painful medical act that was without benefit and might do damage. Few patients would demand it, and even fewer payers would reimburse for it. But in other circumstances, competition for resources poses a dilemma. How does one choose, for example, between a new, effective, but expensive drug of help to only a few, or use of a less-expensive but less-effective drug for a larger number of persons? The necessity for a democratic, open, public debate about rationing in the future seems inevitable.

Even in the absence of agreement on ethical assumptions, and facing diversity and complexity that prohibit easy compromises, we suggest mechanisms for resolving the ethical dilemmas in health care do exist. We explore them in the concluding section of this chapter.

A word of caution: space is short and our topic complex. We cannot explore every dimension of every relevant topic to the satisfaction of all readers. We offer here, instead, an introduction whose goal is to awaken readers—be they practitioners, researchers, students, patients, or consumers—to the ethical dimension of public health. We hope to remind them of the ethical assumptions that underlie their own public health care choices. This chapter, then, is limited to considering selected ethical issues in public health and provision of personal health services. We examine our topic by way of components of the health system: (1) development of health resources, (2) economic support, (3) organization of services, (4) management of services, (5) delivery of care, and (6) assurance of the quality of care.[6]

# Overarching Public Health Principles: Our Assumptions

We argue for these general assumptions of a public health ethic:

- Provision of care on the basis of health need, without regard to race, religion, gender, sexual orientation, or ability to pay
- Equity in distribution of resources, giving due regard to vulnerable groups in the population (ethnic minorities, migrants, children, pregnant women, the poor, the handicapped, and others)
- Respect for human rights—including autonomy, privacy, liberty, health, and well-being—keeping in mind social justice considerations

Central to the solution of ethical problems in health services is the role of law, which sets forth the legislative, regulatory, and judicial controls of society. The development of law in a particular field narrows the discretion of providers in making ethical judgments. At the same time, law sets guidelines for determining policy on specific issues or in individual cases.[7]

## Ethical Issues in Developing Resources

When we talk about developing resources, we mean health personnel, facilities, drugs and equipment, and knowledge. Choices among the kinds of personnel trained, the facilities made available, and the commodities produced are not neutral. Producing and acquiring each of these involve ethical assumptions, and they in turn have public health consequences.

The numbers and kinds of personnel required and their distribution are critical to public health.[8] We need to have an adequate supply of personnel and facilities for a given population in order to meet the ethical requirements of providing health care without discrimination or bias. The proper balance of primary care physicians and specialists is essential to the ethical value of beneficence so as to maximize health status. The ethical imperative of justice requires special measures to protect the economically disadvantaged, such as primary care physicians working in health centers. The imperfect free market mechanisms employed in the United States to date have resulted in far too many specialists relative to generalists. Other modern western countries have achieved some balance, but this has involved closely controlling medical school enrollments and residency programs.

At the same time, the ethical principle of autonomy urges that resource development also be diverse enough to permit consumers some choice of providers and facilities. Absence of choice is a form of coercion. It also reflects an inadequate supply. But it results, as well, from the absence of a range of personnel. Patients should have some freedom—though not unlimited—to choose the type of care they prefer. Midwives, chiropractors, and other effective and proven practitioners should be available if health resources permit it without sacrificing other ethical considerations. The ethical principle of autonomy here might conflict with that of equity, which would limit general access to specialists in the interest of better distribution of health care access to the whole population. The need for ample public health personnel is another ethical priority, necessary for the freedom of all individuals to enjoy a healthful, disease-free environment.

Physician assistants and nurses are needed, and they may serve an expanded role, substituting for primary care providers in some instances to alleviate the shortage of primary care physicians, especially in underserved areas. But too great a reliance on these providers might diminish quality of care if they are required to substitute entirely for physicians, particularly with respect to differential diagnosis.[9] The point of service is also a significant consideration. For example, effective and expanded health care and dental care for children could be achieved by employing the school as a geographic point for monitoring and providing selected services.

Health personnel are not passive commodities, and freedom of individual career choice may conflict with public health needs. Here autonomy of the individual must be balanced with social justice and beneficence. In the past, the individual's decision to become a medical specialist took precedence over society's need for more generalists. A public health ethic appeals to the social justice involved and considers the impact on the population. A balance between individual choice and society's needs is being achieved today by restructuring financial compensation for primary care providers.

Similarly, in the United States an individual medical provider's free choice as to where to practice medicine has resulted in underserved areas, and ways to develop and train health personnel for rural and central city areas are a public health priority. About 20 percent of the U.S. population lives in rural communities, and four in ten do not have adequate access to health care. Progress has been made in the complex problem of ensuring rural health clinics, but providing for the health care of rural America remains a problem. It challenges efforts at health care reform as well.[10] Foreign medical graduates are commonly employed in underserved urban centers and rural areas in the United States today, but this raises other ethics questions. Is it just to deprive the citizens of the country of origin of these practitioners of their services?[11]

An important issue in educating health professionals is the need to ensure racial and ethnic diversity in both the training and practice of health professionals. A series of court decisions and state initiatives have, with one exception, seriously limited admissions of minority students to professional schools.

In 1978, the U.S. Supreme Court in the *Bakke* case invalidated a quota system in admissions to medical schools but provided that race could be considered as one factor among various criteria for admission.[12] In 1996, the Court of Appeals for the Fifth Circuit in the *Hopwood* case, in considering admission policies for the University of Texas Law School, held unconstitutional a preference based on race.[13] In 2003, the U.S. Supreme Court made a sharp turn and in two cases involving affirmative action policies at the University of Michigan upheld an individualized policy of admission to the law school but struck down an undergraduate admission policy based on a point system. It held that the law school had a compelling interest in attaining a diverse student body and that its affirmative action policies were legally sound as evaluating each candidate as an individual.[14] At the same time, the court invalidated the undergraduate admission policy as not providing for individualized consideration of each candidate.[15]

The ethical issues of beneficence and justice involved in these decisions also plague initiatives at the state level. In California, Proposition 209, passed in 1996, banned consideration of race, gender, or national origin in hiring and school admissions. In the state of Washington, Initiative 200, adopted by the voters in 1998, eliminated all preferential treatment based on race or gender in government hiring and school admissions. In Florida, the governor's cabinet enacted in 2000 the "One Florida" program, which ended consideration of race in university admissions and state contracts.[16] These state actions have significant ethical effects on the health system and underserved communities. They contribute to a shortage of physicians in minority communities, and they deny many minority candidates admission to medical school.[17]

Similar ethical public health dilemmas are confronted with respect to health facilities. From a public health point of view, the need for equitable access to quality institutions and for fair distribution of health care facilities takes priority over an individual real estate developer's ends or the preferences of for-profit hospital owners. Offering a range of facilities to maximize choice suggests the need for both public and private hospitals, community clinics and health centers, and in-patient and outpatient mental health facilities, as well as long-term care facilities and hospices. At the same time, not-for-profit providers, on several performance variables, do a better job than the for-profit institutions. Overall, studies since 1980 suggest that nonprofit providers outperform for-profit providers on cost, quality, access, and charity care.[18] For example, the medical loss ratio is much higher in nonprofit health care providers compared to for-profit health care providers. The higher the medical loss ratio, the greater the proportion of revenue received that goes for health care, rather than administration and management. In 1995, for example, Kaiser Foundation Health Plan in California "devoted 96.8 percent of its revenue to health care and retained only 3.2 percent for administration and income."[19] Nonprofits have lower disenrollment rates,[20] offer more community benefits,[21] and feature more preventive services[22] too. How long this can continue to be the case in the highly competitive health care market is unknown because not-for-profits may have to adopt for-profit business practices to survive.[23]

The financial crisis facing public hospitals throughout the nation poses an ethical problem of major proportions. At stake is the survival of facilities that handle an enormous volume of care for the poor, that train a large number of physicians and other health personnel, and that make available specialized services—trauma care, burn units, and others—for the total urban and rural populations they serve.

Research serves a public health purpose too. It has advanced medical technology, and its benefits in new and improved products should be accessible to all members of society. Public health ethics also focuses on the importance of research in assessing health system performance, including equity of access and medical outcomes. Only if what works and is medically effective can be distinguished from what does not work and what is medically ineffective are public health interests best served. Health care resources need to be used wisely and not wasted. Health services research can help ensure this goal. This is especially important in an era in which market competition appears, directly or indirectly, to be having a negative influence on research capacity.[24]

Research is central to developing public health resources. Equity mandates a fair distribution of research resources among the various diseases that affect the public's health because research is costly, resources are limited, and choices have to be made. Research needs both basic and applied orientation to ensure quality. There is a need for research on matters that have been neglected in the past,[25] as has been recognized in the field of women's health. Correction of other gross inequities in allocating research funds is urgent. Recent reports indicate that younger scientists are not sufficiently consulted in the peer review process, and they do not receive their share of research funds. Ethical implications involving privacy, informed consent, and equity affect targeted research grants for AIDS, breast cancer, and other special diseases. The legal and ethical issues in the human genome project, and now stem cell research, involve matters of broad scope—wide use of genetic screening, information control, privacy, and possible manipulation of human characteristics. It is no surprise that Annas has called for "taking ethics seriously."[26]

Federal law in the United States governs conduct of biomedical research involving human subjects. Ethical issues are handled by ethics advisory boards, convened to advise the Department of Health and Human Services on the ethics of biomedical or behavioral research projects, and by institutional review boards of research institutions seeking funding of research proposals. Both kinds of board are charged with responsibility for reviewing clinical research proposals and for ensuring that the legal and ethical rights of human subjects are protected.[27] Finding researchers to serve on IRBs is a growing problem because about half of all researchers have serious conflicts of interest from serving as industry consultants.[28]

An overarching problem is the conflict of interest of scientists who are judging the effectiveness of treatments and drugs and may be, at the same time, employed by or serving as consultants to a pharmaceutical or biotechnology firm. In 2005, several scientists at the National Institutes of Health resigned in the wake of a new regulation banning NIH scientists from accepting funding from pharmaceutical firms.[29]

Among the principal concerns of these boards is assurance of fully informed and unencumbered consent, by patients competent to give it, in order to secure the autonomy of subjects. They are also concerned with protecting the privacy of human subjects and the confidentiality of their relation to the project. An important legal and ethical duty of researchers, in the event that a randomized clinical trial proves beneficial to health, is to terminate the trial immediately and make the benefits available to the control group and to the treated group alike.

The ethical principles that should govern biomedical research involving human subjects are a high priority, but criticism has been leveled at the operation of some institutional review boards. Some say they lack objectivity and are overly identified with the interests of the researcher and the institution. Recommendations to correct this type of problem include appointing patient and consumer advocates to review boards, in addition to physicians and others affiliated with the institution and along with the sole lawyer who is generally a member of the review board; having consumer advocates involved early in drawing up protocols for the research; having third parties interview patients after they have given their consent to make sure that they understood the research and their choices; requiring the institution to include research in its quality assurance monitoring; and establishing a national human experimentation board to oversee the four thousand institutional review boards in the country.[30] Others say the pendulum has moved in the other direction and that IRBs excessively limit researchers' ability to do their studies, and that they increase the cost of research, perhaps making it impossible to carry it out at all in some cases.

Correction of fraud in science and the rights of subjects are important ethical considerations in developing knowledge. Ethical conflict between the role of the physician as caregiver and as researcher is not uncommon inasmuch as what is good for the research project is not always what is good for the patient. Certainly, in some instances society stands to benefit at the expense of the research subject, but respect for the basic worth of the individual means that he or she has a right to be informed before agreeing to participate in an experiment. Only when consent is informed, clear, and freely given can altruism, for the sake of advancing science and humanity, be authentic.

Policy makers concerned with developing resources for health care thus confront tensions between protecting public health and protecting the rights of individual patients and providers. They face issues concerning allocation of scarce resources and use of expensive medical technology. We trust that in resolving these issues their decisions are guided by principles of autonomy, beneficence, and justice as applied to the health of populations.

## Ethical Issues in Economic Support

Nowhere is the public health ethical perspective clearer than on issues of economic support. Personal autonomy and respect for privacy remain essential, as does beneficence. But a public health orientation suggests that the welfare of society merits close regard for justice. It is imperative that everyone in the population have equitable access to health care services with dignity, so as not to discourage necessary utilization; in most cases, this means universal health insurance coverage. Forty-five million Americans lack health insurance, which makes for poorer medical outcomes even though individuals without health insurance do receive care in hospital emergency rooms and community clinics. Most of the uninsured are workers in small enterprises whose employers do not offer health insurance for their workers or dependents.[31] The uninsured are predicted to rise to 56 million, or by 27.8 percent, by 2013.[32] The Institute of Medicine has conducted an up-to-date and thorough analysis of the scope of uninsurance and underinsurance in America.[33] The underinsured, those with coverage that is not sufficient and leaves bills that the individual cannot pay, are also on the rise. This happens when employers shift health insurance costs to employees with greater deductibles and co-pays, for example.[34]

From a public health perspective, financial barriers to essential health care are inappropriate. Yet they exist to a surprising degree. Witness the fact that the cost reached $5,670 per person in the United States in 2003.[35] If each and every human being is to develop to his or her full potential, to participate fully as a productive citizen in our democratic society, then preventive health services and alleviation of pain and suffering due to health conditions that can be effectively treated must be available without financial barriers. Removing economic barriers to health services does not mean that the difference in health status between rich and poor will disappear. But it is a necessary (if not sufficient) condition for this goal.

Economic disparity in society is a public health ethical issue related to justice. Increasing evidence suggests that inequality in terms of income differences between the rich and the poor has a large impact on a population's health.[36] This may be due to psychosocial factors,[37] or a weakened societal social fabric,[38] or loss of social capital,[39] or a range of other factors.[40] Whatever the cause, "income inequality, together with limited access to health care, has serious consequences for the working poor."[41]

From a public health point of view, the economic resources to support health services should be fair and equitable. Any individual's contribution should be progressive, based on ability to pay. This is especially important because the rise of managed care has made it increasingly difficult to provide charity care.[42] This may be because of funding restrictions for a defined population. Although some individual contribution is appropriate—no matter how small—as a gesture of commitment to the larger community, it is also ethically befitting for the nation to take responsibility for a portion of the cost. The exact proportion may vary across nation and time, depending on the country's wealth and the public priority attributed to health services.[43]

Similarly, justice and equity suggest the importance of the ethical principle of social solidarity in any number of forms.[44] By definition, social insurance means that there is wisdom in assigning responsibility for payment by those who are young and working to support the health care of children and older people no longer completely independent. A public health orientation suggests that social solidarity forward and backward in time, across generations, is ethically persuasive. Those in the most productive stages of the life cycle today were once dependent children, and they are likely one day to be dependent older persons.

Institutions such as Social Security and Medicare play a moral role in a democracy. They were established to attain common aims and are fair in that they follow agreed-on rules.[45] Proposals to privatize them undermine these goals. Financing of the Social Security system in part by individual investment accounts, favored by the Bush administration, carries serious risks in case of market failure and certainly does not ensure the subsidy for low-income workers contained in the current government system. With respect to Medicare, the Bush administration's support of a voucher system enabling the beneficiary to buy private insurance will induce the healthy and affluent elderly to opt out of Medicare, leaving Medicare as a welfare program for the sick and the poor. With less income, Medicare will be forced to cut services.

Social solidarity between the young and the elderly is critical. As members of a society made up of overlapping communities, we find our lives intricately linked together. No man or woman is an island; not even the wealthiest or most "independent" can exist alone. The social pact that binds us to live in peace together requires cooperation of such a fundamental nature that we could not travel by car (assuming respect for traffic signals) to the grocery store to purchase food (or assume it is safe for consumption) without appealing to social solidarity. These lessons apply to health care as well.

In 1983, the President's Commission for the Study of Ethical Problems in Medicine and Biomedical and Behavioral Research made as its first and principal recommendation on ethics in medicine that society has an obligation to ensure equitable access to health care for all its citizens.[46] Equitable access, the commission said, requires that all citizens be able to secure an adequate level of care without excessive burden. Implementation of this principle as an ethical imperative is even more urgent all these years later, as an increasing number of people become uninsured and as the price of pharmaceuticals rises dramatically.[47]

## Ethical Issues in Organization of Services

The principal ethical imperative in organization of health services is that services be organized and distributed in accordance with health needs and the ability to benefit. The problem with rationing on the basis of ability to pay is that it encourages the opposite.[48] Issues of geographic and cultural access also illustrate this ethical principle.

To be fair and just, a health system must minimize geographic inequity in distributing care. Rural areas are underserved, as are inner cities. Any number of solutions have been proposed and tried to bring better access in health services to underserved areas. They include mandating a period of service for medical graduates as a condition of licensure, loan forgiveness and expansion of the National Health Service Corps, rural preceptorships, creating economic incentives for establishing a practice in a rural area, and employing physician assistants and nurse practitioners.[49] Telemedicine may make the best medical consultants available to rural areas in the near future,[50] but the technology involves initial start-up costs that are not trivial. Higher Medicare payments to rural hospitals also ensure that they will remain open.[51]

Similarly, the principles of autonomy and beneficence require health services to be culturally relevant to the populations they are designed to serve.[52] This means that medical care professionals need to be able to communicate in the language of those they serve and to understand the cultural preferences of those for whom they seek to furnish care.[53] The probability of success is enhanced if needed health professionals are from the same cultural background as those they serve. This suggests that schools of medicine, nursing, dentistry, and public health should intensify their efforts to reach out and extend educational and training opportunities to qualified and interested members of such populations. To carry out such programs, however, these schools must have the economic resources required to offer fellowships and teaching assistant positions.

The development of various forms of managed care—health maintenance organizations, prepaid group practices, preferred provider organizations, and independent practice associations—raises another set of ethical questions. As experienced in the United States in recent years, managed care is designed more to minimize costs than to ensure that health care is efficient and effective. If managed care ends up constraining costs by depriving individuals of needed medical attention (reducing medically appropriate access to specialists, for instance), then it violates the ethical principle of beneficence because such management interferes with doing good for the patient.[54] If managed care is employed as a cost-containment scheme for Medicaid and Medicare without regard to quality of care, it risks increasing inequity. It could even contribute to a two-tiered health care system in which those who can avoid various forms of managed care by paying privately for their personal health services obtain higher-quality care.

Historically, the advantages of staff-model managed care are clear: team practice, emphasis on primary care, generous use of diagnostic and therapeutic outpatient services, and prudent use of hospitalization. All contribute to cost containment. At the same time, managed care systems have the disadvantage of restricted choice of provider. Today's for-profit managed care companies run the risk of underserving; they may achieve cost containment through cost shifting and risk selection.[55]

The ethical issues in the relationships among physicians, patients, and managed care organizations include denial of care, restricted referral to specialists, and gag rules that bar physicians from telling patients about alternative treatments (which may not be covered by the plan) or from discussing financial arrangements between the physician and the plan (which may include incentives for cost containment).[56] Requiring public disclosure of information about these matters has been proposed as a solution, but there is little evidence that disclosure helps the poor and illiterate choose a better health plan or a less-conflicted health care provider.

The ethical issues in managed care are illustrated most sharply by the question of who decides what is medically necessary: the physician or others, the disease management program, the insurer, the employer, or the state legislature.[57]

This question is not unique to managed care; it has also arisen with respect to insurance companies and Medicaid.[58] On the one hand, the physician has a legal and ethical duty to adhere to the standard of care that any reasonable physician in similar circumstances would employ. On the other hand, insurers have traditionally specified what is covered or not covered as medically necessary in insurance contracts. The courts have sometimes reached contrasting results, depending on the facts of the case, the character of the treatment sought (whether generally accepted or experimental), and the interpretation of medical necessity. With the rise of managed care, the problem becomes an ethical dilemma because, as even those highly favorable to managed care agree, there is a risk of too little health care.[59]

Malpractice suits against managed care organizations in self-insured plans are barred by the provision in the Employee Retirement Income Security Act that preempts or supersedes "any and all state laws insofar as they may now or hereafter relate to any employee benefit plan."[60] As a result of the preemption, employees covered by such plans are limited to the relief provided by ERISA—only the cost of medical care denied—with no compensation for lost wages and pain and suffering.[61] Self-insured health insurance plans that cause injury by denying care or providing substandard care have immunity from suit in state courts because of legal interpretation of ERISA by the U.S. Supreme Court. In view of the fact that 140 million people receive their health care through plans sponsored by employers and covered by ERISA, it is a serious matter of equity to bar them from access to the state courts for medical malpractice.[62]

In June 2004, the Supreme Court "immunized" employer-sponsored health plans against damage suits for wrongful denial of coverage. It thus voided laws that allowed such suits in ten states. This means that the legal risk to health plans for denying coverage will be reduced. The poor will be the greatest losers because they cannot afford to fight such denials through the currently available reviews mandated in forty states. This law is also likely to make for higher malpractice claims as physicians and hospital do not have legal shelter from responsibility.[63]

As more and more integrated health care delivery systems are formed, as more mergers of managed care organizations occur, as pressure for cost containment increases, ethical issues concerning conflict of interest, quality of care choices, and patients' rights attain increasing importance. The principles of autonomy, beneficence, and justice are severely tested in resolving the ethical problems facing a complex, corporate health care system.

If medicine is "for profit," as seems to be the case today and for the near future in the United States, then the ethical dilemma between patients' interests and profits will be a continuing problem.[64] Sometimes the two can both be served, but it is unlikely to be the case in all instances. Surveys of business "executives admit and point out the presence of numerous generally accepted practices in their industry which they consider unethical."[65] As Fisher and Welch conclude, "Stakeholders in the increasingly market-driven U.S. health care system have few incentives to explore the harms of the technologies from which they stand to profit."[66] That both consumers and employers are concerned about quality of care is clear from Paul Ellwood's statement expressing disappointment in the evolution of HMOs because "they tend to place too much emphasis on saving money and not enough on improving quality—and we now have the technical skill to do that."[67]

## Ethical Issues in Management of Health Services

Management involves planning, administration, regulation, and legislation. The style of management depends on the values and norms of the population. Planning involves determining the population's health needs (with surveys and research, for example) and then ensuring that programs are in place to supply these services. A public health perspective suggests that planning is appropriate to the extent that it makes available efficient, appropriate health care (beneficence) to all who seek it (equity and justice). Planning may avoid waste and contribute to rational use of health services. But it is also important that planning not be so invasive as to be coercive and deny the individual any say in his or her health care, unless such intervention is necessary to protect public health interests. The ethical principle of autonomy preserves the right of the individual to refuse care, to determine his or her own destiny, especially when the welfare of others is not involved. A balance between individual autonomy and public health intervention that affords benefit to society is not easy to achieve. But in some cases the resolution of such a dilemma is clear, as with mandatory immunization programs. Equity and beneficence demand that the social burdens and benefits of living in a disease-free environment be shared. Therefore, for example, immunization requirements should cover all those potentially affected.

Health administration has ethical consequences that may be overlooked because they appear ethically neutral: organization, staffing, budgeting, supervision, consultation, procurement, logistics, records and reporting, coordination, and evaluation.[68] But all these activities involve ethical choices. Faced with a profit squeeze, the managed care industry is pressuring providers to reduce costs and services.[69] The result has been downsizing, which means more unlicensed personnel are hired to substitute for nurses.[70] California is the first state to mandate nurse-to-patient staffing ratios.[71] Surveys of doctors suggest patients do not always get needed care from HMOs.[72] Denial of appropriate needed health care is an ethical problem related to beneficence. In addition, the importance of privacy in record-keeping (to take an example) raises once again the necessity to balance the ethical principles of autonomy and individual rights with social justice and protection of society.[73]

Distribution of scarce health resources is another subject of debate. The principle of first come, first served may initially seem equitable. But it also incorporates the "rule of rescue," whereby a few lives are saved at great cost, and this policy results in the "invisible" loss of many more lives. Cost-benefit or cost-effectiveness analysis of health economics attempts to apply hard data to administrative decisions. This approach, however, does not escape ethical dilemmas either, because the act of assigning numbers to years of life, for example, is itself value-laden. If administrative allocation is determined on the basis of the number of years of life saved, then the younger are favored over the older, which may or may not be equitable. If one factors into such an analysis the idea of "quality" years of life, other normative assumptions must be made as to how important quality is and what constitutes quality. Some efforts have been made to assign a dollar value to a year of life as a tool for administering health resources. But here too, we encounter worrisome normative problems. Does ability to pay deform such calculations?[74]

Crucial to management of health services are legal tools—legislation, regulations, and sometimes litigation—necessary for fair administration of programs. Legislation and regulations are essential for authorizing health programs; they also serve to remedy inequity and to introduce innovation into a health service system. Effective legislation depends on a sound scientific base, and ethical questions are especially troubling when the scientific evidence is uncertain.

For example, in a landmark decision in 1976, the Court of Appeals for the District of Columbia upheld a regulation of the Environmental Protection Agency restricting the amount of lead additives in gasoline largely on the basis of epidemiological evidence.[75] Analysis of this case and of the scope of judicial review of the regulatory action of an agency charged by Congress with regulating substances harmful to health underlines the dilemma the court faced: the need of judges trained in the law, not in science, to evaluate the scientific and epidemiological evidence on which the regulatory agency based its ruling.[76] The majority of the court based its upholding of the agency's decision on its own review of the evidence. By contrast, Judge David Bazelon urged an alternative approach: "In cases of great technological complexity, the best way for courts to guard against unreasonable or erroneous administrative decisions is not for the judges themselves to scrutinize the technical merits of each decision. Rather, it is to establish a decision making process that assures a reasoned decision that can be held up to the scrutiny of the scientific community and the public."[77]

The dilemma of conflicting scientific evidence is a persistent ethical minefield, as reflected by a 1993 decision of the U.S. Supreme Court involving the question of how widely accepted a scientific process or theory must be before it qualifies as admissible evidence in a lawsuit. The case involved the issue of whether a drug prescribed for nausea during pregnancy, Bendectin, causes birth defects. Rejecting the test of "general acceptance" of scientific evidence as the absolute prerequisite for admissibility, as applied in the past, the Court ruled that trial judges serve as gatekeepers to ensure that pertinent scientific evidence is not only relevant but reliable. The Court also suggested various factors that might bear on such determinations.[78]

It is significant for the determination of ethical issues in cases where the scientific evidence is uncertain that epidemiological evidence—which is the core of public health—is increasingly recognized as helpful in legal suits.[79] Of course, it should be noted that a court's (or an agency's) refusal to act because of uncertain scientific evidence is in itself a decision with ethical implications.

Enactment of legislation and issuance of regulations are important for management of a just health care system, but these strategies are useless if they are not enforced. For example, state legislation has long banned the sale of cigarettes to minors, but only recently have efforts been made to enforce these statutes rigorously through publicity, "stings" (arranged purchases by minors), and penalties on sellers, threats of license revocation, denial of federal funds under the Synar Amendment, and banning cigarette sales from vending machines.[80] A novel case of enforcement involves a Baltimore ordinance prohibiting billboards promoting cigarettes in areas where children live, recreate, and go to school, enacted in order to enforce a law banning tobacco sales to minors. The Baltimore ordinance has not been overturned despite the fact that a Massachusetts regulation restricting advertising of tobacco and alcohol near schools was struck down as unconstitutional by the U.S. Supreme Court on the ground of preemption.[81]

Thus management of health services involves issues of allocating scarce resources, evaluating scientific evidence, measuring quality of life, and imposing mandates by legislation and regulation. Although a seemingly neutral function, management of health services must rely on principles of autonomy, beneficence, and justice in its decision-making process.

## Ethical Issues in Delivery of Care

Delivery of health services—actual provision of health care services—is the end point of all the other dimensions just discussed. The ethical considerations of only a few of the many issues pertinent to delivery of care are explored here.

Resource allocation in a time of cost containment inevitably involves rationing. At first blush, rationing by ability to pay may appear natural, neutral, and inevitable, but the ethical dimensions for delivery of care may be overlooked. If ability to pay is recognized as a form of rationing, the question of its justice is immediately apparent. The Oregon Medicaid program (Oregon Health Plan) is another example. It is equitable by design and grounded in good part in the efficacy of the medical procedure in question, thus respecting the principle of ethical beneficence. It is structured to extend benefits to a wider population of poor people than those entitled to care under Medicaid. It has been tested for more than ten years in its effort to establish a basic level of care deemed effective and appropriate without overtreatment. The Prioritized List of Health Services continues to be reevaluated and updated in light of new evidence by the Health Services Commission of the Department of Administrative Services' Office for Oregon Health Policy and Research. But the legislature, starting in 2004, was required to reduce benefits as Oregon's economy suffered serious setbacks.[82]

From the start the plan did not qualify as equitable, however, because it did not apply to the whole population of Oregon, but only to those on Medicaid. It denied some services to some people on Medicaid in order to widen the pool of beneficiaries. It has therefore not resolved all the ethical problems in this respect.[83]

Rationing medical care is not always ethically dubious; rather, it may conform to a public health ethic. In some cases, too much medical care is counterproductive and may produce more harm than good. Canada, Sweden, the United Kingdom, and the state of Oregon, among others, have rationing of one sort or another.[84] For example, Canada rations health care, pays one-third less per person than the United States, and offers universal coverage; yet health status indicators do not suggest that Canadians suffer. In fact, on several performance indicators Canada surpasses the United States.[85] Were there better information about medical outcomes and the efficacy of many medical procedures, rationing would actually benefit patients if it discouraged the unneeded and inappropriate treatment that plagues the U.S. health system.[86]

Rationing organ transplants, similarly, is a matter of significant ethical debate because fewer organs are available for transplant than needed for the eighty-five thousand people on waiting lists. Rationing must therefore be used to determine who is given a transplant. Employing tissue match makes medical sense and also seems ethically acceptable. But to the extent that ability to pay is a criterion, ethical conflict is inevitable. It may, in fact, go against scientific opinion and public health ethics if someone who can pay receives a transplant even though the tissue match is not so good as it would be for a patient who is also in need of a transplant but unable to pay the cost. Rationing on this basis seems ethically unfair and medically ill advised. It is no surprise, then, that the National Organ Transplant Act, adopted in 1984, made it illegal to offer or receive payment for organ transplantation. Yet the sale of organs for transplantation still exists. It has even been advocated as a market-friendly, for-profit solution to the current supply problems.[87]

One solution would be to make more organs available through mandatory donation from fatal automobile accidents, without explicit consent of individuals and families. A number of societies have adopted this policy of presumed consent because the public health interest of society and the seriousness of the consequences are so great for those in need of a transplant that it is possible to justify ignoring the individual autonomy (preferences) of the accident victim's friends and relatives. Spain leads other nations regarding organ donation with 33.8 donors per million in 2003 by interpreting an absence of prohibition to constitute a near-death patient's implicit authorization for organ transplantation.[88] This has not been the case in the United States to date.[89]

Delivery of services raises conflict-of-interest questions for providers that are of substantial public health importance. Criminal prosecution of fraud in the health care sector increased threefold between 1993 and 1997.[90] In today's market-driven health system, about half of all doctors report that they have "exaggerated the severity of a patient's condition to get them care they think is medically necessary."[91] Hospitals pressed by competitive forces strain to survive and in some cases do so only by less-than-honest cost shifting—or even direct fraud. A recent survey of hospital bills found that more than 99 percent included "mistakes" that favored the hospital.[92]

Class action suits claim that HMOs are guilty of deceiving patients because they refuse to reveal financial incentives in physician payment structures.[93] Physicians have been found to refer patients to laboratories and medical testing facilities that they co-own to a far greater extent than can be medically justified.[94] As the trend to make medicine a business develops, the AMA's Council on Ethical and Judicial Affairs has adopted guidelines for the sale of nonprescription, health-related products in physicians' offices, but problems remain.[95] The purpose is to "help protect patients and maintain physicians' professionalism."[96] The public health ethic of beneficence is called into question by unnecessary products and inappropriate medical tests.

The practice of medicine and public health screening presents serious ethical dilemmas. Screening for diseases for which there is no treatment, except where such information can be used to postpone onset or prevent widespread population infection, is difficult to justify unless the information is explicitly desired by the patient for personal reasons (life planning and reproduction). In a similar case, screening without provision to treat those discovered to be in need of treatment is unethical. Public health providers need to be sure in advance that they can offer the health services required to care for those found to be affected. These are the ethical principles of beneficence and social justice.

The tragic epidemic of HIV/AIDS has raised serious ethical questions concerning testing, reporting, and partner notification. The great weight of authority favors voluntary and confidential testing, so as to encourage people to come forward for testing, counseling, and behavior change.[97] A study by the U.S. Centers for Disease Control and Prevention (CDC) concludes that confidential name-based reporting of HIV has not deterred testing and treatment.[98] Nevertheless, concern about violation of privacy and possible deterrence of testing and treatment with confidential name-based reporting of HIV persists.

This issue raises sharply the ethical conflict between the individual's right to confidentiality and the needs of public health. Some guidance for resolving ethical questions in this difficult sphere is presented by Stephen Joseph, former commissioner of health for New York City, who states that the AIDS epidemic is a public health emergency involving extraordinary civil liberties issues—not a civil liberties emergency involving extraordinary public health issues.[99]

Partner notification was at first generally disapproved on grounds of nonfeasibility and protection of privacy, but in accordance with CDC guidelines some states have enacted legislation permitting a physician or public health department to notify a partner that a patient is HIV-positive if the physician believes that the patient will not inform the partner.[100]

With the finding that administration of AZT during pregnancy to an HIV-positive woman reduces the risk of transmission of the virus to the infant dramatically, CDC recommends that all pregnant women be offered HIV testing as early in pregnancy as possible because of the available treatments for reducing the likelihood of perinatal transmission and maintaining the health of the woman. CDC also recommends that women should be counseled about their options regarding pregnancy by a method similar to genetic counseling.[101]

The field of reproductive health is a major public health concern, affecting women in their reproductive years. Here the principles of autonomy, beneficence, and justice apply to providing contraceptive services, including long-acting means of contraception, surgical abortion, medical abortion (made possible by development of Mifepristone), sterilization, and use of noncoital technologies for reproduction. The debate on these issues has been wide, abrasive, and divisive. Thirty-two years after abortion was legalized by the U.S. Supreme Court's decision in *Roe* v. *Wade*,[102] protests against abortion clinics have escalated. Violence against clinics and murders of abortion providers threaten access to abortion services and put the legal right to choose to terminate an unwanted pregnancy in jeopardy. The shortage of abortion providers in some states and in many rural areas restricts reproductive health services. The mergers of Catholic hospitals with secular institutions and the insistence that the merged hospital be governed by the Ethical and Religious Directives for Catholic Health Care Services means that not only abortion services are eliminated but also other contraceptive and counseling services (except for "natural family planning"), sterilization procedures, infertility treatments, and emergency postcoital contraception (even for rape victims).[103] The Food and Drug Administration's refusal to approve over-the-counter sales of emergency contraception, despite the approval of two scientific committees, is a particularly troubling ethical decision.

We state our position as strongly favoring the prochoice point of view in order to ensure autonomy of women, beneficence for women and their families faced with unwanted pregnancy, and justice in society. In the highly charged debate on teenage pregnancy, we believe that social realities, the well-being of young women and their children, and the welfare of society mandate access to contraception and abortion and respect for the autonomy of young people. The ethics of parental consent and notification laws, which often stand as a barrier to abortions needed and wanted by adolescents, is highly questionable. Economists estimate the cost of such laws to be around $150 million in Texas alone.[104]

Many other important ethical issues in delivering health care have not been discussed extensively in this chapter because of space limitations. There are three such issues that we want to mention briefly.

First, the end-of-life debate is generally considered a matter of medical ethics involving the patient, his or her family, and the physician. But this issue is also a matter of public health ethics because services at the end of life entail administrative and financial dimensions that are part of public health and management of health services. The Terri Schiavo case is an example where the potential alternative use of societal resources brings to mind the contradictions involved in end-of-life issues.[105]

Second, in the field of mental health, the conflict between the health needs and legal rights of patients on the one hand and the need for protection of society on the other illustrates sharply the ethical problems facing providers of mental health services. This conflict has been addressed most prominently by reform of state mental hospital admission laws to make involuntary admission to a mental hospital initially a medical matter, with immediate and periodic judicial review as to the propriety of hospitalization—review in which a patient advocate participates.[106] The Tarasoff case presents another problem in providing mental health services: the duty of a psychiatrist or psychologist to warn an identified person of a patient's intent to kill the person, despite the rule of confidentiality governing medical and psychiatric practice.[107] In both instances, a public health perspective favors protection of society as against the legal rights of individuals.

Third, basic to public health strategies and effective delivery of preventive and curative services are records and statistics. The moral and legal imperative of privacy to protect an individual's medical record gives way to public health statutes requiring reporting of gunshot wounds, communicable diseases, child abuse, and AIDS.[108] More generally, the right to keep one's medical records confidential conflicts with society's need for epidemiological information to monitor the incidence and prevalence of diseases in the community and to determine responses to this information. At the same time, it is essential, for example, that an individual's medical records be protected from abuse by employers, marketers, and so on.[109] A common resolution of this problem is to make statistics available without identifying information.

Congress adopted HIPAA (the Health Insurance Portability and Accountability Act) in 1996 to protect the privacy of medical records. Only in 2003 did these aspects of the law take effect. HIPAA limits who may see medical records, how the records are stored, and even how they are disposed of when no longer needed. Compliance costs have been enormous.[110]

## Ethical Issues in Ensuring Quality of Care

If a public health ethic requires fair and equitable distribution of medical care, then it is essential that waste and inefficiency be eliminated. Spending scarce resources on useless medical acts is a violation of a public health ethic.[111] To reach this public health goal, knowledge about what is useful and medically efficacious is essential.

As strategies for evaluating the quality of health care become increasingly important, the ethical dimensions of peer review, practice guidelines, report cards, and malpractice suits—all methods of quality assurance—come to the fore. Established in 1972 to monitor hospital services under Medicare to ensure that they were "medically necessary" and delivered in the most efficient manner, professional standards review organizations came under attack as overregulatory and too restrictive.[112] Congress ignored the criticism and in 1982 passed the Peer Review Improvement Act, which did not abolish outside review but consolidated the local peer review agencies, replaced them with statewide bodies, and increased their responsibility.[113] In 1986, Congress passed the Health Care Quality Improvement Act, which established national standards for peer review at the state and hospital levels for all practitioners regardless of source of payment.[114] The act also established a national data bank on the qualifications of physicians and provided immunity from suit for reviewing physicians acting in good faith.

The functions of peer review organizations (PROs) in reviewing the adequacy and quality of care necessarily involve some invasion of the patient's privacy and the physician's confidential relationship with his or her patient. Yet beneficence and justice in an ethical system of medical care mandate a process that controls the cost and quality of care. Finding an accommodation between protection of privacy and confidentiality on the one hand and necessary but limited disclosure on the other has furthered the work of PROs. Physicians whose work is being reviewed are afforded the right to a hearing at which the patient is not present, and patients are afforded the protection of outside review in accordance with national standards.

Practice guidelines developed by professional associations, health maintenance organizations and other organized providers, third-party payers, and governmental agencies are designed to evaluate the appropriateness of procedures. Three states—Maine, Minnesota, and Vermont—have passed legislation permitting practice guidelines to be used as a defense in malpractice actions under certain circumstances.[115] Defense lawyers are reluctant to use this legislation, however, because they fear their case will be caught up in a lengthy constitutional appeal. Such a simplistic solution, however, avoids the question of fairness: whose guidelines should prevail in the face of multiple sets of guidelines issued by different bodies, and how should accommodation be made to evolving and changing standards of practice?[116]

Beneficence and justice are involved in full disclosure of information about quality to patients. Health plan report cards aim to fulfill this role.[117] Employers, too, could use report cards to choose health plans for their employees, though some studies suggest that many employers are interested far more in cost than quality.[118] How well reports actually measure quality is itself subject to debate.[119] These matters are discussed in Part Three of this book.

Malpractice suits constitute one method of regulating the quality of care, although an erratic and expensive system. The subject is fully discussed elsewhere in this volume. Here we raise only the ethical issue of the right of the injured patient to compensation for the injury and the need of society for a system of compensation that is more equitable and more efficient than the current one.

The various mechanisms for ensuring quality of care all pose ethical issues. Peer review requires some invasion of privacy and confidentiality to conduct surveillance of quality, although safeguards have been devised. Practice guidelines involve some interference with physician autonomy but in return afford protection for both the patient and the provider. Malpractice suits raise questions of equity, since many injured patients are not compensated. In the process of developing and improving strategies for quality control, the public health perspective justifies social intervention to protect the population.

# Mechanisms for Resolving Ethical Issues in Health Care

Even in the absence of agreement on ethical assumptions, and in the face of diversity and complexity that prohibit easy compromise, mechanisms for resolving ethical dilemmas in public health do exist. Among them are ombudsmen, institutional review boards, ethics committees, standards set by professional associations, practice guidelines, financing mechanisms, and courts of law. Some of these mechanisms are voluntary; others are legal. None is perfect. Some, such as financing mechanisms, are particularly worrisome.

Although ethics deals with values and morals, the law has been very much intertwined with ethical issues. In fact, the more that statutes, regulations, and court cases decide ethical issues, the narrower is the scope of ethical decision making by providers of health care.[120] For example, the conditions for terminating life support for persons in a persistent vegetative state are clearer when the patient has an up-to-date living will. The scope of decision making by physicians and families is constrained. A court of law is therefore an important mechanism for resolving ethical issues in such cases.

The law deals with many substantive issues in numerous fields, including that of health care. It also has made important procedural contributions to resolving disputes by authorizing, establishing, and monitoring mechanisms or processes for handling claims and disputes. Such mechanisms are particularly useful for resolving ethical issues in health care because they are generally informal and flexible and often involve the participation of all parties. Administrative mechanisms are much less expensive than litigation and in this respect potentially more equitable.

Ombudsmen in health care institutions are a means of supporting patient representation and advocacy. They may serve as channels for expression of ethical concerns of patients and their families.

Ethics committees in hospitals and managed care organizations operate to resolve ethical issues involving specific cases in the institution. They may be composed solely of the institution's staff, or they may include an ethicist specialized in handling such problems.

Institutional review boards, discussed earlier, are required to evaluate research proposals for their scientific and ethical integrity.

Practice guidelines, also discussed earlier, offer standards for ethical conduct and encourage professional behavior that conforms to procedural norms generally recognized by experts in the field.

Finally, financing mechanisms that create incentives for certain procedures and practices have the economic power to encourage ethical conduct. Perhaps the highest ethical priority in health care in the United States is achievement of universal coverage of the population by health insurance. At the same time, financing mechanisms may function to encourage the opposite behavior.[121]

As the health care system continues to deal with budget cuts, the growing number of uninsured, and restructuring into managed care and integrated delivery systems, ethical questions loom large. Perhaps their impact can be softened by imaginative and rational strategies to finance, organize, and deliver health care in accordance with the ethical principles of autonomy, beneficence, and justice.

Ethical issues in public health and health services management are likely to become increasingly complex in the future. New technology and advances in medical knowledge challenge us and raise ethical dilemmas. In the future they will need to be evaluated and applied in a public health context and submitted to a public health ethical analysis. Few of these developments are likely to be entirely new and without precedent, however. Already, current discussions, such as what is presented here, may inform these new developments.

# Notes

1. Beauchamp, T. L., and Childress, J. F. *Principles of Biomedical Ethics.* New York: Oxford University Press, 1989 (esp. Chapters 3, 4, and 5); Beauchamp, T. L., and Walters, L. *Contemporary Issues in Bioethics.* Belmont, Calif.: Wadsworth, 1999 (Chapter 1).

2. Burris, S. "The Invisibility of Public Health: Population-Level Measures in a Politics of Market Individualism." *American Journal of Public Health,* 1997, *87*(10), 1607–1610.

3. Foege, W. H. "Public Health: Moving from Debt to Legacy. 1986 Presidential Address." *American Journal of Public Health,* 1987, *77*(10), 1276–1278.

4. Annas, G. J. *American Bioethics: Crossing Human Rights and Health Law.* New York: Oxford University Press, 2004.

5. Another public health question is how threats to the environment should be reconciled with the need for employment. We acknowledge that issues in environmental control have an enormous impact on public health. Here, however, our focus is on the ethical issues in policy and management of personal health services. For a discussion of equity and environmental matters, see Paehlke, R., and Vaillancourt Rosenau, P. "Environment/Equality: Tensions in North American Politics." *Policy Studies Journal,* 1993, *21*(4), 672–686.

6. This outline is taken from Roemer, M. I. *National Health Systems of the World. Vol. 1: The Countries.* New York: Oxford University Press, 1991. Financial resources are treated later in the section on economic support.

7. For an example of the symbiotic relationship between ethics and law, see Annas, G. J. *Some Choice: Law, Medicine, and the Market.* New York: Oxford University Press, 1998; and Annas, G. I., *American Bioethics: Crossing Human Rights and Health Law Boundaries.* New York: Oxford University Press, 2004.

8. Gebbie, K., Merrill, J., and Tilson, H. H. "The Public Health Workforce." *Health Affairs,* 2002, *21*(6), 57–68.

9. Roemer, M. I. "Primary Care and Physician Extenders in Affluent Countries." *International Journal of Health Services,* 1977, *7*(4), 545–555.

10. Moscovice, I., and Rosenblatt, R. "Quality of Care Challenges for Rural Health." Rural Health Research Centers at University of Minnesota and University of Washington. [http://www.hsr.umn.edu/centers/rhrc/rhrc.html] (accessed Oct. 17, 1999).

11. McMahon, G. T. "Coming to America: International Medical Graduates in the United States." *New England Journal of Medicine,* June 10, 2004; "Outward Bound: Do Developing Countries Gain or Lose When Their Brightest Talents Go Abroad?" *Economist,* Sept. 28, 2002.

12. *Regents of University of California v. Bakke,* 438 U.S. 265, 1978.

13. *University of Texas* v. *Hopwood*, 78 F.3d 932(5th Cir. 1996), cert. denied, 116 S.Ct. 2581, 1996.

14. *Gruntter* v. *Bollinger et al.*, no 02-241, 2003, U.S. Court of Appeals for the sixth circuit.

15. *Gratz* v. *Bollinger.*

16. Steinberg, J. "The Supreme Court: University Admissions; An Admissions Guide, *New York Times*, June 24, 2003, National, p. A25.

17. Komaromy, M. "Affirmative Action and the Health of Californians, UCLA Center for Health Policy Research." (Policy brief.) Oct. 1996.

18. Rosenau, P. V., and Linder, S. "Two Decades of Research Comparing For-Profit and Non-profit Health Provider Performance." *Social Science Quarterly*, 2003, *84*(2), 219–241. Rosenau, P. V., and Linder, S. "A Comparison of the Performance of For-Profit and Nonprofit U.S. Psychiatric Care Providers since 1980." *Psychiatric Services*, 2003, *54*(2), 183–187. Rosenau, P. V. "Performance Evaluations of For-Profit and Nonprofit Hospitals in the U.S. Since 1980." *Nonprofit Management and Leadership*, 2003, *13*(4), 401–423.

19. Bell, J. E. "Saving Their Assets: How to Stop Plunder at Blue Cross and Other Nonprof-its." *American Prospect*, 1996, *26*, 60–66.

20. Dallek, G., and Swirsky, L. *Comparing Medicare HMOs: Do They Keep Their Members?* Washington, D.C.: Families USA Foundation, 1997.

21. Claxton, G., Feder, J., Shactman, D., and Altman, S. "Public Policy Issues in Nonprofit Conversions: An Overview." *Health Affairs*, 1997, *16*(2), 9–27.

22. Himmelstein, D. U., Woolhandler, S., Hellander, I., and Wolfe, S. M. "Quality of Care in Investor-Owned vs. Not-for-Profit HMOs." *Journal of the American Medical Association*, 1999, *282*(2), 159–163.

23. Melnick, G., Keeler, E., and Zwanziger, J. "Market Power and Hospital Pricing: Are Non-profits Different?" *Health Affairs*, 1999, *18*(3), 167–173.

24. Moy, E., and others. "Relationship Between National Institutes of Health Research Awards to US Medical Schools and Managed Care Market Penetration." *Journal of the American Medical Association*, 1997, *278*(3), 217–221.

25. Gross, C. P., Anderson, G. F., and Powe, N. R. "The Relation Between Funding by the National Institutes of Health and the Burden of Disease." *New England Journal of Medicine*, June 17, 1999, *340*, 1881–1887; Varmus, H. "Evaluating the Burden of Disease and Spending the Research Dollars of the National Institutes of Health." *New England Journal of Medicine*, June 17, 1999, *340*, 1914–1915.

26. Annas, G. J. "Who's Afraid of the Human Genome?" *Hastings Center Report*, 1989, *19*(4), 19–21.

27. 422 USCS Secs. 289,289a-1-6, 1994), 21 CFR Secs. 56–58, 1994. See Ladimer, I., and Newman, R. W. (eds.). *Clinical Investigation in Medicine: Legal, Ethical and Moral Aspects, An Anthology and Bibliography.* Boston: Law-Medicine Research Institute, Boston University, 1963.

28. Campbell, E. G., and others. "Characteristics of Medical School Faculty Members Serving on Institutional Review Boards: Results of a National Survey." *Academic Medicine*, 2003, *78*, 831–836.

29. Rosenwald, M. S., and Weiss, R. "New Ethics Rules Cost NIH Another Top Researcher." *Washington Post*, Apr. 2, 2005, p. A01.

30. Hilts, P. J. "Conference Is Unable to Agree on Ethical Limits of Research: Psychiatric Experiment Helped Fuel Debate." *New York Times*, Jan. 15, 1995, p. 12.

31. Schauffler, H. H., Brown, E. R., and Rice, T. *The State of Health Insurance in California, 1996.* Los Angeles: Health Insurance Policy Program, University of California Berkeley School of Public Health, and UCLA Center for Health Policy Research, 1997.

32. Gilmer, T., and Kronick, R. "It's the Premiums, Stupid: Projections of the Uninsured Through 2013." *Health Affairs,* Web special, Apr. 5, 2005, pp. 143–151.

33. Institute of Medicine (U.S.). Committee on the Consequences of Uninsurance. *Insuring America's Health: Principles and Recommendations.* Committee on the Consequences of Uninsurance, Board on Health Care Services, Institute of Medicine of the National Academies. Washington, D.C.: National Academies Press, 2004; Institute of Medicine (U.S.). Committee on the Consequences of Uninsurance. *Hidden Costs, Value Lost: Uninsurance in America.* Committee on the Consequences of Uninsurance, Board on Health Care Services, Institute of Medicine of the National Academies. Washington, D.C.: National Academies Press, 2003; Institute of Medicine (U.S.). Committee on the Consequences of Uninsurance. *A Shared Destiny: Community Effects of Uninsurance.* Committee on the Consequences of Uninsurance, Board on Health Care Services, Institute of Medicine. Washington, D.C.: National Academy Press, 2003; Institute of Medicine (U.S.). Committee on the Consequences of Uninsurance. *Care Without Coverage: Too Little, Too Late.* Committee on the Consequences of Uninsurance, Board on Health Care Services, Institute of Medicine. Washington, D.C.: National Academy Press, 2002; Institute of Medicine (U.S.). Committee on the Consequences of Uninsurance. *Health Insurance Is a Family Matter.* Committee on the Consequences of Uninsurance, Board of Health Care Services, Institute of Medicine. Washington, D.C.: National Academy Press, 2002; Institute of Medicine (U.S.). Committee on the Consequences of Uninsurance. *Coverage Matters: Insurance and Health Care.* Committee on the Consequences of Uninsurance, Board on Health Care Services, Institute of Medicine. Washington, D.C.: National Academy Press, 2001.

34. Finkelstein, J. B. "Underinsured and Overlooked: The Growing Problem of Inadequate Insurance." *MedNews.com:* The Newspaper for America's Physicians, Apr. 18, 2005 [www.ama-assn.org/amednews/2005/04/04/gusa0404.htm].

35. Smith, C., and others. "Health Spending Growth Slows in 2003." *Health Affairs, 24*(1), 155–194.

36. Wilkinson, R. G. *Unhealthy Societies: The Afflictions of Inequality.* London: Routledge, 1996.

37. Kawachi, I., Kennedy, B. P., Lochner, K., and Prothrow-Stith, D. "Social Capital, Income Inequality, and Mortality." *American Journal of Public Health,* 1997, *87,* 1491–1498. Kawachi, I., and Kennedy, B. P. "Income Inequality and Health: Pathways and Mechanisms." *Health Services Research,* 1999, *34*(1), 215–228.

38. Wilkinson (1996).

39. Putnam, R. D. "Bowling Alone: America's Declining Social Capital." *Journal of Democracy,* 1995, *6*(1), 65–78.

40. Evans, R. G., Barer, M. L., and Marmor, T. R. *Why Are Some People Healthy and Others Not? The Determinants of Health of Populations.* Hawthorne, N.Y.: Aldine de Gruyter, 1994.

41. Lynch, J. W., Kaplan, G. A., and Shema, S. J. "Cumulative Impact of Sustained Economic Hardship on Physical, Cognitive, Psychological, and Social Functioning." *New England Journal of Medicine,* 1997, *337*(26), 1889–1895.

42. Winslow, R. "Rise in Health-Care Competition Saps Medical-Research Funds, Charity Care." *Wall Street Journal,* Mar. 24, 1999, p. B6; Cunningham, P. J., Grossman, J. M., St. Peter, R. F., and Lesser, C. S. "Managed Care and Physicians' Provision of Charity Care." *Journal of the American Medical Association,* 1999, *281*(12), 1087–1092; Preston, J. "Hospitals Look on Charity Care as Unaffordable Option of Past." *New York Times,* Apr. 14, 1996, pp. A1 and A15.

43. Roemer (1991).

44. For an explanation of the communitarian form of social solidarity, see "The Responsive Communitarian Platform: Rights and Responsibilities: A Platform." *Responsive Community,*

Winter 1991/1992, pp. 4–20. Robert Bellah, Richard Madsen, William Sullivan, Ann Swindler, and Steven Tipton take a similar view in *Habits of the Heart* (New York: Harper-Collins, 1985). See also Minkler, M. "Intergenerational Equity: Divergent Perspectives." (Paper presented at the annual meeting of the American Public Health Association, Washington, D.C., Nov. 1994); also Minkler, M., and Robertson, A. "Generational Equity and Public Health Policy: A Critique of 'Age/Race War' Thinking." *Journal of Public Health Policy*, 1991, *12*(3), 324–344.

45. Bellah, R., and others. *The Good Society.* New York: Knopf, 1991.

46. President's Commission for the Study of Ethical Problems in Medicine and Biomedical and Behavioral Research (A. M. Capron, exec. dir.). *Securing Access to Health Care: The Ethical Implications of Differences in the Availability of Health Services, Vol. 1.* Washington, D.C.: U.S. Government Printing Office, 1983.

47. Soumerai, S. B., and Ross-Degnan, D. "Inadequate Prescription-Drug Coverage for Medicare Enrollees—A Call to Action." *New England Journal of Medicine*, Mar. 4, 1999, *340*, 722–728.

48. Maynard, A., and Bloor, K. *Our Certain Fate: Rationing in Health Care.* London: Office of New Health Economics, 1998.

49. Lewis, C. E., Fein, R., and Mechanic, D. *The Right to Health: The Problem of Access to Primary Medical Care.* New York: Wiley, 1976.

50. Wheeler, S. V. "TeleMedicine." *BioPhotonics*, Fall 1994, 34–40; and Smothers, R. "150 Miles Away, the Doctor Is Examining Your Tonsils." *New York Times*, Sept. 16, 1992 (Late Edition Final), p. C14.

51. Moscovice, I., Wellever, A., and Stensland, J. "Rural Hospitals: Accomplishments and Present Challenges, July 1999." Rural Health Research Center, School of Public Health, University of Minnesota, July 1999 [www.hsr.umn.edu/centers/rhrc/rhrc.html] (accessed Oct. 18, 1999).

52. Marin, G., and Marin, B. V. *Research with Hispanic Populations.* Thousand Oaks, Calif.: Sage, 1991, chapter 3. See also, for example, Orlandi, M. (ed.). *Cultural Competence for Evaluators.* Rockville, Md.: U.S. Department of Health and Human Services, 1992.

53. Rafuse, J. "Multicultural Medicine." *Canadian Medical Association Journal*, 1993, *148*, 282–284; Maher, J. "Medical Education in a Multilingual and Multicultural World." *Medical Education*, 1993, *27*, 3–5.

54. There is no evidence that prior to 1992 HMOs offered reduced quality of care. Miller, R. H., and Luft, H. S. "Does Managed Care Lead to Better or Worse Quality of Care?" *Health Affairs*, 1997, *16*(5), 7–25. The evidence on HMOs and quality of care in the context of today's market competition is still out. The not-for-profit HMOs seem to provide better quality than do the for-profit HMOs. "How Good Is Your Health Plan?" *Consumer Reports*, Aug., 1996, pp. 40–44; Kuttner, R. "Must Good HMOs Go Bad? The Commercialization of Prepaid Group Health Care." *New England Journal of Medicine*, 1998, *338*(21), 1558–1563; Kuttner, R. "Must Good HMOs Go Bad? The Search for Checks and Balances." *New England Journal of Medicine*, 1998, *338*(22), 1635–1639; Himmelstein, Woolhandler, Hellander, and Wolfe (1999).

55. Rice, T. *The Economics of Health Reconsidered.* Chicago: Health Administration Press, 1998.

56. Miller, T. E., and Sage, W. M. "Disclosing Physician Financial Incentives." *Journal of the American Medical Association*, 1999, *281*(15), 1424–1430.

57. Bodenheimer, T. "Disease Management: Promises and Pitfalls." *New England Journal of Medicine*, 1999, *340*(15), 1202–1205; Mariner, W. K. "Patients' Rights After Health Care

Reform: Who Decides What Is Medically Necessary?" *American Journal of Public Health,* 1994, *84*(9), 1515–1519; Rosenbaum, S., Frankford, D. M., Moore, B., and Borzi, P. "Who Should Determine When Health Care Is Medically Necessary?" *New England Journal of Medicine,* Jan. 21, 1999, *340,* 229–232; *Fox* v. *Health Net of California,* California Superior Court, no. 219692, Dec. 23 and 28, 1993.

58. *Pinneke* v. *Preisser,* 623 F.2d 546 (8th Cir. 1980); *Bush* v. *Barham,* 625 F.2d 1150 (5th Cir. 1980).

59. Danzon, P. M. "Tort Liability: A Minefield for Managed Care?" (Part 2.) *Journal of Legal Studies,* 1997, *26*(2), 491–519.

60. 29 U.S.C. sec. 1144 (a)-(b), 1994.

61. *Shaw* v. *Delta Airlines,* 463 U.S. 85, 1983; *Corcoran* v. *United Healthcare, Inc.,* 965 F.2d 1321 (5th Cir.), cert. denied 506 U.S. 1033, 1992. See Kilcullen, J. K. "Groping for the Reins: ERISA, HMO Malpractice, and Enterprise Liability." *American Journal of Law and Medicine,* 1996, *22*(1), 7.

62. Rosenbaum, Frankford, Moore, and Borzi (1999).

63. *Aetna Health Inc.* v. *Davila,* 124 S. Ct 2488 (2004); Bloche, M. G. "Back to the 90s—The Supreme Court Immunizes Managed Care." *New England Journal of Medicine,* 2004, *351*(13), 1277–1279.

64. Emanuel, E. J. "Choice and Representation in Health Care." *Medical Care Research and Review,* 1999, *56*(1), 113–140.

65. Baumhart, R. C. "How Ethical Are Businessmen?" *Harvard Business Review,* July/Aug. 1961, pp. 6–19, 156–176.

66. Fisher, E. S., and Welch, H. G. "Avoiding the Unintended Consequences of Growth in Medical Care: How Might More Be Worse?" *Journal of the American Medical Association,* 1999, *281*(5), 452; Deyo, R. A., and others. "The Messenger Under Attack: Intimidation of Researchers by Special-Interest Groups." *New England Journal of Medicine,* 1997, *336*(16), 1176–1180.

67. Ellwood, quoted in Noble, H. B. "Quality Is Focus for Health Plans." *New York Times,* July 3, 1995, pp. 1, 7. For discussion of problems in business ethics, see Cederblom, J., and Dougherty, C. J. *Ethics at Work.* Belmont, Calif.: Wadsworth, 1990; Iannone, A. P. (ed.). *Contemporary Moral Controversies in Business.* New York: Oxford University Press, 1989; Bayles, M. D. *Professional Ethics* (2nd ed.). Belmont, Calif.: Wadsworth, 1989; Callahan, J. C. *Ethical Issues in Professional Life.* New York: Oxford University Press, 1988.

68. Roemer (1991).

69. Kuttner, R. "The American Health Care System: Wall Street and Health Care." *New England Journal of Medicine,* Feb. 25, 1999, *340,* 664–668.

70. Shindul-Rothschild, J., Berry, D., and Long-Middleton, E. "Where Have All the Nurses Gone? Final Results of Our Patient Care Survey." *American Journal of Nursing,* Nov. 1996, *96,* 25–39.

71. Rundle, R. L. "California Is the First State to Require Hospital-Wide Nurse-to-Patient Ratios." *Wall Street Journal,* Oct. 12, 1999, p. B6.

72. Kaiser Family Foundation and Harvard University School of Public Health. *Survey of Physicians and Nurses: Randomly Selected Verbatim Descriptions from Physicians and Nurses of Health Plan Decisions Resulting in Declines in Patients' Health Status.* Menlo Park, Calif.: Kaiser Family Foundation, July 1999.

73. See, for example, *Whalen* v. *Roe,* 429 U.S. 589, 1977, upholding the constitutionality of a state law requiring that patients receiving legitimate prescriptions for drugs with potential for abuse have name, address, age, and other information reported to the state department of health.

74. Hillman, A. L., and others. "Avoiding Bias in the Conduct and Reporting of Cost-Effectiveness Research Sponsored by Pharmaceutical Companies." *New England Journal of Medicine*, 1991, *324*, 1362–1365.

75. *Ethyl Corporation* v. *Environmental Protection Agency*, 541 F.2d 1, 1976.

76. Silver, L. "An Agency Dilemma: Regulating to Protect the Public Health in Light of Scientific Uncertainty." In R. Roemer and G. McKray (eds.), *Legal Aspects of Health Policy: Issues and Trends*. Westport, Conn.: Greenwood Press, 1980.

77. Silver (1980), p. 81, quoting this passage from Judge Bazelon's concurring opinion in *International Harvester Company* v. *Ruckelshaus*, 478 F.2d 615, 652, 1973.

78. *Daubert* v. *Merrell Dow Pharmaceuticals, Inc.*, 509 U.S. 579, 113 S. Ct. 2786, 125 L.Ed. 2d 469, 1993.

79. Ginzburg, H. M. "Use and Misuse of Epidemiologic Data in the Courtroom: Defining the Limits of Inferential and Particularistic Evidence in Mass Tort Litigation." *American Journal of Law and Medicine*, 1986, *12*(3 and 4), 423–439.

80. Roemer, R. *Legislative Action to Combat the World Tobacco Epidemic* (2nd ed.). Geneva: World Health Organization, 1993; U.S. Department of Health and Human Services. *Reducing the Health Consequences of Smoking: 25 Years of Progress. A Report of the Surgeon General.* (DHHS publication no. CDC 89-8411.) Washington, D.C.: Office on Smoking and Health, Center for Chronic Disease Prevention and Health Promotion, Centers for Disease Control, Public Health Service, U.S. Department of Health and Human Services, 1989.

81. *Penn Advertising of Baltimore, Inc.* v. *Mayor of Baltimore*, 63 F.3d 1318 (4th Cir. 1995) aff'g 862 F. Supp. 1402 (D. Md. 1994), discussed by Garner, D. W. "Banning Tobacco Billboards: The Case for Municipal Action." *Journal of the American Medical Association*, 1996, *275*(16), 1263–1269. But see *Lorillard Tobacco Company* v. *Thomas Riley, Attorney General of Massachusetts*, 533 US 525 (2001).

82. http://egov.oregon.gov/DAS/OHPPR/HSC/docs/InterMod4-05.pdf and http://www.oregon.gof/DHS/healthplan/priorlist/main.shtml.

83. Annas, G. J. *The Standard of Care: The Law of American Bioethics*. New York: Oxford University Press, 1993; Rosenbaum, S. "Mothers and Children Last: The Oregon Medicaid Experiment." *American Journal of Law and Medicine*, 1992, *18*(1 and 2), 97–126; see also Lamb, E. J. "Rationing of Medical Care: Rules of Rescue, Cost-Effectiveness, and the Oregon Plan." *American Journal of Obstetrics and Gynecology*, 2004, *190*, 1636-1641.

84. Maynard and Bloor (1998).

85. Anderson, G. F., and Poullier, J. P. "Health Spending, Access, and Outcomes: Trends in Industrialized Countries." *Health Affairs*, 1999, *18*(3), 178–182.

86. Schuster, M. A., McGlynn, E. A., and Brook, R. H. "How Good Is the Quality of Health Care in the United States?" *Milbank Quarterly*, 1998, *76*(4), 517–563.

87. Kaserman, D. L., and Barnett, A. H. *The U.S. Organ Procurement System: A Prescription for Reform.* American Enterprise Institute, 2002. The *New England Journal of Medicine* published a "sounding board" article strongly opposed to the sale of organs: Delmonico, F., and others. "Financial Incentives—Not Payment—for Organ Donation." *New England Journal of Medicine*, 2002, *346*(25), 2002–2005.

88. Bosch, X. "Spain Leads World in Organ Donation and Transplantation." *Journal of the American Medical Association*, July 7, 1999, *282*, 17–18.

89. "Legislation, Practice, and Donor Rates." (Postnote.) Council of Europe: National Transplant Organization in Parliamentary Office of Technology. Oct. 2004, no. 231, p. 2.

90. Defino, T. "Mediscare." *Healthcare Business*, 1999, *2*(3), 60–70.

91. Kaiser Family Foundation (1999), pp. 7, 16.

92. The GAO estimate is quoted in Rosenthal, E. "Confusion and Error Are Rife in Hospital Billing Practices." *New York Times,* Jan. 27, 1993; see also Kerr, P. "Glossing over Health Care Fraud." *New York Times,* Apr. 5, 1992, p. F17; U.S. General Accounting Office. *Health Insurance: Remedies Needed to Reduce Losses from Fraud and Abuse—Testimony.* (GAO/T-HRD-9308.) Washington, D.C.: General Accounting Office, Mar. 8, 1993. Alan Hillman, director of the Center for Health Policy at the University of Pennsylvania, suggests that hospital records are so deformed and manipulated for billing and reimbursement purposes that they are no longer of any use for outcomes research (quoted in *New York Times,* Aug. 9, 1994, p. A11).

93. Pear, R. "Stung by Defeat in House, HMO's Seek Compromise." *New York Times,* Oct. 9, 1999, p. A9.

94. Hillman, B., and others. "Physicians' Utilization and Charges for Outpatient Diagnostic Imaging in a Medicare Population." *Journal of the American Medical Association,* Oct. 21, 1992, *268,* 2050–2054; Mitchell, J., and Scott, E. "Physician Ownership of Physical Therapy Services: Effects on Charges, Utilization, Profits, and Service Characteristics." *Journal of the American Medical Association,* Oct. 21, 1992, *268,* 2055–2059; Kolata, G. "Pharmacists Help Drug Promotions; Pharmacists Paid by Companies to Recommend Their Drugs." *New York Times,* July 29, 1994, pp. A1, D2; Hilts, P. J. "FDA Seeks Disclosures by Scientists: Financial Interests in Drugs Are at Issue." *New York Times,* Sept. 24, 1994, p. 7; Winslow, R. "Drug Company's PR Firm Made Offer to Pay for Editorial, Professor Says." *Wall Street Journal,* Sept. 8, 1994, p. B12; U.S. General Accounting Office. *Medicare: Referrals to Physician-Owned Imaging Facilities Warrant HCFA's Scrutiny.* (GAO/HEHS-95-2.) Washington, D.C.: General Accounting Office, 1994.

95. Krimsky, S. *Science in the Private Interest: Has the Lure of Profits Corrupted Biomedical Research?* Lanham, Md.: Rowman and Littlefield, 2003.

96. Prager, L. O. "Selling Products OK—But Not for Profit." *American Medical News,* July 12, 1999, p. 1.

97. WHO Consultation on Testing and Counseling for HIV Infection. (WHO/GPA/NF/93.2.) Geneva: Global Programme on AIDS, World Health Organization, 1993; Field, M. A. "Testing for AIDS: Uses and Abuses." *American Journal of Law and Medicine,* 1990, *16*(1 and 2), 33–106; Fluss, S. S., and Zeegers, D. "AIDS, HIV, and Health Care Workers: Some International Perspectives." *Maryland Law Review,* 1989, *48*(1), 77–92.

98. Nakashima, A. K., and others. "Effects of HIV Reporting by Name on Use of HIV Testing in Publicly Funded Counseling and Testing Programs." *Journal of the American Medical Association,* 1998, *280*(16), 1421–1426.

99. Joseph, S. C. *Dragon Within the Gates: The Once and Future AIDS Epidemic.* New York: Carroll and Graf, 1992.

100. "1998 Guidelines for Treatment of Sexually Transmitted Diseases." *Morbidity and Mortality Weekly Report,* Jan. 23, 1998, *47*(RR-1), 16. See California Health and Safety Code, sec. 199.25 (1990) and the insightful analysis of Bayer, R. "HIV Prevention and the Two Faces of Partner Notification." *American Journal of Public Health,* Aug. 9, 1992, *82,* 1156–1164.

101. "1998 Guidelines . . ." (1998); "Public Health Service Task Force Recommendations for the Use of Antiretroviral Drugs in Pregnant Women Infected with HIV-1 for Maternal Health and for Reducing Perinatal HIV-1 Transmission in the United States." *Morbidity and Mortality Weekly Report,* Jan. 30, 1998, *47*(RR-2).

102. 410 U.S. 113, 1973.

103. United States Conference of Catholic Bishops. *Ethical and Religious Directives for Catholic Health Care Services* (4th ed.). 2001 [http://www.usccb.org/bishops/directives.htm]. See especially directives 36, 45, 48, 53, and 54.

104. Franzini, L., and others. "Projected Economic Costs Due to Health Consequences of Teenagers' Loss of Confidentiality in Obtaining Reproductive Health Care Services in Texas." *Archives of Pediatric Adolescent Medicine*, 2004, *158*, 1140-1146.

105. Kitzhaber, J. "Congress' Implicit Healthcare Rationing." *Christian Science Monitor*, Apr. 4, 2005. For an insightful analysis of how a society's cultural beliefs, concept of autonomy, and informed consent laws influence resource allocation at the end of life, see Annas, G. J., and Miller, F. H. "The Empire of Death: How Culture and Economics Affect Informed Consent in the U.S., the U.K., and Japan." *American Journal of Law and Medicine*, 1994, *20*(4), 359–394.

106. See, for example, N.Y. Mental Hygiene Law, Article 9, Secs 9.01–9.59, 1988 and Supp. 1995); Special Committee to Study Commitment Procedures of the Association of the Bar of the City of New York, in cooperation with the Cornell Law School. *Mental Illness and Due Process: Report and Recommendations on Admission to Mental Hospitals Under New York Law.* Ithaca, N.Y.: Cornell University Press, 1962.

107. *Tarasoff v. Regents of the University of California*, 17 Cal. 3d 425, 551 2d 334, 131 Cal. Rptr. 14, 1976.

108. Grad, F. P. *The Public Health Law Manual* (2nd ed.). Washington, D.C.: American Public Health Association, 1990.

109. Starr, P. "Health and the Right to Privacy." *American Journal of Law and Medicine*, 1999, *25*(2 and 3), 193–201.

110. Conkey, C. "Doctors, Hospitals Act to Safeguard Medical Data." *Wall Street Journal*, Apr. 21, 2003, p. D2.

111. McGlynn, E. A. "Evaluating the Quality of Care," Chapter Nine of this edition; Chassin, M. R., and Galvin, R. W. "The Urgent Need to Improve Health Care Quality: Institute of Medicine National Roundtable on Health Care Quality." *Journal of the American Medical Association*, 1998, *280*(11), 1000–1005; Detsky, A. S. "Regional Variation in Medical Care." *New England Journal of Medicine*, 1995, *333*(9), 589–590; Leape, L. L. "Error in Medicine." *Journal of the American Medical Association*, 1994, *272*, 1851–1857.

112. For a thoughtful discussion of peer review organizations under the law as it existed in November 1979, see Price, S. J. "Health Systems Agencies and Peer Review Organizations: Experiments in Regulating the Delivery of Health Care." In Roemer and McKray (1980). For a more recent analysis, see Luce, G. M. "The Use of Peer Review Organizations to Control Medicare Costs." *ALI-ABA Course Materials-Journal*, 1986, *10*, 111–120; Pear, R. "Clinton to Unveil Rules to Protect Medical Privacy." *New York Times*, Oct. 27, 1999, p. A1.

113. 42 U.S.C. Sec. 1320c et seq.

114. 42 U.S.C. Sec. 11101 et seq.

115. U.S. Congress, Office of Technology Assessment. *Impact of Legal Reform on Medical Malpractice Costs.* (OTA-BP-H-19.) Washington, D.C.: U.S. Government Printing Office, 1993.

116. For analysis of various aspects of practice guidelines, see Capron, A. M. "Practice Guidelines: How Good Are Medicine's New Recipes?" *Journal of Law, Medicine, and Ethics*, 1995, *23*(1), 47–56; Parker, C. W. "Practice Guidelines and Private Insurers." *Journal of Law, Medicine, and Ethics*, 1995, *23*(1), 57–61; Kane, R. L. "Creating Practice Guidelines: The Dangers of Over-Reliance on Expert Judgment." *Journal of Law, Medicine, and Ethics*, 1995, *23*(1), 62–64; Pauly, M. V. "Practice Guidelines: Can They Save Money? Should They?"

*Journal of Law, Medicine, and Ethics*, 1995, *23*(1), 65–74; Halpern, J. "Can the Development of Practice Guidelines Safeguard Patient Values?" *Journal of Law, Medicine, and Ethics*, 1995, *23*(1), 75–81.

117. The Joint Commission on Accreditation of Healthcare Organizations and the National Committee on Quality Assurance make information available to consumers about provider performance and outcomes. See, for example, http://www.ncqa.org/Pages/Main/index. htm. *Consumer Reports, Newsweek,* and *U.S. News & World Report* also publish HMO assessments.

118. McLaughlin, C. G., and Ginsburg, P. B. "Competition, Quality of Care, and the Role of the Consumer." *Milbank Quarterly,* 1998, *76*(4), 737–743; Weinstein, M. M. "Economic Scene: The Grading May Be Too Easy on Health Plans' Report Cards." *New York Times,* Aug. 19, 1999, p. C2.

119. Hofer, T. P., and others. "The Unreliability of Individual Physician 'Report Cards' for Assessing the Costs and Quality of Care of a Chronic Disease." *Journal of the American Medical Association,* 1999, *281*(22), 2098–2105.

120. Grad, F. P. "Medical Ethics and the Law." *Annals of the American Academy of Political and Social Science,* May 1978, *437,* 19–36.

121. See the references in note 94 on conflict of interest and referral.

# INDEX